Cerebral Plasticity

Cerebral Plasticity

New Perspectives

edited by
Leo M. Chalupa
Nicoletta Berardi
Matteo Caleo
Lucia Galli-Resta
Tommaso Pizzorusso

The MIT Press
Cambridge, Massachusetts
London, England

For information about special quantity discounts, please email special_sales@mitpress.mit.edu

This book was set in Times Roman by Toppan Best-set Premedia Limited. Printed and bound in the United States of America.

Library of Congress Cataloging-in-Publication Data

Cerebral plasticity : new perspectives / edited by Leo M. Chalupa [et al.].
  p. ; cm.
Includes bibliographical references and index.
ISBN 978-0-262-01523-3 (hardcover : alk. paper)
1. Neuroplasticity. 2. Cerebral cortex. I. Chalupa, Leo M.
[DNLM: 1. Cerebral Cortex—growth & development. 2. Cerebral Cortex—physiology. 3. Neurodegenerative Diseases. 4. Neuronal Plasticity—physiology. WL 307]
QP363.3.C467   2011
612.8′25—dc22
                                                                    2010030465

10 9 8 7 6 5 4 3 2 1

Contents

Preface

The notion that neurons in the living brain can change in response to experience is denoted by the term "plasticity," which has become a major conceptual theme in basic research as well as a practical focus in the fields of neural rehabilitation and neurodegenerative diseases. Much of the early work in this field dealt with plasticity of the developing brain using a model systems approach. Such studies aptly demonstrated that sensory experience plays a critical role in the normal development of certain fundamental attributes of a given sensory system. As the plasticity field evolved, two broader research themes emerged. One of these concerns plasticity of the adult brain, and indeed, this is one of the hottest areas of current research. The other major focus is the search for underlying mechanisms. Here the challenge is to explain the cellular, molecular, and epigenetic factors controlling plasticity throughout the normal lifespan as well as in response to injury or disease. The prevalent thinking today is that if we can attain a fundamental understanding of what underlies neuronal plasticity, we can ultimately make use of this information in devising strategies for the repair of injuries rendered by myriad neurological disorders and, potentially, even improve the learning capabilities of the normal brain.

The chapters in this volume cover all three of these approaches to the study of cerebral plasticity. A number of chapters deal with issues of normal development and the influence of various environmental manipulations. Others are concerned with cerebral plasticity at maturity. Most chapters also consider underlying mechanisms of plasticity, with some focused primarily on this important topic. The reader will note a rather wide diversity of neuronal systems encompassed in this volume, reflective of the field of cerebral plasticity. Moreover, some chapters do not deal with the topic of plasticity per se; rather, they present an organizational framework upon which future studies of plasticity could be formulated.

Lamberto Maffei, to whom this volume is dedicated, has been a major figure in brain plasticity research for nearly half a century, particularly renowned for his studies of the plasticity of the visual system. The idea for this book originated during a meeting in a villa near Lucca, Lamberto's birthplace, organized by his former students. The invited participants to this meeting were leading researchers in their respective fields who have had a long personal and professional association with Lamberto. It seemed natural to build on this talented group by inviting additional individuals to provide up-to-date accounts of their research topics. Thus originated

Cerebral Plasticity, a volume that we believe will be of interest to students and colleagues in diverse specialties within neuroscience ranging from fundamental neural mechanisms to professional fields such as neurosurgery, neurology, rehabilitation medicine, and computer science.

On behalf of the editors, I would like to express sincere gratitude to the authors that contributed a chapter to this volume. I would also like to thank Robert Prior, Executive Editor of MIT Press, for his keen advice in the planning stages for this volume, as well as Andrea Chalupa for her expert editorial assistance.

1 Introduction

Nicoletta Berardi, Matteo Caleo, Lucia Galli-Resta, and Tommaso Pizzorusso

For all of his professional life, Lamberto Maffei has been a scientific explorer of new trails in uncharted territories. Many of his papers have opened new fields of research and have introduced a new way of thinking about vision research and cerebral plasticity. As his former students, we have been fortunate to gain the benefits of his wisdom and dedication to cutting-edge scientific endeavors.

As a young man, Lamberto studied medicine at the University of Pisa, graduating in 1961. During his medical studies, he was brought into contact with Professor Giuseppe Moruzzi, a neurophysiologist, famous for his research on the reticular formation and the mechanisms governing sleep and wakefulness. Moruzzi's laboratory was international, with scientists frequently visiting from all parts of the globe. In a recent interview, Lamberto recalled that he found this intellectual, international lifestyle—devotion to science, almost secluded from the world—"poetically" attractive. Certainly, this was the feeling that entering Lamberto's laboratory evoked in his students.

In his early work, Lamberto investigated the functions of the mammalian visual system. During this period from the mid 1960s to the early 1980s, he carried out pioneering research on spatial frequency selectivity in primary visual cortex, neural adaptation to contrast, and extrareceptive field influences on visual neurons. He was among the first to rely on multidisciplinary approaches to study neural functions, pursuing parallel experiments in psychophysics and electrophysiology of the visual system with Adriana Fiorentini in the CNR Laboratory of Neurophysiology in Pisa. Some of us have very clear memories of electrophysiological experiments, carried out in the dark late into the night, with the firing of the neurons crackling through the loudspeaker and the quiet, terse exchanges between Lamberto and Adriana. They were so used to thinking and working together that they understood each other completely with only a few spoken words. It was sheer pleasure to participate in those early experiments. The instruments in the laboratory at that time were often "homemade" in the electronic and mechanical shops. Among the items custom built in the laboratory was the first computer to average neuronal electrical signals, spatial frequency generators, optic benches for the psychophysical experiments, and electrode microdrives. We assembled all the psychophysical equipment. It was all very complicated, but for us students, it had the advantage that we knew every single component of the apparatus, why it was there, its function, and its underlying principles of operation.

During those years, Lamberto, working with Fergus Campbell, introduced the technique of recording visual evoked potentials (VEPs) in response to gratings, showing that these were an accurate predictor of psychophysical responses. Subsequently, he demonstrated that the electroretinogram (ERG) evoked by a flash of light (flash ERG), the only type of ERG used in clinic at the time, was not affected by degeneration of retinal ganglion cells following section of the optic nerve. At the same time, he showed that ERG responses to gratings (pattern ERG) disappeared after degeneration of ganglion cells. Thus, the pattern but not flash ERG was discovered to be suitable for investigating retinal ganglion cell function. This finding contributed to the introduction of pattern VEPs and ERG to vision research and to clinical evaluations. Both techniques are still widely used in neurological and ophthalmological clinics as well as in experimental studies of the visual system, both in animals and humans.

Lamberto later moved on to the investigation of the development and plasticity of the brain, using the mammalian visual system as a model, and in particular, introducing the rodent to the study of visual cortical plasticity. His work with Lucia Galli on the presence of spontaneous discharge in visual neurons in prenatal life is another example of an experiment that opened a new field of research. This study, highly challenging from a technical point of view, showed that retinal ganglion cells are spontaneously active in utero, long before photoreceptors are formed. This discovery implied that such early activity carries a position code, which could contribute to building visual maps, allowing a tremendous advance in our understanding of the mechanisms underlying neural development.

Many of us remember the precise moment when Lamberto proposed a new experiment, so novel that we remained silent for a while, thinking "How did he come to think of this?" One of these events was when Lamberto proposed to study the role of neurotrophic factors in the development and plasticity of the visual cortex. At that time, neurotrophic factors were thought to be only survival factors for specific classes of developing neurons. The experiments proposed by Lamberto demonstrated for the first time that neurotrophic factors have a role in visual cortical development and plasticity and might even compensate for the lack of visual experience. The original intuition that neurotrophic factors might be organizers of the development of neural circuits and connections has been progressively better defined on the basis of incoming experimental data. This has changed the way we think about the plasticity process, both during development and in the adult, and has also opened up new brain repair perspectives.

Another memorable event was Lamberto's idea to study the role of environmental enrichment in visual development and in visual cortical plasticity in the adult. At the time these experiments began, nothing was known with respect to the possible role of an enriched environment in visual development. Lamberto's experiments have shown that an enriched environment acts on visual development at very early ages, when animals have yet to interact with the environment through vision or exploration. Thus, nonvisual components of the environment can influence visual development. This has led to recent work on premature babies showing that enriching the environment of the babies in terms of body massage promotes brain development and, in particular, visual development. A molecular factor mediating this effect has been identified.

In his work on the effects of an enriched environment on adult visual cortical plasticity, Lamberto has shown that living in an enriched environment can potentiate visual cortical plasticity in adult rats to the point of allowing complete recovery from amblyopia, acting on the balance between cortical excitation and inhibition. Besides being another experiment that opens an unexplored field, this work has obvious clinical implications for humans. Possible applications to humans of interventions based on the "philosophy" of an enriched environment are also currently being explored by Lamberto in the field of neurodegenerative pathologies, such as Alzheimer's disease.

Lamberto has worked in Tübingen, Cambridge, Boston, Paris, Oxford, and Davis, California, making long-standing friends, some of whom have contributed to this book. In Italy, he has been director of the CNR Laboratory of Neurophysiology (later Institute of Neurophysiology) and then of the Institute of Neuroscience of the National Research Council and Professor of Neurobiology of Scuola Normale Superiore, in Pisa. Recently he was elected President of the Accademia Nazionale dei Lincei, the oldest and most prestigious cultural institution in Italy, so that he can contribute even more to shaping Italian scientific culture. Thus, nowadays, his days in the laboratory intermingle with meetings of the Academia in beautiful Palazzo Corsini in Rome and with his travels on behalf of the academy.

His activities as a scientist have always gone together with his being a great teacher. His attention to his students, the time devoted to their formation, and the never-ending activity devoted to organizing visits of prominent scientists to Pisa so that his students could interact with the very best of the international scientific community are examples of what a great teacher should be. This requires time, patience, and the desire to teach. No matter how busy he was, he always found time to speak with a student, to discuss projects and data, to offer advice, and to direct. He has always encouraged his students to delve deeply into a project, to "let it under your skin," to be ready to understand the message of the data. Over the years, he has contributed to the formation of many independent neuroscientists working both in Italy and abroad, including Ruxandra Sireteanu, Luigi Cervetto, Marco Piccolino, Silvia Bisti, Donatella Spinelli, Luciano Domenici, Giulio Sandini, Paolo M. Rossini, Maria Concetta Morrone, Antonino Cattaneo, David C. Burr, Giorgio Carmignoto, Maria Cristina Cenni, Michela Fagiolini, Graziella Di Cristo, Alessandro Cellerino, Paolo Medini, Claudia Lodovichi, Gimmi Ratto, Yuri Bozzi, Alessandro Sale, and the four of us.

A posteriori, we have understood that Lamberto has applied the concept of enriched environments to his students. Indeed, in addition to providing students with the sensory and cognitive stimulation entailed in being a part of the thinking and experimenting that has taken place in his laboratory, he has always encouraged motor activity, giving himself as the prime example, by swimming and jogging and going to the gym. Most likely, he foresaw that physical exercise is beneficial for brain function before this was demonstrated by scientific studies. Also social, convivial activity was encouraged. We all remember the evenings in Lamberto's house, with

Graziella, Lamberto's wife, preparing homemade pizzas for us famished students, baking them in the big oven under the porch, working with the long iron shovel to put aside the embers so that they did not burn the pizzas. On those occasions, we also often played volleyball with the rather idiosyncratic rules that Lamberto made up to cope with the unique playing field, between the wisteria-covered wall and the flower bushes, rules that he often changed even in midplay. Statistically, the team he was on was victorious more often than the opponents. These evenings would sometimes end with us singing long into the night, particularly if Adriana's niece, a very gifted guitar player and singer, was with us.

Thank you, Lamberto, for creating and maintaining such an enriched environment that has benefited, and is benefiting, generations of students and friends.

2 The Dynamic Building of the Brain

Alessandro Sale, Laura Baroncelli, Maria Spolidoro, and Lamberto Maffei

Nature–Nurture Interplay in the Regulation of Nervous System Development

The relative contribution of nature versus nurture to the construction and maintenance of brain architecture has been a controversial matter for many decades, leading only recently to a widely accepted consensus that genes and environment work in concert in shaping neural circuits and behavior (Krubitzer and Kahn, 2003). In humans, studies on behavioral traits displayed by twins are frequently used to investigate the biological basis of individuality, revealing a role for both genes and environment in the construction of personality. Despite this evidence, genetic and environmental influences have been considered mutually exclusive for a long time in the history of neurobiology. While the contribution of genetic programs was established early on, the influence exerted by the environment on the nervous system's development has for a long time been underestimated, mostly due to methodological limits in quantifying environment-induced changes in the brain. Only since the early 1960s has the assembly of neuronal circuits ceased to be considered as an entirely experience-independent process.

A synthesis of the two theories was made possible by the discovery and characterization of biological processes in which neural plastic rearrangements in response to experience occur under the control of genetically programmed rules. The most compelling example is the "critical period" (CP) concept (for reviews, see Berardi et al., 2000, and Knudsen, 2004). CPs are restricted time windows in early postnatal life during which neural circuits display a heightened sensitivity to acquire instructive and adaptive signals from the external environment. CPs have been identified for brain areas involved in functions as various as sensory perception, motor control, and language, exhibiting different time courses under the control of distinct cellular and molecular mechanisms (Hensch, 2004).

The primary visual cortex (V1) is the election test bed for studying experience-dependent plasticity in the brain. The pioneering experiments performed by Hubel and Wiesel showed how dramatically early sensory deprivation can affect the anatomy and physiology of the visual cortex. They reported that reducing input from one eye by lid suture, a treatment usually referred to as monocular deprivation (MD), early in development disrupts the binocularity (ocular dominance, OD) of V1 with a loss of the cortical response to the deprived eye and a strong increment in the number of neurons driven by the open eye, accompanied by a poor development of visual acuity (VA) and contrast sensitivity for the deprived eye (Wiesel and Hubel, 1963). The same manipulation of visual experience is totally ineffective in the adult (Hubel and Wiesel, 1970).

In parallel to the experiments based on protocols of sensory deprivation, the development of the nature–nurture debate has been strongly driven by the introduction of environmental enrichment (EE) as an experimental paradigm devoted to investigating the influence of environment on brain and behavior. Rosenzweig and colleagues showed that the morphology, chemistry, and physiology of the brain can be modified by increasing the quality and intensity of environmental stimulation (Rosenzweig and Bennett, 1969). Since then, a great number of studies have detailed the effects elicited by EE in the adult brain, spanning from the molecular to the anatomical and functional level (van Praag et al., 2000).

Environmental Enrichment: Definition and Effects on Brain and Behavior

EE has the goal to improve the animals' quality of life by providing them with a combination of multisensory and cognitive stimulation, increased physical activity, and enhanced social interactions and by promoting explorative behavior and attentional processes. Enriched animals live in large groups and in wide environments where a variety of toys, tunnels, stairs, running wheels, and other differently shaped objects are present and changed frequently (see figure 2.1).

It is generally assumed that EE is simply a way of rearing the animals in a setting more similar to life in the wild, but we can speculate that EE offers a challenge-free condition in which exploration and play are stimulated without the dangers and contingent necessities of life. Considering the use of EE as a paradigm for investigating the influence of environmental stimulation on the brain, it is interesting to compare it with MD, the most classic procedure employed in the study of experience-dependent plasticity in the brain. MD is a rather severe experimental protocol that is mostly effective only during a well-defined CP and is focused on the role of altered sensory experience on the maturation and plasticity of specific sensory systems. In contrast, EE is a natural treatment, which has been shown to exert its effects at all ages and which is particularly suitable for eliciting subtle physiological changes in the whole organism—for instance, affecting levels of hormones and growth factors. Since EE gives the opportunity to perform studies "for optimization" rather than "for alteration or reduction" of sensory experience and since EE is able to affect behavior, the results obtained with this paradigm are usually of great interest and applicability for humans in many different fields, from psychology to the medical clinic.

However, given the complexity and variability of the possible EE conditions adopted, concerns have been raised about a lack of standardization and methodological precision affecting the reproducibility of EE experiments. This criticism is not well-founded. In an important study, distinct inbred strains of mice exhibiting well-known differences in some behavioral tasks typically used in drug screening and behavioral phenotyping were tested after a period of

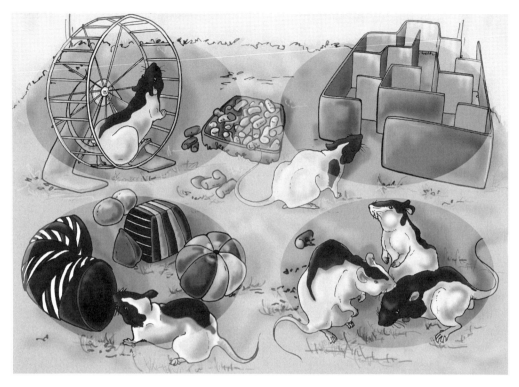

Figure 2.1
Environmental enrichment (EE) for laboratory rodents. EE is a manipulation of the standard rearing setting, improving the quality and intensity of environmental stimulation. Enriched animals receive enhanced multisensory stimulation, attain sustained levels of physical activity, and are provided with increased opportunities for play and for the execution of their spontaneous behavioral repertoire.

differential rearing in either standard or EE conditions and in three different laboratories (Wolfer et al., 2004). EE was found to improve behavioral performances of each strain to the same extent in all the laboratories, thus maintaining the expected behavioral differences between them, and in no case was the within-group variability increased in the EE group with respect to controls (Wolfer et al., 2004). Furthermore, EE is a highly reliable treatment since similar effects on brain measures have been found in several species of mammals, from mice and rats to gerbils, ground squirrels, cats, and monkeys (Rosenzweig and Bennett, 1969). These results underscore the possibility of benefiting from EE's potential without the risk of obtaining conflicting data in replicate studies.

EE exerts a large number of effects on the adult brain. EE modifies the behavior, improving animal performance especially in tasks involving complex cognitive functions (Rampon and Tsien, 2000) and reducing the cognitive decline associated with aging (Mohammed et al., 1993; Mohammed et al., 2002). This outcome is related to a robust facilitation of hippocampal long-term potentiation (LTP), a widely accepted synaptic plasticity model of learning and memory (van Praag et al., 2000). EE also positively affects emotional and stress reactivity, both in normal animals and in strains of mice considered pathologically anxious (Chapillon et al., 2002).

Prominent changes at the anatomical level have been observed in the brains of EE animals, with strong increments in cortical thickness and weight and modifications of neuronal morphology, in terms of enhanced dendritic arborization, number of dendritic spines, synaptic density, and postsynaptic thickening, that are particularly evident in the occipital cortex and in the hippocampus (Mohammed et al., 2002). Moreover, exposure to EE increases hippocampal neurogenesis, reducing apoptotic cell death of proliferating neurons (Young et al., 1999), and promotes the integration of newly born cells into functional circuits (van Praag et al., 2000).

In the search for "enviromimetics," that is, molecules able to reproduce the beneficial effects elicited by the enriched experience, the first studies by Rosenzweig et al. (Rosenzweig et al., 1967) reported an increase in acetylcholinesterase activity, suggesting an effect on the cholinergic system. Subsequent research extended this observation to other neurotransmitter systems which have diffuse projections to the brain, like the serotonergic (Rasmuson et al., 1998) and the noradrenergic systems (Naka et al., 2002). More recently, gene chip analysis revealed that a large number of genes related to neuronal structure, synaptic transmission and plasticity, neuronal excitability, and neuroprotection change their expression levels in response to EE (Rampon et al., 2000). One group of molecules particularly sensitive to experience are neurotrophins, a family of secreted factors critically involved in structural and functional plasticity during development and adulthood (Pham et al., 2002).

An important line of research deals with the potential therapeutic effects of EE. Indeed, it has been shown that enriching the living environment delays the progression of and facilitates recovery from various nervous system dysfunctions, including neurodevelopmental disorders, neurodegenerative diseases, different types of brain injury, and psychiatric disorders (Nithianantharajah and Hannan, 2006).

Environmental Enrichment and Visual System Development

Despite the large literature documenting the effects on the adult brain, until recently the influence of EE on nervous system development has remained scarcely investigated. In the past few years, this gap has been filled with a series of studies focusing on the visual system as a paradigmatic model (see figure 2.2, plate 1).

Acceleration of Visual System Development by Environmental Enrichment

Far from being controlled by rigidly established genetic programs, the development of VA, a very sensitive and predictive index of visual system maturation, is accelerated about one week in animals enriched since birth (see figure 2.3, plate 2). This remarkable effect has been consistently reported in mice and rats using both electrophysiological and behavioral methods

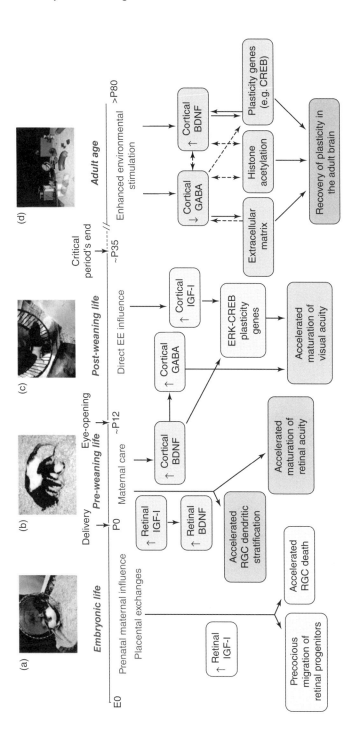

Figure 2.2 (plate 1)

Environmental enrichment (EE) effects on the developing and the adult visual system: an interpretative framework. Three consecutive temporal phases during development are differently controlled by the richness of the environment. (a) The maturation of the nervous system is sensitive to environmental stimulation already during prenatal life, with the mother mediating the influence of the environment through placental exchanges with the fetus. Indeed, exposing pregnant females to EE leads to an acceleration of structural processes critical for retinal maturation in the embryos, an effect mostly due to increased levels of insulin-like growth factor-I (IGF-I). (b) In the early postnatal phase, EE pups receive enhanced maternal care stimulating the expression of experience-dependent factors, such as BDNF, both in the retina and the visual cortex. This drives the accelerated maturation of retinal ganglion cells (RGCs) observed in EE pups and, through an increased GABAergic inhibitory transmission, triggers a faster visual cortex development. (c) Finally, when developing pups are able to autonomously interact with the enriched environment, an increase of cortical IGF-I, which in turn promotes the maturation of the GABAergic system, induces a quite strong acceleration (about one week) in the time course of visual acuity maturation. (d) Recent data have documented a previously unsuspected high potential of neuronal plasticity in the adult visual cortex, with EE in adulthood promoting visual acuity and binocularity recovery from amblyopia. This is due to a decreased intracortical inhibition and to an enhanced BDNF expression. Both the increase in overall cortical activity and BDNF intracellular signaling could in turn induce the activation of other genes promoting plasticity—for instance, through the ERK–CREB pathway. An influence on the epigenetic control of gene transcription has been also suggested for EE. Finally, changes leading to extracellular matrix remodeling may trigger structural modifications at the level of synaptic connectivity. Continuous arrows represent well-documented interactions between boxes; dashed arrows indicate likely interactions in the context of visual cortical plasticity deserving further experimental characterization.

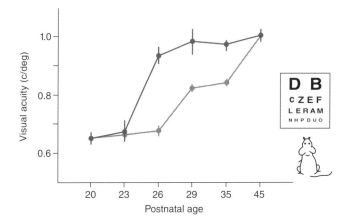

(a)

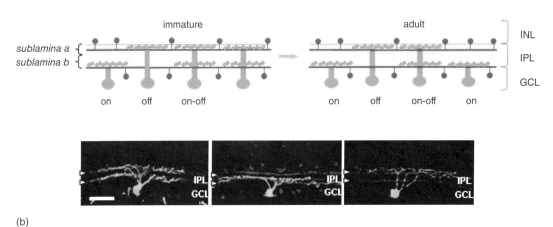

(b)

Figure 2.3 (plate 2)

Acceleration of visual system development by environmental enrichment (EE). (a) Environmental enrichment strongly accelerates visual acuity maturation. Visual acuity measured by visual evoked potentials in non-EE (green) and EE (red) rats during postnatal development is plotted as a function of age to show the leftward shift of the curve for EE animals. (b) Top row: Schematic representation illustrating the passage from immature to adult state during development of retinal ganglion cell (RGC) dendritic stratification (cholinergic amacrine cells in red, RGCs in green). The patterning of cholinergic amacrine cell projections identifies the *a* and *b* sublaminae of the IPL. ON-OFF bistratified RGCs could develop in either ON or OFF RGCs, with dendrites respectively monostratified in the *a* or *b* sublaminae. GCL, ganglion cell layer; IPL, inner plexiform layer; INL, inner nuclear layer. Bottom row: Examples of monostratified or bistratified RGCs. Confocal images are taken from 25-μm vertical retinal sections from P30 transgenic mice expressing the green fluorescent protein. White arrows indicate the sublaminae of the IPL (red bands). Scale bar: 50 μm. Modified from Landi et al. (2007a, 2007b).

(Cancedda et al., 2004; Landi et al., 2007a). In the time scale of human visual development, it is as if a child would reach his final VA at around three years of age, that is, about two years before the age at which children's acuity development normally ends. One crucial molecular factor involved in this process is brain-derived neurotrophic factor (BDNF). Indeed, the acceleration of visual cortical development in EE animals closely resembles that documented in transgenic mice overexpressing BDNF in their forebrain (Huang et al., 1999), and BDNF levels are precociously (P7) raised in the visual cortex of mice reared from birth in EE (Cancedda et al., 2004). BDNF accelerates the development of the inhibitory GABAergic system, which, by affecting receptive field development and synaptic plasticity, could in turn cause the faster maturation of VA. Consistently, enriched pups display at P7 and P15 an increased expression of the GABA biosynthetic enzymes, GAD65/67 (Cancedda et al., 2004; see figure 2.2).

Another molecule that mediates the EE effects on visual system development is insulin-like growth factor-I (IGF-I). IGF-I expression is increased at P18 in the visual cortex of EE rats, and exogenous IGF-I supply mimics, whereas blocking IGF-I action prevents, the EE effects on VA maturation (Ciucci et al., 2007). Also in this case the action of IGF-I on VA development seems to be related to the inhibitory GABAergic system since cortical interneurons respond to IGF-I infusion with a GAD65 enhancement in their synaptic terminals (Ciucci et al., 2007; see figure 2.2). BDNF and IGF-I signaling may eventually converge on the activation of intracellular pathways, leading to the phosphorylation of the transcription factor cyclic AMP response element binding (CREB). The wave of CREB/cyclic AMP responsive element (CRE) mediated gene expression in the visual cortex is accelerated in EE mice, and chronic injections of non-EE animals with rolipram, a pharmacological treatment increasing the phosphorylation of CREB, partially mimic the EE outcome on VA maturation (Cancedda et al., 2004; see figure 2.2).

Environmental Enrichment and Dark Rearing

Given the precociousness of the EE effects on BDNF and GABAergic inhibition, which are clearly evident before eye opening, one could speculate that the acceleration of visual system development does not necessarily require vision. This issue has been addressed in a study where EE and dark rearing (DR) have been combined. Rearing mammals in total darkness from birth affects the maturation of visual cortical circuits, prolonging the duration of the CP and slowing down the progression of developmental VA increase (Timney et al., 1978; Fagiolini et al., 1994). These developmental delays are completely counteracted by coupling DR with EE: dark-reared rats exposed to EE show a normal closure of the CP for OD plasticity and a proper VA development (Bartoletti et al., 2004). The outcome of EE is very similar to that found in BDNF overexpressing mice, where a rescue of DR phenotype has been reported (Gianfranceschi et al., 2003). The similarity between the effects obtained using either genetic engineering techniques to increase neurotrophin expression or conditions of high environmental complexity is a paradigmatic example of how nature and nurture can converge on common molecular pathways involved in the development of sensory systems.

Environmental Enrichment and Retinal Development

It is commonly believed that retinal development is independent from sensory inputs. In marked contrast with visual cortical acuity, indeed, retinal acuity is unresponsive to visual deprivation in cats, rats, and humans (Baro et al., 1990; Fagiolini et al., 1994; Fine et al., 2003).

This view has been challenged by new data showing that the anatomical and physiological retinal maturation is altered by lack of visual experience (Tian and Copenhagen, 2001, 2003). Then, retinal acuity development has also proved to be very sensitive to EE, displaying an acceleration on a time scale equal to that of cortical acuity and even in animals exposed to differential rearing only before eye opening (Landi et al., 2007a). Moreover, a faster process of retinal ganglion cell (RGC) dendrite segregation into ON and OFF sublaminae is evident in enriched rats (Landi et al., 2007b; see figure 2.3). IGF-I and BDNF are key molecular factors in these processes: retinal levels of both proteins are precociously increased in the RGC layer of developing EE rats, and blocking either IGF-I or BDNF action in EE animals counteracts the faster retinal maturation (Landi et al., 2007a, 2007b, 2009). More specifically, BDNF is a downstream target of IGF-I signaling, with the IGF-I increase being necessary and sufficient to mediate the EE effects on retinal BDNF expression (Landi et al., 2009; see figure 2.2).

Strikingly, environmental stimulation also promotes nervous system maturation during pre-natal life. Enriching pregnant female rats during gestation has profound effects on the retinal anatomical development of the embryos, with faster dynamics of neural progenitor migration and spontaneous apoptosis in the RGC layer (see figure 2.2). IGF-I turned out to be a critical factor also in this process: IGF-I levels, indeed, are higher in enriched pregnant rats and in their milk, and this increment is translated into increased IGF-I levels in the retina of the embryos. Furthermore, the neutralization of IGF-I in enriched mothers abolishes the action of maternal enrichment on retinal development, and chronic IGF-I injection to standard-reared females mimics the effects of EE in the fetuses (Sale et al., 2007a; see figure 2.2).

Maternal Enrichment and Visual System Development

It was soon realized that differences in maternal behavior between EE and non-EE conditions could be a fundamental player triggering the earliest effects of EE on visual system development. The first two weeks of life in rodents, indeed, are characterized by a prevalent absence of inter-action between the newborn and the external environment, which is almost completely repre-sented by the mother (Liu et al., 2000). A detailed quantitative analysis of maternal care in EE and standard condition showed that EE pups receive higher levels of maternal care compared to standard-reared pups (Sale et al., 2004). More specifically, EE animals experience a continu-ous physical contact due to the presence of adult females in the nest and are also provided with increased levels of licking and grooming, a fundamental source of tactile stimulation that can directly affect pup brain development. In accordance with this view, it is known that the amount of maternal care received by the developing pup influences hippocampal structure and function, affects molecular factors crucial for plasticity such as BDNF and NMDA receptors, and leaves long-lasting epigenetic marks in the offspring physiology and behavior (Liu et al., 2000; Weaver et al., 2004; Weaver et al., 2006; Champagne and Curley, 2009).

Very recently, a protocol of daily artificial tactile stimulation in the rat has proved to be highly effective in promoting the maturation of physiological visual functions, in particular of VA. This protocol of sensory enrichment increases IGF-I levels in the visual cortex at P18, and blocking IGF-I action prevents its effects on VA development (Guzzetta et al., 2009). Tactile stimulation, mimicking maternal behavior, is also able to compensate for the deleterious effects on pup growth, hormone secretion, hypothalamus–pituitary–adrenal axis and BDNF expression that are typically caused by repeated episodes of maternal separation or by prenatal stress (Schanberg and Field, 1987; Burton et al., 2007; Chatterjee et al., 2007). Altogether, these results provide an example of cross-modal plasticity by which an increased input in a single modality reverberates as a driving force for the whole brain.

Early Sensory Enrichment in Humans

Though EE research has been mostly done on rodents, similar effects occur in primates (Kozorovitskiy et al., 2005), and several epidemiological observations suggest that physical activity and cognitive stimulation have a neuroprotective influence on the human brain, reducing the risk of developing neurodegenerative diseases (Nithianantharajah and Hannan, 2009). Until recently, however, a direct demonstration that an experimental manipulation improving environmental experience causes measurable changes in human brain function was still lacking. In one of the first attempts to study the mechanisms underlying the influence of EE on the human brain, Guzzetta et al. (2009) reported that enriching the environment in terms of body massage ("massage therapy") accelerates brain development in infants. The authors found that a combination of gently stroking and massaging is highly effective in accelerating the maturation of visual functions in healthy preterm babies (gestational age between 30 and 33 weeks; see figure 2.4).

Massaged infants exhibit an earlier shortening of the interburst intervals in the EEG, a reliable index of the developmental stage of the brain, a greater reduction in the latency of flash visual evoked potentials, and an increase in behavioral VA outlasting the end of the treatment. As found in the animal model, massaged infants have increased levels of plasma IGF-I, a result in agreement with previous findings by Kuhn and colleagues (Field et al., 2008), and exhibit reduced levels of circulating cortisol. Thus, massage seems to both decrease stress and provide enriched sensory stimulation, which makes this procedure highly recommendable as an intervention to promote growth and development of preterm and low-birth-weight infants. These results not only underscore the importance of the environment as a driving force in early postnatal development of humans but also suggest that massage therapy could be a good implementation of normal intensive treatment for preterm babies aimed at counteracting the onset of neurological pathologies associated with a precocious delivery. Recent papers have shown that IGF-I and the IGF-I binding protein IGFBP3 could be protective against

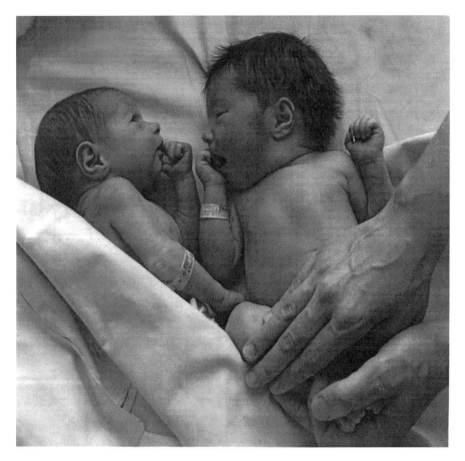

Figure 2.4
Maturation of visual system is accelerated in massaged preterm infants. Massage therapy was begun on day 10 after birth. Sessions were performed three times a day for 10 days. Each treatment session consisted of 10 minutes of tactile stimulation, followed by 5 minutes of kinesthetic stimulation. During tactile stimulation, the infant was placed prone and was given moderate pressure stroking with the flats of the fingers of both hands. In addition, passive flexion/extension movements of the limbs were applied in sequence. Visual acuity in massaged infants was significantly higher than in controls at 3 months. Two monozygotic twins were assigned to different arms of the study. Strikingly, their results confirmed on a single case-control basis the general pattern of results obtained for the entire group.

proliferative retinopathy of prematurity, a severe and relatively frequent visual disorder in preterm infants (Lofqvist et al., 2006, 2007).

Rejuvenating the Adult Brain

Great effort is being put forth by the neuroscience community to develop strategies capable of promoting nervous system plasticity in adulthood, when recovery from injury is poor and functional rehabilitation very hard to achieve. The visual system is the premier model for studying experience-dependent plasticity, with two most classic experimental paradigms: (1) the OD shift of visual cortical neurons after MD and (2) the recovery of visual functions in amblyopic animals. Amblyopia (lazy eye) is a widely diffused pathology of the visual system refractory to treatment in the adult. Amblyopia causes a broad range of disabling perceptual abnormalities, including a dramatic loss of VA in an apparently healthy eye and deficits in stereopsis and contrast sensitivity (Holmes and Clarke, 2006). This severe dysfunction derives from conditions of early abnormal visual experience in which a functional imbalance between the two eyes is predominant due to anisometropia (unequal refractive power in the two eyes), strabismus (abnormal alignment of one or both eyes), congenital cataract, or, in animal models, long-term MD starting during the CP. The traditional therapy consists of patching or penalizing the preferred fellow eye, thus forcing the brain to use the visual input carried by the weaker amblyopic eye (Wu and Hunter, 2006). While it is generally accepted that recovery of visual functions is possible only if normal visual experience is reestablished early in development, recent studies in rodents have shown new therapeutic possibilities for the treatment of adult subjects (see figure 2.5).

Effects of Chondroitinase ABC

The first treatment that proved to be effective in restoring plasticity in the adult visual cortex was the pharmacological degradation of components of the extracellular matrix (ECM; Pizzorusso et al., 2002). ECM represents a substantial fraction of brain volume consisting of a complex network of molecules filling the space between cells. A great number of studies have involved several ECM elements, such as integrins, cadherins, neural cell adhesion molecules, tenascins, and heparin-sulfate proteoglycans, in synaptic plasticity (for a review, see Dityatev and Schachner, 2003). Major components of the ECM are the chondroitin-sulfate proteoglycans (CSPGs) that comprise a core protein and chondroitin-sulfate glycosaminoglycan chains. CSPGs condense during development at high concentration into lattice-like structures, called perineuronal nets (PNNs), completely ensheathing cortical neurons (see figure 2.6). CSPGs exert a powerful repressive control on adult plasticity. Their digestion by means of the enzyme chondroitinase ABC, indeed, reactivates OD plasticity in adult rats and promotes recovery from long-term MD on VA and binocularity of cortical neurons (Pizzorusso et al., 2002, 2006). The action of ECM on cortical plasticity could occur at the level of inhibitory interneurons, around which most of the current studies localize PNNs, or at the level of excitatory neurons,

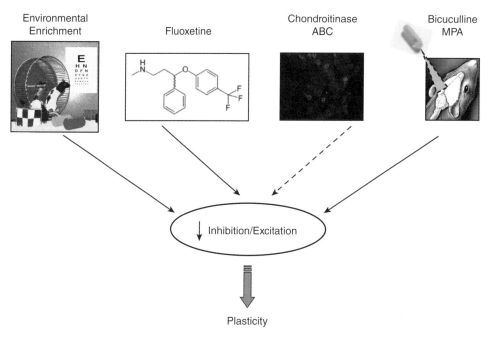

Figure 2.5
Restoring plasticity in the adult visual cortex. Recent data have documented a previously unsuspected high potential of neuronal plasticity in the adult visual cortex. Plasticity can be elicited by exposure to an environmental enrichment setting, chronic administration of antidepressants (fluoxetine), or pharmacological treatment with chondroitinase ABC (which degrades the extracellular matrix chondroitin sulphate proteoglycans) or mercaptopropionic acid (MPA; which decreases the GABAergic tone). We propose a model in which the balance between inhibition and excitation is the central hub triggering plasticity in the adult cortex. Continuous arrows represent well-documented actions on intracortical inhibition; dashed arrow indicates a likely interaction in the context of visual cortical plasticity deserving further experimental characterization.

as suggested by the presence of CSPG-containing nets also around pyramidal neurons (Hockfield et al., 1990). Another appealing explanation could be that the mature ECM is a strongly unfavorable environment for synaptic dynamics forcing neuronal circuits to stability. Consistently, a great number of in vivo two-photon-microscopy studies have showed a developmental decline in experience-dependent spine motility and pruning (Majewska and Sur, 2003; Mataga et al., 2004; Oray et al., 2004), and it has been observed that the removal of CSPGs leads to a recovery of dendritic-spine density in the visual cortex of amblyopic animals (Pizzorusso et al., 2006). These data indicate that ECM degradation sets up a permissive milieu for plasticity modifications facilitating the structural remodeling of synaptic contacts among neurons.

Effects of Enriched Environment
Strikingly, EE is also able to reverse the abnormal function of the visual cortex in adult amblyopic rats. A brief exposure (two to three weeks) to EE promoted a full recovery of VA and

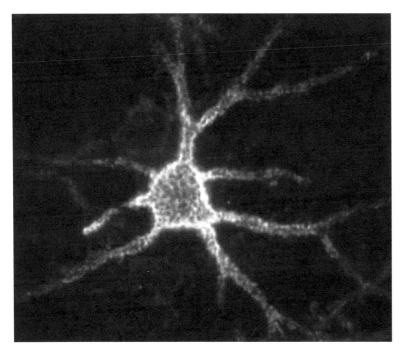

Figure 2.6
Example of a chondroitin-sulfate proteoglycan perineuronal net immunostained for *Wisteria floribunda* (WFA) in the rat primary visual cortex.

binocularity (Sale et al., 2007b), an effect documented with both electrophysiological and behavioral assessments (see figures 2.2 and 2.5). These promising results open new perspectives for clinical application to human patients, given the completely noninvasive nature of the EE approach. Indeed, an increasing number of clinical studies have shown that visual perceptual learning based on sensory enrichment procedures may favor recovery from amblyopia, providing a substantial improvement in a variety of visual tasks (Levi and Li, 2009).

The study of experimental models of amblyopia allows researchers to uncover the molecular mechanisms underlying the therapeutic value of the employed procedures. A three-fold reduction in the basal levels of GABA was detected in the visual cortex contralateral to the amblyopic eye in EE rats (see figure 2.2), and this decrease of intracortical inhibition resulted in a full recovery of white-matter induced LTP, a model of synaptic plasticity that is normally occluded in the visual cortex of adult animals as a result of the maturation of inhibitory circuits (Kirkwood and Bear, 1994). The restoration of plasticity is completely prevented by benzodiazepine cortical infusion during the EE period, demonstrating that the reduction of inhibition is a crucial molecular mechanism underlying the enhancement of plasticity induced by EE (Sale et al., 2007b).

The most direct demonstration that high levels of GABAergic inhibition prevent plasticity in the adult visual cortex comes from the very recent report that a pharmacological reduction of inhibition through intracortical infusion of either MPA (an inhibitor of GABA synthesis) or picrotoxin (a GABAA antagonist) reactivates OD plasticity in response to MD in adult rats (Harauzov et al., 2010; see figure 2.5). It has been suggested that the balance between excitation and inhibition is also impaired during development in amblyopic human subjects and that cortical overinhibition could underlie the degradation of spatial vision abilities (Levi et al., 2002; Polat et al., 2005).

The reduction of GABA release in the visual cortex of EE rats is paralleled by an increased expression of the neurotrophic factor BDNF (Sale et al., 2007b; see figure 2.2). It has been shown that intracortical administration of BDNF reactivates per se neural plasticity in the adult visual cortex (Maya Vetencourt et al., 2008) and that TrkB signaling is required for the recovery of deprived-eye responses subsequent to the reinstatement of binocular vision during development (Kaneko et al., 2008). The increase of cortical activity and BDNF intracellular signaling could in turn induce a transcriptional program that leads to activation of other genes promoting plasticity, acting, for instance, on chromatin remodeling. EE, indeed, leads to increased levels of histone acetylation in the hippocampus and neocortex (Fischer et al., 2007). A similar relationship between histone acetylation and EE could mediate the effects of an enriched experience in the adult visual system (see figure 2.2), where pharmacological treatment with inhibitors of histone deacetylases restores OD plasticity (Putignano et al., 2007). Looking at the brain extracellular milieu, it has been shown that EE in amblyopic rats reduces the density of ECM PNNs in the visual cortex (Sale et al., 2007b). Thus, EE could also affect the synaptic remodeling of visual cortical pyramidal neurons.

Effects of Fluoxetine

It is well-known that EE has a profound effect on those neural systems characterized by diffuse projections in the brain, increasing acetylcholinesterase activity, noradrenalin, and serotonin (Rosenzweig et al., 1967; Rasmuson et al., 1998; Naka et al., 2002). Since these neuromodulators have been reported to influence plasticity in the adult brain and have a fundamental role in regulating the arousal state and attentional processes, it is likely that they are important mediators of the EE experience. Accordingly, one would be able to reproduce the EE effects on adult visual cortex plasticity by an artificial modulation of one or more of these transmitters. We addressed this possibility in a recent study by Maya Vetencourt et al. (2008), showing that the previously unsuspected potential for adult brain plasticity set in motion by EE can also be evoked by administration of fluoxetine, a selective serotonin reuptake inhibitor (SSRI) widely prescribed in the treatment of depression. SSRIs enhance extracellular serotonin and/or noradrenalin levels, but the relationship between acute increases in these neurotransmitters and the clinical antidepressant effect remains unclear. There is evidence that a disturbance of brain plasticity is involved in animal models of depression and that antidepressant treatment may counteract these alterations, stimulating hippocampal neurogenesis, synaptogenesis, and BDNF signaling

(Malberg et al., 2000; Saarelainen et al., 2003; Hajszan et al., 2005). Although these are events that correlate with neuronal plasticity, it is only in a recent paper that the capability of SSRIs to induce functional modifications of neuronal circuitries in the brain was demonstrated for the first time in a direct way (Maya Vetencourt et al., 2008). The authors showed that chronic treatment with fluoxetine delivered in the drinking water induces the reinstatement of OD plasticity in response to MD and a full recovery of visual functions from amblyopia in adult animals. As found for EE rats, these functional effects are associated with a marked reduction of GABAergic inhibition and are completely prevented by cortical diazepam administration (Maya Vetencourt et al., 2008).

Concluding Remarks and Future Research Lines

The data reviewed in this chapter have shown that EE is a powerful tool to modulate the development of the central nervous system and to reopen plasticity gates in the adult cortex in a totally noninvasive way. In particular, the restoration of neural plasticity by EE in adulthood has a multifactorial molecular substrate, with a reduced intracortical inhibition and an enhanced neurotrophin expression which could in turn upregulate the expression of other genes involved in brain plasticity. At the very end of this pathway, changes at the level of chromatin function and synaptic structure may be involved (see figure 2.2).

EE emerges as an elective therapeutic strategy for the treatment of developmental disorders and degenerative diseases in which neuronal plasticity is compromised. One paradigmatic case is that of dementia in the elderly. Among the pathologies which may lead to dementia, Alzheimer's disease (AD) and vascular dementia (VaD) are by far the most frequent. At present, there are no effective therapeutic treatments for AD or VaD, which are still pathologies orphan of treatment. Indeed, current strategies are at best effective in controlling some psychological and behavioral symptoms. In the absence of suitable pharmacological therapies for dementia, substantial interest is starting to be attracted by methods of cognitive stimulation aiming at maintaining—and possibly at least partially recovering—brain functions not yet totally compromised. Several studies have demonstrated that cognitive and motor stimulation reduce from 20% to 50% the risk of developing dementia in aged people (Laurin et al., 2001; Churchill et al., 2002; Fratiglioni et al., 2004; Marx, 2005; Podewils et al., 2005). Therefore, the combination of cognitive stimulation and physical exercise represents a potential protective strategy of intervention to restrain cognitive decline and reduce the progression of brain damage associated with AD.

Scientific studies that rigorously address the effects of EE in patients with dementia are still scarce. The authors have started in the laboratories of CNR in Pisa a new venture specifically devoted to filling this essential gap (figure 2.7). Clinical trials aimed at studying the effects of enhanced environmental stimulation on mild cognitive impairment, predictive of AD onset, are presently going on in our laboratory. The primary endpoint of the present project is to assess the efficacy of a combined protocol of physical exercise and cognitive stimulation on the

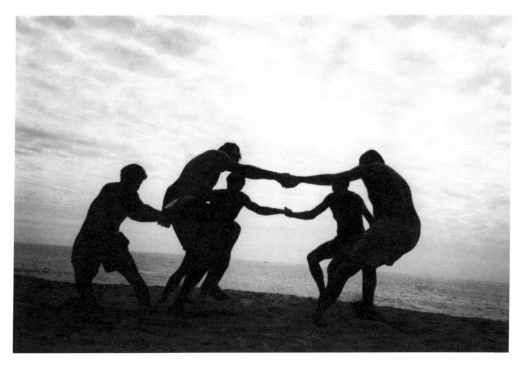

Figure 2.7
A photographic memento portraying Lamberto Maffei with some famous neurobiologists trying to train their brain on a Mexican beach: controversial results. From the left clockwise: Tommaso Pizzorusso, Giorgio Carmignoto, Lamberto Maffei, Stefano Vicini, Gimmi Ratto. Cabo San Lucas, November 1998.

progression of the disease in patients at the earliest phases of AD and VaD, with the final aim of developing a reproducible nonpharmacological therapeutic strategy easily applicable in humans.

References

Baro JA, Lehmkuhle S, Kratz KE. 1990. Electroretinograms and visual evoked potentials in long-term monocularly deprived cats. *Invest Ophthalmol Vis Sci* 31: 1405–1409.

Bartoletti A, Medini P, Berardi N, Maffei L. 2004. Environmental enrichment prevents effects of dark-rearing in the rat visual cortex. *Nat Neurosci* 7: 215–216.

Berardi N, Pizzorusso T, Maffei L. 2000. Critical periods during sensory development. *Curr Opin Neurobiol* 10: 138–145.

Burton CL, Chatterjee D, Chatterjee-Chakraborty M, Lovic V, Grella SL, Steiner M, Fleming AS. 2007. Prenatal restraint stress and motherless rearing disrupts expression of plasticity markers and stress-induced corticosterone release in adult female Sprague-Dawley rats. *Brain Res* 1158: 28–38.

Cancedda L, Putignano E, Sale A, Viegi A, Berardi N, Maffei L. 2004. Acceleration of visual system development by environmental enrichment. *J Neurosci* 24: 4840–4848.

Champagne FA, Curley JP. 2009. Epigenetic mechanisms mediating the long-term effects of maternal care on development. *Neurosci Biobehav Rev* 33: 593–600.

Chapillon P, Patin V, Roy V, Vincent A, Caston J. 2002. Effects of pre- and postnatal stimulation on developmental, emotional, and cognitive aspects in rodents: a review. *Dev Psychobiol* 41: 373–387.

Chatterjee D, Chatterjee-Chakraborty M, Rees S, Cauchi J, de Medeiros CB, Fleming AS. 2007. Maternal isolation alters the expression of neural proteins during development: "Stroking" stimulation reverses these effects. *Brain Res* 1158: 11–27.

Churchill JD, Galvez R, Colcombe S, Swain RA, Kramer AF, Greenough WT. 2002. Exercise, experience and the aging brain. *Neurobiol Aging* 23: 941–955.

Ciucci F, Putignano E, Baroncelli L, Landi S, Berardi N, Maffei L. 2007. Insulin-like growth factor 1 (IGF-1) mediates the effects of enriched environment (EE) on visual cortical development. *PLoS ONE* 2: 475–484.

Dityatev A, Schachner M. 2003. Extracellular matrix molecules and synaptic plasticity. *Nat Rev Neurosci* 4: 456–468.

Fagiolini M, Pizzorusso T, Berardi N, Domenici L, Maffei L. 1994. Functional postnatal development of the rat primary visual cortex and the role of visual experience: dark rearing and monocular deprivation. *Vision Res* 34: 709–720.

Field T, Diego M, Hernandez-Reif M, Dieter JN, Kumar AM, Schanberg S, Kuhn C. 2008. Insulin and insulin-like growth factor-1 increased in preterm neonates following massage therapy. *J Dev Behav Pediatr* 29: 463–466.

Fine I, Wade AR, Brewer AA, May MG, Goodman DF, Boynton GM, Wandell BA, MacLeod DI. 2003. Long-term deprivation affects visual perception and cortex. *Nat Neurosci* 6: 915–916.

Fischer A, Sananbenesi F, Wang X, Dobbin M, Tsai LH. 2007. Recovery of learning and memory is associated with chromatin remodelling. *Nature* 447: 178–182.

Fratiglioni L, Paillard-Borg S, Winblad B. 2004. An active and socially integrated lifestyle in late life might protect against dementia. *Lancet Neurol* 3: 343–353.

Gianfranceschi L, Siciliano R, Walls J, Morales B, Kirkwood A, Huang ZJ, Tonegawa S, Maffei L. 2003. Visual cortex is rescued from the effects of dark rearing by overexpression of BDNF. *Proc Natl Acad Sci USA* 100: 12486–12491.

Guzzetta A, Baldini S, Bancale A, Baroncelli L, Ciucci F, Ghirri P, Putignano E, et al. 2009. Massage accelerates brain development and the maturation of visual function. *J Neurosci* 29: 6042–6051.

Hajszan T, MacLusky NJ, Leranth C. 2005. Short-term treatment with the antidepressant fluoxetine triggers pyramidal dendritic spine synapse formation in rat hippocampus. *Eur J Neurosci* 21: 1299–1303.

Harauzov A, Spolidoro M, Di Cristo G, De Pasquale R, Cancedda L, Pizzorusso T, Viegi A, Berardi N, Maffei L. 2010. Reducing intracortical inhibition in the adult visual cortex promotes ocular dominance plasticity. *J Neurosci* 30: 361–371.

Hensch TK. 2004. Critical period regulation. *Annu Rev Neurosci* 27: 549–579.

Hockfield S, Kalb RG, Zaremba S, Fryer H. 1990. Expression of neural proteoglycans correlates with the acquisition of mature neuronal properties in the mammalian brain. *Cold Spring Harb Symp Quant Biol* 55: 505–514.

Holmes JM, Clarke MP. 2006. Amblyopia. *Lancet* 367: 1343–1351.

Huang ZJ, Kirkwood A, Pizzorusso T, Porciatti V, Morales B, Bear MF, Maffei L, Tonegawa S. 1999. BDNF regulates the maturation of inhibition and the critical period of plasticity in mouse visual cortex. *Cell* 98: 739–755.

Hubel DH, Wiesel TN. 1970. The period of susceptibility to the physiological effects of unilateral eye closure in kittens. *J Physiol* 206: 419–436.

Kaneko M, Hanover JL, England PM, Stryker MP. 2008. TrkB kinase is required for recovery, but not loss, of cortical responses following monocular deprivation. *Nat Neurosci* 11: 497–504.

Kirkwood A, Bear MF. 1994. Hebbian synapses in visual cortex. *J Neurosci* 14: 1634–1645.

Knudsen EI. 2004. Sensitive periods in the development of the brain and behavior. *J Cog Neurosci* 16: 1412–1425.

Kozorovitskiy Y, Gross CG, Kopil C, Battaglia L, McBreen M, Stranahan AM, Gould E. 2005. Experience induces structural and biochemical changes in the adult primate brain. *Proc Natl Acad Sci USA* 102: 17478–17482.

Krubitzer L, Kahn DM. 2003. Nature versus nurture revisited: an old idea with a new twist. *Prog Neurobiol* 70: 33–52.

Landi S, Sale A, Berardi N, Viegi A, Maffei L, Cenni MC. 2007a. Retinal functional development is sensitive to environmental enrichment: a role for BDNF. *FASEB J* 21: 130–139.

Landi S, Cenni MC, Maffei L, Berardi N. 2007b. Environmental enrichment effects on development of retinal ganglion cell dendritic stratification require retinal BDNF. *PLoS ONE* 2: 346–356.

Landi S, Ciucci F, Maffei L, Berardi N, Cenni MC. 2009. Setting the pace for retinal development: environmental enrichment acts through insulin-like growth factor 1 and brain-derived neurotrophic factor. *J Neurosci* 29: 10809–10819.

Laurin D, Verreault R, Lindsay J, MacPherson K, Rockwood K. 2001. Physical activity and risk of cognitive impairment and dementia in elderly persons. *Arch Neurol* 58: 498–504.

Levi DM, Hariharan S, Klein SA. 2002. Suppressive and facilitatory spatial interactions in amblyopic vision. *Vision Res* 42: 1379–1394.

Levi DM, Li RW. 2009. Improving the performance of the amblyopic visual system. *Philos Trans R Soc Lond B Biol Sci* 364: 399–407.

Liu D, Diorio J, Day JC, Francis DD, Meaney MJ. 2000. Maternal care, hippocampal synaptogenesis and cognitive development in rats. *Nat Neurosci* 3: 799–806.

Lofqvist C, Andersson E, Sigurdsson J, Engstrom E, Hard AL, Niklasson A, Smith LE, Hellstrom A. 2006. Longitudinal postnatal weight and insulin-like growth factor I measurements in the prediction of retinopathy of prematurity. *Arch Ophthalmol* 124: 1711–1718.

Lofqvist C, Chen J, Connor KM, Smith AC, Aderman CM, Liu N, Pintar JE, Ludwig T, Hellstrom A, Smith LE. 2007. IGFBP3 suppresses retinopathy through suppression of oxygen-induced vessel loss and promotion of vascular regrowth. *Proc Natl Acad Sci USA* 104: 10589–10594.

Majewska A, Sur M. 2003. Motility of dendritic spines in visual cortex in vivo: changes during the critical period and effects of visual deprivation. *Proc Natl Acad Sci USA* 100: 16024–16029.

Malberg JE, Eisch AJ, Nestler EJ, Duman RS. 2000. Chronic antidepressant treatment increases neurogenesis in adult rat hippocampus. *J Neurosci* 20: 9104–9110.

Marx J. 2005. Alzheimer's disease: play and exercise protect mouse brain from amyloid buildup. *Science* 307: 1547.

Mataga N, Mizuguchi Y, Hensch TK. 2004. Experience-dependent pruning of dendritic spines in visual cortex by tissue plasminogen activator. *Neuron* 44: 1031–1041.

Maya Vetencourt JF, Sale A, Viegi A, Baroncelli L, De Pasquale R, O'Leary OF, Castren E, Maffei L. 2008. The antidepressant fluoxetine restores plasticity in the adult visual cortex. *Science* 320: 385–388.

Mohammed AH, Henriksson BG, Soderstrom S, Ebendal T, Olsson T, Seckl JR. 1993. Environmental influences on the central nervous system and their implications for the aging rat. *Behav Brain Res* 57: 183–191.

Mohammed AH, Zhu SW, Darmopil S, Hjerling-Leffler J, Ernfors P, Winblad B, Diamond MC, Eriksson PS, Bogdanovic N. 2002. Environmental enrichment and the brain. *Prog Brain Res* 138: 109–133.

Naka F, Shiga T, Yaguchi M, Okado N. 2002. An enriched environment increases noradrenaline concentration in the mouse brain. *Brain Res* 924: 124–126.

Nithianantharajah J, Hannan AJ. 2006. Enriched environments, experience-dependent plasticity and disorders of the nervous system. *Nat Rev Neurosci* 7: 697–709.

Nithianantharajah J, Hannan AJ. 2009. The neurobiology of brain and cognitive reserve: Mental and physical activity as modulators of brain disorders. *Prog Neurobiol* 89: 369–382.

Oray S, Majewska A, Sur M. 2004. Dendritic spine dynamics are regulated by monocular deprivation and extracellular matrix degradation. *Neuron* 44: 1021–1030.

Pham TM, Winblad B, Granholm AC, Mohammed AH. 2002. Environmental influences on brain neurotrophins in rats. *Pharmacol Biochem Behav* 73: 167–175.

Pizzorusso T, Medini P, Berardi N, Chierzi S, Fawcett JW, Maffei L. 2002. Reactivation of ocular dominance plasticity in the adult visual cortex. *Science* 298: 1248–1251.

Pizzorusso T, Medini P, Landi S, Baldini S, Berardi N, Maffei L. 2006. Structural and functional recovery from early monocular deprivation in adult rats. *Proc Natl Acad Sci USA* 103: 8517–8522.

Podewils LJ, Guallar E, Kuller LH, Fried LP, Lopez OL, Carlson M, Lyketsos CG. 2005. Physical activity, APOE genotype, and dementia risk: findings from the Cardiovascular Health Cognition Study. *Am J Epidemiol* 161: 639–651.

Polat U, Bonneh Y, Ma-Naim T, Belkin M, Sagi D. 2005. Spatial interactions in amblyopia: effects of stimulus parameters and amblyopia type. *Vision Res* 45: 1471–1479.

Putignano E, Lonetti G, Cancedda L, Ratto G, Costa M, Maffei L, Pizzorusso T. 2007. Developmental downregulation of histone posttranslational modifications regulates visual cortical plasticity. *Neuron* 53: 747–759.

Rampon C, Jiang CH, Dong H, Tang YP, Lockhart DJ, Schultz PG, Tsien JZ, Hu Y. 2000. Effects of environmental enrichment on gene expression in the brain. *Proc Natl Acad Sci USA* 97: 12880–12884.

Rampon C, Tsien JZ. 2000. Genetic analysis of learning behavior-induced structural plasticity. *Hippocampus* 10: 605–609.

Rasmuson S, Olsson T, Henriksson BG, Kelly PA, Holmes MC, Seckl JR, Mohammed AH. 1998. Environmental enrichment selectively increases 5–HT1A receptor mRNA expression and binding in the rat hippocampus. *Brain Res Mol Brain Res* 53: 285–290.

Rosenzweig MR, Bennett EL. 1969. Effects of differential environments on brain weights and enzyme activities in gerbils, rats, and mice. *Dev Psychobiol* 2: 87–95.

Rosenzweig MR, Bennett EL, Diamond MC. 1967. Effects of differential environments on brain anatomy and brain chemistry. *Proc Annu Meet Am Psychopathol Assoc* 56: 45–56.

Saarelainen T, Hendolin P, Lucas G, Koponen E, Sairanen M, MacDonald E, Agerman K, et al. 2003. Activation of the TrkB neurotrophin receptor is induced by antidepressant drugs and is required for antidepressant-induced behavioral effects. *J Neurosci* 23: 349–357.

Sale A, Putignano E, Cancedda L, Landi S, Cirulli F, Berardi N, Maffei L. 2004. Enriched environment and acceleration of visual system development. *Neuropharmacology* 47: 649–660.

Sale A, Cenni MC, Ciucci F, Putignano E, Chierzi S, Maffei L. 2007a. Maternal enrichment during pregnancy accelerates retinal development of the fetus. *PLoS ONE* 2: 1160–1167.

Sale A, Maya Vetencourt JF, Medini P, Cenni MC, Baroncelli L, De Pasquale R, Maffei L. 2007b. Environmental enrichment in adulthood promotes amblyopia recovery through a reduction of intracortical inhibition. *Nat Neurosci* 10: 679–681.

Schanberg SM, Field TM. 1987. Sensory deprivation stress and supplemental stimulation in the rat pup and preterm human neonate. *Child Dev* 58: 1431–1447.

Tian N, Copenhagen DR. 2001. Visual deprivation alters development of synaptic function in inner retina after eye opening. *Neuron* 32: 439–449.

Tian N, Copenhagen DR. 2003. Visual stimulation is required for refinement of ON and OFF pathways in postnatal retina. *Neuron* 39: 85–96.

Timney B, Mitchell DE, Giffin F. 1978. The development of vision in cats after extended periods of dark-rearing. *Exp Brain Res* 31: 547–560.

van Praag H, Kempermann G, Gage FH. 2000. Neural consequences of environmental enrichment. *Nat Rev Neurosci* 1: 191–198.

Weaver IC, Cervoni N, Champagne FA, D'Alessio AC, Sharma S, Seckl JR, Dymov S, Szyf M, Meaney MJ. 2004. Epigenetic programming by maternal behavior. *Nat Neurosci* 7: 847–854.

Weaver IC, Meaney MJ, Szyf M. 2006. Maternal care effects on the hippocampal transcriptome and anxiety-mediated behaviors in the offspring that are reversible in adulthood. *Proc Natl Acad Sci USA* 103: 3480–3485.

Wiesel TN, Hubel DH. 1963. Single-cell responses in striate cortex of kittens deprived of vision in one eye. *J Neurophysiol* 26: 1003–1017.

Wolfer DP, Litvin O, Morf S, Nitsch RM, Lipp HP, Würbel H. 2004. Laboratory animal welfare: Cage enrichment and mouse behaviour. *Nature* 432: 821–822.

Wu C, Hunter DG. 2006. Amblyopia: diagnostic and therapeutic options. *Am J Ophthalmol* 141: 175–184.

Young D, Lawlor PA, Leone P, Dragunow M, During MJ. 1999. Environmental enrichment inhibits spontaneous apoptosis, prevents seizures and is neuroprotective. *Nat Med* 5: 448–453.

3 The Plasticity of Retinal Ganglion Cells

Julie L. Coombs and Leo M. Chalupa

As is made abundantly clear in this volume dedicated to Lamberto Maffei, he has made seminal contributions to vision research and in particular to the fields of visual development and plasticity. For much of his career, Lamberto's studies on visual plasticity have been concerned with the cortex, where visual experience has been found to have profound effects on the functional and structural properties of neurons. Much less is known about plasticity of the retina and of retinal ganglion cells (RGCs), but in this field Lamberto Maffei and his group have also made important contributions, demonstrating for the first time the importance of environmental enrichment (EE) on retinal development. An excellent chapter in this volume summarizes their recent work in this area; thus we are absolved from the duty of reviewing this work in our offering to this book.

Our goal in this chapter is to review the available literature on the plasticity of RGCs. In this context, plasticity can be defined as a change in a cell's established morphology and/or connectivity pattern in response to specific manipulations, whether these occur during early development or at maturation. For the most part, the studies that have dealt with plasticity of RGCs have been concerned with dendritic morphology of these neurons and have focused on manipulations that have led to changes either in the lateral or vertical extent of these processes. Collectively, these studies have implicated neuronal activity as playing a key role in the normal development and plasticity exhibited by developing ganglion cells.

The development of many neurons, including RGCs, is characterized by exuberant growth followed by a paring back of cells and cellular processes during the course of maturation. In all vertebrate species there is an initial overproduction of RGCs followed by a massive loss of cells as the retina develops and dendrites start to expand (Perry et al., 1983; Young, 1984; Williams et al., 1986, Farah and Easter, 2005). This is followed by the exuberant growth of dendrites that are subsequently pruned back during the course of normal development (Ramoa et al., 1988; Sernagor et al., 2001; Coombs et al., 2007). The available evidence indicates that activity can influence different aspects of RGC development, in terms of the choice of which cells die, the lateral spread of dendrites and the consequent cell–cell interactions, and the stratification of RGC dendrites within the inner plexiform layer (IPL).

Cell Spacing and Lateral Growth of RGC Dendrites

Like some other retinal cells, RGCs tile the inner retina in regularly spaced mosaics of homotypic cells (Wässle and Riemann, 1978; Wässle et al., 1981a, 1981b; Cook and Chalupa, 2000; Galli-Resta, 2002). This emerges over a number of days during development and is influenced by two factors: the developmental loss of RGCs and cell–cell interactions between homotypic cells. Both of these factors can be affected by neuronal activity.

Computer models indicate that selective cell death can contribute to the appearance of RGC tiling early in retinal development (Jeyarasasingam et al., 1998; Eglen, 2006). The emergent spacing between RGCs in cat retina is inhibited by stopping electrical activity with intraocular injections of tetrodotoxin (TTX) to block voltage-dependent sodium channels. For this study, the presence of RGC mosaics was determined by tracking the pairing of somas from different types of alpha RGCs, one responding to the onset and the other to the offset of light. Though ON and OFF alpha cells form separate mosaics with regular spaces between homotypes, the heterotype somas tend be located near each other (Wässle et al., 1981b), a pairing that emerges as many RGCs die and mosaics of homotypic cells form across the retina. TTX injected into developing eyes resulted in a decrease in these ON–OFF soma pairings in a dose-dependent manner. However, the density of the mature RGCs remained the same, suggesting that electrical activity regulates the normal patterning of RGCs by disrupting normal pattern of RGC loss. Since TTX had little effect on the total number of cells lost, the disruption of mosaic formation could reflect blocked electrical communication between homotypic RGCs via gap junctions (Jeyarasasingam et al., 1998).

It was suggested many years ago that cell–cell interactions between the dendrites of homotypic cells is responsible for creating and maintaining RGC mosaics (Wässle et al., 1981a). In support of this notion, Perry and Linden (1982) showed that RGCs extend longer than normal dendrites into areas of the retina devoid of other RGCs due to a retinal lesion early in development. This demonstrated that the geometry of dendritic fields is influenced by interactions with other cells. The importance of interactions with cell neighbors was also shown in retinas of cats in which one eye was removed before birth, a procedure that resulted in a larger than normal density of RGCs in the mature untreated eye. Though the mosaics of RGCs remained intact, the size of individual RGC dendritic fields was reduced to match the increased cell density (Kirby and Chalupa, 1986). Conversely, the somas of alpha and beta RGCs were shown to be larger when cell density was decreased by unilateral section of the optic tract (Leventhal et al., 1988). Altered RGC morphologies were also reported in rat retina when retinal cell densities were reduced by the lesioning of brain target regions (Linden and Perry, 1982). These experiments all suggest that RGC size is influenced by cell–cell interactions. In ferrets, it was shown that RGCs interact with homotypic cells, forming short-term fasciculations along their dendrites, but not with heterotypic RGCs (Lohmann and Wong, 2001). The exuberance of dendrites in immature RGCs often includes fine processes not prevalent in mature cells. Wong et al. (1992) showed that these thin processes do not form synapses and are normally transient. They suggested a possible role for these abundant but usually short-lived processes in cell–cell recognition during development.

Contrary to the findings discussed above, a recent study has called into question the influence of homotypic cell interactions on mosaic formation and on dendritic field shape and size. Thus, Lin et al. (2004) reported normal RGC morphologies in Brn3b knockout mice in which 80% of the normal RGC population is lost. It was expected that this greatly reduced density of RGCs would alter RGC morphology and spacing due to the reduction or elimination of interactions between cells; however, the authors found normal shapes and sizes of RGC dendritic fields (see also Badea et al., 2009), suggesting that interactions between RGCs are not required for their normal morphological development. While the somas were distantly located across the retina, the spacing between homotypic cells was still found to be regular! On the basis of these observations, Lin et al. concluded that cell spacing and dendritic spread are regulated separately, but cell–cell interactions may still refine dendrites to avoid overlap as in the case of increased cell density (Kirby and Chalupa., 1986; Logan and Vetter, 2004).

A number of antagonists of retinal neurotransmitters have been found to disrupt the maturation of RGC morphology. In the chick retina, antagonists to acetylcholine and glutamate reduced RGC dendrite motility, but only during the periods when they were responsible for spontaneous retinal waves of activity (Wong et al., 2000; Wong and Wong, 2001). Blocking GABA or voltage-dependent calcium channels also decreased dendrite motility while TTX did not. In turtle retinas, blocking acetylcholine-based spontaneous activity with curare inhibited RGC growth (Mehta and Sernagor, 2006). The neurotransmitter glycine also has an effect on the maturation of RGC dendrites. In *spastic* mice, a mutant strain with knocked down expression of the glycine receptor (GlyR), the dendrites of adult RGCs had immature stratification patterns and altered responses to light stimulations (Xu and Tian, 2008). These results suggest a distinct and specific effect of retinal neurotransmitters on the vertical growth and elaboration of RGC dendrites.

Dendritic Stratification in the Inner Plexiform Layer

Dendrites grow in a three dimensional space, with the processes of RGCs extending toward the outer retina and ramifying in specific sublayers within the IPL. Input to different IPL laminae is correlated with different types of visual information such that dendritic stratification is an indicator of RGC function (Famiglietti and Kolb, 1976; Nelson et al., 1978; Roska and Werblin, 2001). The growth of dendrites into the appropriate synaptic layers of the IPL and the timing of that growth can depend on information from within the retina. It was first shown in the developing cat retina that the dendrites of RGCs are initially multistratified, meaning that they spread across many layers of the IPL, and become restricted to specific IPL laminae as synapses with bipolar cells are formed (Maslim et al., 1986; Maslim and Stone, 1988; Bodnarenko and Chalupa, 1993). Blocking bipolar cell input onto RGCs prevented this retraction of dendrites into specific sublayers of the IPL (Bodnarenko and Chalupa, 1993). The glutamate analog 2-amino-4-phosphonobutyrate (APB) binds the metabotropic glutamate receptor 6 (mGluR6), thus mimicking the effects of darkness and hyperpolarizing ON cone bipolar and rod bipolar cells, which prevents their release of glutamate. When APB was injected into cat retinas, many RGCs failed to narrow their dendritic stratification into either the ON or OFF layers of the IPL, remaining in an immature multistratified state both morphologically and functionally (Bodnarenko and Chalupa, 1993; Bodnarenko et al., 1995; Bisti et al., 1998; Deplano et al., 2004). It should be noted that this finding is not at odds with the normal laminar structure of the IPL seen in retinas of mGluR6 knockout mice (Tagawa et al., 1999). APB does not mimic the loss of mGluR6; rather, it activates the inhibition of a nonselective cation channel which hyperpolarizes the bipolar cell as it would in the dark (Snellman et al., 2008). A loss of mGluR6 should cause ON bipolar cells to remain depolarized.

Amacrine cells may also influence the maturation of RGC morphology. Acetylcholine, a neurotransmitter commonly associated with amacrine cells, has been shown to influence the maturation of dendritic laminar choice in the IPL. Transgenic mice in which the nicotinic acetylcholine receptors on RGCs have been disabled showed delayed RGC stratification (Bansal et al., 2000), and blocking spontaneous acetylcholine-controlled activity with curare inhibited dendritic growth in the RGCs of turtle retina (Mehta and Sernagor, 2006).

Further evidence supporting the idea that inputs from bipolar and amacrine cells dictate RGC dendritic growth and distribution is seen in their real-time effects on dendritic motility. Blocking glutamate signals in chick retina decreased RGC dendrite extension and retraction as did blocking calcium channels, while TTX did not (Wong et al., 2000). The timing of the inputs onto RGCs affected the response of the RGC dendrites. In chick retina, acetylcholine, glutamate, and GABA all were found to affect dendritic motility in RGCs (Wong and Wong, 2001). In sum, these experiments show that inputs from retinal interneurons are required for the normal maturation of RGC dendritic stratification and function.

Role of Visual Experience in Development of Retinal Ganglion Cells

In 1947 A. H. Riesen described behavioral experiments on chimpanzees showing that visual experience was needed for the proper organization of visual perception (Riesen, 1947). The biological basis for this requirement has been debated ever since. Early papers describe profound alterations in the retina (Chow et al., 1957) while others found such differences to be small (Weiskrantz, 1958; Rasch et al., 1961) or nonexistent (Goodman, 1932). The work of Wiesel and Hubel (1963) demonstrated unequivocally that visual input can have profound effects on the wiring of the brain, but until recently little attention has been paid in the modern era of vision research to the role of visual experience on retinal development.

This issue was reopened by Tian and Copenhagen (2001, 2003), who demonstrated a surge of synaptic potentials (both excitatory and inhibitory) occurring in RGCs, beginning around postnatal day 21 (P21), 8–10 days after eye opening. This increase was temporary (gone by about P60) and was not seen when mice were reared in the dark. These researchers also reported that a majority of RGCs (about 80%) responded to both the onset and offset of light before eye opening, a number that dropped to around 20% by about two weeks after eye opening. This developmental refinement of ON/OFF responses to ON or OFF only responses was not seen in dark-reared mice. Mice raised in the dark retained the large percentage of ON/OFF RGCs seen in the normal immature retinas, an indication that visual activity controls the stratification of RGC dendrites. An accompanying change in the morphology of RGCs was also described, with a large percentage of bistratified RGCs reported before eye opening (53%), dropping to 29% by P30 in normal mice. Again dark rearing prevented the decrease in bistratified cells (53% bistratified RGCs at P30 in dark-reared mice). Bistratification was defined as cells with dendrites ramifying in separate (ON and OFF) laminae of the IPL. These findings are reminiscent of the effects Bodnarenko and Chalupa (1993) reported with APB injections, discussed above.

It should be noted that the claim that mouse RGCs are bistratified early and become increasingly monostratified with light stimulation and maturation has been recently modified somewhat. Recent work from the Tian laboratory speaks not of bistratified RGCs becoming monostratified but rather of initially monostratified dendrites from a central IPL location (the border of the ON and OFF sublaminae) moving to more specific layers of the IPL with maturation, with a preponderance of the affected dendrites relocating into OFF layers of the IPL (Xu and Tian, 2007, 2008). Moreover, there are differing accounts about the prevalence of bistratified RGCs in the mouse before eye opening. Some researchers report that large percentages of immature RGCs are bistratified (44%–69%, Landi et al., 2007a; 52%, Liu et al., 2007; 66%, Liu et al., 2009) while others find a much smaller proportion of such cells (10%, Diao et al., 2004; 18%, Coombs et al., 2007; 9%, Xu and Tian, 2007, 2008). The prevalence of ON/OFF functional responses in RGCs before eye opening is also in dispute (Kerschensteiner and Wong, 2008). Finally, there is considerable variation in the estimates of the prevalence of bistratified RGCs in the normal adult mouse retina (22%, Sun et al., 2002; 21%, Badea and Nathans, 2004; 27%, Coombs et al., 2006; 41%, Liu et al., 2007; 39%, Liu et al., 2009). These disagreements over the number of bistratified RGCs in the developing, dark-reared and mature mouse retinas are unsettling. It is unclear what accounts for these differences, but it may have to do with the techniques used to label or record from cells, an issue that deserves further scrutiny.

A mechanistic link between visual activity and plasticity of RGC dendrites appears to involve neurotrophins, particularly brain derived neurotrophic factor (BDNF). In rat retina, BDNF expression was shown to increase in RGCs after eye opening, an upregulation that was not seen if animals were kept in the dark (Seki et al., 2003). In transgenic mice where expression of yellow fluorescent protein is linked to that of thy1, increasing BDNF expression has been reported to accelerate the maturation of RGC dendritic stratification (Landi et al., 2007a, 2009; Liu et al., 2007). In this study a shift from bistratified to monostratified RGCs was found to occur earlier if BDNF was overexpressed and was delayed when the presence and function of the BDNF receptor, TrkB, was decreased (Liu et al., 2007). An increase in BDNF expression was also seen in the retinas of mice raised in environmentally enriched surroundings—larger cages with access to other mice, toys, and exercise. This boost in BDNF has been implicated in controlling the early stratification of RGCs in mice raised in EE cages (Landi et al., 2007a), along with the earlier appearance of a number of other developmental milestones, including enhanced retinal acuity (Landi et al., 2007b).

Recently, a role for visual activity in determining the dendrite morphology and laminar choices of RGCs has been questioned. Transgenic mice were created in which the expression of tetanus toxin (TeNT) was linked to that of mGluR6, specifically targeting ON bipolar cells. TeNT inhibits synaptic vesicle fusion so that neurotransmission between ON bipolar cells and RGCs was nearly eliminated, while that of OFF bipolar cells remained intact. The expectation was that RGC dendrites in the ON laminae of the IPL would be disrupted. In fact, RGC dendritic morphology appeared normal. However, the number of synapses within the ON sublaminae of the IPL was reduced by about 50%, The reduction of ON synapses was most likely due to a reduction in synapse formation since the rate of synapse loss remained unchanged (Kerschensteiner et al., 2009).

Plasticity of Retinal Interneurons

Retinal ganglion cells are not the only cells in the retina suggested to have plastic responses to their environments. The tiling and size of the dendritic fields of horizontal cells have been shown to be dependent on homotypic interactions while their dendritic branching patterns appear to be shaped by afferent inputs from photoreceptors (Reese, et al., 2005; Poche et al., 2008; Raven et al., 2008; Huckfeldt et al., 2009). Functional properties of certain amacrine cells were affected by blocking retinal activity with TTX (Bloomfield, 1996), and dark rearing mice into adulthood resulted in marked decreases in cholinergic amacrine cell numbers (Zhang et al., 2005). Some adult bipolar cells are plastic as well; in aged mice and humans, rod bipolar cells have been reported to have unusual processes extending into the outer nuclear layer (ONL), where they appeared to synapse with rods. This has been postulated to be caused by bipolar cells' "seeking out" rods that have retracted during the course of normal aging into the ONL. There is some disagreement over whether these unusual processes (few are seen in younger adults) are the result of normal aging or caused by pathology (Liets et al., 2006; Eliasieh et al., 2007; Sullivan et al., 2007).

Concluding Remarks

While there is general agreement that developing RGCs are plastic, a number of key issues in this field remain to be resolved. Much of the recent work in this field has relied on transgenic mice. A number of these studies have found no (or a limited) role for interactions between RGCs or RGCs and ON bipolar cells in determining RGC structure, though connectivity may be altered (Lin et al., 2004; Kerschensteiner et al., 2009). These reports call into question a suite of previous work on other species. However, others working with transgenic mice have shown a strong influence of visual activity as well as activity-dependent production of neurotrophins on RGC morphology and function (Tian and Copenhagen, 2001, 2003; Landi et al., 2007a, 2007b, 2009;

Liu et al., 2007, 2009). Clearly, more work is needed to clarify the role of retinal activity on RGC structure and connectivity.

References

Badea TC, Cahill H, Ecker J, Hattar S, Nathans J. 2009. Distinct roles of transcription factors brn3a and brn3b in controlling the development, morphology, and function of retinal ganglion cells. *Neuron* 61(6): 852–864.

Badea TC, Nathans J. 2004. Quantitative analysis of neuronal morphologies in the mouse retina visualized by using a genetically directed reporter. *J Comp Neurol* 480(4): 331–351.

Bansal A, Singer JH, Hwang BJ, Xu W, Beaudet A, Feller MB. 2000. Mice lacking specific nicotinic acetylcholine receptor subunits exhibit dramatically altered spontaneous activity patterns and reveal a limited role for retinal waves in forming ON and OFF circuits in the inner retina. *J Neurosci* 20(20): 7672–7681.

Bisti S, Gargini C, Chalupa LM. 1998. Blockade of glutamate-mediated activity in the developing retina perturbs the functional segregation of ON and OFF pathways. *J Neurosci* 18(13): 5019–5025.

Bloomfield SA. 1996. Effect of spike blockade on the receptive-field size of amacrine and ganglion cells in the rabbit retina. *J Neurophysiol* 75(5): 1878–1893.

Bodnarenko SR, Chalupa LM. 1993. Stratification of ON and OFF ganglion cell dendrites depends on glutamate-mediated afferent activity in the developing retina. *Nature* 364(6433): 144–146.

Bodnarenko SR, Jeyarasasingam G, Chalupa LM. 1995. Development and regulation of dendritic stratification in retinal ganglion cells by glutamate-mediated afferent activity. *J Neurosci* 15(11): 7037–7045.

Chow KL, Riesen AH, Newell FW. 1957. Degeneration of retinal ganglion cells in infant chimpanzees reared in darkness. *J Comp Neurol* 107(1): 27–42.

Cook JE, Chalupa LM. 2000. Retinal mosaics: new insights into an old concept. *Trends Neurosci* 23(1): 26–34.

Coombs J, van der List D, Wang GY, Chalupa LM. 2006. Morphological properties of mouse retinal ganglion cells. *Neuroscience* 140(1): 123–136.

Coombs JL, Van Der List D, Chalupa LM. 2007. Morphological properties of mouse retinal ganglion cells during postnatal development. *J Comp Neurol* 503(6): 803–814.

Deplano S, Gargini C, Maccarone R, Chalupa LM, Bisti S. 2004. Long-term treatment of the developing retina with the metabotropic glutamate agonist APB induces long-term changes in the stratification of retinal ganglion cell dendrites. *Dev Neurosci* 26(5–6): 396–405.

Diao L, Sun W, Deng Q, He S. 2004. Development of the mouse retina: emerging morphological diversity of the ganglion cells. *J Neurobiol* 61(2): 236–249.

Eglen SJ. 2006. Development of regular cellular spacing in the retina: theoretical models. *Math Med Biol* 23(2): 79–99.

Eliasieh K, Liets LC, Chalupa LM. 2007. Cellular reorganization in the human retina during normal aging. *Invest Ophthalmol Vis Sci* 48(6): 2824–2830.

Famiglietti EV, Jr, Kolb H. 1976. Structural basis for ON- and OFF-center responses in retinal ganglion cells. *Science* 194(4261): 193–195.

Farah MH, Easter SS, Jr. 2005. Cell birth and death in the mouse retinal ganglion cell layer. *J Comp Neurol* 489(1): 120–134.

Galli-Resta L. 2002. Putting neurons in the right places: local interactions in the genesis of retinal architecture. *Trends Neurosci* 25(12): 638–643.

Goodman L. 1932. Effect of total absence of function of the optic system of rabbits. *Am J Physiol* 100(1): 46–63.

Huckfeldt RM, Schubert T, Morgan JL, Godinho L, Di Cristo G, Huang ZJ, Wong RO. 2009. Transient neurites of retinal horizontal cells exhibit columnar tiling via homotypic interactions. *Nat Neurosci* 12(1): 35–43.

Jeyarasasingam G, Snider CJ, Ratto GM, Chalupa LM. 1998. Activity-regulated cell death contributes to the formation of ON and OFF alpha ganglion cell mosaics. *J Comp Neurol* 394(3): 335–343.

Kerschensteiner D, Morgan JL, Parker ED, Lewis RM, Wong RO. 2009. Neurotransmission selectively regulates synapse formation in parallel circuits in vivo. *Nature* 460(7258): 1016–1020.

Kerschensteiner D, Wong RO. 2008. A precisely timed asynchronous pattern of ON and OFF retinal ganglion cell activity during propagation of retinal waves. *Neuron* 58(6): 851–858.

Kirby MA, Chalupa LM. 1986. Retinal crowding alters the morphology of alpha ganglion cells. *J Comp Neurol* 251(4): 532–541.

Landi S, Cenni MC, Maffei L, Berardi N. 2007a. Environmental enrichment effects on development of retinal ganglion cell dendritic stratification require retinal BDNF. *PLoS ONE* 2(4): 1–11.

Landi S, Ciucci F, Maffei L, Berardi N, Cenni MC. 2009. Setting the pace for retinal development: environmental enrichment acts through insulin-like growth factor 1 and brain-derived neurotrophic factor. *J Neurosci* 29(35): 10809–10819.

Landi S, Sale A, Berardi N, Viegi A, Maffei L, Cenni MC. 2007b. Retinal functional development is sensitive to environmental enrichment: a role for BDNF. *FASEB J* 21(1): 130–139.

Leventhal AG, Schall JD, Ault SJ. 1988. Extrinsic determinants of retinal ganglion cell structure in the cat. *J Neurosci* 8(6): 2028–2038.

Liets LC, Eliasieh K, van der List DA, Chalupa LM. 2006. Dendrites of rod bipolar cells sprout in normal aging retina. *Proc Natl Acad Sci USA* 103(32): 12156–12160.

Lin B, Wang SW, Masland RH. 2004. Retinal ganglion cell type, size, and spacing can be specified independent of homotypic dendritic contacts. *Neuron* 43(4): 475–485.

Linden R, Perry VH. 1982. Ganglion cell death within the developing retina: a regulatory role for retinal dendrites? *Neuroscience* 7(11): 2813–2827.

Liu X, Grishanin RN, Tolwani RJ, Renteria RC, Xu B, Reichardt LF, Copenhagen DR. 2007. Brain-derived neurotrophic factor and TrkB modulate visual experience-dependent refinement of neuronal pathways in retina. *J Neurosci* 27(27): 7256–7267.

Liu X, Robinson ML, Schreiber AM, Wu V, Lavail MM, Cang J, Copenhagen DR. 2009. Regulation of neonatal development of retinal ganglion cell dendrites by neurotrophin-3 overexpression. *J Comp Neurol* 514(5): 449–458.

Logan MA, Vetter ML. 2004. Do-it-yourself tiling: dendritic growth in the absence of homotypic contacts. *Neuron* 43(4): 439–440.

Lohmann C, Wong RO. 2001. Cell-type specific dendritic contacts between retinal ganglion cells during development. *J Neurobiol* 48(2): 150–162.

Maslim J, Stone J. 1988. Time course of stratification of the dendritic fields of ganglion cells in the retina of the cat. *Brain Res Dev Brain Res* 44(1): 87–93.

Maslim J, Webster M, Stone J. 1986. Stages in the structural differentiation of retinal ganglion cells. *J Comp Neurol* 254(3): 382–402.

Mehta V, Sernagor E. 2006. Early neural activity and dendritic growth in turtle retinal ganglion cells. *Eur J Neurosci* 24(3): 773–786.

Nelson R, Famiglietti EV, Jr, Kolb H. 1978. Intracellular staining reveals different levels of stratification for on- and off-center ganglion cells in cat retina. *J Neurophysiol* 41(2): 472–483.

Perry VH, Henderson Z, Linden R. 1983. Postnatal changes in retinal ganglion cell and optic axon populations in the pigmented rat. *J Comp Neurol* 219(3): 356–368.

Perry VH, Linden R. 1982. Evidence for dendritic competition in the developing retina. *Nature* 297(5868): 683–685.

Poche RA, Raven MA, Kwan KM, Furuta Y, Behringer RR, Reese BE. 2008. Somal positioning and dendritic growth of horizontal cells are regulated by interactions with homotypic neighbors. *Eur J Neurosci* 27(7): 1607–1614.

Ramoa AS, Campbell G, Shatz CJ. 1988. Dendritic growth and remodeling of cat retinal ganglion cells during fetal and postnatal development. *J Neurosci* 8(11): 4239–4261.

Rasch E, Swift H, Riesen AH, Chow KL. 1961. Altered structure and composition of retinal cells in dark-reared mammals. *Exp Cell Res* 25: 348–363.

Raven MA, Orton NC, Nassar H, Williams GA, Stell WK, Jacobs GH, Bech-Hansen NT, Reese BE. 2008. Early afferent signaling in the outer plexiform layer regulates development of horizontal cell morphology. *J Comp Neurol* 506(5): 745–758.

Reese BE, Raven MA, Stagg SB. 2005. Afferents and homotypic neighbors regulate horizontal cell morphology, connectivity, and retinal coverage. *J Neurosci* 25(9): 2167–2175.

Riesen AH. 1947. The development of visual perception in man and chimpanzee. *Science* 106(2744): 107–108.

Roska B, Werblin F. 2001. Vertical interactions across ten parallel, stacked representations in the mammalian retina. *Nature* 410(6828): 583–587.

Seki M, Nawa H, Fukuchi T, Abe H, Takei N. 2003. BDNF is upregulated by postnatal development and visual experience: quantitative and immunohistochemical analyses of BDNF in the rat retina. *Invest Ophthalmol Vis Sci* 44(7): 3211–3218.

Sernagor E, Eglen SJ, Wong RO. 2001. Development of retinal ganglion cell structure and function. *Prog Retin Eye Res* 20(2): 139–174.

Snellman J, Kaur T, Shen Y, Nawy S. 2008. Regulation of ON bipolar cell activity. *Prog Retin Eye Res* 27(4): 450–463.

Sullivan RK, Woldemussie E, Pow DV. 2007. Dendritic and synaptic plasticity of neurons in the human age-related macular degeneration retina. *Invest Ophthalmol Vis Sci* 48(6): 2782–2791.

Sun W, Li N, He S. 2002. Large-scale morphological survey of mouse retinal ganglion cells. *J Comp Neurol* 451(2): 115–126.

Tagawa Y, Sawai H, Ueda Y, Tauchi M, Nakanishi S. 1999. Immunohistological studies of metabotropic glutamate receptor subtype 6-deficient mice show no abnormality of retinal cell organization and ganglion cell maturation. *J Neurosci* 19(7): 2568–2579.

Tian N, Copenhagen DR. 2001. Visual deprivation alters development of synaptic function in inner retina after eye opening. *Neuron* 32(3): 439–449.

Tian N, Copenhagen DR. 2003. Visual stimulation is required for refinement of ON and OFF pathways in postnatal retina. *Neuron* 39(1): 85–96.

Wässle H, Peichl L, Boycott BB. 1981a. Dendritic territories of cat retinal ganglion cells. *Nature* 292(5821): 344–345.

Wässle H, Peichl L, Boycott BB. 1981b. Morphology and topography of on- and off-alpha cells in the cat retina. *Proc R Soc Lond B Biol Sci* 212(1187): 157–175.

Wässle H, Riemann HJ. 1978. The mosaic of nerve cells in the mammalian retina. *Proc R Soc Lond B Biol Sci* 200(1141): 441–461.

Weiskrantz L. 1958. Sensory deprivation and the cat's optic nervous system. *Nature* 181(4615): 1047–1050.

Wiesel TN, Hubel DH. 1963. Effects of visual deprivation on morphology and physiology of cells in the cat's lateral geniculate body. *J Neurophysiol* 26: 978–993.

Williams RW, Bastiani MJ, Lia B, Chalupa LM. 1986. Growth cones, dying axons, and developmental fluctuations in the fiber population of the cat's optic nerve. *J Comp Neurol* 246(1): 32–69.

Wong RO, Yamawaki RM, Shatz CJ. 1992. Synaptic contacts and the transient dendritic spines of developing retinal ganglion cells. *Eur J Neurosci* 4(12): 1387–1397.

Wong WT, Faulkner-Jones BE, Sanes JR, Wong RO. 2000. Rapid dendritic remodeling in the developing retina: dependence on neurotransmission and reciprocal regulation by Rac and Rho. *J Neurosci* 20(13): 5024–5036.

Wong WT, Wong RO. 2001. Changing specificity of neurotransmitter regulation of rapid dendritic remodeling during synaptogenesis. *Nat Neurosci* 4(4): 351–352.

Xu HP, Tian N. 2007. Retinal ganglion cell dendrites undergo a visual activity-dependent redistribution after eye opening. *J Comp Neurol* 503(2): 244–259.

Xu HP, Tian N. 2008. Glycine receptor-mediated synaptic transmission regulates the maturation of ganglion cell synaptic connectivity. *J Comp Neurol* 509(1): 53–71.

Young RW. 1984. Cell death during differentiation of the retina in the mouse. *J Comp Neurol* 229(3): 362–373.

Zhang J, Yang Z, Wu SM. 2005. Development of cholinergic amacrine cells is visual activity-dependent in the postnatal mouse retina. *J Comp Neurol* 484(3): 331–343.

4 Using Indelible Transgenic Markers to Identify, Analyze, and Manipulate Neuronal Subtypes: Examples from the Retina

In-Jung Kim and Joshua R. Sanes

Processing of information by circuits of interconnected neurons underlies our perceptions, decisions, and behaviors. Neurobiologists are therefore eager to learn how circuits form. The task is a formidable one: our brain consists of some 10^{11} neurons connected by some 10^{14} synapses; even that of a mouse contains some 10^8 neurons. Moreover, mammals, unlike many invertebrates and some lower vertebrates, do not have unique neurons that can be identified from individual to individual. To make headway in circuit analysis, therefore, it is essential to divide neurons into discrete groups. Only in this way is it possible to relate results obtained from multiple individuals and to generalize results obtained from a few neurons to many (or many millions). The most revealing neuronal groups, generally called types and subtypes, are those that share patterns of connectivity and function. Most often, however, types and subtypes are initially defined based on their structure, which then serves as a basis for analysis of function, connectivity, development, relationship to disease, and, most recently, patterns of gene expression.

Until recently, neuronal subtypes were generally identified by labeling cells one at a time with nonselective methods. Class-specific labeling became possible with immunohistochemical methods, but these could, with rare exceptions, be applied only to fixed tissue. Recently, the introduction of genetically encoded reporters such as the green fluorescent protein (GFP), combined with new methods for introducing these reporters in vivo, have led to revolutionary advances in our ability to mark, identify, analyze, and manipulate neuronal subtypes. It is now possible to mark meaningful group of cells in live animals, allowing direct correlation of structure with gene expression or function. Moreover, these methods can be readily modified to permit manipulation of neurons in subtype-specific sets. This suite of methods has been reviewed comprehensively in the past few years (Dymecki and Kim, 2007; Luo et al., 2008). In this chapter, therefore, we review them only briefly and then discuss their application to one specific system, the mouse retina.

Traditional Methods for Studying Neuronal Subtypes

In most studies prior to the 1970s, neurons were classified based on images obtained by non-selective delivery of labeling dyes. Best known is the work of Santiago Ramon y Cajal, who used the "dark reaction" of Golgi. This technique produces dark precipitates in labeled cells, revealing their detailed structure. By analyzing numerous labeled cells, Cajal was able to classify them into numerous subtypes, based on their appearance. These studies essentially founded the field of neurobiology but had several major limitations. First, the Golgi stain labels neurons quasirandomly, so huge data sets must be accumulated prior to any attempt at classification. Second, the Golgi stain is capricious even in the hands of experts, and there may be biases in which neurons are labeled. Third, the stain cannot be targeted to cells that have been studied in other ways, such as electrophysiologically. Thus, it is poorly suited for relating structure to function. Finally, it can only be applied to fixed tissue, so live imaging is out of the question.

A modern variation of this method uses a ballistic "gene gun" to deliver tungsten particles coated with reporter genes or fluorescent dyes to neurons (Lo et al., 1994; Gan et al., 2000). This strategy provides some control over the number of cells labeled and permits multicolor labeling, but it is essentially random and therefore subject to the same limitations as the Golgi method. In addition, limited penetration of tungsten particles restricts use of the method to thin tissues or slices, and bleaching and phototoxicity restrict use of some organic fluorescent dyes with which particles are most readily coated.

Some of these limitations were circumvented by the introduction of methods for intracellular injection of neurons with a glass micropipette. With this strategy, it is possible to assess the physiological properties of a neuron and then reveal its structure following introduction of a dye (Lynch et al., 1974; Nelson et al., 1978; Gilbert and Wiesel, 1979; Stewart, 1981; Gerfen and Sawchenko, 1984). The ability to correlate structure with function is a great strength of this strategy. However, classification of neuronal subtypes by this method, as with the Golgi stain, requires injection of many cells. In that the method is extremely labor-intensive and requires great technical expertise, such data sets have been obtained in rather few cases (Volgyi et al., 2009).

A major advance in the 1970s was the introduction of immunohistochemical methods that allowed labeling of neurons based on their molecular properties, providing a way to define neuronal subtypes based on shared molecular profiles. By now, a wide variety of molecular features have been used to define subtypes, including neurotransmitters, receptors, and transcriptional factors. However, antibodies seldom stain a whole cell and often stain overlapping cells. As a result, it has been challenging to examine morphologies and spatial distribution of labeled cells.

The Green Revolution

The introduction of GFP as a genetically encoded reporter in the mid-1990s dramatically changed the way we examine biological phenomena (Chalfie, 2009). GFP and its derivatives are less phototoxic and more photostable than many other fluorescent dyes that had been used, but their greatest advantage is that they are genetically encoded. They can therefore be introduced noninvasively, they can label many cells per animal, and they do not need to be replenished.

Moreover, it soon became possible to expand the palette of fluorescent colors by mutating GFP and isolating photopigments from other organisms (Shaner et al., 2005). By using spectrally distinct fluorophores in combination one could therefore mark distinct neurons or neuronal populations—first by breeding together transgenic animals each expressing a single fluorophore ("XFP" lines: Feng et al., 2000) and eventually by expressing XFPs combinatorially from a single transgene in "Brainbow" lines (Livet et al., 2007). In the Brainbow method, differential and stochastic expression of each XFP in different neurons enables labeling individual cells with one of ~100 distinct colors. The advent of a multicolor labeling method makes it conceivable to reconstruct neuronal connections comprehensively, since many individual neurons can be followed from location to location through their unique tags.

Finally, the value of XFPs is enhanced because they can be fused to many other proteins without significantly affecting either the activity of the fusion partner or the fluorescence of the XFP. As we shall see below, such fusion proteins provide a useful way to combine marking with manipulation: effects of introducing proteins that affect the activity of neurons are best interpreted when one can be sure of where and when the protein is present.

Transgenesis

Successful use of XFPs to mark and manipulate neuronal subtypes—as opposed to individual neurons—depends critically on cell type-specific expression. Expression, in turn, depends on the regulatory elements linked to the cDNA that encodes the XFP (or an XFP fusion). Several strategies have been used to obtain specific expression. We review several of them here:

(a) Transgenes can be linked to fragments of a gene expressed in an appropriate spatiotemporal pattern. The expression vector is injected into the fertilized oocyte to generate transgenic mice. In the best of cases, the transgene is expressed in a pattern corresponding to that of the endogenous gene.

(b) Method (a) sometimes fails because small fragments (1–10kb) are used, but regulatory elements that restrict gene expression to specific subtypes may extend for a hundred kilobases or more. To circumvent this problem, methods have been developed to link transgenes to larger genomic segments, often derived from bacterial artificial chromosomes (BACs). These transgenes are more difficult to construct and inject, but "recombineering" methods for manipulating BACs are now well developed (Gong et al., 2002; Chan et al., 2007).

(c) In some cases, transgenic mice generated by either method (a) or (b) exhibit transgene expression that differs markedly from expectations. This ectopic expression may result from genomic sequences near the site of transgene integration. BAC transgenics were initially believed to be immune from these "integration site-dependent" influences, but this turns out not to be the case. In these cases, the transgene sometimes fortuitously marks a neuronal subtype of interest (Haverkamp et al., 2009; Kim et al., 2010).

(d) To avoid unexpected influence of insertion sites, transgenes can be targeted into designated loci in the genome to replace endogenous genes (knockin; Capecchi, 1989). Homologous recombination swaps targeting vectors with endogenous genes in embryonic stem cells that are then used to generate mice. Thus, this method enables transgene expression to faithfully follow that of endogenous genes.

(e) Recombinant viral vectors or electroporation can be used to directly deliver expression vectors to neurons. In some cases this is done because it is simpler and cheaper than generating transgenic mice; in other cases it is preferable because it allows spatial and temporal control over expression. Popular viral vectors include lentivirus, adeno-associated virus, and herpes simplex virus (Kootstra et al., 2003; Verma and Weitzman, 2005). Viral vectors used for injection and expression vectors used for electroporation can both employ regulatory elements from characterized genes to restrict expression to specific neuronal subtypes (Matsuda and Cepko, 2007).

(f) Expression of reporter genes decided by strength of endogenous promoters or enhancers is often too weak to be detected. This problem has been overcome by utilizing a binary system in which highly specific regulatory elements from one gene lead to expression of a protein that in turn activates strong XFP expression from a second transgene. In other words, distinct regulatory elements determine selectivity and strength of expression. Binary strategies were originally developed in yeast and flies (Gal4-UAS; Fischer et al., 1988; Brand and Perrimon, 1993), and several versions have now been used successfully in mice. In one, a transcription factor regulated by the drug tetracycline (tetracycline-controlled transactivator) activates expression of a second transgene controlled by a promoter to which the transactivator binds (tetO; Gossen and Bujard, 1992; Berens and Hillen, 2004). In a second, the site-specific DNA recombinases, Cre or Flp, excise inhibitory sequences from a second gene, activating its expression (Dymecki and Kim, 2007).

Binary systems not only facilitate strong expression of reporter genes but also provide other advantages. First, once transgenic lines that express recombinases are established, they can be crossed to other mice in which expression of different effectors is controlled by the recombinases. The effectors that control cellular activity or survival (e.g., channelrhodopsin and toxins) have been successfully used to assess neuronal connectivity and behavioral aspects (Breitman et al., 1987; Grieshammer et al., 1998; Yamamoto et al., 2003; Zemelman et al., 2003; Boyden et al., 2005; Lerchner et al., 2007; Zhang et al., 2007b). Second, specificity can be enhanced by an "intersectional" strategy in which the two components are expressed under the control of separate regulatory elements such that activation occurs only in the subset of cells that express both transgenes (Dymecki and Kim, 2007). Alternatively, specificity can be enhanced by using viral vectors to deliver one component to specific sites in transgenic mice that express the second component. Third, the tetracycline system is intrinsically drug sensitive, and recombinases have been synthesized that are made drug sensitive by fusion to a modified ligand-activated estrogen receptor. Therefore, the extent and timing of gene activation can be controlled by adjusting activities of the first gene product (the transactivator or recombinase; Dymecki and Kim, 2007).

The Retina

The retina senses light, processes visual signals, and transfers salient information to the brain (see figure 4.1a). Although its neural circuits are complex, its geometric regularity, accessibility, and well-defined function have made the retina an excellent model for studying the structure, function, and development of neuronal connections.

The retina contains five types of neurons: sensory neurons (photoreceptors) in the outer nuclear layer, three types of interneurons (horizontal, bipolar, and amacrine cells) in the inner nuclear layer, and projection neurons that send information to the brain (retinal ganglion cells; RGCs) in the ganglion cell layer (Wässle, 2004). The photoreceptors transfer information to bipolar and horizontal cells at synapses in the outer synaptic or plexiform layer. The bipolar cells, in turn, form synapses with amacrine cells and RGCs in the inner plexiform layer. Thus, a vertical pathway through the retina comprises three cells: photoreceptors, bipolar cells, and RGCs. Responses through the vertical pathway are modified by two sets of lateral interactions, mediated by horizontal cells in the outer plexiform layer and amacrine cells in the inner plexiform layer (Masland, 2001; Wässle, 2004).

Response properties of RGCs are determined by the synapses they receive from bipolar and amacrine cells. Multiple bipolar and amacrine subtypes send afferent processes to specific sublaminae within the inner plexiform layer, where they form synapses on lamina-restricted dendrites of RGCs. The particular properties of bipolar and amacrine subtypes, and the specific connections they form in the inner plexiform sublaminae, play a predominant role in tuning RGC subtypes to particular visual features, such as increases or decreases in light intensity (ON and OFF cells, respectively), color, or moving objects (Kuffler, 1953; Roska and Werblin, 2001). Indeed, studies in which RGCs were characterized physiologically and then filled with dye for structural analysis have shown a striking correspondence between the visual features to which an RGC is tuned and the inner plexiform sublamina in which its dendrites arborize. Because of this correspondence between structure and function, understanding how layer-specific neuronal connections in the retina are established will provide general insights into how proper functional circuits are organized.

Retinal Neuronal Subtypes

The complexity of retinal processing arises from the existence of multiple, structurally distinct and functionally specialized, subtypes of bipolar, amacrine, and RGCs. With few exceptions, classification into subtypes has been based on analysis of large sets of neurons labeled nonselectively with Golgi stains, organic dyes, or XFPs (Pu and Amthor, 1990; Rockhill et al., 2002; Dacey et al., 2003; Kong et al., 2005; Volgyi et al., 2009). Such surveys have been reported

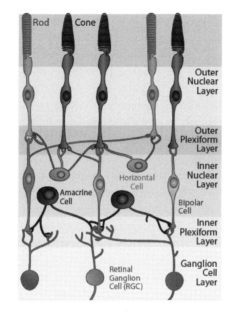

(a)

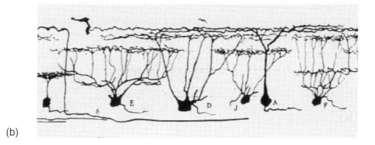

(b)

Figure 4.1
Vertebrate retina. (a) Schematic of retina. Visual signals activate photoreceptors in the outer nuclear layer, are processed by interneurons (horizontal, bipolar, and amacrine cells) in the inner nuclear layer, and are integrated by retinal ganglion cells (RGCs) in the ganglion cell layer. Photoreceptors, horizontal cells, and bipolar cells make synapses in the outer plexiform layer. Bipolar, amacrine, and RGCs make synapses in the inner plexifrom layer. (b) Cajal's drawing of RGCs, showing restriction of distinct subtypes to discrete sublaminae within the inner plexiform layer.

for several mammalian species, including mouse, rat, rabbit, cat, and monkey, as well as nonmammalian vertebrates such as chicken and zebrafish (Kolb et al., 1981; Amthor et al., 1989; Rodieck and Watanabe, 1993; Dacey, 1994; Mangrum et al., 2002; Sun et al., 2002a, 2002b; Naito and Chen, 2004; Isayama et al., 2009). Main criteria include laminar restriction of processes in the inner plexiform layer and arbor size. Numbers of subtypes vary among species and even among surveys within a species, but in general there appear to be ~10 subtypes of bipolar cells, ~25 subtypes of amacrine cells, and ~20 subtypes of RGCs in the mouse retina (Sun et al., 2002a; Badea and Nathans, 2004; Ghosh et al., 2004; Coombs et al., 2006; Volgyi et al., 2009).

But what is a subtype? In the morphological surveys reported to date, subdivisions are arbitrary. One would imagine that natural subtypes share not only histological characteristics such as size, arbor shape, and laminar restriction but also molecular features and functional properties. It remains unclear, however, whether these diverse characteristics cosegregate. For example, even within a subtype, patterns of gene expression can vary with physiological state, morphology can vary with retinal eccentricity, and physiological properties can vary with prior experience. Given these uncertainties, patterns of transgenes expression cannot on their own be used to define subtype but can provide important clues as well as facilitate structural and functional studies that may, in turn, reveal more profound similarities among the marked cells.

It is noteworthy, however, that there is one criterion for defining a neuronal subtype that can be applied uniquely to the retina. Cells of a particular subtype are spaced more evenly than would be expected by chance alone, as measured by the diminished frequency of finding two cells of the same subtype as near neighbors (Novelli et al., 2005; Eglen, 2006). This arrangement, called a mosaic, can be viewed as a means of ensuring that all regions of the visual world are sampled by each set of processors. Mosaic arrangements have been documented for subtypes of photoreceptors (rods and cones), amacrines, bipolars, and RGCs. Importantly, mosaics are independent of each other (Rockhill et al., 2000), suggesting that spacing is mediated by cell type-specific interactions. Thus, arrangement of cells marked by expression of an endogenous gene or a transgene in a mosaic indicates that the retina deals with those cells as a natural cell type.

Over the past few years, the XFP and transgenic technologies outlined above have been combined to mark several groups of retinal neurons, many of which comprise subtypes as defined by structure, function, gene expression, or mosaic arrangement. A selection of those reported to date is listed in table 4.1. In what follows, we briefly describe three studies that illustrate the power of these methods to aid in identification, manipulation, and developmental analysis of retinal subtypes.

Identification and Characterization of a Novel Subtype

In initial studies of the chick retina, we found a set of four immunoglobulin superfamily (IgSF) adhesion molecules that label nonoverlapping subsets of retinal interneurons and RGCs and

Table 4.1

Transgenic mice used in retinal subtype-specific studies

Purposes	Labeled Neurous	Transgenes	Methods to Generate Transgenics	References
Dendritic development of RGC subtypes	RGCs	YFP	Tg	Tian and Copenhagen, 2003
Morphological survey of RGC subtypes	RGCs	GFP	Tg	Kong et al., 2005
Morphological survey of RGC subtypes	RGCs	YFP	Tg	Coombs et al., 2006
Mark ON BPs for developmental study	ON BPs	GFP	Tg	Morgan et al., 2006
Morphological survey of AC & RGC subtypes	ACs, RGCs	GFP	Tg	Sarthy et al., 2007
Mark doparminergic ACs for functional study	ACs	RFP	Tg	Zhang et al., 2007a
ChR2-induced restoration of visual responses in *rd1* mice	ON BPs	ChR2 YFP	Tg	Lagali et al., 2008
Effect of neurotransmission on synpase formation	ON BPs	TeNT XFPs	Tg	Kerschensteiner et al., 2009
Characterize RGC subtype (tOFF-αRGCs)	ACs, RGCs	GFP	BAC	Huberman et al., 2008
Characterize RGC subtype (ON/OFF DSGCs)	RGCs	GFP	BAC	Huberman et al., 2009
Morphological survey of retinal subtypes	various	GFP	BAC	Haverkamp et al., 2009
Development of horizontal cells	Horizontal	GFP	BAC	Huckfeldt et al., 2009
Morphological survey of retinal subtypes	various	GFP	BAC	Siegert et al., 2009
Characterize RGC subtype (melanopsin-RGCs)	RGCs	LacZ	KI	Hattar et al., 2002
Characterize RGC subtype (ON DSGCs)	RGCs	GFP	KI	Yonehara et al., 2008 & 2009
Characterize RGC subtype (Brn3-RGCs)	RGCs	AP	KI	Badea and Nathans, 2009
Transneuronal tracing of synpatic connections	various	WGA	Binary: Tg (Cre) × Tg (floxed)	Braz et al., 2002
Morphological survey of retina subtypes	various	AP	Binary: KI (CreER) × Tg (floxed)	Badea and Nathans, 2004
Characterize RGC subtype (J-RGCs)	ACs, RGCs	YFP	Binary: BAC (CreER) × Tg (floxed)	Kim et al., 2008
Analyze RGC development	RGC	YFP	Binary: BAC (CreER) × Tg (floxed) & Tg	Kim et al., 2010
Characterize RGC subtype (melanopsin-RGCs)	RGCs	GFP DTR	Binary: KI (Cre) × Tg (floxed)	Hatori et al., 2008
Morphological survey of retinal subtypes	various	AP	Binary: KI (CreER) × Tg (floxed)	Rotolo et al., 2008
Model for study of RGCs death and optic nerve	RGCs	DTX	Binary: Tg (CreER) × KI (floxed)	Cho et al., 2009
Characterize AC subtype	various	GFP	Binary: BAC (Cre) × KI (floxed)	Dedek et al., 2009
Characterize RGC subtype (Looming detector)	RGCs	YFP	Binary: KI (Cre) × Tg (floxed)	Münch et al., 2009
Morphological survey of retinal subtypes	various	XFPs	Binary: Tg, BAC, KI (Cre) × KI (floxed)	Ivanova et al., 2009

AC, amacrine cell; AP, alkaline phosphatase; BAC, bacterial artificial chromosome; BP, bipolar cell; ChR2, channelrhodopsin-2; DSGC, direction-selective ganglion cell; DTR, diphtheria toxin receptor; DTX, diphtheria toxin; Floxed, flanked by LoxP site; KI, knock-in; LacZ, β-galactosidase; RGC, retinal ganglion cell; TeNT, tetanoux toxin; Tg, transgenic; WGA, wheat germ agglutinin.

promote lamina-specific connections between pre- and postsynaptic cells that express the same IgSF member (Yamagata et al., 2002; Yamagata and Sanes, 2008). Based on these results, we asked whether any other IgSF genes were expressed by RGC subsets in the mouse (Kim et al., 2008, 2010). We found that Junctional Adhesion Molecule B (JAM-B) was expressed by a set of RGCs that were arranged in a mosaic, as defined above. To mark JAM-B expressing cells for structural and functional studies, we generated mice that express a ligand-activated Cre recombinase-estrogen receptor fusion protein (CreER) under control of regulatory elements from the JAM-B gene. These mice were then mated to Thy1-Stop-YFP transgenic mice to visualize JAM-B expressing cells (J-RGCs; see figure 4.2).

Dendrites of J-RGCs arborize in the outer part of the inner plexiform layer and are markedly asymmetrical; all extend in a ventral direction from the soma. Such cells had been noted in previous surveys, but because they were encountered rarely and in isolation, their striking directional preference had not been noted. Electrical recording showed that J-RGCs respond to decreased light intensity (OFF cells) and to objects moving in the direction in which their

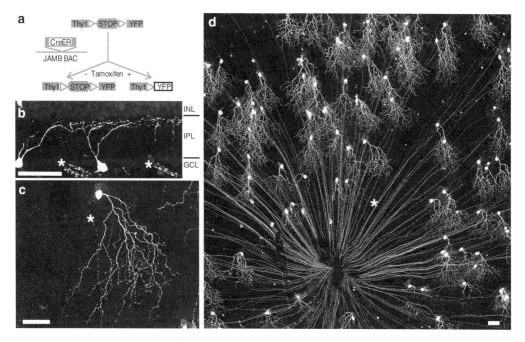

Figure 4.2
Unique morphology of junctional adhesion molecule B (JAM-B) expressing retinal ganglion cells (J-RGCs). (a) Transgenic strategy for labeling J-RGCs with yellow fluorescent protein (YFP). Triangles, Cre recognition (loxP) sites; CreER, Cre recombinase-estrogen receptor fusion protein; BAC, bacterial artificial chromosome. (b) Dendrites of J-RGCs are confined to the outer part of the inner plexiform layer (IPL). INL, inner nuclear layer; GCL, ganglion cell layer. (c) Dendritic asymmetry of J-RGC. (d) A whole-mounted retina revealing that J-RGCs point their dendrites in the same direction. Asterisks in b, c, and d mark RGC axons. Scale bar: 50 μm in b and 20 μm in c and d.

dendrites point. Because the eye's lens reverses images (like a camera), J-RGCs would respond to objects moving up in the real world. Thus, J-RGCs represent a novel subtype of RGCs characterized by unique morphological, physiological, and molecular properties.

The use of a binary system involving CreER to mark these cells will facilitate future studies of J-RGCs. For example, one can cross JAM-B-CreER mice to transgenic lines expressing Cre-activated transsynaptic tracers to identify their inputs and targets, or to lines expressing Cre-activated channels or toxins to assess the role of J-RGCs in visually evoked behavior.

Manipulation of a Retinal Subtype

Genetic delivery of effectors makes it possible to assess the role of specific neuronal subtypes in information processing within complex circuits. One recently developed effector is channel-rhodopsin (ChR2), a light-gated cation channel that activates neurons through depolarization when cells expressing the channel are illuminated. A recent study by Lagali et al. (2008) used subtype-specific expression of ChR2 to test the idea that visual stimuli could be delivered to the brain even in the absence of photoreceptors. They used *rd1* mutants, a popular model of retinal degeneration in which photoreceptors are lost and the mice become insensitive to light. Lagali et al. (2008) targeted expression of ChR2 to ON type of bipolar cells, placing ChR2 under control of regulatory elements from the metabotropic receptor, mGluR6, which is specifically expressed in ON bipolar cells. The DNA construct included ChR2 as well as YFP to visualize ON bipolar cells so that they could be targeted for electrical recording. The transgene was introduced by in vivo electroporation. *Rd1* mice specifically expressing ChR2 in ON bipolar cells showed restoration of ganglion cell activity, increased cortical activity, and visually evoked behavior responses, indicating that the retinas lacking photoreceptors are able to process visual information. This work provides a new approach to gene therapy for cases of blindness in which photoreceptors have been irreversibly damaged.

Development of Subtype-Specific Circuitry

Refinement of circuits is thought to involve initial overproduction of branches and synapses followed by activity-dependent elimination of inappropriate ones (Katz and Shatz, 1996). In only a few cases, however, has refinement of connections of a specific subtype been documented. In a recent paper, Kerschensteiner et al. (2009) asked whether activity affects the targeting of ON bipolar cell processes to the ON sublaminae of the inner plexiform layer, within which they selectively synapse on dendrites of ON RGCs. To this end, they made use of the fact that ON but not OFF bipolar cells express the metabotropic glutamate receptor, mGluR6; indeed this receptor is critical for their function. They generated transgenic mice in which a tetanus toxin-fluorescent protein fusion was expressed under the control of regulatory elements from the mGluR6 gene. The active subunit of tetanus toxin is an enzyme that cleaves proteins required for synaptic vesicle exocytosis, thereby blocking neurotransmitter release. Fusion to a fluorescent protein made it straightforward to monitor the bipolar processes in which blockade had occurred. One critical result was that the intoxicated ON bipolar cells made fewer synapses than control ON bipolars onto ON RGCs, indicating that in this instance activity appears to enhance specificity by promoting formation of synapses on appropriate partners rather than by promoting elimination of synapses on inappropriate partners. Interestingly, ON/OFF RGCs, which receive inputs from ON and OFF bipolars in distinct inner plexiform sublaminae, were depleted of ON but not OFF bipolar inputs. Thus, changes in synaptic activity appear to act locally, modifying individual connections rather than inducing large-scale structural rearrangements. Together, these results provide an intriguing counterpoint to the prevailing view on roles of activity in circuit development.

Concluding Remarks

Understanding the development and function of neural circuits are two key goals of basic neuroscience over the next few decades. Transgenic mice have already been useful in moving toward this goal, and the rapidly expanding molecular genetic toolbox makes it a near certainty that their utility will continue to increase. Nonetheless, the task remains a daunting one. We suggest that using well-defined model systems such as the retina, and focusing on well-defined neuronal subtypes, will be critical in speeding progress.

References

Amthor FR, Takahashi ES, Oyster CW. 1989. Morphologies of rabbit retinal ganglion cells with complex receptive fields. *J Comp Neurol* 280: 97–121.

Badea TC, Nathans J. 2004. Quantitative analysis of neuronal morphologies in the mouse retina visualized by using a genetically directed reporter. *J Comp Neurol* 480: 331–351.

Badea TC, Cahill H, Ecker J, Hattar S, Nathans J. 2009. Distinct roles of transcription factors brn3a and brn3b in controlling the development, morphology, and function of retinal ganglion cells. *Neuron* 61: 852–864.

Berens C, Hillen W. 2004. Gene regulation by tetracyclines. *Genet Eng (NY)* 26: 255–277.

Boyden ES, Zhang F, Bamberg E, Nagel G, Deisseroth K. 2005. Millisecond-timescale, genetically targeted optical control of neural activity. *Nat Neurosci* 8: 1263–1268.

Brand AH, Perrimon N. 1993. Targeted gene expression as a means of altering cell fates and generating dominant phenotypes. *Development* 118: 401–415.

Braz JM, Rico B, Basbaum AI. 2002. Transneuronal tracing of diverse CNS circuits by Cremediated induction of wheat germ agglutinin in transgenic mice. *Proc Natl Acad Sci USA* 99: 15148–15153.

Breitman ML, Clapoff S, Rossant J, Tsui LC, Glode LM, Maxwell IH, Bernstein A. 1987. Genetic ablation: targeted expression of a toxin gene causes microphthalmia in transgenic mice. *Science* 238: 1563–1565.

Capecchi MR. 1989. Altering the genome by homologous recombination. *Science* 244: 1288–1292.

Chalfie M. 2009. GFP: Lighting up life. *Proc Natl Acad Sci USA* 106: 10073–10080.

Chan W, Costantino N, Li R, Lee SC, Su Q, Melvin D, Court DL, Liu P. 2007. A recombineering based approach for high-throughput conditional knockout targeting vector construction. *Nucleic Acids Res* 35: e64.

Cho JH, Mu X, Wang SW, Klein WH. 2009. Retinal ganglion cell death and optic nerve degeneration by genetic ablation in adult mice. *Exp Eye Res* 88: 542–552.

Coombs J, van der List D, Wang GY, Chalupa LM. 2006. Morphological properties of mouse retinal ganglion cells. *Neuroscience* 140: 123–136.

Dacey DM. 1994. Physiology, morphology and spatial densities of identified ganglion cell types in primate retina. *Ciba Found Symp* 184:12–28; discussion 28–34, 63–70.

Dacey DM, Peterson BB, Robinson FR, Gamlin PD. 2003. Fireworks in the primate retina: in vitro photodynamics reveals diverse LGN-projecting ganglion cell types. *Neuron* 37: 15–27.

Dedek K, Breuninger T, de Sevilla Muller LP, Maxeiner S, Schultz K, Janssen-Bienhold U, Willecke K, Euler T, Weiler R. 2009. A novel type of interplexiform amacrine cell in the mouse retina. *Eur J Neurosci* 30: 217–228.

Dymecki SM, Kim JC. 2007. Molecular neuroanatomy's "Three Gs": a primer. *Neuron* 54: 17–34.

Eglen SJ. 2006. Development of regular cellular spacing in the retina: theoretical models. *Math Med Biol* 23: 79–99.

Feng G, Mellor RH, Bernstein M, Keller-Peck C, Nguyen QT, Wallace M, Nerbonne JM, Lichtman JW, Sanes JR. 2000. Imaging neuronal subsets in transgenic mice expressing multiple spectral variants of GFP. *Neuron* 28: 41–51.

Fischer JA, Giniger E, Maniatis T, Ptashne M. 1988. GAL4 activates transcription in Drosophila. *Nature* 332: 853–856.

Gan WB, Grutzendler J, Wong WT, Wong RO, Lichtman JW. 2000. Multicolor "DiOlistic" labeling of the nervous system using lipophilic dye combinations. *Neuron* 27: 219–225.

Gerfen CR, Sawchenko PE. 1984. An anterograde neuroanatomical tracing method that shows the detailed morphology of neurons, their axons and terminals: immunohistochemical localization of an axonally transported plant lectin, Phaseolus vulgaris leucoagglutinin (PHA-L). *Brain Res* 290: 219–238.

Ghosh KK, Bujan S, Haverkamp S, Feigenspan A, Wassle H. 2004. Types of bipolar cells in the mouse retina. *J Comp Neurol* 469: 70–82.

Gilbert CD, Wiesel TN. 1979. Morphology and intracortical projections of functionally characterised neurones in the cat visual cortex. *Nature* 280: 120–125.

Gong S, Yang XW, Li C, Heintz N. 2002. Highly efficient modification of bacterial artificial chromosomes (BACs) using novel shuttle vectors containing the R6Kgamma origin of replication. *Genome Res* 12: 1992–1998.

Gossen M, Bujard H. 1992. Tight control of gene expression in mammalian cells by tetracycline-responsive promoters. *Proc Natl Acad Sci USA* 89: 5547–5551.

Grieshammer U, Lewandoski M, Prevette D, Oppenheim RW, Martin GR. 1998. Musclespecific cell ablation conditional upon Cre-mediated DNA recombination in transgenic mice leads to massive spinal and cranial motoneuron loss. *Dev Biol* 197: 234–247.

Hatori M, Le H, Vollmers C, Keding SR, Tanaka N, Buch T, Waisman A, Schmedt C, Jegla T, Panda S. 2008. Inducible ablation of melanopsin-expressing retinal ganglion cells reveals their central role in non-image forming visual responses. *PLoS ONE* 3: e2451.

Hattar S, Liao HW, Takao M, Berson DM, Yau KW. 2002. Melanopsin-containing retinal ganglion cells: architecture, projections, and intrinsic photosensitivity. *Science* 295: 1065–1070.

Haverkamp S, Inta D, Monyer H, Wassle H. 2009. Expression analysis of green fluorescent protein in retinal neurons of four transgenic mouse lines. *Neuroscience* 160: 126–139.

Huberman AD, Wei W, Elstrott J, Stafford BK, Feller MB, Barres BA. 2009. Genetic identification of an On–Off direction-selective retinal ganglion cell subtype reveals a layerspecific subcortical map of posterior motion. *Neuron* 62: 327–334.

Huberman AD, Manu M, Koch SM, Susman MW, Lutz AB, Ullian EM, Baccus SA, Barres BA. 2008. Architecture and activity-mediated refinement of axonal projections from a mosaic of genetically identified retinal ganglion cells. *Neuron* 59: 425–438.

Huckfeldt RM, Schubert T, Morgan JL, Godinho L, Di Cristo G, Huang ZJ, Wong RO. 2009. Transient neurites of retinal horizontal cells exhibit columnar tiling via homotypic interactions. *Nat Neurosci* 12: 35–43.

Isayama T, O'Brien BJ, Ugalde I, Muller JF, Frenz A, Aurora V, Tsiaras W, Berson DM. 2009. Morphology of retinal ganglion cells in the ferret (Mustela putorius furo). *J Comp Neurol* 517: 459–480.

Ivanova E, Hwang GS, Pan ZH. 2009. Characterization of transgenic mouse lines expressing Cre-recombinase in the retina. *Neuroscience*.

Katz LC, Shatz CJ. 1996. Synaptic activity and the construction of cortical circuits. *Science* 274: 1133–1138.

Kerschensteiner D, Morgan JL, Parker ED, Lewis RM, Wong RO. 2009. Neurotransmission selectively regulates synapse formation in parallel circuits in vivo. *Nature* 460: 1016–1020.

Kim IJ, Zhang Y, Yamagata M, Meister M, Sanes JR. 2008. Molecular identification of a retinal cell type that responds to upward motion. *Nature* 452: 478–482.

Kim IJ, Zhang Y, Meister M, Sanes JR. 2010. Laminar restriction of retinal ganglion cell dendrites and axons: Subtype-specific developmental patterns revealed with transgenic markers. *J Neurosci* 30: 1452–1462.

Kolb H, Nelson R, Mariani A. 1981. Amacrine cells, bipolar cells and ganglion cells of the cat retina: a Golgi study. *Vision Res* 21: 1081–1114.

Kong JH, Fish DR, Rockhill RL, Masland RH. 2005. Diversity of ganglion cells in the mouse retina: unsupervised morphological classification and its limits. *J Comp Neurol* 489: 293–310.

Kootstra NA, Matsumura R, Verma IM. 2003. Efficient production of human FVIII in hemophilic mice using lentiviral vectors. *Mol Ther* 7: 623–631.

Kuffler SW. 1953. Discharge patterns and functional organization of mammalian retina. *J Neurophysiol* 16: 37–68.

Lagali PS, Balya D, Awatramani GB, Munch TA, Kim DS, Busskamp V, Cepko CL, Roska B. 2008. Light-activated channels targeted to ON bipolar cells restore visual function in retinal degeneration. *Nat Neurosci* 11: 667–675.

Lerchner W, Xiao C, Nashmi R, Slimko EM, van Trigt L, Lester HA, Anderson DJ. 2007. Reversible silencing of neuronal excitability in behaving mice by a genetically targeted, ivermectin-gated Cl- channel. *Neuron* 54: 35–49.

Livet J, Weissman TA, Kang H, Draft RW, Lu J, Bennis RA, Sanes JR, Lichtman JW. 2007. Transgenic strategies for combinatorial expression of fluorescent proteins in the nervous system. *Nature* 450: 56–62.

Lo DC, McAllister AK, Katz LC. 1994. Neuronal transfection in brain slices using particle mediated gene transfer. *Neuron* 13: 1263–1268.

Luo L, Callaway EM, Svoboda K. 2008. Genetic dissection of neural circuits. *Neuron* 57: 634–660.

Lynch G, Gall C, Mensah P, Cotman CW. 1974. Horseradish peroxidase histochemistry: a new method for tracing efferent projections in the central nervous system. *Brain Res* 65: 373–380.

Mangrum WI, Dowling JE, Cohen ED. 2002. A morphological classification of ganglion cells in the zebrafish retina. *Vis Neurosci* 19: 767–779.

Masland RH. 2001. Neuronal diversity in the retina. *Curr Opin Neurobiol* 11: 431–436.

Matsuda T, Cepko CL. 2007. Controlled expression of transgenes introduced by in vivo electroporation. *Proc Natl Acad Sci USA* 104: 1027–1032.

Morgan JL, Dhingra A, Vardi N, Wong RO. 2006. Axons and dendrites originate from neuroepithelial-like processes of retinal bipolar cells. *Nat Neurosci* 9: 85–92.

Münch TA, da Silveira RA, Siegert S, Viney TJ, Awatramani GB, Roska B. 2009. Approach sensitivity in the retina processed by a multifunctional neural circuit. *Nat Neurosci* 12: 1308–1316.

Naito J, Chen Y. 2004. Morphologic analysis and classification of ganglion cells of the chick retina by intracellular injection of Lucifer Yellow and retrograde labeling with DiI. *J Comp Neurol* 469: 360–376.

Nelson R, Famiglietti EV, Jr, Kolb H. 1978. Intracellular staining reveals different levels of stratification for on- and off-center ganglion cells in cat retina. *J Neurophysiol* 41: 472–483.

Novelli E, Resta V, Galli-Resta L. 2005. Mechanisms controlling the formation of retinal mosaics. *Prog Brain Res* 147: 141–153.

Pu ML, Amthor FR. 1990. Dendritic morphologies of retinal ganglion cells projecting to the lateral geniculate nucleus in the rabbit. *J Comp Neurol* 302: 675–693.

Rockhill RL, Euler T, Masland RH. 2000. Spatial order within but not between types of retinal neurons. *Proc Natl Acad Sci USA* 97: 2303–2307.

Rockhill RL, Daly FJ, MacNeil MA, Brown SP, Masland RH. 2002. The diversity of ganglion cells in a mammalian retina. *J Neurosci* 22: 3831–3843.

Rodieck RW, Watanabe M. 1993. Survey of the morphology of macaque retinal ganglion cells that project to the pretectum, superior colliculus, and parvicellular laminae of the lateral geniculate nucleus. *J Comp Neurol* 338: 289–303.

Roska B, Werblin F. 2001. Vertical interactions across ten parallel, stacked representations in the mammalian retina. *Nature* 410: 583–587.

Rotolo T, Smallwood PM, Williams J, Nathans J. 2008. Genetically-directed, cell type-specific sparse labeling for the analysis of neuronal morphology. *PLoS ONE* 3: e4099.

Sarthy V, Hoshi H, Mills S, Dudley VJ. 2007. Characterization of green fluorescent protein-expressing retinal cells in CD 44-transgenic mice. *Neuroscience* 144: 1087–1093.

Shaner NC, Steinbach PA, Tsien RY. 2005. A guide to choosing fluorescent proteins. *Nat Methods* 2: 905–909.

Siegert S, Scherf BG, Del Punta K, Didkovsky N, Heintz N, Roska B. 2009. Genetic address book for retinal cell types. *Nat Neurosci*.

Stewart WW. 1981. Lucifer dyes—highly fluorescent dyes for biological tracing. *Nature* 292: 17–21.

Sun W, Li N, He S. 2002a. Large-scale morphological survey of mouse retinal ganglion cells. *J Comp Neurol* 451: 115–126.

Sun W, Li N, He S. 2002b. Large-scale morophological survey of rat retinal ganglion cells. *Vis Neurosci* 19: 483–493.

Tian N, Copenhagen DR. 2003. Visual stimulation is required for refinement of ON and OFF pathways in postnatal retina. *Neuron* 39: 85–96.

Verma IM, Weitzman MD. 2005. Gene therapy: twenty-first century medicine. *Annu Rev Biochem* 74: 711–738.

Volgyi B, Chheda S, Bloomfield SA. 2009. Tracer coupling patterns of the ganglion cell subtypes in the mouse retina. *J Comp Neurol* 512: 664–687.

Wässle H. 2004. Parallel processing in the mammalian retina. *Nat Rev Neurosci* 5: 747–757.

Yamagata M, Sanes JR. 2008. Dscam and Sidekick proteins direct lamina-specific synaptic connections in vertebrate retina. *Nature* 451: 465–469.

Yamagata M, Weiner JA, Sanes JR. 2002. Sidekicks: synaptic adhesion molecules that promote lamina-specific connectivity in the retina. *Cell* 110: 649–660.

Yamamoto M, Wada N, Kitabatake Y, Watanabe D, Anzai M, Yokoyama M, Teranishi Y, Nakanishi S. 2003. Reversible suppression of glutamatergic neurotransmission of cerebellar granule cells in vivo by genetically manipulated expression of tetanus neurotoxin light chain. *J Neurosci* 23: 6759–6767.

Yonehara K, Shintani T, Suzuki R, Sakuta H, Takeuchi Y, Nakamura-Yonehara K, Noda M. 2008. Expression of SPIG1 reveals development of a retinal ganglion cell subtype projecting to the medial terminal nucleus in the mouse. *PLoS ONE* 3: e1533.

Yonehara K, Ishikane H, Sakuta H, Shintani T, Nakamura-Yonehara K, Kamiji NL, Usui S, Noda M. 2009. Identification of retinal ganglion cells and their projections involved in central transmission of information about upward and downward image motion. *PLoS ONE* 4: e4320.

Zemelman BV, Nesnas N, Lee GA, Miesenbock G. 2003. Photochemical gating of heterologous ion channels: remote control over genetically designated populations of neurons. *Proc Natl Acad Sci USA* 100: 1352–1357.

Zhang DQ, Zhou TR, McMahon DG. 2007a. Functional heterogeneity of retinal dopaminergic neurons underlying their multiple roles in vision. *J Neurosci* 27: 692–699.

Zhang F, Wang LP, Brauner M, Liewald JF, Kay K, Watzke N, Wood PG, Bamberg E, Nagel G, Gottschalk A, Deisseroth K. 2007b. Multimodal fast optical interrogation of neural circuitry. *Nature* 446: 633–639.

5 Vision-Dependent Plasticity at the Retinogeniculate Synapse

Chinfei Chen

One of the most compelling issues in the field of neuroscience is the question of how proper neuronal circuits are formed and how they adapt in response to experience. Dr. Lamberto Maffei has been at the forefront of advancing our knowledge on this subject. Among many notable achievements, he has contributed tremendously to our understanding of experience-dependent plasticity, the importance of the enriched environment in the maturation of the nervous system, and the molecular mechanisms underlying these processes. Much of his work has focused on the visual cortex as a model system to study experience-dependent plasticity. The cortex, however, is not an isolated region of the brain but part of a larger neuronal circuit. Visual information is encoded in firing patterns of retinal ganglion cells (RGCs), transmitted to the visual thalamus, the lateral geniculate nucleus (LGN), via the retinogeniculate synapse (see figure 5.1). In this chapter, I will summarize some of the recent work examining plasticity at this synapse, including our own work that points to a role of experience-dependent plasticity in the visual thalamus.

The retinogeniculate synapse has served as a powerful model for studying synaptic plasticity during development in the central nervous system. This connection offers ease of manipulating activity along with the ability to monitor subsequent changes in synaptic structure and function. The accumulated knowledge from many investigators working in a variety of species has led to a current view that circuit development between the retina and the thalamus involves a sequence of at least three distinct periods of plasticity (Huberman, 2007; Kano and Hashimoto, 2009). The first phase occurs soon after the mapping of RGC axons to the LGN when there is coarse rearrangement of axon terminals into eye-specific regions. This is followed by a phase of fine-scale remodeling of synaptic function. Finally, a third phase of synapse development involves further refinement of neuronal circuits to visual experience and the maintenance of the optimized circuitry.

Segregation of Eye-Specific Layers

One valuable feature of the retinogeniculate synapse is that changes in large-scale anatomical mapping of axons to the LGN can be monitored by labeling of RGCs from the two eyes with

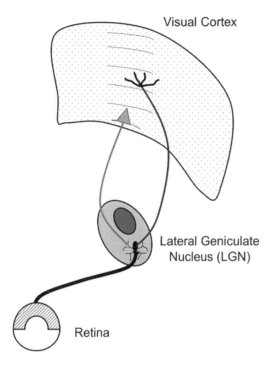

Figure 5.1
The retinothalamocortical circuit.

different fluorophores. This feature has allowed the visualization of normal developmental refinement of bulk axon terminals during the first phase of refinement. Initially, RGC axons map broadly to both contralateral and ipsilateral LGN. Over development, these axon arbors segregate into eye-specific regions of the LGN as some segments of the axons elaborate and others, in inappropriate regions of the LGN, retract and disappear (Shatz and Kirkwood, 1984; Sretavan and Shatz, 1984; Sretavan and Shatz, 1986). This refinement can be disrupted by continuous infusion of tetrodotoxin or *N*-methyl-D-aspartate receptor antagonist into the cerebral spinal fluid, suggesting an activity-dependent mechanism (Hahm et al., 1991; Shatz and Stryker, 1988; Sur et al., 1982). Yet, for many years, the source of this activity was debated. In the cat, eye-specific segregation occurs prior to birth (Shatz, 1983), while in ferret, rat, and mice, the majority of segregation is complete by the time of eye opening (Godement et al., 1984; Jeffery, 1984; Linden et al., 1981). Thus, vision is not the source of activity that drives this process. Lamberto Maffei and Lucia Galli identified a likely source of activity when they succeeded in performing technically challenging experiments that entailed recording from the retina of embryonic rat pups. These studies revealed that even in utero, neurons of the retina fired in ensemble, resulting in enormous compound action potentials (Galli and Maffei, 1988; Maffei and Galli-Resta, 1990). Subsequent studies demonstrating that this spontaneous activity is synchronized and spreads across the retina in waves supported a Hebbian explanation for how axons from the same eye might segregate together (Butts et al., 2007; Meister et al., 1991; Wong et al., 1995). However, the features of retinal activity that drive and maintain eye-specific segregation are still the subject of intense interest and debate (Demas et al., 2006; Huberman et al., 2003; Sun et al., 2008; Torborg et al., 2005).

In addition to activity-dependent processes, molecular cues are important for the mapping and refinement of retinal axons to their proper targets. Guidance cues such as ephrin/Eph receptors are though to place the axon terminal in the general region of potentially appropriate targets in the LGN (Feldheim et al., 1998; Huberman et al., 2005; Lyckman et al., 2001). Notably, retinal waves and axon guidance cues appear to have distinct roles in dictating the final location of RGC axon terminals as eye-specific layering defects are greater in mice lacking both waves and ephrin molecules than in mice lacking ephrin A proteins alone, or in mice with abnormal retinal waves (Pfeiffenberger et al., 2005; Pfeiffenberger et al., 2006). Recent studies have also identified a variety of molecules associated with the immune system, such as MHC I, pentraxins, and the complement protein C1q, as playing a role in eye-specific segregation in the LGN (Bjartmar et al., 2006; Huh et al., 2000; Stevens et al., 2007).

Synaptic Refinement Once Retinal Axons Reach Their Proper Target

The bulk of eye-specific lamination is complete by postnatal day (P) 0 in cat and P8–12 in ferret, rat, and mouse (Linden et al., 1981; Muir-Robinson et al., 2002; Shatz, 1983; Ziburkus and Guido, 2006). At this point in development, connections between RGCs and relay neurons are already functional, although very weak (Chen and Regehr, 2000; Ramoa and McCormick, 1994; Shatz and Kirkwood, 1984). Over the subsequent weeks spanning eye opening, synaptic strength and connectivity change dramatically (Chen and Regehr, 2000; Jaubert-Miazza et al., 2005). In mice, the retinogeniculate synapse strengthens more than 20-fold, while during the same time period the number of retinal inputs that innervate a given LGN neuron is pruned from greater than ten inputs to approximately one to three inputs (Chen and Regehr, 2000; see figure 5.2). The functional output resulting in these synaptic changes is still not clear; however, the developmental timing of these changes in synaptic strength and connectivity corresponds temporally to a sharpening of the geniculate neuron receptive fields described in cat, monkey, and ferret (Blakemore and Vital-Durand, 1986; Daniels et al., 1978; Tavazoie and Reid, 2000).

The strength of a retinal input is dictated by the probability of release of the connection, the quantal size (the response to the release of a single vesicle), and the number of release sites. Thus, one can assess whether changes in any of these features contribute to the developmental strengthening observed at this synapse. Electrophysiological recordings demonstrate that probability of release does not change dramatically between P8 and P32 at the mouse retinogeniculate synapse. A doubling of quantal size from 6 pA to 12 pA also cannot account for the 20-fold increase in synaptic strength. Thus, an increase in the number of synaptic release sites is thought to underlie the developmental strengthening of individual retinal inputs (Chen and Regehr,

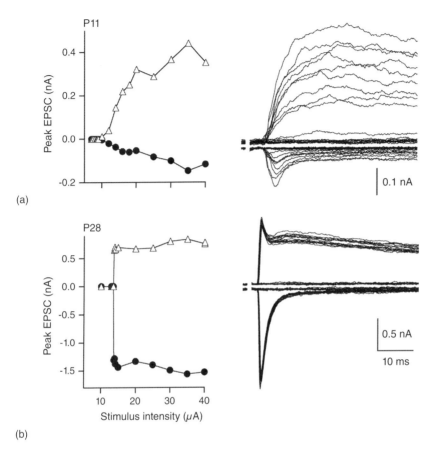

Figure 5.2
Representative excitatory synaptic responses to incremental increases in stimulus intensities from mice of different ages: (a) P11, (b) P28. (Left) Plots of the peak amplitudes of the AMPAR (closed symbols) and NMDAR (open symbols) peak currents as a function of stimulus intensities while alternating between holding potentials of +40 mV (outward currents, NMDAR) and −70 mV (inward currents, AMPAR). All recordings are performed in the presence of the GABA$_A$ receptor blocker, bicuculline. From these experiments, synaptic connectivity is assessed by the strength of a retinal input and the convergence. The strength of retinal inputs can be assessed by measuring the response to minimal stimulation, called the single-fiber response. In addition, the average number of inputs that innervate a given relay neuron can be estimated by assessing the ratio of the peak amplitude of the single-fiber response to that of the maximal current elicited by activating as many retinal inputs as possible (modified from Hooks and Chen, 2006). P, postnatal day; EPSC, excitatory postsynaptic current.

2000). Based on the synaptic response to pairs of stimuli, the probability of release is estimated to be about 0.3–0.4 (Dittman and Regehr, 1998). Thus, a simple back-of-the-envelope calculation, using a quantal size of 6 pA and an average single-fiber strength of 40 pA, estimates that the average immature retinal axon makes about 20 release sites or contacts onto a given relay neuron. In contrast, a similar calculation at mature synapses, with an average single-RGC input strength of 800 pA and quantal size of 12 pA yields an estimate of approximately 190 release sites. These numbers are consistent with the elegant electron microscopy data in the adult cat showing that a single retinal axon can make as many as 200 contacts on the proximal dendrites of a single relay neuron (Hamos et al., 1987). Taken together, these numbers suggest that fine-scale refinement during this phase of development involves changes in the distribution of release sites between afferent inputs and postsynaptic relay neurons.

Although synaptic refinement at the retinogeniculate synapse spans the developmental time point of eye opening, vision does not appear to influence this process. Dark rearing around the time of eye opening or from birth does not alter eye-specific lamination (Garraghty et al., 1987), synaptic strengthening, or input elimination (Hooks and Chen, 2006). Instead, as with eye-specific layering, spontaneous activity plays an important role in driving this later developmental period of synapse remodeling that occurs around the time of eye opening.

Are the mechanisms underlying the period of eye-specific layering and that of synaptic refinement between P12 and P16 the same? The two phases of development share common features. Both depend on spontaneous activity and not vision. Moreover, a few genetically altered mice, such as the C1q null mice, exhibit disruptions in both eye-specific layering and synaptic connectivity (Stevens et al., 2007). However, there are other mice, such as the β2 nAChR knockout mice and ephrin-A2/A5 knockout mice, that exhibit disruption of eye-specific targeting or segregation but do not exhibit obvious defects in synapse pruning and strengthening when tested at mature ages (Feldheim et al., 1998; Muir-Robinson et al., 2002; unpublished data). Thus, it appears that while the developmental stages of eye-specific layering and fine synaptic remodeling may share some mechanisms, other mechanisms are distinct.

Vision-Dependent Plasticity in the Visual Thalamus

While synaptic forms of plasticity involving neuromodulation and short-term plasticity persist throughout life, it was generally believed that large-scale changes in synaptic connectivity in the thalamus diminish once axon rearrangement, synapse strengthening, and elimination of connections are complete early in development (Fox et al., 2000). In the mammalian visual system, for example, subcortical regions such as the LGN were thought to develop before eye opening in a vision-independent manner (Katz and Shatz, 1996).

Once retinal connections in the LGN stabilize, it was thought that the center of plasticity moves to the cortex, where sensory experience sculpts neuronal circuits during a later developmental critical period (Daw et al., 1992; Hensch, 2005; Hubel and Wiesel, 1970). Recent studies at the mouse retinogeniculate synapse, however, have revealed that visual experience can

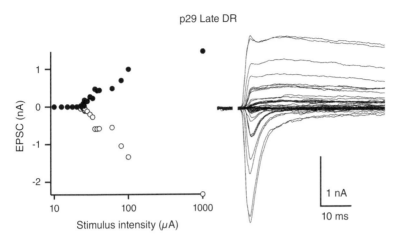

Figure 5.3
Representative response to incremental increase in stimulus intensity in a mouse dark reared from postnatal day (P) 20 for 7 days (late DR). When this mouse is compared to normally reared P20 mice, the average number of inputs increases and average strength of the inputs decreases with late DR (Hooks and Chen, 2008). Symbols as in figure 5.2.

influence synaptic circuits in the visual thalamus (Hooks and Chen, 2006). Dark rearing from P20, referred to as late DR, results in a robust reorganization of synaptic connections. After 7 days of late DR, the number of inputs to a relay neuron more than doubles, while the average strength of a single RGC input decreases to less than half of that observed in normally reared mice at P20 (see figure 5.3).

These findings would suggest that visual experience is necessary for the maintenance of refined retinogeniculate connections during a later phase of development, much like that described for orientation selectivity in the cortex (Crair et al., 1998) and receptive fields in the superior colliculus (Carrasco et al., 2005). However, the relationship between vision and remodeling of the retinogeniculate synapse is more complex than just maintenance, as reflected by the synaptic response to dark rearing from birth (chronic dark rearing). In mice chronically dark reared from P1 to P32, the RGC afferent pruning and input strengthening do not appear to be significantly different from that which occurs in normally reared mice even though after the age of P20 the condition is identical to that of late DR (see figure 5.4). An alternative perspective on these findings, however, is that in the case of late DR, plasticity is elicited in response to deprivation, while in chronic DR, no change in synaptic connectivity occurs. In other words, the response to late DR is desirable and reflects a normal adaptive response to the environment, and the response to chronic DR is abnormal.

Thus, the timing of dark rearing appears to be important in eliciting plasticity at this subcortical connection (Hooks and Chen, 2008). The retinogeniculate synapse does not simply become sensitive to vision because eyes open (at P12). Dark rearing from P15 does not evoke the same degree of plasticity as that from P20 (see figure 5.4). Single-fiber strength and estimated number

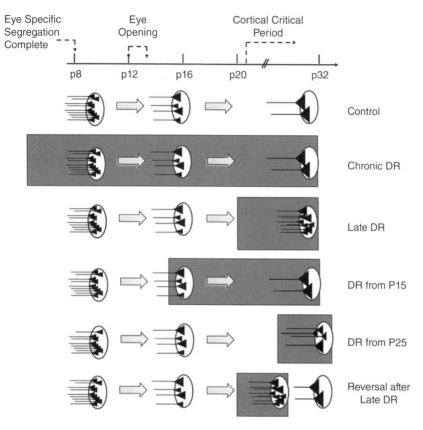

Figure 5.4
Schematic summary of developmental retinogeniculate synaptic remodeling. After the initial phase of axon mapping and coarse rearrangement of axon arbors (before postnatal day [P] 8), the second phase of synapse development involves synapse remodeling that is dependent on spontaneous activity (P8–16). This is followed by a third phase of development when synapse remodeling is dependent on visual experience (>P17). Conditions: control, 12-hr light/dark cycle; chronic DR, dark reared from birth; late DR, dark reared from P20+, test P27–32; DR P15+, test P27–32; DR P25+, test P32–34; reversal, dark reared from P20–27 and then exposed to normal light/dark cycle for 3–5 days, test P30–32.

of inputs do not significantly change with the former condition, while the latter manipulation results in robust changes. The late developmental plasticity at the retinogeniculate synapse meets the criteria of a critical period—that is, a period of plasticity with a distinct onset and end. If deprivation is shifted 5 days later, to P25, the synaptic response is different. As with late DR, the average strength of an RGC input decreases; however, the average number of afferent inputs to a given relay neuron does not change. One interpretation for these findings is that there is a small window of time during development where the pairings of pre- and postsynaptic partners can change in response to a change in the environment or experience. After that period, changes in the strength of connections between RGC and relay neurons can still be regulated by vision, but the possibility of recruiting additional afferent inputs to relay neurons is diminished.

These studies in the visual thalamus suggest that even after the connections between RGC and thalamic relay neurons have undergone the normal developmental synapse strengthening, elimination, and refinement, there is the potential to rewire and reorganize the thalamic circuitry around the developmental time point of P20 in mice. Strikingly, this time coincides with the onset of the cortical critical period for ocular dominance plasticity as well as other forms of synaptic plasticity in cortical layer 2/3 of rodents (Desai et al., 2002; Fagiolini et al., 1994; Gordon and Stryker, 1996). Yet the kinetics of plasticity in the thalamus differs from that of the cortex. In the case of the cortex, monocular deprivation or dark rearing can result in robust changes in synaptic strength, single-unit responses, visual evoked potentials, and ocular dominance within 1–4 days (Desai et al., 2002; Gordon and Stryker, 1996; Heynen et al., 2003). In contrast, dark rearing for three to four days elicits some changes in total synaptic current evoked by retinal inputs but does not significantly alter the strength or number of connections between RGC and relay neurons. Instead, four to seven days of deprivation are required for changes in connectivity. Thus, experience-dependent changes at the retinogeniculate synapse are not likely to influence the initial rapid cortical response to visual deprivation. It remains to be seen, however, whether alterations in retinothalamic connectivity drive rearrangements in thalamocortical axon arbors and subsequent changes in cortical function in response to longer periods of deprivation (Antonini et al., 1999; Antonini and Stryker, 1993; Dursteler et al., 1976).

Other features that distinguish cortical and thalamic critical periods include reversibility. Restoring light to mice that have undergone late DR for 7 days results in rapid pruning of excess number of afferent inputs and strengthening of remaining retinogeniculate connections. Thus, the pairings between RGCs and relay neurons appear to be malleable during the thalamic critical period. In contrast, deprivation-induced shifts in ocular dominance are not easily or rapidly reversed by reopening the eye (Blakemore and Van Sluyters, 1974; Hubel and Wiesel, 1970; Malach et al., 1984; Wiesel and Hubel, 1965). However, other forms of cortical critical periods, such as that of homeostatic plasticity, exhibit reversibility similar to that of the retinogeniculate synapse (Desai et al., 2002; Maffei et al., 2004).

Generalizability of Subcortical Experience-Dependent Plasticity

Vision-dependent synaptic plasticity in thalamic circuits had not been previously recognized; however, work in other regions of the visual system have demonstrated that experience-dependent remodeling of neuronal circuits exists outside of the cortex. Much like the LGN, mapping of retinal axons to the superior colliculus depends on spontaneous retinal activity and not vision (Chalupa and Rhoades, 1978; Chandrasekaran et al., 2005; Chow and Spear, 1974; Pfeiffenberger et al., 2006; Rhoades and Chalupa, 1978). In the colliculus, initial receptive field refinement does not require vision; however, with prolonged visual deprivation, collicular receptive fields gradually become larger with age (Carrasco et al., 2005). At the synaptic level, in vitro studies of rat colliculus demonstrate that visual experience can accelerate the normal process of synaptic refinement during development, although the exact synaptic connection that is altered is not clear (Lu and Constantine-Paton, 2004). Vision has also been shown to play a role in the refinement of RGC dendritic arbors into ON and OFF regions of the inner plexiform layer, a process that can be blocked by dark rearing (Tian and Copenhagen, 2003). Thus, vision may be playing similar roles in the refinement and maintenance of synapses and synaptic circuits at many regions of the visual system (Carrasco et al., 2005; Crair et al., 1998; Hooks and Chen, 2008). It is still not clear whether plasticity in the retina or the superior colliculus satisfies the criteria of a critical period, and how periods of plasticity in different subcortical regions relate to each other.

Why the vision-sensitive phase of thalamic development has not previously been observed is still not clear. However, there are few studies in cat, ferret, or monkey LGN that examine the physiological consequences of dark rearing after the animals have experienced vision. Other possible explanations include differences in experimental techniques, with single-cell synaptic recordings revealing finer changes in circuit connectivity than receptive field recording. Finally, species differences and the proportion of monocular versus binocular innervation could play a role in the effects of various forms of deprivation.

Following the discovery of an experience-dependent period of plasticity in the LGN, studies in the somatosensory thalamus also showed a similar period of sensory-dependent plasticity (Wang and Zhang, 2008). These studies revealed that whisker plucking at P12–13 altered the normal synapse elimination of the leminscal inputs onto VPm relay neurons only during a specific period of development. Much as in the visual system, this experience-dependent period of plasticity in the somatosensory thalamus overlaps with the period of sensory-dependent plasticity in the cortex. Therefore, accumulating observations support a new view of thalamic critical periods during development (Kano and Hashimoto, 2009) and raise new questions about the relationship between thalamic and cortical plasticity.

A Proposed Model for Retinogeniculate Plasticity

Based on our current understanding of plasticity at the retinogeniculate synapse, we put forth a model to be tested in the future. We propose that following the first phase of large-scale axon rearrangement that results in the segregation of retinal axons into proper eye-specific layers, there is a second, vision-independent phase of robust synapse elimination and strengthening of remaining inputs. By P15–16, the afferent inputs have pruned to approximately three to five inputs and the average strength is about 50% of the mature retinogeniculate synapse. We hypothesize that refinement during this phase results in a coarse approximation of the final synaptic circuit—that is, retinotopy, as assayed by labeling of terminal zones (Pfeiffenberger et al., 2005; Pfeiffenberger et al., 2006), has refined and RGCs are connected to a subset of the possible postsynaptic partners that are in the proper target area.

With eye opening, visual information is transmitted from the eye to LGN and activates a third phase of plasticity. We know that vision triggers this late phase of development, but the features of vision, and the cellular mechanisms involved in the activation of this phase, have yet to be identified. During this later period, there is an increase in the plasticity of the connection between the retina and LGN as further refinement of synaptic connections occurs in response to visual information. Some connections continue to strengthen, while others are eliminated, and sometimes, new connections in the same target area are made. As rearrangement of these connections occur, they are stabilized into the final mature circuit through mechanisms that depend on vision. In the case of late dark rearing, loss of vision results in a destabilization of the synaptic circuit and an increase in the turnover of synapses between RGC and relay neurons, resulting in the weakening of previously strengthened connections and recruitment of new connections. In the case of chronic dark rearing, the late phase of experience-dependent refinement is not activated and thus the retinogeniculate circuit is stabilized in the coarse experience-independent form. From the perspective of the postsynaptic neuron, it is innervated by one to three RGCs, but they are not necessarily the optimal presynaptic partners.

In the future, a number of approaches can be taken to test this model. Identification of distinct mechanisms that differentiate one period of refinement from another will help to confirm or modify this model. In addition, understanding the axon arbor structural changes that underlie the late experience-dependent thalamic plasticity will shed light on how neuronal connections can rewire during late development. While detailed changes in the morphological rearrangement of axon terminals during this later developmental period have not been documented in mice, insight into the possible structural correlate of the changes in synaptic function may be obtained from elegant microscopy studies in the cat that suggest that the axon structure in adults is much broader than functionally necessary (Hamos et al., 1987; Sur et al., 1984). Perhaps there is a potential for the remnants of arbor development to be harnessed for plasticity at a later age.

As we delve deeper into future questions regarding experience-dependent plasticity, we can look to Lamberto Maffei as an example of how a curiosity for the unknown, combined with a fearlessness in exploring new territories, opened doors to new avenues of work and tantalizing ideas.

Acknowledgments

This work was supported by NIH RO1 EY013613 and the Children's Hospital Boston Mental Retardation and Developmental Disabilities Research Center NIH PO1 HD18655.

References

Antonini A, Fagiolini M, Stryker MP. 1999. Anatomical correlates of functional plasticity in mouse visual cortex. *J Neurosci* 19: 4388–4406.

Antonini A, Stryker MP. 1993. Rapid remodeling of axonal arbors in the visual cortex. *Science* 260: 1819–1821.

Bjartmar L, Huberman AD, Ullian EM, Renteria RC, Liu X, Xu W, Prezioso J, et al. 2006. Neuronal pentraxins mediate synaptic refinement in the developing visual system. *J Neurosci* 26: 6269–6281.

Blakemore C, Van Sluyters RC. 1974. Reversal of the physiological effects of monocular deprivation in kittens: further evidence for a sensitive period. *J Physiol* 237: 195–216.

Blakemore C, Vital-Durand F. 1986. Organization and post-natal development of the monkey's lateral geniculate nucleus. *J Physiol* 380: 453–491.

Butts DA, Kanold PO, Shatz CJ. 2007. A burst-based "Hebbian" learning rule at retinogeniculate synapses links retinal waves to activity-dependent refinement. *PLoS Biol* 5: 0651–0661.

Carrasco MM, Razak KA, Pallas SL. 2005. Visual experience is necessary for maintenance but not development of receptive fields in superior colliculus. *J Neurophysiol* 94: 1962–1970.

Chalupa LM, Rhoades RW. 1978. Directional selectivity in hamster superior colliculus is modified by strobe-rearing but not by dark-rearing. *Science* 199: 998–1001.

Chandrasekaran AR, Plas DT, Gonzalez E, Crair MC. 2005. Evidence for an instructive role of retinal activity in retinotopic map refinement in the superior colliculus of the mouse. *J Neurosci* 25: 6929–6938.

Chen C, Regehr WG. 2000. Developmental remodeling of the retinogeniculate synapse. *Neuron* 28: 955–966.

Chow KL, Spear PD. 1974. Morphological and functional effects of visual deprivation on the rabbit visual system. *Exp Neurol* 42: 429–447.

Crair MC, Gillespie DC, Stryker MP. 1998. The role of visual experience in the development of columns in cat visual cortex. *Science* 279: 566–570.

Daniels JD, Pettigrew JD, Norman JL. 1978. Development of single-neuron responses in kitten's lateral geniculate nucleus. *J Neurophysiol* 41: 1373–1393.

Daw NW, Fox K, Sato H, Czepita D. 1992. Critical period for monocular deprivation in the cat visual cortex. *J Neurophysiol* 67: 197–202.

Demas J, Sagdullaev BT, Green E, Jaubert-Miazza L, McCall MA, Gregg RG, Wong RO, Guido W. 2006. Failure to maintain eye-specific segregation in nob, a mutant with abnormally patterned retinal activity. *Neuron* 50: 247–259.

Desai NS, Cudmore RH, Nelson SB, Turrigiano GG. 2002. Critical periods for experience-dependent synaptic scaling in visual cortex. *Nat Neurosci* 5: 783–789.

Dittman JS, Regehr WG. 1998. Calcium dependence and recovery kinetics of presynaptic depression at the climbing fiber to Purkinje cell synapse. *J Neurosci* 18: 6147–6162.

Dursteler MR, Garey LJ, Movshon JA. 1976. Reversal of the morphological effects of monocular deprivation in the kitten's lateral geniculate nucleus. *J Physiol* 261: 189–210.

Fagiolini M, Pizzorusso T, Berardi N, Domenici L, Maffei L. 1994. Functional postnatal development of the rat primary visual cortex and the role of visual experience: dark rearing and monocular deprivation. *Vision Res* 34: 709–720.

Feldheim DA, Vanderhaeghen P, Hansen MJ, Frisen J, Lu Q, Barbacid M, Flanagan JG. 1998. Topographic guidance labels in a sensory projection to the forebrain. *Neuron* 21: 1303–1313.

Fox K, Glazewski S, Schulze S. 2000. Plasticity and stability of somatosensory maps in thalamus and cortex. *Curr Opin Neurobiol* 10: 494–497.

Galli L, Maffei L. 1988. Spontaneous impulse activity of rat retinal ganglion cells in prenatal life. *Science* 242: 90–91.

Garraghty PE, Frost DO, Sur M. 1987. The morphology of retinogeniculate X- and Y-cell axonal arbors in dark-reared cats. *Exp Brain Res* 66: 115–127.

Godement P, Salaun J, Imbert M. 1984. Prenatal and postnatal development of retinogeniculate and retinocollicular projections in the mouse. *J Comp Neurol* 230: 552–575.

Gordon JA, Stryker MP. 1996. Experience-dependent plasticity of binocular responses in the primary visual cortex of the mouse. *J Neurosci* 16: 3274–3286.

Hahm JO, Langdon RB, Sur M. 1991. Disruption of retinogeniculate afferent segregation by antagonists to NMDA receptors. *Nature* 351: 568–570.

Hamos JE, Van Horn SC, Raczkowski D, Sherman SM. 1987. Synaptic circuits involving an individual retinogeniculate axon in the cat. *J Comp Neurol* 259: 165–192.

Hensch TK. 2005. Critical period plasticity in local cortical circuits. *Nat Rev Neurosci* 6: 877–888.

Heynen AJ, Yoon BJ, Liu CH, Chung HJ, Huganir RL, Bear MF. 2003. Molecular mechanism for loss of visual cortical responsiveness following brief monocular deprivation. *Nat Neurosci* 6: 854–862.

Hooks BM, Chen C. 2006. Distinct roles for spontaneous and visual activity in remodeling of the retinogeniculate synapse. *Neuron* 52: 281–291.

Hooks BM, Chen C. 2008. Vision triggers an experience-dependent sensitive period at the retinogeniculate synapse. *J Neurosci* 28: 4807–4817.

Hubel DH, Wiesel TN. 1970. The period of susceptibility to the physiological effects of unilateral eye closure in kittens. *J Physiol* 206: 419–436.

Huberman AD. 2007. Mechanisms of eye-specific visual circuit development. *Curr Opin Neurobiol* 17: 73–80.

Huberman AD, Murray KD, Warland DK, Feldheim DA, Chapman B. 2005. Ephrin-As mediate targeting of eye-specific projections to the lateral geniculate nucleus. *Nat Neurosci* 8: 1013–1021.

Huberman AD, Wang GY, Liets LC, Collins OA, Chapman B, Chalupa LM. 2003. Eye-specific retinogeniculate segregation independent of normal neuronal activity. *Science* 300: 994–998.

Huh GS, Boulanger LM, Du HP, Riquelme PA, Brotz TM, Shatz CJ. 2000. Functional requirement for class I MHC in CNS development and plasticity. *Science* 290: 2155–2159.

Jaubert-Miazza L, Green E, Lo FS, Bui K, Mills J, Guido W. 2005. Structural and functional composition of the developing retinogeniculate pathway in the mouse. *Vis Neurosci* 22: 661–676.

Jeffery G. 1984. Retinal ganglion cell death and terminal field retraction in the developing rodent visual system. *Brain Res* 315: 81–96.

Kano M, Hashimoto K. 2009. Synapse elimination in the central nervous system. *Curr Opin Neurobiol* 19: 154–161.

Katz LC, Shatz CJ. 1996. Synaptic activity and the construction of cortical circuits. *Science* 274: 1133–1138.

Linden DC, Guillery RW, Cucchiaro J. 1981. The dorsal lateral geniculate nucleus of the normal ferret and its postnatal development. *J Comp Neurol* 203: 189–211.

Lu W, Constantine-Paton M. 2004. Eye opening rapidly induces synaptic potentiation and refinement. *Neuron* 43: 237–249.

Lyckman AW, Jhaveri S, Feldheim DA, Vanderhaeghen P, Flanagan JG, Sur M. 2001. Enhanced plasticity of retinothalamic projections in an ephrin-A2/A5 double mutant. *J Neurosci* 21: 7684–7690.

Maffei A, Nelson SB, Turrigiano GG. 2004. Selective reconfiguration of layer 4 visual cortical circuitry by visual deprivation. *Nat Neurosci* 7: 1353–1359.

Maffei L, Galli-Resta L. 1990. Correlation in the discharges of neighboring rat retinal ganglion cells during prenatal life. *Proc Natl Acad Sci USA* 87: 2861–2864.

Malach R, Ebert R, Van Sluyters RC. 1984. Recovery from effects of brief monocular deprivation in the kitten. *J Neurophysiol* 51: 538–551.

Meister M, Wong RO, Baylor DA, Shatz CJ. 1991. Synchronous bursts of action potentials in ganglion cells of the developing mammalian retina. *Science* 252: 939–943.

Muir-Robinson G, Hwang BJ, Feller MB. 2002. Retinogeniculate axons undergo eye-specific segregation in the absence of eye-specific layers. *J Neurosci* 22: 5259–5264.

Pfeiffenberger C, Cutforth T, Woods G, Yamada J, Renteria RC, Copenhagen DR, Flanagan JG, Feldheim DA. 2005. Ephrin-As and neural activity are required for eye-specific patterning during retinogeniculate mapping. *Nat Neurosci* 8: 1022–1027.

Pfeiffenberger C, Yamada J, Feldheim DA. 2006. Ephrin-As and patterned retinal activity act together in the development of topographic maps in the primary visual system. *J Neurosci* 26: 12873–12884.

Ramoa AS, McCormick DA. 1994. Enhanced activation of NMDA receptor responses at the immature retinogeniculate synapse. *J Neurosci* 14: 2098–2105.

Rhoades RW, Chalupa LM. 1978. Receptive field characteristics of superior colliculus neurons and visually guided behavior in dark-reared hamsters. *J Comp Neurol* 177: 17–32.

Shatz CJ. 1983. The prenatal development of the cat's retinogeniculate pathway. *J Neurosci* 3: 482–499.

Shatz CJ, Kirkwood PA. 1984. Prenatal development of functional connections in the cat's retinogeniculate pathway. *J Neurosci* 4: 1378–1397.

Shatz CJ, Stryker MP. 1988. Prenatal tetrodotoxin infusion blocks segregation of retinogeniculate afferents. *Science* 242: 87–89.

Sretavan D, Shatz CJ. 1984. Prenatal development of individual retinogeniculate axons during the period of segregation. *Nature* 308: 845–848.

Sretavan DW, Shatz CJ. 1986. Prenatal development of retinal ganglion cell axons: segregation into eye-specific layers within the cat's lateral geniculate nucleus. *J Neurosci* 6: 234–251.

Stevens B, Allen NJ, Vazquez LE, Howell GR, Christopherson KS, Nouri N, Micheva KD, et al. 2007. The classical complement cascade mediates CNS synapse elimination. *Cell* 131: 1164–1178.

Sun C, Warland DK, Ballesteros JM, van der List D, Chalupa LM. 2008. Retinal waves in mice lacking the beta2 subunit of the nicotinic acetylcholine receptor. *Proc Natl Acad Sci USA* 105: 13638–13643.

Sur M, Humphrey AL, Sherman SM. 1982. Monocular deprivation affects X- and Y-cell retinogeniculate terminations in cats. *Nature* 300: 183–185.

Sur M, Weller RE, Sherman SM. 1984. Development of X- and Y-cell retinogeniculate terminations in kittens. *Nature* 310: 246–249.

Tavazoie SF, Reid RC. 2000. Diverse receptive fields in the lateral geniculate nucleus during thalamocortical development. *Nat Neurosci* 3: 608–616.

Tian N, Copenhagen DR. 2003. Visual stimulation is required for refinement of ON and OFF pathways in postnatal retina. *Neuron* 39: 85–96.

Torborg CL, Hansen KA, Feller MB. 2005. High frequency, synchronized bursting drives eye-specific segregation of retinogeniculate projections. *Nat Neurosci* 8: 72–78.

Wang H, Zhang ZW. 2008. A critical window for experience-dependent plasticity at whisker sensory relay synapse in the thalamus. *J Neurosci* 28: 13621–13628.

Wiesel TN, Hubel DH. 1965. Extent of recovery from the effects of visual deprivation in kittens. *J Neurophysiol* 28: 1060–1072.

Wong RO, Chernjavsky A, Smith SJ, Shatz CJ. 1995. Early functional neural networks in the developing retina. *Nature* 374: 716–718.

Ziburkus J, Guido W. 2006. Loss of binocular responses and reduced retinal convergence during the period of retinogeniculate axon segregation. *J Neurophysiol* 96: 2775–2784.

6 Is Half a Loaf Worse than No Bread?: The Role of Normal and Abnormal Patterns of Neuronal Activity in the Development of the Visual System

Barbara Chapman

In the adult mammalian visual system, information from the two eyes is kept anatomically and physiologically segregated into ipsilateral and contralateral lateral geniculate nucleus (LGN) layers and into ocular dominance columns in the input layers of primary visual cortex. The development of these eye-specific connections has served as a model system for studying the development of precise connections in the brain and has influenced many fields within neurobiology, including the study of learning and memory and of adult plasticity.

Historically, it has been thought that eye-specific projections emerge during development from an immature state where axons serving the two eyes are initially intermingled in both LGN and cortex, and that they segregate during development by an activity-dependent, competitive process following a Hebbian learning rule (Hebb, 1949) where "neurons that fire together, wire together" (Katz and Shatz, 1996). Recently, however, new data have brought this view into question. Therefore, the basic intellectual scaffolding underlying our understanding of the development of eye-specific connections is now open to debate. In particular, questions remain about the initial state of ocular dominance columns early in development, about whether retinal activity actually drives eye-specific segregation during normal development, and about what features of activity are important for normal versus abnormal development of connections.

Are Eye-Specific Connections Initially Segregated or Overlapping Early in Normal Development?

There is good agreement that the projections from the two eyes to the LGN do start out overlapping and only segregate into eye-specific layers over time during development. This pattern has been seen anatomically in mouse (Godement et al., 1984), ferret (Linden et al., 1981; Speer et al., 2010), cat (Shatz, 1983), monkey (Rakic, 1976; Huberman et al., 2005), and human (Hevner, 2000). Physiological recordings have also confirmed that early in development individual LGN neurons receive functional synapses from both eyes and then become monocular in their responses as the retinogeniculate arbors from the two eyes segregate (mouse: Jaubert-Miazza et al., 2005; cat: Shatz and Kirkwood, 1984).

The normal pattern of development of ocular dominance columns, however, has recently become controversial. Early studies of ocular dominance column development relied on transneuronal tracers injected into one eye to label geniculocortical afferents and thus visualize ocular dominance columns. In these studies, transneuronal labeling in layer IV of primary visual cortex appeared uniform early in development; ocular dominance columns (seen as periodic labeling) appeared later in development and became more distinct over time (ferret: Ruthazer et al., 1999; cat: LeVay et al., 1978; monkey: Rakic, 1976). A potential problem with the use of transneuronal labeling is that the uniformity of label seen in young animals could be due to "spillover" of the label into the LGN layer serving the noninjected eye (LeVay et al., 1978) rather than to actual overlap of the arbors serving the two eyes. Recent experiments using optical imaging, physiological recording, and retrograde tracing from cortex to LGN, as well as transneuronal labeling visualized in horizontal sections through flattened primary visual cortex (which provides a more sensitive measure of periodic labeling than do the cross sections used in earlier studies), all show that ocular dominance columns in cat are actually present at least one week earlier in development than was previously thought (Crair et al., 1998, 2001). These same studies did still show that at an even earlier time in development, cortex was visually responsive but no ocular dominance columns were seen either with optical imaging or with transneuronal label. It is not clear whether the lack of visible ocular dominance columns very early in development in these studies indicates that columns are actually not present at that time. The lack of columns seen in transneuronal label at the earliest ages could still be due to spillover, and the lack of columns seen in optical imaging could be due to a lack of sensitivity of that technique in very young animals (this has been seen in studies of the development of orientation selectivity in visual cortex, where development of orientation selectivity can be seen several days earlier in electrophysiological recordings than it can be seen in optical imaging; Chapman et al., 1996).

The idea that ocular dominance columns form by refinement of initially overlapping axons serving the two eyes has been challenged. Experiments injecting a tracer into a contralateral or ipsilateral LGN layer showed patchy connections to primary visual cortex at very early stages of development, almost as early as the axons grow into the cortical plate (Crowley and Katz, 2000). The spatial arrangement of these patchy connections resembled adult ocular dominance columns. These experiments have been interpreted to show that axons serving the two eyes initially grow into cortex already segregated, and that the overlap of axons inferred from earlier studies was an artifact due to spillover (Crowley and Katz, 2000). However, these experiments themselves have been criticized as potentially not really revealing ocular dominance column development (Huberman, 2007). Careful studies of the arbors of individual geniculocortical afferents during development have been performed (Ghosh and Shatz, 1992; Antonini and Stryker, 1993). These studies show that geniculocortical axon arbors are sparse early in development and elaborate over time, but such studies cannot resolve the issue of whether sparse axons early in development are arranged into ocular dominance columns or not (Crair et al., 2001).

Does the Initial Formation of Eye-Specific Connections Require Neuronal Activity?

The idea that the normal development of eye-specific connections in the visual system is dependent on retinal activity grew out of the finding that monocular deprivation during the critical period causes ocular dominance plasticity, with the deprived eye columns shrinking and the open eye columns expanding (Wiesel and Hubel, 1965). Plasticity during the critical period appears to be due to competition between the two eyes; binocular deprivation does not cause shrinking of both eyes' ocular dominance columns (LeVay et al., 1980). It was therefore an attractive hypothesis that competition between the two eyes could also be driving the initial segregation of afferents into columns (Stryker and Harris, 1986).

Conceptually it is very easy to test whether the development of eye-specific LGN layers and ocular dominance columns is activity dependent; one need only block activity and observe whether layers or columns form. This approach has been taken by several labs in the past, but the conclusions drawn from the experiments have had to be reinterpreted due to new data. The sodium channel blocker tetrodotoxin (TTX) was used to block retinal ganglion cell action potentials in young kittens. Following the activity blockade, ocular dominance columns were not seen using transneuronal labeling, which was interpreted to mean that ocular dominance column formation is in fact activity dependent (Stryker and Harris, 1986). Unfortunately, in these studies the TTX treatment was started at an age where columns were at that time thought not to have formed (LeVay et al., 1978) but at which age we now know columns are present (Crair et al., 1998, 2001). Therefore, it is necessary to reinterpret these experiments as showing that activity is necessary to maintain geniculocortical afferent segregation rather than that activity is necessary for the initial establishment of the columns (Huberman et al., 2008). The need for activity to maintain eye-specific connections has also been seen in the LGN, where blockade or alterations of activity after afferents have segregated into eye-specific layers can cause desegregation (Chapman, 2000; Demas et al., 2006). A second approach has been to physically remove the eyes early in development. This binocular enucleation does not affect the pattern of patchy connections seen when a small tracer injection is made into an LGN layer, which as been interpreted to mean that ocular dominance column development is not activity dependent (Crowley and Katz, 1999). This conclusion, however, may not be justified, given that in the absence of eyes retinogeniculate cells are still more correlated within a layer than between layers (Weliky and Katz, 1999). This correlation structure could be sufficient to drive ocular dominance column formation by an activity-dependent process (Crair et al., 2001). It is also important to note that, at least in rodents, retinal wave activity is able to drive cortical activity very early in development (Hanganu et al., 2006). Therefore the question of whether the initial formation of ocular dominance columns is activity dependent remains open.

TTX has also been used to block activity during the period of segregation of afferents from the two eyes in the LGN. Experiments using TTX to block brain activity in utero in kittens showed profound effects on eye-specific retinogeniculate projections (Shatz and Stryker, 1988;

Sretavan et al., 1988). However, using TTX to block retinal activity postnatally in the retinas in ferrets had little effect (Cook et al., 1999). It is not clear why these two experiments yielded different results. It is possible that the prenatal effects of TTX were more severe because activity was blocked throughout the brain, not only in the retinas. It is also possible that the prenatal TTX might have caused side effects, slowing the overall maturation of the fetuses. On the other hand, it is possible that the postnatal TTX did not actually provide a continuous blockade of retinal activity. Another approach to blocking retinal activity was to use the acetylcholine analog epibatidine, which was thought to block ganglion cell activity based on patch clamp recordings. Segregation was found not to occur in the presence of epibatidine (Penn et al., 1998). Unfortunately, as was later shown using multielectrode array recordings, epibatidine only blocks activity in some retinal ganglion cells while altering patterns of activity in cells that remain active (Cang et al., 2005; Pfeiffenberger et al., 2005; Sun et al., 2008). Therefore, the question of whether activity blockade prevents retinogeniculate axon segregation into eye-specific layers is also unresolved.

What Features of the Spatiotemporal Patterns of Retinal Activity Drive Normal versus Abnormal Segregation of Eye-Specific Connections?

Although it is not yet clear whether the normal development of eye-specific LGN layers and ocular dominance columns requires that retinal ganglion cells are firing action potentials (see above), it is clear that altering the patterns of retinal activity can disrupt the normal development and/or the maintenance of eye-specific connections. This could be because normal patterns of activity actually instruct the proper development of connections. On the other hand, it could be that connections can form without activity, but abnormal patterns of activity disrupt normal development. The dogma in the field has been that eye-specific connections form through an activity-dependent, competitive process, and that normal development requires balanced levels of activity in the two eyes and requires high correlation of retinal ganglion cell action potentials within one eye and low correlations between eyes (for reviews, see Katz and Shatz, 1996; Crair, 1999; Wong, 1999; Sur et al., 1999; Cohen-Cory, 2002; Feller, 2002; Sengpiel and Kind, 2002; Torborg and Feller, 2005; Huberman, 2007; Huberman et al., 2008).

The idea that the initial development of eye-specific connections occurs through a Hebbian process has been challenged in recent years (Crowley and Katz, 2002; Chalupa, 2007). The fact that patchy connections between an LGN layer and visual cortex are seen very early in development (Crowley and Katz, 2000) and are not altered by monocular enucleation (Crowley and Katz, 1999) argues against the classical view that development occurs by refinement of initially diffuse projections, where postsynaptic cells would initially receive input from both eyes and only later weaken or lose one connection by a competitive process. The clear existence of a "precritical" period (during which monocular deprivation has no effect on ocular dominance columns) in all animals studied (for a review, see Feller and Scanziani, 2005) suggests that competition between the two eyes may not be important for the initial development of columns which occurs before the critical period. The fact that there is a strong dominance of the contralateral eye throughout primary visual cortex early in development also poses a problem for a purely Hebbian process of column development which would suggest that due to this bias the contralateral eye would win all of the territory in the cortex (Crair et al., 2001). Therefore, there remains debate in the field not only over whether activity is involved in the normal development of eye-specific segregation but also over whether or not activity plays an instructive role causing segregation to occur based on a correlation-based learning rule.

There is good agreement in the field that altering levels of activity in the two eyes during development results in plasticity of eye-specific connections. This was first shown by monocular deprivation studies that resulted in profound changes in the width of ocular dominance columns, with the deprived eye columns shrinking and open eye columns expanding (Wiesel and Hubel, 1965). Such changes were not seen when both eyes were deprived of vision, highlighting the competitive nature of the interaction (LeVay et al., 1980). Similar results have been seen in the development of LGN layers in experiments altering the levels of activity in one eye using pharmacological methods. If the levels of activity are lowered in one eye, that eye's projection to the LGN shrinks (Penn et al., 1998). If the levels of activity are increased in one eye, however, that eye's projection to the LGN expands (Stellwagen and Shatz, 2002). It should be noted that interpreting the results of these experiments does require some caution, as both visual deprivation and the pharmacological agents used in the experiments do alter the patterns of activity in the affected eye as well as the levels of activity.

There is less agreement in the field about the role that correlations of activity within one eye and lack of correlations between the two eyes play in the normal development of connections. The degree of correlation between the two eyes can be decreased by altering visual experience in animals raised with surgically induced strabismus. Strabismus does result in an increase in cortical cell monocularity, and in sharpened ocular dominance column borders, as would be expected if relative within- and between-eye correlations are important for normal development (Wiesel and Hubel, 1963; Shatz et al., 1977; Löwel, 1994). Artificially decreasing or increasing correlation of the two eyes by alternate or synchronous electrical stimulation of the optic nerves also has the expected result: alternating stimulation (which decorrelates the activity of the two eyes) results in more segregation of eye-specific connections to the cortex while synchronous stimulation results in less segregation (Stryker and Strickland, 1984). Unfortunately, all of these experiments were done during the critical period for plasticity, not during the period of initial establishment of ocular dominance columns, so the results support the hypothesis that correlations are important for plasticity but do not address whether they are important for the initial establishment of segregated eye-specific connections.

The fact that the formation of eye-specific LGN layers occurs before eye opening in all species studied (Rakic, 1976; Linden et al., 1981; Godement et al., 1984; Shatz, 1983; Hevner, 2000; Huberman et al., 2005; Speer et al., 2010), and that ocular dominance columns form before birth in the monkey (Horton and Hocking, 1996), indicate that if patterns of retinal activity are important for the initial development of eye-specific connections, that retinal activity must be spontaneous rather than visually driven. The discovery and characterization of retinal waves (Galli and Maffei, 1988; Maffei and Galli-Resta, 1990; Meister et al., 1991; Feller et al., 1996; Zhou, 1998) led many in the field to propose that this early pattern of spontaneous activity was the perfect pattern to increase within-eye correlations and decrease between-eye correlations, and thus that retinal waves are necessary for the development of eye-specific connections (Eglen, 1999; Wong, 1999; Butts, 2002).

It is clear that some manipulations that alter the patterns of retinal activity, such as epibatidine treatment (Penn et al., 1998), and knockout of the beta-2 acetylcholine receptor (Bansal et al., 2000; Rossi et al., 2001; Muir-Robinson et al., 2002) prevent the normal segregation of axons from the two eyes in the LGN. On the other hand, other manipulations that dramatically alter retinal activity patterns such as knockout of connexin36 (Torborg et al., 2005), manipulations of cyclic AMP (cAMP) levels (Stellwagen and Shatz, 2002), and treatment with an immunotoxin that targets starburst amacrine cells (Huberman et al., 2003) do not affect the normal segregation of retinal ganglion cell axons in the LGN. Because each of these manipulations affects many aspects of retinal activity, it is hard to know from these experiments what might be the crucial features of activity patterns that allow or prevent normal segregation of eye-specific connections. Generally, the three features of activity that have gained the most attention are the overall level of activity, the degree of correlation between nearby cells, and the presence of bursts of action potentials. If levels of activity are the key feature, this would tend to indicate that activity is playing a permissive rather than an instructive role in the development of eye-specific layers. Both epibatidine treatment (Sun et al., 2008) and knockout of the beta-2 receptor (Feller, 2002) do greatly increase the number of retinal ganglion cells that are not firing action potentials, thus lowering the overall level of activity in the retina. On the other hand, knockout of connexin36 (Torborg et al., 2005), alterations of cAMP levels (Stellwagen and Shatz, 2002), and low-dose vesicular acetylcholine transporter immunotoxin (Huberman et al., 2003) all either increase or do not affect overall levels of firing. This is consistent with activity levels being the important feature for segregation and, therefore, with activity playing a permissive role in the process. The degree of correlation among neighboring cells is diminished in epibatidine-treated (Sun et al., 2008) and beta-2 knockout (Torborg et al., 2005) animals, but not in connexin36 knockouts (Torborg et al., 2005) or animals with altered levels of cAMP in the retina (Stellwagen and Shatz, 2002). These findings support a role for within-eye correlations in normal development of eye-specific connections and thus support the Hebbian model. Counter to this hypothesis, however, is the finding that immunotoxin treatment, which does not disrupt normal development of retinogeniculate projections, does radically reduce nearest neighbor correlations in firing (Huberman et al., 2003). Because multielectrode array recordings were not performed in the characterizations of the activity in immunotoxin-treated retinas (Huberman et al., 2003), it is possible that there might be some residual correlations remaining in these retinas, and that those low levels of correlation might be enough to drive normal segregation. Finally, the amount of time that retinal ganglion cells fire high-frequency (over 10 Hz) bursts of action potentials has been identified as a potentially important feature of retinal activity. In fact, a burst-timing dependent learning rule has been demonstrated at the developing retinogeniculate synapse, suggesting that if patterns of activity are important for development of eye-specific segregation, it may be the presence and timing of bursts, rather than of spikes, that is the crucial factor (Butts and Rokhsar, 2001; Butts et al., 2007). Consistent with this theory, epibatidine-treated (Sun et al., 2008) and beta-2 knockout (Torborg et al., 2005) retinas have decreased bursts with firing over 10 Hz, while connexin36 knockouts (Torborg et al., 2005) and retinas with altered levels of cAMP (Stellwagen and Shatz, 2002) do not. However, all of the manipulations of activity that have been studied so far alter many aspects of the spatiotemporal pattern of retinal ganglion cell action potential firing, making it difficult to determine exactly which feature may be important for normal development.

Is Half a Loaf Worse than No Bread?

From the extant data, one could argue that abnormal segregation occurs when aspects of retinal activity needed for normal segregation are missing. However, it is also possible that normal segregation can occur with no information from retinal activity, but abnormal patterns of activity drive plasticity in the system. Ocular dominance plasticity in cortex and LGN is clearly driven by abnormal activity (Wiesel and Hubel, 1965; Penn et al., 1998; Stellwagen and Shatz, 2002). Increasing correlations between the two eyes by electrical stimulation can lead to desegregation of ocular dominance columns (Stryker and Strickland, 1984), while decreasing correlations by strabismus leads to increased segregation (Wiesel and Hubel, 1963; Shatz et al., 1977; Löwel, 1994). These studies were all performed after the initial establishment of columns and, therefore, show that altered patterns of activity can drive plasticity of segregation in the cortex. In studies of the LGN, increased correlations between the two eyes might be expected if waves were more frequent. Increasing wave frequency in both eyes by altering cAMP levels did not alter the normal initial development of the retinogeniculate pathway (Stellwagen and Shatz, 2002). Increased frequency of waves after normal segregation occurred in the *nob* mouse, however, did lead to desegregation of the eye-specific retinogeniculate projections (Demas et al., 2006). It is not clear whether this difference in results reflects a real difference between the mechanisms of the initial development of connections versus the mechanisms of plasticity of those connections later in development, or whether the difference could be explained by differences in the degree to which the two manipulations cause increased correlations between the two eyes, or whether there is some other alteration in activity patterns in the *nob* retinas that is not seen in the cAMP-treated retinas that actually caused the desegregation. It therefore remains an open question whether manipulations of retinal activity that result in a lack of eye-specific segregation act through the loss of information in the pattern of normal activity that is needed for segregation to occur or whether they act through abnormal patterns of activity causing plasticity of connections.

Lessons from Studies of Cortical Orientation and Direction Selectivity

Interestingly, the development of orientation and direction selectivity, which have been less extensively studied than the development of eye-specific segregation, provide the best evidence in favor of an instructive role for activity in the development of specific connections in the visual system. Cortical activity blockade with TTX has been shown to prevent the maturation of orientation selectivity in visual cortex, showing that activity is needed for normal development to occur (Chapman and Stryker, 1993). Alterations in the correlation structure of retinal activity also prevent the development of orientation selectivity (Weliky and Katz, 1997; Chapman and Gödecke, 2000) although it is not clear whether this is due to the system's remaining in an immature state in the absence of information needed for development or whether it is caused by plasticity of connections in response to abnormal activity. Interestingly, binocular deprivation proves more detrimental to development of orientation specificity than does dark rearing (White et al., 2001), suggesting that the abnormal pattern of retinal activity due to vision through the eyelid may cause plasticity of connections (although it could also be argued that spontaneous activity has information needed for normal development that is lost in the pattern of activity experienced through the eyelid). Finally, studies of the development of direction selectivity provide the most solid evidence that patterns of retinal activity instruct normal development. Direction selectivity fails to develop in the absence of visual stimulation, and specific directions of motion of visual stimuli drive the development of selectivity for that direction (Li et al., 2006, 2008). It can only be hoped that further study of the development of orientation and direction selectivity will not make this field as uncertain and confusing as the field of development of eye-specific connections has become!

References

Antonini A, Stryker MP. 1993. Development of individual geniculocortical arbors in cat striate cortex and effects of binocular impulse blockade. *J Neurosci* 13(8): 3549–3573.

Bansal A, Singer JH, Hwang BJ, Xu W, Beaudet A, Feller MB. 2000. Mice lacking specific nicotinic acetylcholine receptor subunits exhibit dramatically altered spontaneous activity patterns and reveal a limited role for retinal waves in forming ON and OFF circuits in the inner retina. *J Neurosci* 20: 7672–7681.

Butts DA. 2002. Retinal waves: implications for synaptic learning rules during development. *Neuroscientist* 8: 243–253.

Butts DA, Kanold PO, Shatz CJ. 2007. A burst-based "Hebbian" learning rule at retinogeniculate synapses links retinal waves to activity-dependent refinement. *PLoS Biol* 5: e61.

Butts DA, Rokhsar DS. 2001. The information content of spontaneous retinal waves. *J Neurosci* 21(3): 961–973.

Cang J, Renteria RC, Kaneko M, Liu X, Copenhagen DR, Stryker MP. 2005. Development of precise maps in visual cortex requires patterned spontaneous activity in the retina. *Neuron* 48: 797–809.

Chalupa LM. 2007. A reassessment of the role of activity in the formation of eye-specific retinogeniculate projections. *Brain Res Brain Res Rev* 55(2): 228–236.

Chapman B. 2000. Necessity for afferent activity to maintain eye-specific segregation in ferret lateral geniculate nucleus. *Science* 287: 2479–2482.

Chapman B, Gödecke I. 2000. Cortical cell orientation selectivity fails to develop in the absence of ON-center retinal ganglion cell activity. *J Neurosci* 20: 1922–1930.

Chapman B, Stryker MP. 1993. Development of orientation selectivity in ferret visual cortex and effects of deprivation. *J Neurosci* 13: 5251–5262.

Chapman B, Stryker MP, Bonhoeffer T. 1996. Development of orientation preference maps in ferret primary visual cortex. *J Neurosci* 16: 6443–6453.

Cohen-Cory S. 2002. The developing synapse: construction and modulation of synaptic structures and circuits. *Science* 298: 770–776.

Cook PM, Prusky G, Ramoa AS. 1999. The role of spontaneous retinal activity before eye opening in the maturation of form and function in the retinogeniculate pathway of the ferret. *Vis Neurosci* 16: 491–501.

Crair MC. 1999. Neuronal activity during development: permissive or instructive? *Curr Opin Neurobiol* 9: 88–93.

Crair MC, Gillespie DC, Stryker MP. 1998. The role of visual experience in the development of columns in cat visual cortex. *Science* 279: 566–570.

Crair MC, Horton JC, Antonini A, Stryker MP. 2001. Emergence of ocular dominance columns in cat visual cortex by 2 weeks of age. *J Comp Neurol* 430: 235–249.

Crowley JC, Katz LC. 1999. Development of ocular dominance columns in the absence of retinal input. *Nat Neurosci* 2: 1125–1130.

Crowley JC, Katz LC. 2000. Early development of ocular dominance columns. *Science* 290: 1321–1324.

Crowley JC, Katz LC. 2002. Ocular dominance development revisited. *Curr Opin Neurobiol* 12: 104–109.

Demas J, Sagdullaev BT, Green E, Jaubert-Miazza L, McCall MA, Gregg RG, Wong RO, Guido W. 2006. Failure to maintain eye-specific segregation in nob, a mutant with abnormally patterned retinal activity. *Neuron* 50: 247–259.

Eglen SJ. 1999. The role of retinal waves and synaptic normalization in retinogeniculate development. *Philos Trans R Soc London B Biol Sci* 354: 497–506.

Feller MB. 2002. The role of nAChR-mediated spontaneous retinal activity in visual system development. *J Neurobiol* 53: 556–567.

Feller MB, Scanziani M. 2005. A precritical period for plasticity in visual cortex. *Curr Opin Neurobiol* 15: 94–100.

Feller MB, Wellis DP, Stellwagen D, Werblin FS, Shatz CJ. 1996. Requirement for cholinergic synaptic transmission in the propagation of spontaneous retinal waves. *Science* 272: 1182–1187.

Galli L, Maffei L. 1988. Spontaneous impulse activity of rat retinal ganglion cells in prenatal life. *Science* 242: 90–91.

Ghosh A, Shatz CJ. 1992. Pathfinding and target selection by developing geniculocortical axons. *J Neurosci* 12: 39–55.

Godement P, Salaun J, Imbert M. 1984. Prenatal and postnatal development of retinogeniculate and retinocollicular projections in the mouse. *J Comp Neurol* 230: 552–575.

Hanganu IL, Ben-Ari Y, Khazipov R. 2006. Retinal waves trigger spindle bursts in the neonatal rat visual cortex. *J Neurosci* 26: 6728–6736.

Hebb DO. 1949. *The Organization of Behavior*. New York: Wiley.

Hevner RF. 2000. Development of connections in the human visual system during fetal mid-gestation: a DiI-tracing study. *J Neuropathol Exp Neurol* 59: 385–392.

Horton JC, Hocking DR. 1996. An adult-like pattern of ocular dominance columns in striate cortex of newborn monkeys prior to visual experience. *J Neurosci* 16: 1791–1807.

Huberman AD. 2007. Mechanisms of eye-specific visual circuit development. *Curr Opin Neurobiol* 17: 73–80.

Huberman AD, Dehay C, Berland M, Chalupa LM, Kennedy H. 2005. Early and rapid targeting of eye-specific axonal projections to the dorsal lateral geniculate nucleus in the fetal macaque. *J Neurosci* 25: 4014–4023.

Huberman AD, Feller MB, Chapman B. 2008. Mechanisms underlying development of visual maps and receptive fields. *Annu Rev Neurosci* 31: 479–509.

Huberman AD, Wang GY, Liets LC, Collins OA, Chapman B, Chalupa LM. 2003. Eye-specific retinogeniculate segregation independent of normal neuronal activity. *Science* 300: 994–998.

Jaubert-Miazza L, Green E, Lo FS, Bui K, Mills J, Guido W. 2005. Structural and functional composition of the developing retinogeniculate pathway in the mouse. *Vis Neurosci* 22: 661–676.

Katz LC, Shatz CJ. 1996. Synaptic activity and the construction of cortical circuits. *Science* 274: 1133–1138.

LeVay S, Stryker MP, Shatz CJ. 1978. Ocular dominance columns and their development in layer IV of the cat's visual cortex: a quantitative study. *J Comp Neurol* 179: 223–244.

LeVay S, Wiesel TN, Hubel DH. 1980. The development of ocular dominance columns in normal and visually deprived monkeys. *J Comp Neurol* 191: 1–51.

Li Y, Van Hooser SD, Mazurek M, White LE, Fitzpatrick D. 2008. Experience with moving visual stimuli drives the early development of cortical direction selectivity. *Nature* 456: 952–956.

Li Y, Fitzpatrick D, White LE. 2006. The development of direction selectivity in ferret visual cortex requires early visual experience. *Nat Neurosci* 9: 676–681.

Linden DC, Guillery RW, Cucchiaro J. 1981. The dorsal lateral geniculate nucleus of the normal ferret and its postnatal development. *J Comp Neurol* 203: 189–211.

Löwel S. 1994. Ocular dominance column development: strabismus changes the spacing of adjacent columns in cat visual cortex. *J Neurosci* 14: 7451–7468.

Maffei L, Galli-Resta L. 1990. Correlation in the discharges of neighboring rat retinal ganglion cells during prenatal life. *Proc Natl Acad Sci USA* 87: 2861–2864.

Meister M, Wong RO, Baylor DA, Shatz CJ. 1991. Synchronous bursts of action potentials in ganglion cells of the developing mammalian retina. *Science* 252: 939–943.

Muir-Robinson G, Hwang BJ, Feller MB. 2002. Retinogeniculate axons undergo eye-specific segregation in the absence of eye-specific layers. *J Neurosci* 22: 5259–5264.

Penn AA, Riquelme PA, Feller MB, Shatz CJ. 1998. Competition in retinogeniculate patterning driven by spontaneous activity. *Science* 279: 2108–2112.

Pfeiffenberger C, Cutforth T, Woods G, Yamada J, Renteria RC, Feldheim DA. 2005. Ephrin-As and neural activity are required for eye-specific patterning during retinogeniculate mapping. *Nat Neurosci* 8: 1022–1027.

Rakic P. 1976. Prenatal genesis of connections subserving ocular dominance in the rhesus monkey. *Nature* 261: 467–471.

Rossi FM, Pizzorusso T, Porciatti V, Marubio LM, Maffei L, Changeux JP. 2001. Requirement of the nicotinic acetyl-choline receptor beta 2 subunit for the anatomical and functional development of the visual system. *Proc Natl Acad Sci USA* 98: 6453–6458.

Ruthazer ES, Baker GE, Stryker MP. 1999. Development and organization of ocular dominance bands in primary visual cortex of the sable ferret. *J Comp Neurol* 407: 151–165.

Sengpiel F, Kind PC. 2002. The role of activity in development of the visual system. *Curr Biol* 12: R818–R826.

Shatz CJ. 1983. The prenatal development of the cat's retinogeniculate pathway. *J Neurosci* 3: 482–499.

Shatz CJ, Kirkwood PA. 1984. Prenatal development of functional connections in the cat's retinogeniculate pathway. *J Neurosci* 4: 1378–1397.

Shatz CJ, Lindström S, Wiesel TN. 1977. The distribution of afferents representing the right and left eyes in the cat's visual cortex. *Brain Res* 131(1): 103–116.

Shatz CJ, Stryker MP. 1988. Prenatal tetrodotoxin infusion blocks segregation of retinogeniculate afferents. *Science* 242: 87–89.

Speer CM, Mikula S, Huberman AD, Chapman B. 2010. The developmental remodeling of eye-specific afferents in the ferret dorsal lateral geniculate nucleus. *Anat Rec* 293: 1–24.

Sretavan DW, Shatz CJ, Stryker MP. 1988. Modification of retinal ganglion cell axon morphology by prenatal infusion of tetrodotoxin. *Nature* 336: 468–471.

Stellwagen D, Shatz CJ. 2002. An instructive role for retinal waves in the development of retinogeniculate connectivity. *Neuron* 33: 357–367.

Stryker MP, Harris WA. 1986. Binocular impulse blockade prevents the formation of ocular dominance columns in cat visual cortex. *J Neurosci* 6: 2117–2133.

Stryker MP, Strickland S. 1984. Physiological segregation of ocular dominance columns depends on the pattern of afferent electrical activity. *Invest Ophthal Vis Sci (Suppl.)* 25: 278.

Sun C, Speer CM, Wang G-Y, Chapman B, Chalupa LM. 2008. Epibatidine application in vitro blocks retinal waves without silencing all retinal ganglion cell action potentials in developing retina of the mouse and ferret. *J Neurophysiol* 100: 3253–3263.

Sur M, Angelucci A, Sharma J. 1999. Rewiring cortex: the role of patterned activity in development and plasticity of neocortical circuits. *J Neurobiol* 41: 33–43.

Torborg CL, Feller MB. 2005. Spontaneous patterned retinal activity and the refinement of retinal projections. *Prog Neurobiol* 76(4): 213–235.

Torborg CL, Hansen KA, Feller MB. 2005. High frequency, synchronized bursting drives eye-specific segregation of retinogeniculate projections. *Nat Neurosci* 8: 72–78.

Weliky M, Katz LC. 1997. Disruption of orientation tuning in visual cortex by artificially correlated neuronal activity. *Nature* 386: 680–685.

Weliky M, Katz LC. 1999. Correlational structure of spontaneous neuronal activity in the developing lateral geniculate nucleus in vivo. *Science* 285: 599–604.

Wiesel TN, Hubel DH. 1963. Effects of visual deprivation on morphology and physiology of cells in the cat's lateral geniculate body. *J Neurophysiol* 26: 978–993.

Wiesel TN, Hubel DH. 1965. Comparison of the effects of unilateral and bilateral eye closure on cortical unit responses in kittens. *J Neurophysiol* 28: 1029–1040.

White LE, Coppola DM, Fitzpatrick D. 2001. The contribution of sensory experience to the maturation of orientation selectivity in ferret visual cortex. *Nature* 411: 1049–1052.

Wong RO. 1999. Retinal waves and visual system development. *Annu Rev Neurosci* 22: 29–47.

Zhou ZJ. 1998. Direct participation of starburst amacrine cells in spontaneous rhythmic activities in the developing mammalian retina. *J Neurosci* 18: 4155–4165.

7 Determinants of Synaptic and Circuit Plasticity in the Cerebral Cortex: Implications for Neurodevelopmental Disorders

Nathan R. Wilson and Mriganka Sur

"Cortical plasticity" encompasses a broad set of mechanisms through which cortical circuits adapt their responsiveness to their history of input. In several brain systems, the field has now distilled robust regimes for examining and demonstrating plasticity at the circuit level. In recent years there has also been a rough consensus on cellular and signaling changes which can account for circuit plasticity. In contrast, the control signals that command adjustments in the circuit's "plasticity status" remain largely unknown, as do the specific cues that they monitor—candidate frameworks for these are emerging and are detailed below. A clear articulation of the phenomena, rules, and mechanisms that govern cortical plasticity during development is critical for understanding their misregulation in specific neurodevelopmental disorders. This far-reaching vision, that mechanisms of developmental plasticity can be used to reveal mechanisms of brain disorders and even treat them, owes much to the work and scientific insights of Lamberto Maffei, whom this volume honors.

The Visual Cortex as a Model System for Experience-Dependent Plasticity

Many critical observations on plasticity in the nervous system have been made in the visual cortex. Wiesel and Hubel (1963) had the original insight that the two eyes represent distinct input sources which can be driven differentially with light to evaluate how a circuit responds over time. In a sense, it remains the most straightforward junction for probing the complex circuitry of the cerebral cortex with well-characterized sensory stimuli. More recently, progress in detailing the phenomena and mechanisms of cortical plasticity has been augmented through transgenic mice, which has allowed for the elucidation of a growing network of proteins and pathways, isolated to specific regions and distinct cell types.

Another useful property of the visual cortex for studies of plasticity is the enormous dynamic range of plasticity that it expresses during the course of development and with experience (Katz and Callaway, 1992). Over the life span of cortical circuits, synaptic refinement leads to an increase in organization and correlated activity, while the malleability of the circuit is decreased concomitantly. Through cell-specific rules of plasticity (Desai et al., 2002), a large number of weak synapses with motile spines (the sites of excitatory synapses on cortical neurons) are sculpted into a refined number of strong synapses with stable spines (Majewska and Sur, 2003; Oray et al., 2004). As excitatory transmission is consolidated, it contributes to the release of feedback signals such as brain-derived neurotrophic factor (BDNF; Bonhoeffer, 1996), which eventually attains a critical level for the activation of inhibitory signaling (Buonomano and Merzenich, 1998). This onset of inhibition initiates a brief time frame of exceptional plasticity known as the "critical period" in which the pattern of cortical input is particularly important for organizing and strengthening a functional architecture for future processing (Hensch, 2004). As the synaptic architecture underlying this organization stabilizes, it comes to resist further change (Abraham and Bear, 1996; Bi and Poo, 1998), the specific balance of excitation and inhibition becomes important for delimiting plasticity (Artola and Singer, 1987; Maya Vetencourt et al., 2008), and a network of extracellular matrix proteins begins to entangle the entire circuit to provide an additional measure of circuit stability (Berardi et al., 2004).

Parameterizing Cortical Plasticity

Across development, circuit plasticity itself is modulated by the level of input drive, which stimulates key molecular pathways to reconfigure circuit properties. Received activity is coupled to downstream and intercellular molecular events, and this allows activity at input locations to impact circuit function and plasticity at multiple loci. Here we will review several "feedforward" mechanisms that can initiate circuit change, together with a host of emerging "feedback" network processes that respond to those changes.

Feedforward Synaptic Plasticity

Feedforward changes are initiatory events where input activity to a circuit triggers direct synaptic changes across its synapses, with subsequent reverberatory consequences elsewhere in the circuit. A cardinal example of a feedforward change is long-term potentiation (LTP), in which a pattern of robust input activity triggers the long-term strengthening of that same input to further stabilize its postsynaptic influence over the circuit (Bliss et al., 2003). LTP also provides a link between synaptic changes and the formation and maintenance of cortical maps (Buonomano and Merzenich, 1998). Its sister process is long-term depression (LTD), in which weak activity across a synapse leads to the long-term weakening of that synapse, and loss of influence over the circuit. LTD has also been advanced as a basis for cortical phenomena such as ocular dominance plasticity (Smith et al., 2009). LTP and LTD are further complemented by mechanisms such as spike-timing dependent plasticity, which trigger synaptic plasticity based on how well matched the timing of an input is to firing of the postsynaptic cell (and circuit) on which it impinges (Song and Abbott, 2001; Dan and Poo, 2006). Together these canonical mechanisms lay a foundation for focal circuit changes upon and between cells that depend only on the magnitude and timing of the input itself, independent of the other inputs in the circuit. However, as we will see below, inputs across the cortical circuit are intimately connected via multiple pathways and time courses which add richness to a simple "push–pull" dissection of cortical plasticity phenomena.

Molecular Pathways of Feedforward Plasticity

Modifications to the strengths of excitatory synapses are likely to be enacted via postsynaptic changes in AMPA receptor number and conductance (Malenka and Bear, 2004), and/or presynaptic changes in probability of release (Bolshakov and Siegelbaum, 1995) and vesicular glutamate content (Edwards, 2007). Input strength can also be adjusted via synaptogenesis and synaptic elimination. However, the degree to which such plasticity occurs is gated by a host of molecular pathways that determine the "plasticity status" of the synapse, cell, and circuit.

The NR2B/NR2A Switch   Plasticity is prominently gated by the activation of N-methyl-D-aspartate (NMDA) receptors, which respond to excitatory synaptic transmission by enabling calcium flux into the target synapse and its neuron, with more calcium triggering more plasticity and rearrangement. However, the receptor's capacity to drive plasticity depends on its subunit composition. Some receptors are built from "NR2B" subunits, which enable a high calcium permeability and thus enhanced plasticity, and some are built from "NR2A" subunits, which have a reduced calcium flux (Flint et al., 1997). The ratio of NR2B/NR2A receptors in the synapse and the neuron thus has a pivotal effect on the overall calcium flux upon synaptic activation and determines the capacity for plasticity in response to arriving input.

Here again, a crucial determinant of plasticity is itself regulated by the activity level of the circuit. As animals are exposed to visual experience, the NR2B/NR2A ratio declines (Quinlan et al., 1999), thus reducing the capacity for further plasticity, whereas placing animals in the dark for extended periods recovers the NR2B/NR2A ratio (Chen and Bear, 2007), thereby restoring the capacity for plasticity. Thus, the molecular composition of NMDA receptors is a critical determinant of calcium-mediated cellular plasticity that is directly responsive to activity levels.

Calcium-Calmodulin Kinase II Signaling   Calcium entry at synaptic sites upon activation leads to eventual synaptic change, prominently via calcium-calmodulin kinase II (CaMKII), which is extraordinarily abundant and accounts for 1% to 2% of the total protein found in neurons (Fink and Meyer, 2002). CaMKII is spatially positioned in the synaptic spine to directly sense NMDA-mediated calcium fluxes (Bayer et al., 2001) and respond by mobilizing additional AMPA receptors to synapses (Hayashi et al., 2000). Moreover, its binding and activation is directly specified by the NR2B/NR2A subunit composition described above (Barria and Malinow, 2005). α-CaMKII has been shown to be critical for cortical LTP, as well as for the consolidation of cortical memory traces (Frankland et al., 2001). It also has the interesting property of autophosphorylation, which allows it to undergo long-term modification, and has led to the proposal that it could provide a sort of "molecular memory" of synaptic activity (Lisman, 1994): persistently active CaMKII can indeed bring about LTP effects (Pettit et al., 1994). Interestingly, CaMKII seems be critical for synaptic plasticity yet without impacting large-scale cortical architecture, as its mutations prevent the consolidation of sensory plasticity without disrupting the topography of sensory cortex (Glazewski et al., 1996; Gordon et al., 1996).

The ERK/MAPK Pathway   Stimulation at the synaptic and cellular level drives the Raf/MEK/ ERK pathway, which also serves to promote synapse stabilization (Sweatt, 2001). A direct link has been established between its downstream effector, extracellular signal-regulated kinase 1,2 (ERK, also called p42/44 mitogen-activated protein kinase) and insertion of AMPA receptors into activated synapses (Zhu et al., 2002). The degree of ERK activation also determines the magnitude of LTP in visual cortex and is required for ocular dominance plasticity (Di Cristo et al., 2001). As with several of the plasticity cues described above, the ERK pathway is responsive to activity levels (Fiore et al., 1993), as well as NMDA receptor-mediated calcium levels (Hardingham et al., 2001), and plasticity cues such as BDNF (Patterson et al., 2001). Its downstream targets include critical plasticity triggers such as cyclic AMP response element binding protein (CREB; Impey et al., 1998) and Arc (Ying et al., 2002), and transcription factors that regulate the expression of activity-dependent immediate early genes (Xia et al., 1996). Activity within the ERK pathway therefore offers a number of channels through which NMDA activation can stimulate cell-wide changes in synaptic function, thus promoting coherent integration of inputs between cells and networks (Thomas and Huganir, 2004).

The PI3K/Akt/mTOR Pathway   Along with the now-canonical plasticity pathways listed above, increasing attention has been paid to another protein kinase called mammalian target of rapamycin (mTOR). It is driven by both synaptic stimulation (Cammalleri et al., 2003) and PI3K/ Akt activation (Jaworski and Sheng, 2006), which is known to strengthen synapses by delivering PSD-95 (a critical post-synaptic density protein) into dendrites (Yoshii and Constantine-Paton, 2007). Functionally, increased mTOR activity has been linked to larger and fewer spines with larger AMPA currents (Tavazoie et al., 2005) and seems to serve to facilitate and accentuate LTP (Ehninger et al., 2008b; Hoeffer et al., 2008). Consequently, mTOR signaling seems well placed for stimulating growth, elevating excitatory drive, and forging stronger and more stable synaptic circuits.

Feedback/Homeostatic Plasticity

When a change is exerted at one or more synaptic pathways via the mechanisms described above, a concurrent group of normative processes may arise to rebalance the net function of the circuit. These mechanisms are considered "homeostatic" or "feedback" events because they appear aimed at restoring the net excitability of the circuit back toward its original state prior to plasticity induction (Turrigiano and Nelson, 2000; Davis and Bezprozvanny, 2001).

Sites of Feedback Regulation

Feedback processes that rebalance the strength of excitatory synapses have been identified which operate postsynaptically, via AMPA receptor number and conductance (Turrigiano, 2008), and presynaptically, via probability of release (Murthy et al., 2001) and vesicular glutamate content (Wilson et al., 2005), among others. An input may also be renormalized by scaling its number of connections. Feedback processes that might rebalance at a network level beyond the excitatory synapse include modifications to inhibitory synapses (Maffei et al., 2006), homeostatic modifications to a cell's intrinsic excitability (Pratt and Aizenman, 2007), and changes to the excitatory drive onto inhibitory neurons (Wilson et al., 2007). Feedback regulation within cortical circuits has even been demonstrated to extend from one sensory modality to another (Goel et al., 2006).

Positive Feedback Regulation via TNF-Alpha

What are the signals that control feedback regulation? One molecule that has been shown to be both necessary and sufficient for the activity-dependent scaling up of AMPA receptor function is the tumor necrosis factor TNF-alpha (Stellwagen and Malenka, 2006). Still more recently, the scaling up of open-eye responses following light deprivation in visual cortex was shown to require TNF-alpha (Kaneko et al., 2008). A particularly intriguing possibility is that the excitatory/inhibitory balance is coordinated via a few or even a single molecular control point. Indeed, increases to TNF-alpha signaling have been shown to coordinately increase AMPA receptor surface expression while simultaneously decreasing GABA receptor surface expression (Stellwagen et al., 2005).

Negative Feedback Regulation via CDK5 and Arc

What is responsible for the scaling down of excitability? One pathway that is emerging for rebalancing high levels of activity is CDK5/Polo-like kinase 2 (Plk2; Seeburg et al., 2008). Another likely possibility is the immediate-early gene Arc, the expression of which is regulated by activity, triggers AMPA receptor endocytosis (Chowdhury et al., 2006) and is required for synaptic scaling (Shepherd et al., 2005). Perhaps through its known homeostatic role, Arc has been found to be important for organizing representations in visual cortex (Wang et al., 2006) and has recently been found to underpin the loss of cortical responses that occurs during ocular dominance plasticity (McCurry et al., 2010). The scaling down of input strength mediated by Arc could also lead to the functional elimination of extraneous inputs during cortical refinement; indeed, mice that lack Arc exhibit visual cortical neurons that are less precisely tuned (Wang et al., 2006).

Inhibition as a Plasticity Gate

Inhibitory neurons are widespread in the cortex and may be even more diverse in morphology and function than excitatory neurons (Markram et al., 2004). The balance of excitation and inhibition appears to be dynamically maintained at the level of dendritic branches (Liu, 2004) and neurons (Cline, 2005). In cortical dynamics, stimuli that elicit maximal excitation to neurons also elicit maximal inhibition at those same neurons (Marino et al., 2005; Okun and Lampl, 2008), ensuring that functional responses always result from a precise balance of excitatory and inhibitory drive.

In addition to balancing the firing rates of circuits, inhibition may have a complementary role in controlling the plasticity of circuits. Preventing the activation of inhibition prevents the critical period of plasticity from happening until inhibition is enabled (Hensch et al., 1998). Conversely, augmenting inhibitory signaling prematurely launches the critical period prematurely (Iwai et al., 2003). Once inhibition is developed to adult levels, however, it may become an obstacle to cortical plasticity. Inhibition in the cortex has long been claimed to gate adult LTP, wherein robust LTP was only observable when suppressing inhibition pharmacologically with bicuculline (Artola and Singer, 1987). In the adult visual system of the rat, ocular dominance plasticity is greatly reduced compared to juvenile levels but can be restored to juvenile levels by suppressing inhibition with the antidepressant fluoxetine (Maya Vetencourt et al., 2008).

The Role of Neurotrophins

Neurotrophins such as BDNF have emerged as an ideal candidate for communicating the status of activity across the circuit to regulate plasticity. Neuronal activity has a positive feedback relationship with the transcription of the BDNF gene, the transport of its protein into dendrites, and its secretion at synapses (Lu, 2003). At the cellular level, BDNF is known to support growth and strengthening of synapses during development (Cellerino and Maffei, 1996) and is critical for the proper establishment of excitatory synaptic transmission (Schuman, 1999).

BDNF also seems to play an instructive role in a host of processes relevant to circuit development. BDNF triggers the maturation of inhibition that initiates the critical period as described above (Huang et al., 1999), and expressing it prematurely accelerates the timing of the critical period (Hanover et al., 1999). BDNF also triggers the release of tPA (Fiumelli et al., 1999), which as described below is important for liberating structural plasticity. In homeostatic plasticity, BDNF has been identified as a signal that triggers the reactive scaling of excitatory and inhibitory synapses to offset recent elevations in activity levels (Rutherford et al., 1998).

Extraneuronal Influences: Astrocytes and Perineuronal Nets

Astrocytes constitute more than half of all cortical cells (Nedergaard et al., 2003) and have now been shown to exhibit functional responses to stimuli and organize into maps that are just as exquisitely defined as those of the neurons (Schummers et al., 2008). Astrocytes receive synaptic inputs, express neurotransmitter receptors, and can directly modulate the reliability of neuronal synapses (Perea and Araque, 2007). Furthermore, many of the factors critical for circuit plasticity may be stored by astrocytes and released onto neurons in response to functional events. For example, the TNF alpha described above as a potentially pivotal homeostatic signal is expressed in and released by astrocytes (Stellwagen and Malenka, 2006).

Extraneuronal circuit changes are also reinforced by "perineuronal nets" (PNNs), which are lattice-like structures, comprised of chondroitin-sulfate proteoglycans (CSPGs) and other extra-cellular components, that condense and entangle cortical cells and synapses. These lattices restrict further movement and growth and provide an obstacle to structural and functional plasticity (Berardi et al., 2004). Compounds that degrade CSPGs, such as chondroitinase ABC, have been shown to restore ocular dominance plasticity to adult mice (Pizzorusso et al., 2002). Similarly, the extracellular protease tissue-type plasminogen activator (tPA), which also target CSPGs, has been shown to be most highly expressed at periods of maximal plasticity (Mataga et al., 2004) and play a key permissive role in enabling circuit remodeling during ocular dominance plasticity (Muller and Griesinger, 1998; Mataga et al., 2002; Oray et al., 2004). Recently, it has been shown that fear memories in adult mice, which are typically permanent features that are resilient to erasure, can be made susceptible to erasure via degradation of PNNs (Gogolla et al., 2009). These studies suggest that PNNs provide a form of "hard wiring" that can be dissolved or strengthened in order to modulate circuit flexibility.

Together, these findings demonstrate a rich array of mechanisms by which changes in input activity lead to changes in the structure and function of synapses, cells, and circuits of the cortex. Some of these same mechanisms come into play during disorders of brain development—which can thus be understood as disorders of cortical plasticity.

Disorders of Brain Development

Rett Syndrome

Rett syndrome (RTT) is a subset of autism and an X-linked neurological disorder affecting 1 in every 10,000–15,000 live births (Chahrour and Zoghbi, 2007). Unlike many neurodevelopmental disorders, the basis of RTT is straightforward and in approximately 90% of patients suffering from RTT has been traced to a single gene coding for methyl CpG-binding protein 2 (*MeCP2*; Amir et al., 1999; Guy et al., 2001). Combining a molecular understanding of RTT with a circuit perspective that links activity levels to plasticity could help pave the way for effective treatments (Zoghbi, 2003).

RTT is characterized by a profound reduction in cortical circuit activity (Dani et al., 2005), owing to a negative tilt in the balance of excitatory and inhibitory transmission (Dani et al., 2005; Chao et al., 2007; Tropea et al., 2009). Neurons are smaller (Chen et al., 2001), dendrites exhibit reduced elaboration (Armstrong et al., 1998; Kishi and Macklis, 2004), and spine density is reduced in key areas (Chao et al., 2007; Tropea et al., 2009). Plasticity, meanwhile, remains in an immature state, with impairments to LTP (Moretti and Zoghbi, 2006), and ocular domi-nance plasticity that aberrantly persist into adulthood (Tropea et al., 2009).

Viewed through this lens, RTT seems to arise from a failure of brain circuitry to mature or sustain a mature phenotype (Magee and Johnston, 1997; Moretti and Zoghbi, 2006). This failure has been shown to be reversible by driving pathways that promote circuit maturation and stabi-lization such as BDNF (Guy et al., 2007), which stimulates synaptic strengthening via PI3K/

pAkt/PSD-95 and MAPK signaling (Carvalho et al., 2008). A similar stimulus to circuit maturation may also be derived through the systemic delivery of other neurotrophic factors such as insulin-like growth factor 1 (Tropea et al., 2009) that are capable of crossing the blood-brain barrier (Aberg et al., 2000; Lopez-Lopez et al., 2004; Jaworski et al., 2005) and which stimulate these same pathways (Zheng and Quirion, 2004; Tropea et al., 2006). Thus, RTT offers a prime example for how an understanding of circuit plasticity may aid in elucidating pathways for targeted intervention.

Tuberous Sclerosis

Tuberous sclerosis (TSC) is another neurodevelopmental disorder associated with cognitive impairment, seizures, perseverative behavior, and other disabilities similar to autism (Ehninger et al., 2008a). It has been linked to specific heterozygous mutations in 2 genes—*TSC1* and *TSC2*. TSC may offer an excellent model for how too much synaptic potentiation can lead to cortical rigidity. Disruption of *TSC1/2* brings about a fundamental shift in spine morphology—converting numerous small spines into fewer large spines, with stronger excitatory transmission (Tavazoie et al., 2005). A likely reason for this is that TSC results in enhanced mTOR signaling (Ehninger et al., 2008a; Meikle et al., 2008), which lowers the threshold for plasticity and makes long-lasting LTP more likely to occur, thus pathologically stabilizing synaptic pathways (Hoeffer et al., 2008). Compatible with this interpretation, application of mTOR inhibitors in a mouse model of TSC suppresses seizures, rescues the aberrantly stable synaptic potentiation, and reverses neurocognitive deficits (Ehninger et al., 2008b).

Fragile X

Fragile X is a condition of moderate to severe mental retardation (Loesch et al., 2002) that has been methodically linked to pathologies in cortical circuits (Bear, 2005). In mouse models of the disorder, circuits are characterized by an increased spine density (Grossman et al., 2006), comprised of weaker spines (Hinton et al., 1991; Irwin et al., 2001) with fewer AMPA receptors (Li et al., 2002) that are functionally "hyperplastic" in terms of synaptic changes (Bear et al., 2004) and cortical plasticity (Dolen et al., 2007). According to one hypothesis, increased translation of fragile X mental retardation protein (FMRP) underlies enhanced LTD in the mouse model for the disorder, and blockade of metabotropic glutamate receptors would act as a corrective. Indeed, a genetic rescue of multiple phenotypes of fragile X in the mouse model demonstrates the feasibility of this hypothesis (Dolen et al., 2007).

Conclusion and Future Directions

The development of effective interventions for disorders of cortical plasticity will require tools for rapidly assessing the plasticity status of a circuit in a manner that goes beyond single synapse measures to take into account the host of network influences described above. Promisingly, new imaging methods are allowing more subtle changes in circuit function to be measured optically, including in the intact animal (Grinvald and Hildesheim, 2004; Pologruto et al., 2004; Schummers et al., 2008). Another promising tool is the advent of optical probes of plasticity (Wang et al., 2006; Hayashi et al., 2009), which offer the potential of reporting either the plasticity event or the plasticity status of cells within a circuit. Assays are also becoming available that can detect changes in protein levels in response to specific activity paradigms or plasticity and connect those into functional pathways that might drive or be driven by the plasticity (Tropea et al., 2006). Finally, advances in virally mediated gene transfer and optogenetics continue to provide increasingly pinpointed experimental control over specific cells' genetic makeup and electrical input (Zhang et al., 2007).

As these tools are brought into play, they are revealing that plasticity is not merely a synaptic phenomenon but one that results from the coordinated interplay of excitatory, inhibitory, and glial cells, operating in tandem via feedforward and feedback mechanisms to regulate the plasticity tone of the circuit. Perhaps the greatest challenge in the coming years will be to devise methods for selectively understanding these network components to comprehend how they give rise to the choreographed processes of development and disease.

References

Aberg MA, Aberg ND, Hedbacker H, Oscarsson J, Eriksson PS. 2000. Peripheral infusion of IGF-I selectively induces neurogenesis in the adult rat hippocampus. *J Neurosci* 20: 2896–2903.

Abraham WC, Bear MF. 1996. Metaplasticity: the plasticity of synaptic plasticity. *Trends Neurosci* 19: 126–130.

Amir RE, Van den Veyver IB, Wan M, Tran CQ, Francke U, Zoghbi HY. 1999. Rett syndrome is caused by mutations in X-linked MECP2, encoding methyl-CpG-binding protein 2. *Nat Genet* 23: 185–188.

Armstrong DD, Dunn K, Antalffy B. 1998. Decreased dendritic branching in frontal, motor and limbic cortex in Rett syndrome compared with trisomy 21. *J Neuropathol Exp Neurol* 57: 1013–1017.

Artola A, Singer W. 1987. Long-term potentiation and NMDA receptors in rat visual cortex. *Nature* 330: 649–652.

Barria A, Malinow R. 2005. NMDA receptor subunit composition controls synaptic plasticity by regulating binding to CaMKII. *Neuron* 48: 289–301.

Bayer KU, De Koninck P, Leonard AS, Hell JW, Schulman H. 2001. Interaction with the NMDA receptor locks CaMKII in an active conformation. *Nature* 411: 801–805.

Bear MF. 2005. Therapeutic implications of the mGluR theory of fragile X mental retardation. *Genes Brain Behav* 4: 393–398.

Bear MF, Huber KM, Warren ST. 2004. The mGluR theory of fragile X mental retardation. *Trends Neurosci* 27: 370–377.

Berardi N, Pizzorusso T, Maffei L. 2004. Extracellular matrix and visual cortical plasticity: freeing the synapse. *Neuron* 44: 905–908.

Bi GQ, Poo MM. 1998. Synaptic modifications in cultured hippocampal neurons: dependence on spike timing, synaptic strength, and postsynaptic cell type. *J Neurosci* 18: 10464–10472.

Bliss TV, Collingridge GL, Morris RG. 2003. Introduction. Long-term potentiation and structure of the issue. *Philos Trans R Soc Lond B Biol Sci* 358: 607–611.

Bolshakov VY, Siegelbaum SA. 1995. Regulation of hippocampal transmitter release during development and long-term potentiation. *Science* 269: 1730–1734.

Bonhoeffer T. 1996. Neurotrophins and activity-dependent development of the neocortex. *Curr Opin Neurobiol* 6: 119–126.

Buonomano DV, Merzenich MM. 1998. Cortical plasticity: from synapses to maps. *Annu Rev Neurosci* 21: 149–186.

Cammalleri M, Lutjens R, Berton F, King AR, Simpson C, Francesconi W, Sanna PP. 2003. Time-restricted role for dendritic activation of the mTOR-p70S6K pathway in the induction of late-phase long-term potentiation in the CA1. *Proc Natl Acad Sci USA* 100: 14368–14373.

Carvalho AL, Caldeira MV, Santos SD, Duarte CB. 2008. Role of the brain-derived neurotrophic factor at glutamatergic synapses. *Br J Pharmacol* 153 (Suppl. 1): S310–324.

Cellerino A, Maffei L. 1996. The action of neurotrophins in the development and plasticity of the visual cortex. *Prog Neurobiol* 49(1): 53–71.

Chahrour M, Zoghbi HY. 2007. The story of Rett syndrome: from clinic to neurobiology. *Neuron* 56: 422–437.

Chao HT, Zoghbi HY, Rosenmund C. 2007. MeCP2 controls excitatory synaptic strength by regulating glutamatergic synapse number. *Neuron* 56: 58–65.

Chen RZ, Akbarian S, Tudor M, Jaenisch R. 2001. Deficiency of methyl-CpG binding protein-2 in CNS neurons results in a Rett-like phenotype in mice. *Nat Genet* 27: 327–331.

Chen WS, Bear MF. 2007. Activity-dependent regulation of NR2B translation contributes to metaplasticity in mouse visual cortex. *Neuropharmacology* 52(1): 200–214.

Chowdhury S, Shepherd JD, Okuno H, Lyford G, Petralia RS, Plath N, Kuhl D, Huganir RL, Worley PF. 2006. Arc/Arg3.1 interacts with the endocytic machinery to regulate AMPA receptor trafficking. *Neuron* 52: 445–459.

Cline H. 2005. Synaptogenesis: a balancing act between excitation and inhibition. *Curr Biol* 15: R203–R205.

Dan Y, Poo MM. 2006. Spike timing-dependent plasticity: from synapse to perception. *Physiol Rev* 86: 1033–1048.

Dani VS, Chang Q, Maffei A, Turrigiano GG, Jaenisch R, Nelson SB. 2005. Reduced cortical activity due to a shift in the balance between excitation and inhibition in a mouse model of Rett syndrome. *Proc Natl Acad Sci USA* 102: 12560–12565.

Davis GW, Bezprozvanny I. 2001. Maintaining the stability of neural function: a homeostatic hypothesis. *Annu Rev Physiol* 63: 847–869.

Desai NS, Cudmore RH, Nelson SB, Turrigiano GG. 2002. Critical periods for experience-dependent synaptic scaling in visual cortex. *Nat Neurosci* 5: 783–789.

Di Cristo G, Berardi N, Cancedda L, Pizzorusso T, Putignano E, Ratto GM, Maffei L. 2001. Requirement of ERK activation for visual cortical plasticity. *Science* 292: 2337–2340.

Dolen G, Osterweil E, Rao BS, Smith GB, Auerbach BD, Chattarji S, Bear MF. 2007. Correction of fragile X syndrome in mice. *Neuron* 56: 955–962.

Edwards RH. 2007. The neurotransmitter cycle and quantal size. *Neuron* 55: 835–858.

Ehninger D, Li W, Fox K, Stryker MP, Silva AJ. 2008a. Reversing neurodevelopmental disorders in adults. *Neuron* 60: 950–960.

Ehninger D, Han S, Shilyansky C, Zhou Y, Li W, Kwiatkowski DJ, Ramesh V, Silva AJ. 2008b. Reversal of learning deficits in a Tsc2+/- mouse model of tuberous sclerosis. *Nat Med* 14: 843–848.

Fink CC, Meyer T. 2002. Molecular mechanisms of CaMKII activation in neuronal plasticity. *Curr Opin Neurobiol* 12: 293–299.

Fiore RS, Murphy TH, Sanghera JS, Pelech SL, Baraban JM. 1993. Activation of p42 mitogen-activated protein kinase by glutamate receptor stimulation in rat primary cortical cultures. *J Neurochem* 61: 1626–1633.

Fiumelli H, Jabaudon D, Magistretti PJ, Martin JL. 1999. BDNF stimulates expression, activity and release of tissue-type plasminogen activator in mouse cortical neurons. *Eur J Neurosci* 11: 1639–1646.

Flint AC, Maisch US, Weishaupt JH, Kriegstein AR, Monyer H. 1997. NR2A subunit expression shortens NMDA receptor synaptic currents in developing neocortex. *J Neurosci* 17: 2469–2476.

Frankland PW, O'Brien C, Ohno M, Kirkwood A, Silva AJ. 2001. Alpha-CaMKII-dependent plasticity in the cortex is required for permanent memory. *Nature* 411: 309–313.

Glazewski S, Chen CM, Silva A, Fox K. 1996. Requirement for alpha-CaMKII in experience-dependent plasticity of the barrel cortex. *Science* 272: 421–423.

Goel A, Jiang B, Xu LW, Song L, Kirkwood A, Lee HK. 2006. Cross-modal regulation of synaptic AMPA receptors in primary sensory cortices by visual experience. *Nat Neurosci* 9: 1001–1003.

Gogolla N, Caroni P, Luthi A, Herry C. 2009. Perineuronal nets protect fear memories from erasure. *Science* 325: 1258–1261.

Gordon JA, Cioffi D, Silva AJ, Stryker MP. 1996. Deficient plasticity in the primary visual cortex of alpha-calcium/calmodulin-dependent protein kinase II mutant mice. *Neuron* 17: 491–499.

Grinvald A, Hildesheim R. 2004. VSDI: a new era in functional imaging of cortical dynamics. *Nat Rev Neurosci* 5: 874–885.

Grossman AW, Aldridge GM, Weiler IJ, Greenough WT. 2006. Local protein synthesis and spine morphogenesis: fragile X syndrome and beyond. *J Neurosci* 26: 7151–7155.

Guy J, Hendrich B, Holmes M, Martin JE, Bird A. 2001. A mouse Mecp2-null mutation causes neurological symptoms that mimic Rett syndrome. *Nat Genet* 27: 322–326.

Guy J, Gan J, Selfridge J, Cobb S, Bird A. 2007. Reversal of neurological defects in a mouse model of Rett syndrome. *Science* 315: 1143–1147.

Hanover JL, Huang ZJ, Tonegawa S, Stryker MP. 1999. Brain-derived neurotrophic factor overexpression induces precocious critical period in mouse visual cortex. *J Neurosci* 19: RC40.

Hardingham GE, Arnold FJ, Bading H. 2001. A calcium microdomain near NMDA receptors: on switch for ERK-dependent synapse-to-nucleus communication. *Nat Neurosci* 4: 565–566.

Hayashi Y, Shi SH, Esteban JA, Piccini A, Poncer JC, Malinow R. 2000. Driving AMPA receptors into synapses by LTP and CaMKII: requirement for GluR1 and PDZ domain interaction. *Science* 287: 2262–2267.

Hayashi Y, Mower AF, Kwok S, Yu H, Majewska A, Okamoto K, Sur M. 2009. Eye domain-specific synaptic CaMKII activation during ocular dominance plasticity in vivo. In: *Society for Neuroscience Abstracts*, p. 167.116/V135. Annual Meeting: Chicago.

Hensch TK. 2004. Critical period regulation. *Annu Rev Neurosci* 27: 549–579.

Hensch TK, Fagiolini M, Mataga N, Stryker MP, Baekkeskov S, Kash SF. 1998. Local GABA circuit control of experience-dependent plasticity in developing visual cortex. *Science* 282: 1504–1508.

Hinton VJ, Brown WT, Wisniewski K, Rudelli RD. 1991. Analysis of neocortex in three males with the fragile X syndrome. *Am J Med Genet* 41: 289–294.

Hoeffer CA, Tang W, Wong H, Santillan A, Patterson RJ, Martinez LA, Tejada-Simon MV, Paylor R, Hamilton SL, Klann E. 2008. Removal of FKBP12 enhances mTOR-Raptor interactions, LTP, memory, and perseverative/repetitive behavior. *Neuron* 60: 832–845.

Huang ZJ, Kirkwood A, Pizzorusso T, Porciatti V, Morales B, Bear MF, Maffei L, Tonegawa S. 1999. BDNF regulates the maturation of inhibition and the critical period of plasticity in mouse visual cortex. *Cell* 98: 739–755.

Impey S, Obrietan K, Wong ST, Poser S, Yano S, Wayman G, Deloulme JC, Chan G, Storm DR. 1998. Cross talk between ERK and PKA is required for Ca2+ stimulation of CREB-dependent transcription and ERK nuclear translocation. *Neuron* 21: 869–883.

Irwin SA, Patel B, Idupulapati M, Harris JB, Crisostomo RA, Larsen BP, Kooy F, et al. 2001. Abnormal dendritic spine characteristics in the temporal and visual cortices of patients with fragile-X syndrome: a quantitative examination. *Am J Med Genet* 98: 161–167.

Iwai Y, Fagiolini M, Obata K, Hensch TK. 2003. Rapid critical period induction by tonic inhibition in visual cortex. *J Neurosci* 23: 6695–6702.

Jaworski J, Sheng M. 2006. The growing role of mTOR in neuronal development and plasticity. *Mol Neurobiol* 34: 205–219.

Jaworski J, Spangler S, Seeburg DP, Hoogenraad CC, Sheng M. 2005. Control of dendritic arborization by the phosphoinositide-3′-kinase-Akt-mammalian target of rapamycin pathway. *J Neurosci* 25: 11300–11312.

Kaneko M, Stellwagen D, Malenka RC, Stryker MP. 2008. Tumor necrosis factor-alpha mediates one component of competitive, experience-dependent plasticity in developing visual cortex. *Neuron* 58: 673–680.

Katz LC, Callaway EM. 1992. Development of local circuits in mammalian visual cortex. *Annu Rev Neurosci* 15: 31–56.

Kishi N, Macklis JD. 2004. MECP2 is progressively expressed in post-migratory neurons and is involved in neuronal maturation rather than cell fate decisions. *Mol Cell Neurosci* 27: 306–321.

Li J, Pelletier MR, Perez Velazquez JL, Carlen PL. 2002. Reduced cortical synaptic plasticity and GluR1 expression associated with fragile X mental retardation protein deficiency. *Mol Cell Neurosci* 19: 138–151.

Lisman J. 1994. The CaM kinase II hypothesis for the storage of synaptic memory. *Trends Neurosci* 17: 406–412.

Liu G. 2004. Local structural balance and functional interaction of excitatory and inhibitory synapses in hippocampal dendrites. *Nat Neurosci* 7: 373–379.

Loesch DZ, Huggins RM, Bui QM, Epstein JL, Taylor AK, Hagerman RJ. 2002. Effect of the deficits of fragile X mental retardation protein on cognitive status of fragile X males and females assessed by robust pedigree analysis. *J Dev Behav Pediatr* 23: 416–423.

Lopez-Lopez C, LeRoith D, Torres-Aleman I. 2004. Insulin-like growth factor I is required for vessel remodeling in the adult brain. *Proc Natl Acad Sci USA* 101: 9833–9838.

Lu B. 2003. BDNF and activity-dependent synaptic modulation. *Learn Mem* 10: 86–98.

Maffei A, Nataraj K, Nelson SB, Turrigiano GG. 2006. Potentiation of cortical inhibition by visual deprivation. *Nature* 443: 81–84.

Magee JC, Johnston D. 1997. A synaptically controlled, associative signal for Hebbian plasticity in hippocampal neurons. *Science* 275: 209–213.

Majewska A, Sur M. 2003. Motility of dendritic spines in visual cortex in vivo: changes during the critical period and effects of visual deprivation. *Proc Natl Acad Sci USA* 100: 16024–16029.

Malenka RC, Bear MF. 2004. LTP and LTD: an embarrassment of riches. *Neuron* 44: 5–21.

Marino J, Schummers J, Lyon DC, Schwabe L, Beck O, Wiesing P, Obermayer K, Sur M. 2005. Invariant computations in local cortical networks with balanced excitation and inhibition. *Nat Neurosci* 8: 194–201.

Markram H, Toledo-Rodriguez M, Wang Y, Gupta A, Silberberg G, Wu C. 2004. Interneurons of the neocortical inhibitory system. *Nat Rev Neurosci* 5: 793–807.

Mataga N, Nagai N, Hensch TK. 2002. Permissive proteolytic activity for visual cortical plasticity. *Proc Natl Acad Sci USA* 99: 7717–7721.

Mataga N, Mizuguchi Y, Hensch TK. 2004. Experience-dependent pruning of dendritic spines in visual cortex by tissue plasminogen activator. *Neuron* 44: 1031–1041.

Maya Vetencourt JF, Sale A, Viegi A, Baroncelli L, De Pasquale R, O'Leary OF, Castren E, Maffei L. 2008. The anti-depressant fluoxetine restores plasticity in the adult visual cortex. *Science* 320: 385–388.

McCurry CL, Shepherd JD, Tropea D, Wang KH, Bear MF, Sur M. 2010. Loss of Arc renders the visual cortex impervious to the effects of sensory experience or deprivation. *Nat Neurosci* 13: 450–457.

Meikle L, Pollizzi K, Egnor A, Kramvis I, Lane H, Sahin M, Kwiatkowski DJ. 2008. Response of a neuronal model of tuberous sclerosis to mammalian target of rapamycin (mTOR) inhibitors: effects on mTORC1 and Akt signaling lead to improved survival and function. *J Neurosci* 28: 5422–5432.

Moretti P, Zoghbi HY. 2006. MeCP2 dysfunction in Rett syndrome and related disorders. *Curr Opin Genet Dev* 16: 276–281.

Muller CM, Griesinger CB. 1998. Tissue plasminogen activator mediates reverse occlusion plasticity in visual cortex. *Nat Neurosci* 1: 47–53.

Murthy VN, Schikorski T, Stevens CF, Zhu Y. 2001. Inactivity produces increases in neurotransmitter release and synapse size. *Neuron* 32: 673–682.

Nedergaard M, Ransom B, Goldman SA. 2003. New roles for astrocytes: redefining the functional architecture of the brain. *Trends Neurosci* 26: 523–530.

Okun M, Lampl I. 2008. Instantaneous correlation of excitation and inhibition during ongoing and sensory-evoked activities. *Nat Neurosci* 11: 535–537.

Oray S, Majewska A, Sur M. 2004. Dendritic spine dynamics are regulated by monocular deprivation and extracellular matrix degradation. *Neuron* 44: 1021–1030.

Patterson SL, Pittenger C, Morozov A, Martin KC, Scanlin H, Drake C, Kandel ER. 2001. Some forms of cAMP-mediated long-lasting potentiation are associated with release of BDNF and nuclear translocation of phospho-MAP kinase. *Neuron* 32: 123–140.

Perea G, Araque A. 2007. Astrocytes potentiate transmitter release at single hippocampal synapses. *Science* 317: 1083–1086.

Pettit DL, Perlman S, Malinow R. 1994. Potentiated transmission and prevention of further LTP by increased CaMKII activity in postsynaptic hippocampal slice neurons. *Science* 266: 1881–1885.

Pizzorusso T, Medini P, Berardi N, Chierzi S, Fawcett JW, Maffei L. 2002. Reactivation of ocular dominance plasticity in the adult visual cortex. *Science* 298: 1248–1251.

Pologruto TA, Yasuda R, Svoboda K. 2004. Monitoring neural activity and [Ca2+] with genetically encoded Ca2+ indicators. *J Neurosci* 24: 9572–9579.

Pratt KG, Aizenman CD. 2007. Homeostatic regulation of intrinsic excitability and synaptic transmission in a developing visual circuit. *J Neurosci* 27: 8268–8277.

Quinlan EM, Philpot BD, Huganir RL, Bear MF. 1999. Rapid, experience-dependent expression of synaptic NMDA receptors in visual cortex in vivo. *Nat Neurosci* 2: 352–357.

Rutherford LC, Nelson SB, Turrigiano GG. 1998. BDNF has opposite effects on the quantal amplitude of pyramidal neuron and interneuron excitatory synapses. *Neuron* 21: 521–530.

Schuman EM. 1999. Neurotrophin regulation of synaptic transmission. *Curr Opin Neurobiol* 9: 105–109.

Schummers J, Yu H, Sur M. 2008. Tuned responses of astrocytes and their influence on hemodynamic signals in the visual cortex. *Science* 320: 1638–1643.

Seeburg DP, Feliu-Mojer M, Gaiottino J, Pak DT, Sheng M. 2008. Critical role of CDK5 and Polo-like kinase 2 in homeostatic synaptic plasticity during elevated activity. *Neuron* 58: 571–583.

Shepherd GM, Stepanyants A, Bureau I, Chklovskii D, Svoboda K. 2005. Geometric and functional organization of cortical circuits. *Nat Neurosci* 8: 782–790.

Smith GB, Heynen AJ, Bear MF. 2009. Bidirectional synaptic mechanisms of ocular dominance plasticity in visual cortex. *Philos Trans R Soc Lond B Biol Sci* 364: 357–367.

Song S, Abbott LF. 2001. Cortical development and remapping through spike timing-dependent plasticity. *Neuron* 32: 339–350.

Stellwagen D, Malenka RC. 2006. Synaptic scaling mediated by glial TNF-alpha. *Nature* 440: 1054–1059.

Stellwagen D, Beattie EC, Seo JY, Malenka RC. 2005. Differential regulation of AMPA receptor and GABA receptor trafficking by tumor necrosis factor-alpha. *J Neurosci* 25: 3219–3228.

Sweatt JD. 2001. The neuronal MAP kinase cascade: a biochemical signal integration system subserving synaptic plasticity and memory. *J Neurochem* 76(1): 1–10.

Tavazoie SF, Alvarez VA, Ridenour DA, Kwiatkowski DJ, Sabatini BL. 2005. Regulation of neuronal morphology and function by the tumor suppressors Tsc1 and Tsc2. *Nat Neurosci* 8: 1727–1734.

Thomas GM, Huganir RL. 2004. MAPK cascade signalling and synaptic plasticity. *Nat Rev Neurosci* 5: 173–183.

Tropea D, Kreiman G, Lyckman A, Mukherjee S, Yu H, Horng S, Sur M. 2006. Gene expression changes and molecular pathways mediating activity-dependent plasticity in visual cortex. *Nat Neurosci* 9: 660–668.

Tropea D, Giacometti E, Wilson NR, Beard C, McCurry C, Fu DD, Flannery R, Jaenisch R, Sur M. 2009. Partial reversal of Rett syndrome-like symptoms in MeCP2 mutant mice. *Proc Natl Acad Sci USA* 106: 2029–2034.

Turrigiano GG. 2008. The self-tuning neuron: synaptic scaling of excitatory synapses. *Cell* 135: 422–435.

Turrigiano GG, Nelson SB. 2000. Hebb and homeostasis in neuronal plasticity. *Curr Opin Neurobiol* 10: 358–364.

Wang KH, Majewska A, Schummers J, Farley B, Hu C, Sur M, Tonegawa S. 2006. In vivo two-photon imaging reveals a role of Arc in enhancing orientation specificity in visual cortex. *Cell* 126: 389–402.

Wiesel TN, Hubel DH. 1963. Single-cell responses in striate cortex of kittens deprived of vision in one eye. *J Neurophysiol* 26: 1003–1017.

Wilson NR, Ty MT, Ingber DE, Sur M, Liu G. 2007. Synaptic reorganization in scaled networks of controlled size. *J Neurosci* 27: 13581–13589.

Wilson NR, Kang J, Hueske EV, Leung T, Varoqui H, Murnick JG, Erickson JD, Liu G. 2005. Presynaptic regulation of quantal size by the vesicular glutamate transporter VGLUT1. *J Neurosci* 25: 6221–6234.

Xia Z, Dudek H, Miranti CK, Greenberg ME. 1996. Calcium influx via the NMDA receptor induces immediate early gene transcription by a MAP kinase/ERK-dependent mechanism. *J Neurosci* 16: 5425–5436.

Ying SW, Futter M, Rosenblum K, Webber MJ, Hunt SP, Bliss TV, Bramham CR. 2002. Brain-derived neurotrophic factor induces long-term potentiation in intact adult hippocampus: requirement for ERK activation coupled to CREB and upregulation of Arc synthesis. *J Neurosci* 22: 1532–1540.

Yoshii A, Constantine-Paton M. 2007. BDNF induces transport of PSD-95 to dendrites through PI3K-AKT signaling after NMDA receptor activation. *Nat Neurosci* 10: 702–711.

Zhang F, Aravanis AM, Adamantidis A, de Lecea L, Deisseroth K. 2007. Circuit-breakers: optical technologies for probing neural signals and systems. *Nat Rev Neurosci* 8: 577–581.

Zheng WH, Quirion R. 2004. Comparative signaling pathways of insulin-like growth factor-1 and brain-derived neurotrophic factor in hippocampal neurons and the role of the PI3 kinase pathway in cell survival. *J Neurochem* 89: 844–852.

Zhu JJ, Qin Y, Zhao M, Van Aelst L, Malinow R. 2002. Ras and Rap control AMPA receptor trafficking during synaptic plasticity. *Cell* 110: 443–455.

Zoghbi HY. 2003. Postnatal neurodevelopmental disorders: meeting at the synapse? *Science* 302: 826–830.

8 Activity-Dependent Development of Inhibitory Synapses and Innervation Pattern in the Visual Cortex: From BDNF to GABA Signaling

Z. Josh Huang

I first came to know the work of Professor Lamberto Maffei when I was starting my postdoctoral research at MIT in 1994. I was in the laboratory of Professor Susumu Tonegawa, who was championing a mouse genetic approach to neuroscience. At the time there was considerable excitement in the hypothesis that neurotrophic factors function beyond neuronal survival and play important roles in neural activity-dependent synaptic plasticity. Lamberto's provocative report that exogenous infusion of nerve growth factor prevents the shift in ocular dominance (OD) distribution of visual cortical neurons following monocular deprivation (Maffei et al., 1992), a prime model for experience-dependent neural plasticity, captured my imagination. I first met Lamberto at the Neural Plasticity Gordon Research Conference in New Hampshire in 1995. The following spring, Professor Emilio Bizzi in the Department of Brain and Cognitive Sciences at MIT invited Lamberto to give two lectures on the study of neurotrophins in neural plasticity. Despite his low-key style and soft voice, I was inspired by his creative mind. It also became clear to me that Lamberto was leading a productive team who excelled in the use of rodent models to study visual cortical plasticity and was open to new approaches, including genetic engineering in mice. With common interest and complementary expertise, I proposed a collaboration to examine the role of brain-derived neurotrophic factor (BDNF) in OD plasticity and its critical period using a genetic approach. I was generating a transgenic mouse line to overexpress BDNF and accelerate its natural rise in pyramidal neurons in visual cortex during the postnatal period. Our hypothesis was that BDNF acts as an activity-dependent retrograde signal to regulate synapse growth; thus, overexpression of BDNF in cortical pyramidal neurons should prevent competition between inputs representing the left and right eye pathway and thus prevent OD plasticity following monocular deprivation. This genetic strategy has an advantage over pharmacological infusion of neurotrophins because it elevates BDNF levels from the endogenous source and engages the endogenous BDNF releasing mechanism. It only became apparent to us subsequently that although our genetic strategy was elegant, it still may not have the necessary spatial and temporal precision to directly test our hypothesis. Nonetheless, our experiments led to unexpected results and insights: together with Alfredo Kirkwood and Mark Bear at Brown University, we discovered that BDNF overexpression led to a precocious critical period of OD plasticity, which was correlated with an accelerated maturation of GABAergic inhibitory circuitry in visual cortex (Huang et al., 1999). These results suggested to us that, in addition to functioning as a putative retrograde signal at excitatory synapses, BDNF mediates activity-dependent regulation of inhibitory synapses, thereby influencing the plasticity of neural circuits in visual cortex. This study in part led to my increased interest in the GABAergic inhibitory neurons and contributed to shaping my future research direction. Indeed, since starting my own laboratory at Cold Spring Harbor in New York in 2000, we have focused on taking a genetic approach to studying the organization, development, and function of GABA inhibitory neurons and circuits.

Experience- and Activity-Dependent Development of Inhibitory Innervation in Visual Cortex

In mammalian neocortex, neural circuits rely on inhibition mediated by γ-aminobutyric acid (GABA) from diverse cell types to control the spatiotemporal patterns of electrical signaling (Markram et al., 2004). The inhibitory output of GABAergic neurons is distributed in the network through their axons and synapses, which constitute elaborate and cell type-specific innervation patterns (Huang et al., 2007). A prominent feature of GABAergic axon arbors in the neocortex is their local exuberance: a single interneuron often elaborates extensive local arbors that innervate hundreds of neurons in its vicinity and form multiple clustered synapses onto each target neuron (Tamas et al., 1997; Wang et al., 2002). Such an innervation pattern likely contributes to their efficient control over the activity patterns in local cell populations. For example, a single parvalbumin-containing (PV) basket interneuron innervates hundred of pyramidal neurons at the soma and proximal dendrites and controls the output and synchrony of pyramidal neurons (see figure 8.1, plate 3; Cobb et al., 1995; Tamas et al., 1997). Furthermore, PV baskets cells form extensive mutual innervation (Tamas et al., 2000) and, together with their unique physiological properties, contribute to the generation of coherent network oscillations that might organize functional neural ensembles (Bartos et al., 2007).

The development of a mature GABAergic innervation pattern is often a prolonged process, extending well into the postnatal period. In primary visual cortex, the maturation of perisomatic inhibition by basket interneurons proceeds into the fifth postnatal week and may contribute to the regulation of the critical period of plasticity (Morales et al., 2002; Huang et al., 1999). Importantly, the maturation of inhibitory innervation in visual and somatosensory cortex is regulated by sensory experience (Chattopadhyaya et al., 2004; Jiao et al., 2006; Morales et al., 2002). Such activity-dependent development of inhibitory synapses and innervation pattern is a major component of neural circuit assembly, yet the underlying cellular and molecular mechanisms are poorly understood.

GABA Signaling Regulates Inhibitory Synapse Development

As key mediators of neural activity, neurotransmitters are particularly well suited to couple synaptic signaling with synaptic wiring (Hua and Smith, 2004; Zhang and Poo, 2001; Malinow

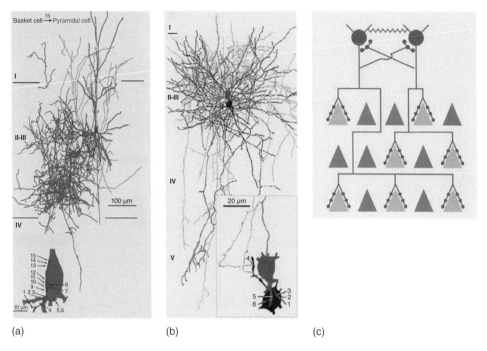

Figure 8.1 (plate 3)
(a) Highly exuberant axonal arborization of a neocortical basket interneuron (blue) and one of its many postsynaptic pyramidal cells (red). Although the basket axon overlaps with a large part of the pyramidal basal dendritic tree, all 15 electron microscopically verified synaptic junctions (bottom panel, right) are clustered around the soma or the most proximal dendrites (bottom left panel) (adapted from Tamas et al., 1997). (b) Reconstructions of the two parvalbumin-containing basket cells connected by both chemical and electrical synapses (presynaptic cell: soma and dendrites, red; axon, green; postsynaptic cell: soma, dendrites, black; axon, blue). Cortical layers (I–V) are indicated on the left. The electron-microscopically identified synaptic junctions (1–4) and gap junctions (5, 6) mediating the interaction between the coupled cells were found nearby on the soma and a proximal dendrite (insert) (adapted from Tamas et al., 2000). (c) A schematic showing prominent features of the innervation pattern of cortical basket interneurons. A single basket cell axon (green) innervating the many pyramidal neurons (red) in its vicinity with clusters of perisomatic synapses (green dots). Basket cells also innervate other basket cells via chemical and electrical (zigzagged lines) synapses. Gray triangles represent pyramidal neurons that are not innervated by these basket cells.

and Malenka, 2002; Cline and Haas, 2008). Initially discovered as an inhibitory transmitter, GABA has since been implicated in multiple processes of neural development, from cell proliferation to circuit formation (Owens and Kriegstein, 2002). The trophic effects of GABA on neuronal migration and neurite growth during the embryonic and perinatal period are largely explained by its depolarizing action in immature neurons, resulting from chloride ion efflux through the $GABA_A$ receptors (Ben-Ari et al., 1989; Leinekugel et al., 1995). During the postnatal period, the upregulation of the chloride transporter potassium chloride cotransporter 2 in neurons results in increased extrusion of intracellular chloride (Rivera et al., 1999), and GABA assumes its classic role as an inhibitory transmitter (Ben-Ari et al., 2007).

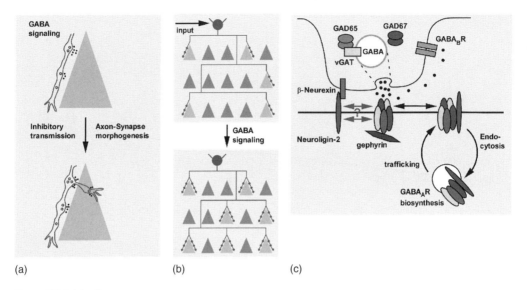

Figure 8.2 (plate 4)
Glutamic acid decaboxylase (GAD) 67 and GABA act beyond inhibitory transmission and regulate inhibitory synapse development and innervation patterns. (a) GABA signaling may regulate the morphogenesis of inhibitory synapses. (b) Since synapse formation is an integral part of axon growth and branching, activity-dependent GABA signaling may further influence the development of GABAergic axon arbor and innervation patterns. (c) A hypothetical model depicting how GABA–GABA receptor signaling and neuroligin–neurexin adhesion may interact and cooperate to regulate the development of inhibitory synapses. Pentameric GABA$_A$ receptors (GABA$_A$Rs) are assembled in the endoplasmic reticulum. Most GABA$_A$Rs are first delivered to extrasynaptic locations; they then either diffuse to and become trapped at postsynaptic sites or undergo endocytosis. Neuroligin 2 (NL2) and synaptic GABA$_A$R stabilize each other, either through intracellular reciprocal interactions aided by scaffolding proteins such as gephyrin or through extracellular cis interaction. In addition, GABA activation of GABA$_A$Rs might further stabilize synaptic GABA$_A$Rs through structural changes or signaling mechanisms. Such activity- and GABA-mediated stabilization of GABA$_A$R might further increase the levels of NL2 at cell–cell contacts and, in turn, stabilize presynaptic terminals through transsynaptic interactions with neurexins.

    Recently, several studies converged and suggest that, in addition to mediating synaptic inhibition in more mature circuits, GABA signaling promotes and coordinates pre- and postsynaptic maturation during activity-dependent development of inhibitory synapses and innervation (see figure 8.2, plate 4).
    A main line of evidence came from our study of the effects of altering GABA synthesis on the development of perisomatic synapses from PV basket interneurons in the visual cortex. The maturation of many features of basket cell axon arbors and perisomatic synapses can be recapitulated in cortical organotypic cultures (Di Cristo et al., 2004) and is strongly regulated by neuronal activity (Chattopadhyaya et al., 2004; Klostermann and Wahle, 1999). Genetic knockdown of GABA synthesis implicates GABA signaling itself in the development of perisomatic synapses (Chattopadhyaya et al., 2007). GABA is synthesized by two glutamate decarboxylases, GAD67 and GAD65 (Soghomonian and Martin, 1998). Among the two enzymes, GAD67 is the rate-limiting enzyme and influences cellular GABA contents in a dosage-dependent manner

(Asada et al., 1997; Ji et al., 1999). Knockdown of GAD67 in single GABAergic interneurons, which should have minimum impact on circuit activity levels, results in profound cell autonomous deficits in synapse formation, axon branching, and innervation field in cortical organotypic cultures; such deficits were partially rescued by blocking GABA reuptake or enhancing GABA$_A$ or GABA$_B$ receptor function (Chattopadhyaya et al., 2007). Similar deficits were found in visual cortex of Gad67 germline heterozygotes, which show ~40% reduction of GABA levels (Chattopadhyaya et al., 2007). These results demonstrate that GABA acts beyond inhibitory transmission in the juvenile and adolescent brain and regulates the maturation of inhibitory synapses and innervation patterns (see figure 8.2), thus revealing a new facet of GABA function distinct from its early tropic action in the neonatal brain.

GABA$_A$ Receptors: Coupling Transmission to Synapse Maturation and Stability

Another line of evidence supporting a role of GABA on the development of inhibitory synapses came from studying the effects of manipulating GABA$_A$ receptor (GABA$_A$R) subunits. GABA$_A$Rs are heteropentameric chloride channels composed of several classes of subunits (Michels and Moss, 2007). Although over 19 subunits have been identified, giving rise to a large number of possible subunit combinations, the vast majority of GABA$_A$Rs consist of α, β, and $\gamma2$ subunits in a 2:2:1 stoichiometry. In the mature brain, GABA$_A$Rs are primarily localized at postsynaptic and extrasynaptic membranes where they mediate phasic and tonic inhibition, respectively.

The $\gamma2$ subunit is essential for accumulation of cell surface GABA$_A$Rs at postsynaptic sites (Essrich et al., 1998; Schweizer et al., 2003). Acute suppression of $\gamma2$ expression in cultured hippocampal neurons not only disrupts GABA$_A$R clustering but also results in a profound reduction of GABAergic innervation of $\gamma2$-deficient neurons (Fang et al., 2006; Li et al., 2005). Moreover, when palmitoylation of the $\gamma2$ subunit was suppressed by knockdown of the DHHC-family palmitoyltransferase GODZ, trafficking of GABA$_A$Rs to postsynaptic sites was perturbed and GABAergic innervation was reduced (Fang et al., 2006). Because both presynaptic GABA and postsynaptic GABA$_A$ receptors influence GABAergic synapse development, a simple hypothesis is that activity-dependent GABA signaling promotes the differentiation of pre- and postsynaptic sites and coordinates the maturation and stabilization of inhibitory synapses. In addition, studies in the cerebellum suggests that GABA$_A$ receptors contribute activity-dependent regulation of synapse density, possibly through promoting the stabilization of transient axodendritic contact into mature synapses.

The mechanism linking GABA signaling to synapse maturation are still unclear. Activation of GABA$_A$Rs may result in the local release of trophic factors which promote inhibitory synapse maturation and/or act as protective signals that prevent synapses elimination. The failure to stabilize presynaptic terminals after postsynaptic loss of GABA$_A$Rs suggests the presence of a retrograde signal that is regulated by synaptic activity or by association with postsynaptic GABA$_A$Rs. Among the molecular mechanisms that may contribute to such an activity-regulated transsynaptic signal, the neuroligin and neurexin complex represents one of the plausible candidates.

From GABA$_A$ Receptors to Synaptic Adhesion and Activity-Dependent Retrograde Signaling

Neuroligins and neurexins are heterophilic synaptic adhesion molecules broadly expressed in the central nervous system (Brose, 1999; Sudhof, 2008). Cell biological studies have revealed potent "synaptogenic" or synapse-organizing activities for these proteins (recently reviewed in Craig and Kang, 2007; Levinson and El-Husseini, 2005). Postsynaptic neuroligins promote assembly of functional presynaptic specializations in axons, while presynaptic neurexins—through interaction with neuroligins—recruit postsynaptic scaffolding proteins and transmitter receptors in dendrites.

While neuroligin–neurexin complexes are common building blocks of glutamatergic and GABAergic synapses, analysis of mutant mice so far supports their particularly critical roles in the organization of GABAergic synapses. Triple or double knockout of alpha-neurexin genes results in significant reduction in the density of GABAergic synapses (Missler et al., 2003; Dudanova et al., 2007). As for neuroligins, mice lacking the three major isoforms (neuroligins [NLs] 1, 2, and 3) are perinatal lethal and show a severe loss of GABA$_A$Rs and the scaffolding protein gephyrin from postsynaptic sites (Varoqueaux et al., 2006). Among the different isoforms, NL2 is exclusively localized to GABAergic synapses. NL2–/– mice display a selective decrease in the number of inhibitory synapses in the postnatal neocortex (Chubykin et al., 2007). In addition, Layer 2/3 neurons in acute cortical slices from NL2 –/– mice show a selective impairment of GABAergic transmission whereas glutamatergic transmission is normal. Overexpression of NL2 in cultured neurons increases the density GABAergic terminals (Chih et al., 2005) and the amplitude of inhibitory postsynaptic currents (Chubykin et al., 2007). Notably, this overexpression-induced increase in GABAergic transmission is blocked by pharmacologically reducing network activity in the culture. Therefore, neuronal and synaptic activity might regulate either the presynaptic response to NL2 or postsynaptic stabilization induced by NL2.

How do GABA/GABA$_A$R-mediated synaptic signaling and neuroligin/neurexin-mediated synaptic adhesion interact and cooperate to regulate activity-dependent development of inhibitory synapses? It is currently unknown at what stage of their biosynthetic pathway GABA$_A$Rs first interact with neuroligins and how such interactions might be regulated. One possibility is NL2 and synaptic GABA$_A$Rs would stabilize each other, either through intracellular reciprocal interactions aided by scaffolding proteins such as gephyrin or through extracellular cis interactions (see figure 8.2). In addition, GABA activation of GABA$_A$Rs might further stabilize GABA$_A$Rs at synapses through as yet unknown structural or signaling mechanisms. Such activity- and GABA-mediated stabilization of GABA$_A$Rs might further increase the levels of NL2 at postsynaptic sites; this, in turn, would stabilize the presynaptic terminals through transsynaptic interactions with neurexins. Evidence consistent with this model includes the following: (1) in vitro studies demonstrated a coaggregation of NL2 and the $GABA_A R\alpha 2$ subunit in heterologous cells (Dong et al., 2007), (2) the residence time of $GABA_A Rs$ on the plasma membrane and their targeting to synapses is regulated by synaptic activity (Saliba et al., 2007), (3) pharmacological blockade of neuronal activity in cultured neurons diminishes the synaptogenic activity of NL2 (Chubykin et al., 2007), and (4) reduced GABA synthesis and release result in a reduction of inhibitory synapses (Chattopadhyaya et al., 2007). Moreover, there is precedent for such mechanisms in activity-dependent recruitment of glutamate receptor and transsynaptic signaling at glutamatergic synapses. Local spontaneous activity and glutamate release reduce diffusion exchange of glutamate receptor 1 (GluR1) between synaptic and extrasynaptic domains, resulting in postsynaptic accumulation of GluR1 (Ehlers et al., 2007). In addition, postsynaptic density protein 95 and NL1 retrogradely modulate presynaptic release probability and may coordinate post- and presynaptic morphological changes (Ehrlich et al., 2007; Futai et al., 2007). It remains to be seen whether analogous mechanisms for GABA and NL2 signaling exist at inhibitory synapses.

Activity-Regulated GAD67 Transcription as a Cell-Wide Mechanism for Modulating GABA Signaling and Innervation Pattern

A mechanism unique to GABAergic neurons is activity-dependent GABA synthesis. Unlike glutamate, which is both the precursor and product of many essential metabolic and signaling processes in the cell, GABA can only be synthesized by two glutamate decarboxylases, and the main function of GABA is intercellular signaling (Soghomonian and Martin, 1998). In most brain regions, GAD67 activity is rate limiting for GABA synthesis (Asada et al., 1996; Kash et al., 1997). Because GAD67 is produced at a limiting level in the brain (Asada et al., 1997), alterations in GAD67 levels influence cellular and vesicular GABA content (Engel et al., 2001; Murphy et al., 1998). Unlike GAD65, which is relatively stable, GAD67 protein has a rather quick turnover rate, with a half-life of several hours (Christgau et al., 1991; Pinal and Tobin, 1998). The major step in the physiological regulation of GAD67 activity is *Gad1* transcription, which is dynamically regulated during development (Kiser et al., 1998) by neural activity (Kinney et al., 2006; Patz et al., 2003) and experience (Benevento et al., 1995; Benson et al., 1989; Gierdalski et al., 2001; Kobori and Dash, 2006; Liang et al., 1996). Therefore, activity-dependent transcription may result in adjustment of GAD67 levels and intracellular GABA pool for release. Because alterations in GAD67 and GABA levels profoundly influence interneuron axon growth and synapse formation during the development of inhibitory circuits, neuronal activity might shape the pattern of inhibitory synaptic innervation through GAD67-mediated GABA synthesis (see figure 8.3, plate 5). Such activity-dependent and cell-wide regulation of a "transmitter resource" implies a novel logic for the maturation of inhibitory synapses and innervation patterns. This hypothesis needs to be tested by disrupting the activity regulation of GAD67 transcription in GABAergic neurons and examining the impact on inhibitory synapse development.

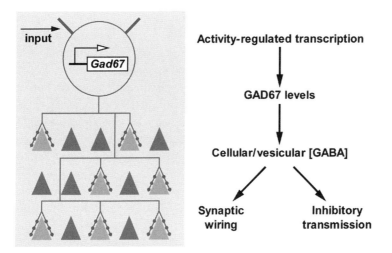

Figure 8.3 (plate 5)
A scheme showing that the level and pattern of neuronal activity may regulate inhibitory synaptic morphogenesis and innervation patterns through glutamic acid decaboxylase (GAD) 67-mediated GABA synthesis and signaling.

More Questions than Answers

The converging findings that GABA and GABA receptor signaling regulate inhibitory synapse development raise numerous questions regarding the underlying mechanisms and their functional implications. The many steps from GABA signaling to receptor trafficking/stability and neuroligin–neurexin function remain to be defined. In addition, it is unknown whether and how postsynaptic activity in pyramidal neurons might influence the action of GABA signaling on inhibitory synapse development. Furthermore, because cortical GABAergic neurons innervate not only pyramidal neurons but also other GABAergic neurons, an obvious question is whether and how GABA signaling might regulate the development of inhibitory synapses onto inhibitory neurons. Addressing such questions will require methods to visualize inhibitory synapses onto inhibitory neurons. Finally, although activity regulation of GAD67 transcription has been well demonstrated in numerous developmental and plasticity paradigms, its impact on GABA signaling and inhibitory synapse development and plasticity remains to be established in vivo. Compared with our understanding of the role of glutamate in excitatory synapse development, we are only beginning to scratch the surface of the role of GABA in the development of inhibitory synapses. Progress in this area will not only enhance our understanding of activity-dependent development of inhibitory synapses, axon arbors, and innervation patterns but also might have implications in the construction of cortical subnetworks, such as reciprocally connected groups of excitatory and inhibitory neurons (Yoshimura and Callaway, 2005).

References

Asada H, Kawamura Y, Maruyama K, Kume H, Ding R, Ji FY, Kanbara N, Kuzume H, Sanbo M, Yagi T, Obata K. 1996. Mice lacking the 65 kDa isoform of glutamic acid decarboxylase (GAD65) maintain normal levels of GAD67 and GABA in their brains but are susceptible to seizures. *Biochem Biophys Res Commun* 229: 891–895.

Asada H, Kawamura Y, Maruyama K, Kume H, Ding RG, Kanbara N, Kuzume H, Sanbo M, Yagi T, Obata K. 1997. Cleft palate and decreased brain gamma-aminobutyric acid in mice lacking the 67-kDa isoform of glutamic acid decarboxylase. *Proc Natl Acad Sci USA* 94: 6496–6499.

Bartos M, Vida I, Jonas P. 2007. Synaptic mechanisms of synchronized gamma oscillations in inhibitory interneuron networks. *Nat Rev Neurosci* 8: 45–56.

Ben-Ari Y, Cherubini E, Corradetti R, Gaiarsa JL. 1989. Giant synaptic potentials in immature rat CA3 hippocampal neurones. *J Physiol* 416: 303–325.

Ben-Ari Y, Gaiarsa JL, Tyzio R, Khazipov R. 2007. GABA: A pioneer transmitter that excites immature neurons and generates primitive oscillations. *Physiol Rev* 87: 1215–1284.

Benevento LA, Bakkum BW, Cohen RS, Port JD. 1995. gamma-aminobutyric acid and somatostatin immunoreactivity in the visual cortex of normal and dark-reared rats. *Brain Res* 689: 172–182.

Benson DL, Isackson PJ, Hendry SH, Jones EG. 1989. Expression of glutamic acid decarboxylase mRNA in normal and monocularly deprived cat visual cortex. *Brain Res Mol Brain Res* 5: 279–287.

Brose N. 1999. Synaptic cell adhesion proteins and synaptogenesis in the mammalian central nervous system. *Naturwissenschaften* 86: 516–524.

Chattopadhyaya B, Di Cristo G, Higashiyama H, Knott GW, Kuhlman SJ, Welker E, Huang ZJ. 2004. Experience and activity-dependent maturation of perisomatic GABAergic innervation in primary visual cortex during a postnatal critical period. *J Neurosci* 24: 9598–9611.

Chattopadhyaya B, Di Cristo G, Wu CZ, Knott G, Kuhlman S, Fu Y, Palmiter RD, Huang ZJ. 2007. GAD67-mediated GABA synthesis and signaling regulate inhibitory synaptic innervation in the visual cortex. *Neuron* 54: 889–903.

Chih B, Engelman H, Scheiffele P. 2005. Control of excitatory and inhibitory synapse formation by neuroligins. *Science* 307: 1324–1328.

Christgau S, Schierbeck H, Aanstoot HJ, Aagaard L, Begley K, Kofod H, Hejnaes K, Baekkeskov S. 1991. Pancreatic beta cells express two autoantigenic forms of glutamic acid decarboxylase, a 65-kDa hydrophilic form and a 64-kDa amphiphilic form which can be both membrane-bound and soluble. *J Biol Chem* 266: 21257–21264.

Chubykin AA, Atasoy D, Etherton MR, Brose N, Kavalali ET, Gibson JR, Sudhof TC. 2007. Activity-dependent validation of excitatory versus inhibitory synapses by neuroligin-1 versus neuroligin-2. *Neuron* 54: 919–931.

Cline H, Haas K. 2008. The regulation of dendritic arbor development and plasticity by glutamatergic synaptic input: a review of the synaptotrophic hypothesis. *J Physiol* 586: 1509–1517.

Cobb SR, Buhl EH, Halasy K, Paulsen O, Somogyi P. 1995. Synchronization of neuronal activity in hippocampus by individual GABAergic interneurons. *Nature* 378: 75–78.

Craig AM, Kang Y. 2007. Neurexin–neuroligin signaling in synapse development. *Curr Opin Neurobiol* 17: 43–52.

Di Cristo G, Wu C, Chattopadhyaya B, Ango F, Knott G, Welker E, Svoboda K, Huang ZJ. 2004. Subcellular domain-restricted GABAergic innervation in primary visual cortex in the absence of sensory and thalamic inputs. *Nat Neurosci* 7: 1184–1186.

Dong N, Qi J, Chen G. 2007. Molecular reconstitution of functional GABAergic synapses with expression of neuroligin-2 and GABAA receptors. *Mol Cell Neurosci* 35: 14–23.

Dudanova I, Tabuchi K, Rohlmann A, Sudhof TC, Missler M. 2007. Deletion of alpha-neurexins does not cause a major impairment of axonal pathfinding or synapse formation. *J Comp Neurol* 502: 261–274.

Ehlers MD, Heine M, Groc L, Lee MC, Choquet D. 2007. Diffusional trapping of GluR1 AMPA receptors by input-specific synaptic activity. *Neuron* 54: 447–460.

Ehrlich I, Klein M, Rumpel S, Malinow R. 2007. PSD-95 is required for activity-driven synapse stabilization. *Proc Natl Acad Sci USA* 104: 4176–4181.

Engel D, Pahner I, Schulze K, Frahm C, Jarry H, Ahnert-Hilger G, Draguhn A. 2001. Plasticity of rat central inhibitory synapses through GABA metabolism. *J Physiol* 535: 473–482.

Essrich C, Lorez M, Benson JA, Fritschy JM, Luscher B. 1998. Postsynaptic clustering of major GABAA receptor subtypes requires the gamma 2 subunit and gephyrin. *Nat Neurosci* 1: 563–571.

Fang C, Deng L, Keller CA, Fukata M, Fukata Y, Chen G, Luscher B. 2006. GODZ-mediated palmitoylation of GABA(A) receptors is required for normal assembly and function of GABAergic inhibitory synapses. *J Neurosci* 26: 12758–12768.

Futai K, Kim MJ, Hashikawa T, Scheiffele P, Sheng M, Hayashi Y. 2007. Retrograde modulation of presynaptic release probability through signaling mediated by PSD-95-neuroligin. *Nat Neurosci* 10: 186–195.

Gierdalski M, Jablonska B, Siucinska E, Lech M, Skibinska A, Kossut M. 2001. Rapid regulation of GAD67 mRNA and protein level in cortical neurons after sensory learning. *Cereb Cortex* 11: 806–815.

Hua JY, Smith SJ. 2004. Neural activity and the dynamics of central nervous system development. *Nat Neurosci* 7: 327–332.

Huang ZJ, Di Cristo G, Ango F. 2007. Development of GABA innervation in the cerebral and cerebellar cortices. *Nat Rev Neurosci* 8: 673–686.

Huang ZJ, Kirkwood A, Pizzorusso T, Porciatti V, Morales B, Bear MF, Maffei L, Tonegawa S. 1999. BDNF regulates the maturation of inhibition and the critical period of plasticity in mouse visual cortex. *Cell* 98: 739–755.

Ji F, Kanbara N, Obata K. 1999. GABA and histogenesis in fetal and neonatal mouse brain lacking both the isoforms of glutamic acid decarboxylase. *Neurosci Res* 33: 187–194.

Jiao Y, Zhang C, Yanagawa Y, Sun QQ. 2006. Major effects of sensory experiences on the neocortical inhibitory circuits. *J Neurosci* 26: 8691–8701.

Kash SF, Johnson RS, Tecott LH, Noebels JL, Mayfield RD, Hanahan D, Baekkeskov S. 1997. Epilepsy in mice deficient in the 65-kDa isoform of glutamic acid decarboxylase. *Proc Natl Acad Sci USA* 94: 14060–14065.

Kinney JW, Davis CN, Tabarean I, Conti B, Bartfai T, Behrens MM. 2006. A specific role for NR2A-containing NMDA receptors in the maintenance of parvalbumin and GAD67 immunoreactivity in cultured interneurons. *J Neurosci* 26: 1604–1615.

Kiser PJ, Cooper NG, Mower GD. 1998. Expression of two forms of glutamic acid decarboxylase (GAD67 and GAD65) during postnatal development of rat somatosensory barrel cortex. *J Comp Neurol* 402: 62–74.

Klostermann O, Wahle P. 1999. Patterns of spontaneous activity and morphology of interneuron types in organotypic cortex and thalamus-cortex cultures. *Neuroscience* 92: 1243–1259.

Kobori N, Dash PK. 2006. Reversal of brain injury-induced prefrontal glutamic acid decarboxylase expression and working memory deficits by D1 receptor antagonism. *J Neurosci* 26: 4236–4246.

Leinekugel X, Tseeb V, Ben-Ari Y, Bregestovski P. 1995. Synaptic GABAA activation induces Ca2+ rise in pyramidal cells and interneurons from rat neonatal hippocampal slices. *J Physiol* 487(Pt 2): 319–329.

Levinson JN, El-Husseini A. 2005. Building excitatory and inhibitory synapses: balancing neuroligin partnerships. *Neuron* 48: 171–174.

Li RW, Yu W, Christie S, Miralles CP, Bai J, Loturco JJ, De Blas AL. 2005. Disruption of postsynaptic GABA receptor clusters leads to decreased GABAergic innervation of pyramidal neurons. *J Neurochem* 95: 756–770.

Liang F, Isackson PJ, Jones EG. 1996. Stimulus-dependent, reciprocal up- and downregulation of glutamic acid decarboxylase and Ca2+/calmodulin-dependent protein kinase II gene expression in rat cerebral cortex. *Exp Brain Res* 110: 163–174.

Maffei L, Berardi N, Domenici L, Parisi V, Pizzorusso T. 1992. Nerve growth factor (NGF) prevents the shift in ocular dominance distribution of visual cortical neurons in monocularly deprived rats. *J Neurosci* 12: 4651–4662.

Malinow R, Malenka RC. 2002. AMPA receptor trafficking and synaptic plasticity. *Annu Rev Neurosci* 25: 103–126.

Markram H, Toledo-Rodriguez M, Wang Y, Gupta A, Silberberg G, Wu C. 2004. Interneurons of the neocortical inhibitory system. *Nat Rev Neurosci* 5: 793–807.

Michels G, Moss SJ. 2007. GABAA receptors: properties and trafficking. *Crit Rev Biochem Mol Biol* 42: 3–14.

Missler M, Zhang W, Rohlmann A, Kattenstroth G, Hammer RE, Gottmann K, Sudhof TC. 2003. Alpha-neurexins couple Ca2+ channels to synaptic vesicle exocytosis. *Nature* 423: 939–948.

Morales B, Choi SY, Kirkwood A. 2002. Dark rearing alters the development of GABAergic transmission in visual cortex. *J Neurosci* 22: 8084–8090.

Murphy DD, Cole NB, Greenberger V, Segal M. 1998. Estradiol increases dendritic spine density by reducing GABA neurotransmission in hippocampal neurons. *J Neurosci* 18: 2550–2559.

Owens DF, Kriegstein AR. 2002. Is there more to GABA than synaptic inhibition? *Nat Rev Neurosci* 3: 715–727.

Patz S, Wirth MJ, Gorba T, Klostermann O, Wahle P. 2003. Neuronal activity and neurotrophic factors regulate GAD-65/67 mRNA and protein expression in organotypic cultures of rat visual cortex. *Eur J Neurosci* 18: 1–12.

Pinal CS, Tobin AJ. 1998. Uniqueness and redundancy in GABA production. *Perspect Dev Neurobiol* 5: 109–118.

Rivera C, Voipio J, Payne JA, Ruusuvuori E, Lahtinen H, Lamsa K, Pirvola U, Saarma M, Kaila K. 1999. The K+/Cl– co-transporter KCC2 renders GABA hyperpolarizing during neuronal maturation. *Nature* 397: 251–255.

Saliba RS, Michels G, Jacob TC, Pangalos MN, Moss SJ. 2007. Activity-dependent ubiquitination of GABA(A) receptors regulates their accumulation at synaptic sites. *J Neurosci* 27: 13341–13351.

Schweizer C, Balsiger S, Bluethmann H, Mansuy IM, Fritschy JM, Mohler H, Luscher B. 2003. The gamma 2 subunit of GABA(A) receptors is required for maintenance of receptors at mature synapses. *Mol Cell Neurosci* 24: 442–450.

Soghomonian JJ, Martin DL. 1998. Two isoforms of glutamate decarboxylase: why? *Trends Pharmacol Sci* 19: 500–505.

Sudhof TC. 2008. Neuroligins and neurexins link synaptic function to cognitive disease. *Nature* 455: 903–911.

Tamas G, Buhl EH, Lorincz A, Somogyi P. 2000. Proximally targeted GABAergic synapses and gap junctions synchronize cortical interneurons. *Nat Neurosci* 3: 366–371.

Tamas G, Buhl EH, Somogyi P. 1997. Fast IPSPs elicited via multiple synaptic release sites by different types of GABAergic neurone in the cat visual cortex. *J Physiol* 500: 715–738.

Varoqueaux F, Aramuni G, Rawson RL, Mohrmann R, Missler M, Gottmann K, Zhang W, Sudhof TC, Brose N. 2006. Neuroligins determine synapse maturation and function. *Neuron* 51: 741–754.

Wang Y, Gupta A, Toledo-Rodriguez M, Wu CZ, Markram H. 2002. Anatomical, physiological, molecular and circuit properties of nest basket cells in the developing somatosensory cortex. *Cereb Cortex* 12: 395–410.

Yoshimura Y, Callaway EM. 2005. Fine-scale specificity of cortical networks depends on inhibitory cell type and connectivity. *Nat Neurosci* 8: 1552–1559.

Zhang LI, Poo MM. 2001. Electrical activity and development of neural circuits. *Nat Neurosci* 4: 1207–1214.

9 Molecular Factors Controlling Inhibitory Circuit Maturation and Onset of Critical Period Plasticity: Implications for Developmental Diseases

Graziella Di Cristo and Bidisha Chattopadhyaya

Have you ever felt frustrated while learning a new language as an adult and observed in awe when children of parents with different origins speak not just parental languages but the local languages too, with a flawless accent? This common challenge faced by anyone who starts anew in a foreign country as an adult highlights that while it is possible to learn certain tasks throughout life, usually the younger you start, the better. More than four decades of research have demonstrated that although the brain remains plastic throughout life, continuously reorganizing its connections in the face of new experiences, childhood represents a specific phase in the development of the synaptic network that is characterized by overall remarkable plasticity. During these epochs of heightened brain plasticity, commonly called critical periods, experience can produce permanent, large-scale changes in neuronal circuits. But what are the mechanisms governing the ability of young brains to be shaped by the environment around them? The question of what mechanisms underlie activation and regulation of critical periods in the central nervous system (CNS) is a seminal one in neuroscience, the underlying motive being that manipulation of such mechanisms may potentially allow reactivation of neural circuit plasticity during times when the adult brain is less plastic. On one hand, this could aid in designing strategies aimed to increase adaptive circuit rewiring following insult, such as stroke. On the other hand, this knowledge may help us to understand and, hopefully, develop rational pharmacological approaches to correct alterations in the brain of children with neurodevelopmental disorders, such as mental retardation.

Although we know that each system—sensory, motor, auditory, and also higher cognitive systems—shows its own critical periods, much of our knowledge of the cellular and molecular mechanisms initiating and operating during and eventually terminating these periods derive from studies on the visual system. Wiesel and Hubel (1963) first introduced the term "critical period" in the context of the developing mammalian visual system in their studies in the cat. They showed that neurons in primary visual cortex are activated to different degrees by visual stimuli presented to one eye or the other, a property termed ocular dominance (OD). Closing one eye during a specific postnatal time period starts a cascade of events leading to synaptic reorganization of neural circuits in visual cortex, which results in the lifelong, irreversible reduction of the ability of the deprived eye to drive neuronal responses in the cortex and a dramatic increase in the number of neurons responding best to stimuli presented to the open eye. The change in which eye is best able to excite neurons in visual cortex is called ocular dominance plasticity. Markedly in contrast to the profound effects in young animals, prolonged eye closure in adults has little to no effect (Hubel and Wiesel, 1970). Behaviorally, animals monocularly deprived during the critical period lose visual acuity in the deprived eye, and no amount of subsequent experience can completely reverse the effects of early deprivation (Berardi et al., 2000). This is consistent with human studies; for example, in 2005 a U.S. nationwide randomized clinical trial showed that the treatment of amblyopia in children between 7 and 17 years of age was effective only in a fourth of the patients, and to a lesser degree than treatment in younger children (Scheiman et al., 2005). To date, OD plasticity remains the best studied experimental model for experience-dependent refinement of neuronal circuits because of the ease of manipulating visual experience independently in the two eyes. In this review, we will focus on the mechanisms regulating the onset of OD plasticity. We will then briefly discuss how alteration in the timing of the critical period can be implicated in neurodevelopmental diseases.

Mechanisms Regulating the Onset of Critical Period Plasticity

Maturation of GABAergic Inhibition

What dictates the time window of a period of heightened plasticity in the brain? Recently, it has been shown that the development of inhibitory circuitry in the cortex plays a pivotal role in controlling the onset and time course of critical periods (Fagiolini and Hensch, 2000; Hensch, 2005). Cortical inhibitory neurons, or interneurons, comprise approximately 20% to 30% of all cortical neurons and use gamma-aminobutyric acid (GABA) as a neurotransmitter. GABAergic interneurons control several aspects of neuronal circuit function from neuronal excitability (Swadlow, 2003) and integration (Pouille and Scanziani, 2001) to the generation of temporal synchrony and oscillation among networks of excitatory neurons (Somogyi and Klausberger, 2005). In addition, GABAergic interneurons also regulate key developmental steps, from cell migration and differentiation to experience-dependent refinement of neuronal connections (Ben-Ari, 2002; Hensch, 2005). In particular, two elegant studies demonstrated a direct role of GABA in the onset of OD plasticity. In a first study, Hensch and collaborators (1998) showed that mice lacking the synaptic isoform of GABA-producing enzyme, glutamic acid decaboxylase (GAD65) show no OD plasticity. This deficit can be rescued by cortical infusion of the GABAa receptor agonist diazepam, demonstrating that a decrease in inhibition effectively abolished the critical period and impaired plasticity mechanisms. In the second study, Fagiolini and Hensch (2000) showed that the early enhancement of GABA-mediated inhibition by diazepam application triggers the precocious onset of OD plasticity.

Cortical GABAergic interneurons are by no means a homogeneous population; in fact, they show striking heterogeneity in morphology, physiological properties, and protein expression (Huang et al., 2007). The hypothesis that different interneuron subtypes play different roles in cortical development, function, and plasticity is therefore a tantalizing one. Fagiolini et al. (2004) showed that GABA transmission mediated by the α1 subunit-containing GABAa receptors is required for the induction of critical period OD plasticity. Because different classes of inhibitory synapses preferentially signal through GABAa receptors with different subunit composition (Ali and Thomson, 2008), these results suggest that maturation of specific subclasses of GABA interneurons is crucial to initiate critical period plasticity. More recent data indicate that site-specific optimization of GABAa receptor numbers on the soma-proximal dendritic compartment of pyramidal cells triggers the onset of OD plasticity (Katagiri et al., 2007). The soma-proximal dendritic compartment of pyramidal cells is preferentially innervated by parvalbumin (PV) positive basket interneurons. Taken altogether, these data suggest a critical role for basket cell interneuron maturation in the onset of critical period plasticity.

What are the molecular mechanisms controlling GABAergic interneuron maturation? The functional maturation of GABA-mediated inhibition, studied in the visual cortex, is a prolonged process that extends well into adolescence, both in rodents and primates (Chattopadhyaya et al., 2004; Lewis et al., 2005; Morales et al., 2002) and correlates with the time course of the critical period for OD plasticity (Chattopadhyaya et al., 2004; Morales et al., 2002). Moreover, the inhibitory maturation process strongly depends on sensory experience since sensory deprivation, induced either by dark rearing or by intraocular tetradotoxin (TTX) injection, significantly retards the morphological and functional maturation of GABAergic synapses (Chattopadhyaya et al., 2004; Morales et al., 2002). This dependence of GABAergic synapse maturation on sensory experience is not limited to visual cortex; indeed, similar results have been found in the somatosensory cortex (Jiao et al., 2006).

Molecular Factors Promoting Inhibitory Circuit Maturation and Onset of Critical Period Plasticity

What are the cellular and molecular mechanisms linking sensory experience to the maturation of GABAergic synapses? Brain derived neurotrophic factor (BDNF), an activity-dependent molecule shown to be upregulated following light stimulation in the visual cortex (Bozzi et al., 1995; Castrén et al., 1992), is one of the first molecules implicated in the formation of GAB-Aergic synapses in hippocampal and cortical cultures (Rutherford et al., 1997; Vicario-Abejon et al., 1998). Most importantly, in transgenic mice with precocious BDNF expression, a marked increase in perisomatic inhibitory innervation in the visual cortex is correlated with a premature onset and closure of OD plasticity, further supporting the link between GABAergic synapse maturation and onset of critical period plasticity (Huang et al., 1999; Hanover et al., 1999). Since BDNF is produced only by pyramidal cells, it could work as an intercellular signaling factor that translates pyramidal cell activity to GABAergic synapse density.

Another factor that has been shown to positively regulate GABAergic synapse maturation is GABA itself. Chattopadhyaya and collaborators (2007) used a transgenic mouse where the GAD67 gene is floxed so as to knock down GAD67 in single inhibitory basket cells. Since GAD67 is the main isoform of GABA synthesizing enzyme, its deletion reduces GABA levels by 90% (Asada et al., 1997). Even a partial reduction in GAD67 caused major defects in basket interneuron axon branching and synapse density in the adolescent brain (Chattopadhyaya et al., 2007). Different aspects of this deficit were rescued by treatment with either GABAa or GABAb agonists, suggesting a receptor-specific effect of GABA-mediated signaling during GABAergic synapse maturation (Chattopadhyaya et al., 2007). This study demonstrates that GABA acts beyond its classical role as an inhibitory neurotransmitter to regulate GABAergic circuit development, which, in turn, regulates critical period plasticity.

A recent study by Fiorentino et al. (2009) proposes that a link between BDNF and GABA signaling influences GABAergic synapse maturation. The authors demonstrate that activation of metabotropic GABAb receptor triggers secretion of BDNF and promotes the development of GABAergic synapses, in particular the perisomatic GABAergic synapses, onto CA3 pyramidal neurons in the hippocampus of newborn mice (Fiorentino et al., 2009). Whether a similar mechanism is at play in the visual cortex is still unknown; however, the picture so far indicates a positive interplay between sensory experience, BDNF, and GABA signaling, to induce GABAergic synapse maturation and, in turn, promote the onset of OD plasticity.

A novel mechanism explaining how visual input is coupled to the onset of OD plasticity has been proposed by Sugiyama et al. (2008). The molecular signals linking visual experience to maturation of GABA interneurons were thought to be recruited from within the cortex itself, such as the activity-dependent synthesis and release of BDNF by pyramidal neurons (Huang et al., 1999). Instead, Sugiyama et al. (2008) demonstrated that a retina-derived homeoprotein, Otx2, is first transferred into the primary visual cortex via a visual experience-dependent mechanism. Once in the cortex, Otx2 then nurtures GABAergic interneurons and promotes critical period plasticity. The investigation of the target genes and proteins of Otx2 will reveal further insights into the mechanisms linking experience, GABAergic circuit maturation, and critical period plasticity.

Molecular Factors Inhibiting Inhibitory Circuit Maturation and Onset of Critical Period Plasticity: Polysialic Acid

In addition to factors promoting GABAergic synapse maturation, recent studies have revealed inhibitory mechanisms that set the appropriate time course for establishment of mature GABAergic innervation patterns and the onset of critical period plasticity. In particular, polysialic acid (PSA), linked to the neural cell adhesion molecule (NCAM), acts as a negative signal to suppress the formation of inhibitory synapses and the onset of OD plasticity in the developing visual cortex (see figure 9.1; Di Cristo et al., 2007). In the mammalian brain, NCAM is a predominant carrier of the unusual long-chain, polyanionic carbohydrate, PSA, although outside the nervous system more carriers of PSA are known, including neuropilin-2 (Curreli et al., 2007). PSA is a long linear homopolymer of α-2,8-linked sialic acid that is synthesized in the Golgi by two polysialyltransferases, PST (also known as ST8SiaIV) and STX (also known as ST8SiaII), either of which is sufficient for the complete synthesis of PSA chain on a standard asparaginyl-linked core carbohydrate attached to NCAM (reviewed by Angata and Fukuda, 2003, and by Rutishauser, 2008).

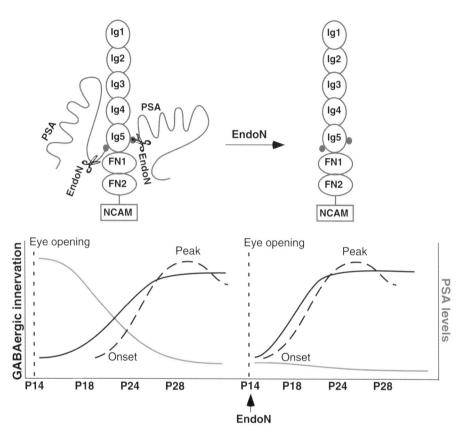

Figure 9.1
Early polysialic acid (PSA) removal promotes precocious inhibitory maturation and onset of critical period plasticity. Top panel: endoneuramidase N (EndoN) specifically removes PSA moiety from neural cell adhesion molecule (NCAM). Left bottom panel: the time course of the decline of PSA expression levels (gray line) correlates with the maturation of GABAergic innervation (black line) in the mouse visual cortex. Dashed line represents the time course of the critical period for ocular dominance plasticity. Right bottom panel: enzymatic removal of PSA by EndoN application at eye opening postnatal day (P) 14 accelerates the maturation of GABAergic innervation and the onset of critical period.

One of the most studied characteristics of PSA is its ability to act as a de-adhesive factor, causing steric hindrance, between cellular membranes. PSA is heavily hydrated because of the large negative charge of PSA. Due to its large size, its high hydration degree, and its ability to rotate around its glycosidic bonds, PSA occupies a large volume. Therefore, cell surface expression of PSA constricts intercellular space between apposing cells (Johnson et al., 2005), which in turn, decreases homophilic binding between NCAM and other cell adhesion molecules including Cadherins, L1 family, and Integrins (Fujimoto et al., 2001). Because of its ability to regulate distance between cell membranes, and therefore their ability to interact, PSA is thought to act as a permissive regulating factor rather than a specific instructive cue. PSA affects distinct developmental processes depending on the location and timing of its expression. For example, in the developing nervous system PSA creates conditions permissive for postmitotic migration of precursor cells. In the adult, migrating cells still retain PSA, such as progenitor cells migrating along rostral migratory stream from the subventricular zone (SVZ) to the olfactory bulb (Hu et al., 1996), and newborn granule cells in the hippocampus (Burgess et al., 2008). In addition, PSA plays a role in axon fasciculation and branching during axon pathfinding, axon myelination, synapse formation, and activity-dependent synaptic plasticity (reviewed by Rutishauser, 2008).

Recent studies show the ability of PSA to regulate OD plasticity (Di Cristo et al., 2007). Although PSA expression is highest in the embryonic stages, it is expressed in the postnatal brain at different levels depending on brain region and age. In the mouse visual cortex PSA expression declines to almost undetectable levels shortly after eye opening, and this decline is attenuated by visual deprivation (Di Cristo et al., 2007). Indeed, PSA levels in visual cortex are higher in mice dark reared from birth compared to littermates reared in a normal light–dark cycle. This effect is echoed in the visual cortex contralateral to the eye that receives daily intra-ocular injection of TTX compared to the ipsilateral cortex (Di Cristo et al., 2007). Since the developmental and activity-regulated expression of PSA inversely correlates with the maturation of GABAergic innervation (Chattopadhyaya et al., 2004), it is thus possible that PSA decline might be sufficient for GABAergic synapse maturation. Indeed, premature enzymatic removal of PSA in the developing visual cortex resulted in precocious maturation of perisomatic innervation by basket interneurons and enhanced inhibitory synaptic transmission. Most importantly, the same treatment causes an earlier onset of critical period plasticity in the visual cortex (Di Cristo et al., 2007). Since PSA removal promotes GABAergic synapse formation, and GABA signaling, in turn, further promotes the maturation of GABAergic innervation (Chattopadhyaya et al., 2007), together GABA signaling and PSA removal may constitute a positive feedback mechanism to accelerate GABAergic synapse formation once sensory experience begins and, consequently, to induce the onset of critical period plasticity in the visual cortex. PSA also regulates glutamatergic synapse formation (Dityatev et al., 2004; Muller et al., 1996) and affects neuron–glia interactions (Theodosis et al., 1999); thus, the possibility of additional mechanisms by which PSA influences OD plasticity cannot be excluded.

What is the precise role of PSA in GABAergic circuit maturation? One possibility is that developmental and activity-dependent removal of PSA might coordinate the timing of axon and synapse morphogenesis during the maturation of GABAergic innervation. Basket interneurons in visual cortex show characteristic axon arbor morphology and exuberant local innervation of the perisomatic region of pyramidal neurons. This pattern of innervation is established during an extended postnatal period involving sequential and overlapping progression of axon growth, branching, and synapse formation (Chattopadhyaya et al., 2004). The increase in exuberant local axon branching and perisomatic synapse number is most pronounced in fourth postnatal week, concurrent with the maturation of functional GABAergic innervation (Chattopadhyaya et al., 2004; Morales et al., 2002). However, it is clear that basket neurons are in fact able to form synapses at least a week earlier; indeed precocious perisomatic synapse formation can be triggered by premature removal of PSA. Excessive, premature synapse formation might constrain axon growth. Higher expression of PSA during the early postnatal weeks might attenuate interactions between basket cell axons and pyramidal neurons, thereby holding off synapse formation and promoting the elaboration of axon arbors. Subsequent activity-dependent removal of PSA might unmask mechanisms that are already in place along the basket cell axon, allowing fast responses to local synaptogenic cues. A similar example of PSA regulating the timing of a biological process comes from studies of migrating neuronal precursor. When PSA is enzymatically removed from newly generated cells in the SVZ, they form neuronal processes and begin to express neuronal molecular markers. This premature developmental transition is dependent on cell contact and appears to involve signaling through NCAM and p59Fyn kinase (Petridis et al., 2004).

Why is such a mechanism in place and what could be its purpose? Interestingly, long polymers of sialic acid are not found in invertebrates (Rutishauser, 2008), where neural circuits are to a large extent genetically determined. This raises the possibility that PSA might have evolved to regulate vertebrate-specific developmental processes. An example is the role of PSA in cell migration and differentiation. In invertebrates, the differentiation of neuronal precursors occurs close to the region of their birth and involves interactions with its immediate neighbor cells. On the other hand, in vertebrates, newly generated precursors often migrate long distances before acquiring their fate and, thus, need to delay their differentiation until they reach their destination. Here, PSA plays a dual role whereby it (1) promotes cell migration by reducing cell–cell adhesion and (2) blocks differentiation by interfering with contact-dependent signaling until the cells arrive at their final location.

Such multifaceted roles for PSA are well suited for the complex experience-dependent neural circuit fine-tuning that occurs in vertebrate CNS. It is interesting to note that vision-dependent critical period plasticity does not start at the onset of eye opening. Instead, it is hypothesized that the critical period cannot start until the input to the circuit has developed reliability and precision (Knudsen, 2004). Thus, cellular mechanisms underlying critical period are not simply an activity-dependent process; instead, it's a sequence of timed events that appears to be important. PSA might then act as a "brake" that holds off the onset of critical period plasticity until input information can be reliably relayed to the cortex. The challenge is to understand what happens if and when this timing is altered, whether onset of critical period before the appropriate time might lead to incorrect refinement of neural circuit based on unreliable or nonoptimal inputs, and whether and how this would, in turn, affect behavior.

Summary and Perspectives for Neurodevelopmental Disorders

Multiple convergent studies show that maturation of GABAergic inhibition regulates onset of the critical period for OD plasticity in the visual cortex. This maturation of GABAergic inhibition is, in turn, regulated by sensory experience. Efforts to explore molecular mechanisms linking sensory experience to GABAergic circuit maturation have revealed several players that include both GABAergic synapse promoting factors (BDNF, Otx2, and GABA itself) and GABAergic synapse inhibiting factors (PSA). It has become increasingly clear that mechanisms are in place to tightly time events leading to the onset of critical period plasticity. The questions to raise then are, what may be the correct or most permissible sequence of events and whether the onset of critical period at a time when circuits are not "ready" could lead to an altered developmental trajectory.

GABA synthesis and signaling has been shown to regulate the maturation of GABAergic innervation in visual cortex and the onset of critical period plasticity (Fagiolini and Hensch, 2000; Chattopadhyaya et al., 2007). These findings further highlight the possible deleterious action of drugs acting on GABA signaling, such as benzodiazepines, during brain development. Recent evidence from both clinical and animal studies suggests that certain anti-epileptic drugs could interfere with normal cognitive development (Marsh et al., 2006). Further studies are required to understand if GABA-targeting drugs could have long-term consequences in young children by interfering, among other things, with critical period plasticity.

Aberrant development and function of the GABAergic system has been implicated in various neurodevelopmental and psychiatric disorders such as schizophrenia (Lewis et al., 2005) and autism (Belmonte et al., 2004; Dani et al., 2005). In particular, reduced *Gad1* mRNA expression in the dorsal lateral prefrontal cortex is one of the most consistent molecular pathological findings in individuals with schizophrenia (Lewis et al., 2005). Further, the homeodomain transcription factor Dlx5, which regulates the differentiation and maturation of forebrain GABAergic interneurons, has been identified as a direct target of MeCP2 (Horike et al., 2005), which is linked to Rett's syndrome. Interestingly, critical period OD plasticity is altered in MeCP2 mutant mice, a well-recognized model for Rett's syndrome (Tropea et al., 2009).

Altered PSA levels are associated with various neuropathological conditions including schizo-phrenia (Barbeau et al., 1995) and temporal lobe epilepsy (Mikkonen et al., 1998). In particular, a decrease in polysialylation of hippocampal neurons in schizophrenic brains correlates with early disease incidence (Barbeau et al., 1995; Vicente et al., 1997). Moreover, ST8SIA2, the human STX-encoding gene, is located in a schizophrenia-susceptible chromosomal region (Tao et al., 2007), raising the possibility that developmental abnormalities associated with defective polysialylation may be involved in schizophrenia.

There is thus increasing evidence that alterations in molecular pathways involved in regulating critical period plasticity are associated with neurodevelopmental diseases. Further detailed studies are essential to understand how critical period plasticity is affected in these diseases and whether therapeutic intervention is possible. Encouragingly, recent papers have revealed some effective strategies to reopen plasticity in a mature brain (Pizzorusso et al., 2002; Sale et al., 2007; Maya-Vetencourt et al., 2008). Altogether, this knowledge will further our understanding of the regulation of developmental plasticity in the brain and could aid in designing strategies aimed to increase adaptive circuit rewiring following insult, such as stroke, and in developing rational pharmacological approaches to correct alterations in the brain of children with neuro-developmental disorders.

Dedication

This chapter is dedicated to Lamberto Maffei, who first introduced me to neuroscience and to the fascinating question of how brain plasticity works. During our recording experiments, it was a common occurrence for Professor Maffei to come into the room and ask how it was going, independently from how busy he was with other things. He taught us passion for the "big" questions in science.

References

Ali AB, Thomson AM. 2008. Synaptic alpha 5 subunit-containing GABAA receptors mediate IPSPs elicited by dendrite-preferring cells in rat neocortex. *Cereb Cortex* 18: 1260–1271.

Angata K, Fukuda M. 2003. Polysialyltransferases: major players in polysialic acid synthesis on the neural cell adhesion molecule. *Biochimie* 85: 195–206.

Asada H, Kawamura Y, Maruyama K, Kume H, Ding RG, Kanbara N, Kuzume H, Sanbo M, Yagi T, Obata K. 1997. Cleft palate and decreased brain gamma-aminobutyric acid in mice lacking the 67-kDa isoform of glutamic acid decarboxylase. *Proc Natl Acad Sci USA* 94: 6496–6499.

Barbeau D, Liang JJ, Robitaille Y, Quirion R, Srivastava LK. 1995. Decreased expression of the embryonic form of the neural cell adhesion molecule in schizophrenic brains. *Proc Natl Acad Sci USA* 92: 2785–2789.

Belmonte MK, Cook EH, Jr, Anderson GM, Rubenstein JL, Greenough WT, Beckel-Mitchener A, Courchesne E, et al. 2004. Autism as a disorder of neural information processing: directions for research and targets for therapy. *Mol Psychiatry* 9: 646–663.

Ben-Ari Y. 2002. Excitatory actions of GABA during development: the nature of the nurture. *Nat Rev Neurosci* 3: 728–739.

Berardi N, Pizzorusso T, Maffei L. 2000. Critical periods during sensory development. *Curr Opin Neurobiol* 10: 138–145.

Bozzi Y, Pizzorusso T, Cremisi F, Rossi FM, Barsacchi G, Maffei L. 1995. Monocular deprivation decreases the expression of messenger RNA for brain-derived neurotrophic factor in the rat visual cortex. *Neuroscience* 69: 1133–1144.

Burgess A, Wainwright SR, Shihabuddin LS, Rutishauser U, Seki T, Aubert I. 2008. Polysialic acid regulates the clustering, migration, and neuronal differentiation of progenitor cells in the adult hippocampus. *Dev Neurobiol* 68: 1580–1590.

Castrén E, Zafra F, Thoenen H, Lindholm D. 1992. Light regulates expression of brain-derived neurotrophic factor mRNA in rat visual cortex. *Proc Natl Acad Sci USA* 89: 9444–9448.

Chattopadhyaya B, Di Cristo G, Higashiyama H, Knott GW, Kuhlman SJ, Welker E, Huang ZJ. 2004. Experience and activity-dependent maturation of perisomatic GABAergic innervation in primary visual cortex during a postnatal critical period. *J Neurosci* 24: 9598–9611.

Chattopadhyaya B, Di Cristo G, Wu CZ, Knott G, Kuhlman S, Fu Y, Palmiter RD, Huang ZJ. 2007. GAD67-mediated GABA synthesis and signalling regulate inhibitory synaptic innervation in the visual cortex. *Neuron* 54: 889–903.

Curreli S, Arany Z, Gerardy-Schahn R, Mann D, Stamatos NM. 2007. Polysialylated neuropilin-2 is expressed on the surface of human dendritic cells and modulates dendritic cell-T lymphocyte interactions. *J Biol Chem* 282: 30346–30356.

Dani VS, Chang Q, Maffei A, Turrigiano GG, Jaenisch R, Nelson SB. 2005. Reduced cortical activity due to a shift in the balance between excitation and inhibition in a mouse model of Rett syndrome. *Proc Natl Acad Sci USA* 102: 12560–12565.

Di Cristo G, Chattopadhyaya B, Kuhlman SJ, Fu Y, Bélanger MC, Wu CZ, Rutishauser U, Maffei L, Huang ZJ. 2007. Activity-dependent PSA expression regulates inhibitory maturation and onset of critical period plasticity. *Nat Neurosci* 10: 1569–1577.

Dityatev A, Dityateva G, Sytnyk V, Delling M, Toni N, Nikonenko I, Muller D, Schachner M. 2004. Polysialylated neural cell adhesion molecule promotes remodeling and formation of hippocampal synapses. *J Neurosci* 24: 9372–9382.

Fagiolini M, Hensch TK. 2000. Inhibitory threshold for critical-period activation in primary visual cortex. *Nature* 404: 183–186.

Fagiolini M, Fritschy JM, Löw K, Möhler H, Rudolph U, Hensch TK. 2004. Specific GABAA circuits for visual cortical plasticity. *Science* 303: 1681–1683.

Fiorentino H, Kuczewski N, Diabira D, Ferrand N, Pangalos MN, Porcher C, Gaiarsa JL. 2009. GABA(B) receptor activation triggers BDNF release and promotes the maturation of GABAergic synapses. *J Neurosci* 29: 11650–11661.

Fujimoto I, Bruses JL, Rutishauser U. 2001. Regulation of cell adhesion by polysialic acid, effects on cadherin, immunoglobulin cell adhesion molecule, and integrin function and independence from neural cell adhesion molecule binding or signaling activity. *J Biol Chem* 276: 31745–31751.

Hanover JL, Huang ZJ, Tonegawa S, Stryker MP. 1999. Brain-derived neurotrophic factor overexpression induces precocious critical period in mouse visual cortex. *J Neurosci* 19: RC40.

Hensch TK, Fagiolini M, Mataga N, Stryker MP, Baekkeskov S, Kash SF. 1998. Local GABA circuit control of experience-dependent plasticity in developing visual cortex. *Science* 282: 1504–1508.

Hensch TK. 2005. Critical period plasticity in local cortical circuits. *Nat Rev Neurosci* 6: 877–888.

Horike S, Cai S, Miyano M, Cheng JF, Kohwi-Shigematsu T. 2005. Loss of silent-chromatin looping and impaired imprinting of DLX5 in Rett syndrome. *Nat Genet* 37: 31–40.

Huang ZJ, Kirkwood A, Pizzorusso T, Porciatti V, Morales B, Bear MF, Maffei L, Tonegawa S. 1999. BDNF regulates the maturation of inhibition and the critical period of plasticity in mouse visual cortex. *Cell* 98: 739–755.

Huang ZJ, Di Cristo G, Ango F. 2007. Development of GABA innervation in the cerebral and cerebellar cortices. *Nat Rev Neurosci* 8: 673–686.

Hu H, Tomasiewicz H, Magnuson T, Rutishauser U. 1996. The role of polysialic acid in migration of olfactory bulb interneuron precursors in the subventricular zone. *Neuron* 16: 735–743.

Hubel DH, Wiesel TN. 1970. The period of susceptibility to the physiological effects of unilateral eye closure in kittens. *J Physiol* 206: 419–436.

Jiao Y, Zhang C, Yanagawa Y, Sun QQ. 2006. Major effects of sensory experiences on the neocortical inhibitory circuits. *J Neurosci* 26: 8691–8701.

Johnson CP, Fujimoto I, Rutishauser U, Leckband DE. 2005. Direct evidence that neural cell adhesion molecule (NCAM) polysialylation increases intermembrane repulsion and abrogates adhesion. *J Biol Chem* 280: 137–145.

Katagiri H, Fagiolini M, Hensch TK. 2007. Optimization of somatic inhibition at critical period onset in mouse visual cortex. *Neuron* 53: 805–812.

Knudsen EI. 2004. Sensitive periods in the development of the brain and behavior. *J Cogn Neurosci* 16: 1412–1425.

Lewis DA, Hashimoto T, Volk DW. 2005. Cortical inhibitory neurons and schizophrenia. *Nat Rev Neurosci* 6: 312–324.

Marsh ED, Brooks-Kayal AR, Porter BE. 2006. Seizures and antiepileptic drugs: does exposure alter normal brain development? *Epilepsia* 47: 1999–2010.

Maya-Vetencourt JF, Sale A, Viegi A, Baroncelli L, De Pasquale R, O'Leary OF, Castrén E, Maffei L. 2008. The antidepressant fluoxetine restores plasticity in the adult visual cortex. *Science* 320: 385–388.

Mikkonen M, Soininen H, Kälviänen R, Tapiola T, Ylinen A, Vapalahti M, Paljärvi L, Pitkänen A. 1998. Remodeling of neuronal circuitries in human temporal lobe epilepsy: increased expression of highly polysialylated neural cell adhesion molecule in the hippocampus and the entorhinal cortex. *Ann Neurol* 44: 923–934.

Morales B, Choi SY, Kirkwood A. 2002. Dark rearing alters the development of GABAergic transmission in visual cortex. *J Neurosci* 22: 8084–8090.

Muller D, Wang C, Skibo G, Toni N, Cremer H, Calaora V, Rougon G, Kiss JZ. 1996. PSA-NCAM is required for activity-induced synaptic plasticity. *Neuron* 17: 413–422.

Petridis AK, El-Maarouf A, Rutishauser U. 2004. Polysialic acid regulates cell contact-dependent neuronal differentiation of progenitor cells from the subventricular zone. *Dev Dyn* 230: 675–684.

Pizzorusso T, Medini P, Berardi N, Chierzi S, Fawcett JW, Maffei L. 2002. Reactivation of ocular dominance plasticity in the adult visual cortex. *Science* 298: 1248–1251.

Pouille F, Scanziani M. 2001. Enforcement of temporal fidelity in pyramidal cells by somatic feed-forward inhibition. *Science* 293: 1159–1163.

Rutherford LC, DeWan A, Lauer HM, Turrigiano GG. 1997. Brain-derived neurotrophic factor mediates the activity-dependent regulation of inhibition in neocortical cultures. *J Neurosci* 17: 4527–4535.

Rutishauser U. 2008. Polysialic acid in the plasticity of the developing and adult vertebrate nervous system. *Nat Rev Neurosci* 9: 26–35.

Sale A, Maya Vetencourt JF, Medini P, Cenni MC, Baroncelli L, De Pasquale R, Maffei L. 2007. Environmental enrichment in adulthood promotes amblyopia recovery through a reduction of intracortical inhibition. *Nat Neurosci* 10: 679–681.

Scheiman MM, Hertle RW, Beck RW, Edwards AR, Birch E, Cotter SA, Crouch ER, Jr, et al., and the Pediatric Eye Disease Investigator Group. 2005. Randomized trial of treatment of amblyopia in children aged 7 to 17 years. *Arch Ophthalmol* 123: 437–447.

Somogyi P, Klausberger T. 2005. Defined types of cortical interneurone structure space and spike timing in the hippocampus. *J Physiol* 562: 9–26.

Sugiyama S, Di Nardo AA, Aizawa S, Matsuo I, Volovitch M, Prochiantz A, Hensch TK. 2008. Experience-dependent transfer of Otx2 homeoprotein into the visual cortex activates postnatal plasticity. *Cell* 134: 508–520.

Swadlow HA. 2003. Fast-spike interneurons and feedforward inhibition in awake sensory neocortex. *Cereb Cortex* 13: 25–32.

Tao R, Li C, Zheng Y, Qin W, Zhang J, Li X, Xu Y, Shi YY, Feng G, He L. 2007. Positive association between SIAT8B and schizophrenia in the Chinese Han population. *Schizophr Res* 90: 108–114.

Theodosis DT, Bonhomme R, Vitiello S, Rougon G, Poulain DA. 1999. Cell surface expression of polysialic acid on NCAM is a prerequisite for activity-dependent morphological neuronal and glial plasticity. *J Neurosci* 19: 10228–10236.

Tropea D, Giacometti E, Wilson NR, Beard C, McCurry C, Fu DD, Flannery R, Jaenisch R, Sur M. 2009. Partial reversal of Rett syndrome-like symptoms in MeCP2 mutant mice. *Proc Natl Acad Sci USA* 106: 2029–2034.

Vicario-Abejon C, Collin C, McKay RD, Segal M. 1998. Neurotrophins induce formation of functional excitatory and inhibitory synapses between cultured hippocampal neurons. *J Neurosci* 18: 7256–7271.

Vicente AM, Macciardi F, Verga M, Bassett AS, Honer WG, Bean G, Kennedy JL. 1997. NCAM and schizophrenia: genetic studies. *Mol Psychiatry* 2: 65–69.

Wiesel TN, Hubel DH. 1963. Single-responses in striate cortex of kittens deprived of vision in one eye. *J Neurophysiol* 26: 1003–1017.

10 Neuron–Astrocyte Partnership in Brain Function and Dysfunction

Giorgio Carmignoto and Marta Gómez-Gonzalo

The observation that cultured glial cell astrocytes can respond to chemical transmitters released by neurons with intracellular Ca^{2+} elevations (Cornell-Bell et al., 1990) was the discovery that triggered a blossoming in the experimental research on these cells over the last decades and fueled a revolution in our basic understanding of how the brain works. Following this initial observation, a small group of neuroscientists began, indeed, to feel that these glial cells may play in the brain roles that are far more important than those that their name hints at. The term glia originates, in fact, from the Greek word for glue, and for many years it was fully consistent with the common belief that these cells serve exclusively a neuron-supportive role. Such a role is more specifically exerted by astrocytes, that is, the most populous cell in the mammalian brain. Astrocytes provide neurons with energy substrates to satisfy their metabolic requirements and exert housekeeping roles by removing, through specific transporters and channels, neurotransmitters and K^+ ions that would otherwise disrupt neuronal function if their concentration in the synaptic cleft became excessive.

While the relevance of these classical actions of astrocytes in normal brain function are not underestimated, the most recent studies unraveled roles of astrocytes that are somewhat more consistent with their starlike shape. The studies that demonstrated the ability of astrocytes to listen and talk to synapses by exerting both excitatory and inhibitory actions on neurons (Araque et al., 1999; Brockhaus and Deitmer, 2002; Zhang et al., 2003; Pascual et al., 2005; Panatier et al., 2006; Serrano et al., 2006; Jourdain et al., 2007; Perea and Araque, 2007) are, indeed, literally revolutionizing our view of brain functions based "only" (!) on billions of neurons interacting dynamically in the neuronal network. On the other hand, clues for a distinct contribution of astrocytes to the increasing complexity of brain cortical networks during phylogeny are the remarkable increase in the complexity and size of protoplasmic astrocytes with respect to the unchanged features of cortical neurons, and the relative expansion in the number of astrocytes with respect to that of neurons (Oberheim et al., 2006). Indeed, while in the cortex of lower mammals, such as rats and mice, the astrocyte-to-neuron ratio is 1:3, in the human cortex it is 1.4:1. As suggested in a recent article, astrocytes are "stars at last" (Ransom et al., 2003).

Those interested in comprehensive overviews of the progress made over the last decades in the glial cell research field are referred to a number of reviews recently appeared in the literature

(Volterra and Meldolesi, 2005; Haydon and Carmignoto, 2006; Iadecola and Nedergaard, 2007; Halassa et al., 2009a; Perea et al., 2009). The specific aim of this article is to provide, on the one hand, a brief overview of the "historical" findings and, on the other, some of the most relevant observations that advance our understanding of the amazing complexity of neuron–astrocyte partnership in the function of the brain.

Astrocytes Are Excitable Cells

The development of the fluorescence dyes for the measurement of the intracellular Ca^{2+} changes in living cells was essential for the discovery that astrocytes, since then considered nonexcitable cells, possess a form of excitability based on variations in the concentrations of the cytosolic Ca^{2+} rather than on membrane potential changes as in neurons. After loading hippocampal cell cultures with an indicator of Ca^{2+} changes, it was found that the application of the chemical transmitter glutamate induced Ca^{2+} oscillations and Ca^{2+} waves between astrocytes (Cornell-Bell et al., 1990; Charles et al., 1991; Finkbeiner, 1992). A large number of experiments in brain slice preparations were then performed, and results obtained revealed that Ca^{2+} elevations could be evoked in astrocytes by the synaptic release of various neurotransmitters, such as glutamate (Porter and McCarthy, 1996; Pasti et al., 1997), GABA (Kang et al., 1998), noradrenaline (Duffy and MacVicar, 1995; Kulik et al., 1999), and acetylcholine (Shelton and McCarthy, 2000; Araque et al., 2002), and also by cannabinoids released by neurons upon activation (Navarrete and Araque, 2008). These transient, often repetitive, Ca^{2+} elevations primarily depend on activation of metabotropic neurotransmitter receptors coupled (Verkhratsky and Kettenmann, 1996; Verkhratsky et al., 1998) to phospholipase C, production of inositol 1,4,5-trisphosphate (InsP3), activation of InsP3 receptors, and, finally, release of Ca^{2+} from intracellular Ca^{2+} compartments (Berridge, 1993; Pozzan et al., 1994). All these studies proved beyond doubt that a specific neuron-to-astrocyte signaling pathway exists in the brain in which neurons "excite" astrocytes through the same signals that allow neurons to transfer information to the postsynaptic neuron. Astrocytes are now recognized to be intrinsic elements of the neuronal circuit that compose a tripartite synapse with the pre-and postsynaptic neuronal membrane (Araque et al., 1999; Carmignoto, 2000; Haydon and Carmignoto, 2006; Halassa et al., 2009a; Perea et al., 2009).

Astrocyte-to-Neuron Signaling Pathway

The Ca^{2+} elevations that the synaptic signals evoke in astrocytes have important functional consequences. The most important of these is the activation of Ca^{2+}-dependent release of neuroactive molecules, including classical neurotransmitters (Pasti et al., 1997; Bezzi et al., 1998; Bezzi et al., 2004). Initial evidence that Ca^{2+} elevations in astrocytes result in glutamate release from these cells was obtained in 1994 by two independent studies (Nedergaard, 1994; Parpura et al., 1994). In both studies, experimentally evoked Ca^{2+} elevations in astrocytes were observed to trigger Ca^{2+} elevations in adjacent neurons through either a gap junctional communication between activated astrocytes and neurons or a Ca^{2+}-dependent release of glutamate that, in turn, activated neuronal glutamate receptors. Over time, through the use of a variety of experimental approaches, including biochemical, amperometric, and capacitance methods, as well as single-vesicle imaging (Araque et al., 2000; Pasti et al., 2001; Kržan et al., 2003; Bezzi et al., 2004; Bowser and Khakh, 2004; Evanko et al., 2004; Kreft et al., 2004; Zhang et al., 2004a; Zhang et al., 2004b; Bowser and Khakh, 2007; Jaiswal et al., 2007), it became clear that astrocytes have, indeed, the ability to release vesicles through a Ca^{2+}-dependent exocitotic mechanism. However, the increase in intracellular Ca^{2+} per se might not be sufficient for the release of astroglial glutamate. Other factors such as the spatial relation between the Ca^{2+} increase and the release site, submembrane and cytoplasmic Ca^{2+} microdomains (Reyes and Parpura, 2008), or different modes of exocytosis might be of critical importance (Agulhon et al., 2008; Shigetomi et al., 2008). It is worth underlining that other Ca^{2+}-independent release mechanisms, including a reverse-operation of glutamate transporters (Szatkowski et al., 1990; Attwell et al., 1993), connexin hemichannels, P2X7-like receptors (Cotrina et al., 1998; Duan et al., 2003; Ye et al., 2003), or swelling-induced opening of anion channels (that can form in the astrocytic membrane large conductance pores for a passive efflux of cytosolic glutamate; Kimelberg et al., 1990; Nedergaard et al., 2002; Kimelberg et al., 2006), can also mediate glutamate release in astrocytes. However, whether these release pathways are operative only under pathological brain conditions or rather exist under normal circumstances in parallel to an exocytotic pathway is still unclear (Fellin and Carmignoto, 2004; Takano et al., 2005).

Besides glutamate, astrocytes release other molecules that are now termed, in general, gliotransmitters, such as GABA, D-serine, ATP, adenosine, prostaglandins, cytokines, and neuropeptides, through mechanisms that may also rely, at least in part, on cytosolic Ca^{2+} changes. Although the physiological consequences of gliotransmission have been extensively investigated over the last years, we are only beginning to understand how deep and wide its impact might be on neuronal functions.

Astrocyte-to-Neuron Signaling: Presynaptic Actions

Glutamate, the most intensively studied among gliotransmitters, has a profound impact on synaptic transmission and neuronal excitability (see figure 10.1). Studies from different laboratories showed that by acting on presynaptic metabotropic glutamate (mGlu) type I or N-methyl-D-aspartate (NMDA) receptors, astrocytic glutamate modifies the probability of neurotransmitter release (thus increasing the frequency of spontaneous events and potentiating the evoked excitatory synaptic response), while by acting on presynaptic kainate or mGlu type II and III receptors, it potentiates or depresses inhibitory transmission, respectively. Gliotrasmitters such as D-serine that are possibly released upon the same stimuli that trigger the release of glutamate sustain the excitatory action of glutamate, while others, such as adenosine (see below), have opposite actions. While it is not easy to reconcile these different effects into a coherent picture of the astrocyte role, it is likely that the ultimate effect of gliotransmission on synaptic transmission likely depends on the specific "contact" between the two cells, the timing of the release process, and the type of receptor involved. An additional, remarkable example of the complexity of astrocyte-to-neuron signaling is represented by ATP that is most likely released from astrocytes through both Ca^{2+}-dependent and Ca^{2+}-independent mechanisms (Abraham et al., 1993; Cotrina et al., 1998; Queiroz et al., 1999; Coco et al., 2003; Anderson et al., 2004). By acting on puringeric ionotropic (P2X) and metabotropic (P2Y) receptors of the neuronal membrane, ATP of astrocytic origin represents an excitatory stimulus for neurons (see figure 10.1; North and Barnard, 1997; Khakh, 2001). Activation of P2Y1 receptors on CA1 interneurons and astrocytes from hippocampal slices by ATP, probably released by both neurons and astrocytes, was also found to cause an interneuron excitation that leads to increased GABAergic synaptic inhibition onto pyramidal neurons (Bowser and Khakh, 2004). On the other hand, by triggering Ca^{2+} oscillations in other astrocytes, ATP also serves as an excitatory signal for astrocytes that coordinates the activity of these cells in the brain network (Guthrie et al., 1999; Cotrina et al., 2000; Fam et al., 2000). Most interestingly, ATP is rapidly degraded by the action of extracellular ectonucleotidases (Dunwiddie et al., 1997), and after its conversion to adenosine, it activates presynaptic A1 receptors to inhibit synaptic transmission (Dunwiddie and Masino, 2001). The inhibitory action of adenosine of glia origin was first revealed in the retina by E. Newman and collaborators. These authors found that light-mediated Ca^{2+} elevations in Muller glial cells triggered a release of ATP that after its conversion to adenosine and A1 receptor activation from these cells caused the activation of K^+ currents that hyperpolarized retinal ganglion neurons and reduced action potential firing rate in these cells. By using a cell type-specific molecular genetic approach that allowed selective inhibition of the release of ATP from astrocytes, it was unequivocally demonstrated that it is the adenosine deriving from astrocytic ATP that through A1 receptor activation exerts the tonic inhibition of transmitter release in the brain, and also the phenomenon of heterosynaptic depression (Zhang et al., 2003; Pascual et al., 2005; Serrano et al., 2006), a phenomenon that was previously considered to be mediated by adenosine released from interneurons (Manzoni et al., 1994). In addition, a remarkable study (from Halassa et al., 2009b) demonstrated that by modulating neuronal A1 receptor activation, adenosine deriving from the degradation of astrocytic ATP regulates sleep homeostasis. This finding represents the first demonstration of an astrocyte role in behavior and opens interesting perspectives for the development of a new therapeutic approach for sleep disorders.

Noteworthy is that the excitatory action of glutamate, D-serine, and also of ATP clearly opposes the inhibitory action of adenosine that derives from ATP. The clarification of this apparent paradigmatic dichotomy in the action of astrocytes represents an engaging challenge for future studies.

Astrocyte-to-Neuron Signaling: Postsynaptic Actions

Astrocytic glutamate affects neuronal excitability also by acting on the postsynaptic membrane (see figure 10.1). The first evidence for such an action was obtained in cell cultures, where

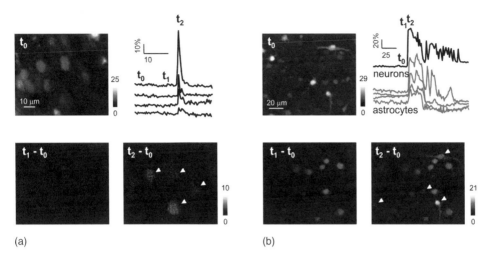

Figure 10.1
The Ca^{2+} signal change in brain slices allows evaluation of synchronous activities in neurons and astrocytes. (a) Basal levels of the Ca^{2+} signal in neurons from a hippocampal slice, as measured by Oregon Green Bapta-1 fluorescence (left), and time course of the transient and synchronous Ca^{2+} elevation activated by astrocytic glutamate in four neurons (right). This "domain" response (arrows) is also clearly illustrated by the difference image obtained by subtracting the fluorescence image at rest (t0) from that obtained before (t1) and after (t2) astrocyte stimulation. (b) Ca^{2+} fluorescence signal from cortical neurons at rest (left), and time course of Ca^{2+} changes in neurons and astrocytes that characterize an ictal discharge evoked by slice perfusion with 0 mM Mg^{2+}/50 µM picrotoxin. The synchronous activity of neurons and the massive Ca^{2+} elevation of astrocytes (arrows) that accompanied the ictal discharge is also illustrated by the difference images.

astrocytic glutamate released from activated astrocytes was observed to trigger NMDA receptor-mediated inward currents with very slow kinetics. Different stimuli that trigger Ca^{2+} elevations in astrocytes evoked in pyramidal neurons from hippocampal slices similar slow inward currents (SICs) with a rise and decay times much slower than the synaptic currents. SICs resulted to be typically mediated by the N-methyl-D-aspartate glutamate receptor (NMDAR) subtype, mainly located at extrasynaptic sites (Fellin et al., 2004). Because of their insensitivity to tetrodotoxin (TTX), they could not be due to action potential-mediated neurotransmitter release (Angulo et al., 2004; Fellin et al., 2004) and are rather due to glutamate released from astrocytes as demonstrated by a series of experiments which included photolysis of a Ca^{2+}-caged compound in single astrocytes (Fellin et al., 2004). Patch-clamp recording experiments then revealed that astrocyte-evoked SICs could occur synchronously in two pyramidal neurons of the hippocampal CA3, CA1, or cortical region when their cell bodies were within about 100 µm of one another (Angulo et al., 2004; Fellin et al., 2004). Calcium imaging experiments reveal that astrocytic glutamate can trigger NMDA receptor-mediated episodes of synchronous Ca^{2+} elevations in small groups of adjacent neurons, thus suggesting that synchronous SICs can occur in more than two neurons (Fellin et al., 2004). Noteworthy also is that the initial activation by astrocytic glutamate of two, or more, neurons may spread significantly to many other neurons since SICs can depolarize the neuronal membrane sufficiently to action potential threshold (Fellin et al., 2006).

In this action of glutamate the ability of astrocytes to release D-serine, probably the endogenous ligand that acts as a co-agonist with glutamate on the so-called "glycine site" of the NMDAR to open the channel (Mothet et al., 2000), can also be important (Schell et al., 1995). Ca^{2+} elevations have been reported to be both necessary and sufficient for triggering D-serine release in astrocytes (Mothet et al., 2005). Given that the "glycine site" on the NMDAR is not saturated, the hypothesis could be advanced that following stimuli that trigger Ca^{2+} oscillations in astrocytes, a corelease of D-serine and glutamate enhances the NMDAR activation, thus expanding astrocyte-mediated neuronal synchrony.

The transient synchronization of groups of neurons is believed to underlie the processing of external sensory signals as well as the dynamics of cognitive processes. The ability of astrocytes to evoke neuronal synchrony represents a clue for the involvement of these glial cells in these fundamental phenomena in brain function. To clarify this issue, a great help is provided by 2-photon microscopy techniques (such as fast z-dimension scanning) that allow researchers to study network activities in the living brain by monitoring the Ca^{2+} signal from hundreds of neurons and astrocytes in three-dimensional space with 20–30 Hz temporal resolution (Gobel et al., 2007).

Astrocytes and Epilepsy

Given the importance of astrocytes in the function of the normal brain, it is not surprising that an involvement of these cells in certain brain diseases is now gradually emerging (Maragakis and Rothstein, 2006; Seifert et al., 2006; Blackburn et al., 2009). Among these diseases is epilepsy, which can be considered a disorder of excess synchronization of neurons, fundamentally linked to an imbalance between excitatory and inhibitory activities that produces hyperexcitability. Epilepsy is, indeed, characterized by intense discharges that occur synchronously in neurons from a relatively small region (i.e., the epileptogenic area) and recruit over time other neuronal populations (Traub and Wong, 1982; Jefferys, 1990; Avoli et al., 2002; Pinto et al., 2005; Trevelyan et al., 2006).

The role of astrocytes as modulators of epileptogenesis was initially proposed over 20 years ago, and for a long period, this role focused on the ability of astrocytes to buffer extracellular K^+ or neurotransmitters (released in excess during epileptic discharges). While studies performed over the last decade, in both animal models and human epilepsy, demonstrated that a dysregulation of K^+ buffering in the astrocyte network is associated with a predisposition to neuronal hyperexcitability and seizures (Wallraff et al., 2006), a more direct role of astrocytes in the generation of epileptiform activities was proposed more recently.

The first clue for such a role was the demonstration that through glutamate release, astrocytes can directly excite groups of neighboring neurons and favor synchronized activities (see figure 10.1a). Studies in brain slice preparation and in vivo then described a significant increase in the frequency of Ca^{2+} oscillations in astrocytes during epileptiform activity (Tian et al., 2005; Fellin et al., 2006) and its reduction in the presence of anticonvulsant drugs (Tian et al., 2005). In animal models of temporal lobe epilepsy, it was also found that the astrocytic expression of metabotropic glutamate receptors that mediates Ca^{2+} oscillations was increased (Aronica et al., 2000; Ulas et al., 2000). These observations suggest that the excessive synchronization of neuronal activity that characterizes the epileptic discharge might derive, at least in part, from an astrocyte hyperactivity. In support of an astrocyte role in epileptogenesis, it has been reported that the paroxysmal depolarizing shifts, that is, the cellular correlate of interictal events recorded between seizures, are TTX resistant and mediated by glutamate released from astrocytes (Tian et al., 2005). This conclusion was, however, disputed by others (Fellin and Haydon, 2005; Fellin et al., 2006) and fueled a controversial debate on the role of these glial cells in focal epileptogenesis (D'Ambrosio, 2006; Seifert et al., 2006; Wetherington et al., 2008). More recent results suggest that astrocytes might contribute to focal seizures rather than to interictal discharges (Gomez-Gonzalo et al., 2010). In a slice model of epilepsy, the ictal, seizure-like discharge was, indeed, regularly accompanied by massive Ca^{2+} elevations in astrocytes (see figure 10.1b) whereas a similar astrocyte activation was never observed during interictal discharges.

Our knowledge of the astrocyte role in epilepsy is thus still primitive, and a number of important issues remain to be clarified. For example, the potential impact on seizure activity of gliotransmitters other than glutamate has been not specifically addressed. The observations that under physiological conditions adenosine derived from astrocytic ATP leads to inhibition of transmitter release and heterosynaptic depression by acting on presynaptic A1 receptors (Pascual et al., 2005; Serrano et al., 2006; Zhang et al., 2003) hint at an anticonvulsant role of astrocytes. In support of such a role, it has been found that in experimental epilepsy, seizure induction decreases adenosine extracellular concentration through an upregulation of astrocytic enzyme adenosine kinase that controls ambient adenosine levels (Boison, 2005) while genetic reduction of adenosine kinase prevents seizures (Li et al., 2008). These findings gave rise to the adenosine kinase hypothesis of epileptogenesis, which considers this enzyme both a diagnostic marker and a potential therapeutic target to prevent epileptogenesis (Boison, 2008).

By releasing glutamate and ATP, astrocytes may thus potentially exert pro- or anticonvulsive actions, respectively. Full clarification of the functional significance of these different astrocyte-to-neuron signaling pathways represents an intriguing challenge in future studies. A great help to these studies can be provided by molecular genetic tools that allow researchers to affect selectively the different pathways that mediate astrocyte-to-neuron signaling. It can be predicted that gliotransmission may soon be recognized as target for developing new antiepileptic therapies.

It is worth underlining that the changes occurring in astrocyte signaling in the epileptic tissue may resemble the dysregulation of molecules and pathways that occurs in other brain disorders. Indeed, astroglial glutamate receptors and transporters, water channels (aquaporins), potassium (Kir) channels, and connexins were found to be dysregulated not only in epilepsy but also in motor neuron disease, stroke, hepatic encephalopathy, schizophrenia, Huntington's disease, and Alzheimer's disease (Maragakis and Rothstein, 2006; Seifert et al., 2006; Blackburn et al., 2009).

All in all, these findings strongly suggest that astrocytes might hold the key to understanding the pathogenesis of these disorders. Thus, it is now time for a detailed investigation of the distinct role of neuron–astrocyte reciprocal signaling in brain dysfunctions.

Neuron to Astrocyte Signaling in the Control of Neurovascular Coupling

Functional hyperemia reflects the dilation of cerebral blood vessels from a restricted brain region activated by a local episode of high neuronal activity. This fundamental phenomenon in brain function was first discovered by A. Mosso in the late 1800s (Mosso, 1880) and later confirmed by Roy and Sherrington (1890). Besides being spatially restricted, this event occurs within a few seconds after the onset of an episode of intense neuronal activity ensuring that active neurons can be sustained by adequate amounts of oxygen and metabolic substrates.

Astrocytes have long been proposed to contribute to functional hyperemia. Besides their role as local modulators of neuronal excitability and synaptic transmission, astrocytes may, indeed, serve a hublike function by integrating the signal received from thousands of synapses and then transferring it to other cells in the neuron–astrocyte network, including the cerebral vasculature that is intimately enwrapped by the astrocytic processes, the so-called endfeet (Peters et al., 1991; Ventura and Harris, 1999).

While the first hypothesis on the putative role of astrocytes in directly regulating CBF was proposed in 1998 (Harder et al., 1998), direct experimental evidence for a distinct role of these cells in neurovascular coupling was provided only a few years later in brain slice preparations (Zonta et al., 2003b). Results obtained from these slice experiments showed that an episode of high neuronal activity activated metabotropic glutamate receptor-mediated Ca^{2+} elevations in astrocyte processes that propagated to perivascular endfeet with a timing correlated with an increase in the diameter of the cerebral blood vessels (see figure 10.2). In both slice preparations and in vivo experiments astrocyte-mediated vasodilation was found to depend mainly on arachidonic acid metabolites, such as prostaglandin E 2 (PGE2; Zonta et al., 2003a; Zonta et al., 2003b).

The results obtained from subsequent studies in brain slice (Filosa et al., 2004; Mulligan and MacVicar, 2004; Lovick et al., 2005; Gordon et al., 2008) and whole-mounted retina preparations (Metea and Newman, 2006), as well as in in vivo experiments in the olfactory bulb (Petzold et al., 2008), somatosensory (Takano et al., 2006) and visual cortex (Schummers et al., 2008), and cerebellum (Nimmerjahn et al., 2009), essentially confirmed the role of astrocytes in the control of neurovascular coupling. The demonstrations of the vasoconstrictive and vasodilating responses of blood vessels to activation of specific populations of interneurons (Cauli et al., 2004) and of a direct link between the metabolic state of the brain tissue and astrocyte signaling (Gordon et al., 2008) suggest at the basis of this complex phenomenon is a sequence of events that involves besides neuron-to-astrocyte signaling interneurons, vascular architecture, and metabolic factors (Iadecola and Nedergaard, 2007). We suggest the reader to refer to a number of recent excellent reviews that provide a comprehensive overview of the astrocyte role in the

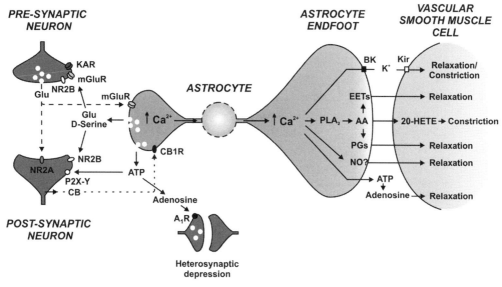

Figure 10.2
Schematic view of a polarized astrocyte and the signaling pathways that control synaptic transmission and neurovascular coupling. We schematically reported the different astrocyte signals that, on the site of the processes in contact with the synapse (left), modulate synaptic transmission by acting on either pre- or postsynaptic neuronal membranes while, on the site of the endfeet in contact with blood vessels (right), they mediate the astrocyte control of neurovascular coupling.

mechanisms at the basis of functional hyperemia (Filosa and Blanco, 2007; Iadecola and Nedergaard, 2007; Koehler et al., 2009; Carmignoto and Gómez-Gonzalo, 2010).

Conclusions

A coherent behavioral response is generated in the brain by neuronal network activities dictated by synaptic connectivity. Studies performed over the last decade provided significant support for the view that the glial cell astrocytes may be equally ranked players with neurons in a number of fundamental events in brain function, including the processing of sensory information. Against this background, it is not surprising that an integrated view of the role of astrocytes not only in the processing of sensory information but also in the genesis of brain disorders is now gradually emerging. Its full understanding represents a formidable challenge in neurobiological research.

Dedication

What I would like to tell you, Lamberto, is that being with you, breathing the same air as you, one cannot but feel your enormous passion for the beauty of Life in all its multiple forms (and science is merely one of these). And that is why your proximity was, and will always be, so rewarding to me. I would also like to thank you, Lamberto, for having immediately understood that astrocytes are not really "glue" in the brain—even when you ironically made fun of me by saying "Giorgio, *are you still wasting your time with those stupid cells?"...* Ironically?...

Acknowledgments

We thank Paulo Magalhães for a critical reading of this chapter. The original work was supported by grants from the European Community 7th Framework Program (NeuroGlia, HEALTH-F2–2007202167), Telethon Italy (GGP07278), and the CARIPARO Foundation.

References

Abraham EH, Prat AG, Gerweck L, Seneveratne T, Arceci RJ, Kramer R, Guidotti G, Cantiello HF. 1993. The multidrug resistance (mdr1) gene product functions as an ATP channel. *Proc Natl Acad Sci USA* 90: 312–316.

Agulhon C, Petravicz J, McMullen AB, Sweger EJ, Minton SK, Taves SR, Casper KB, Fiacco TA, McCarthy KD. 2008. What is the role of astrocyte calcium in neurophysiology? *Neuron* 59: 932–946.

Anderson CM, Bergher JP, Swanson RA. 2004. ATP-induced ATP release from astrocytes. *J Neurochem* 88: 246–256.

Angulo MC, Kozlov AS, Charpak S, Audinat E. 2004. Glutamate released from glial cells synchronizes neuronal activity in the hippocampus. *J Neurosci* 24: 6920–6927.

Araque A, Parpura V, Sanzgiri RP, Haydon PG. 1999. Tripartite synapses: glia, the unacknowledged partner. *Trends Neurosci* 22: 208–215.

Araque A, Li N, Doyle RT, Haydon PG. 2000. SNARE protein-dependent glutamate release from astrocytes. *J Neurosci* 20: 666–673.

Araque A, Martín ED, Perea G, Arellano JI, Buño W. 2002. Synaptically released acetylcholine evokes Ca^{2+} elevations in astrocytes in hippocampal slices. *J Neurosci* 22: 2443–2450.

Aronica E, van Vliet EA, Mayboroda OA, Troost D, da Silva FH, Gorter JA. 2000. Upregulation of metabotropic glutamate receptor subtype mGluR3 and mGluR5 in reactive astrocytes in a rat model of mesial temporal lobe epilepsy. *Eur J Neurosci* 12: 2333–2344.

Attwell D, Barbour B, Szatkowski M. 1993. Nonvesicular release of neurotransmitter. *Neuron* 11: 401–407.

Avoli M, D'Antuono M, Louvel J, Kohling R, Biagini G, Pumain R, D'Arcangelo G, Tancredi V. 2002. Network and pharmacological mechanisms leading to epileptiform synchronization in the limbic system in vitro. *Prog Neurobiol* 68: 167–207.

Berridge MJ. 1993. Inositol trisphosphate and calcium signalling. *Nature* 361: 315–325.

Bezzi P, Gundersen V, Galbete JL, Seifert G, Steinhäuser C, Pilati E, Volterra A. 2004. Astrocytes contain a vesicular compartment that is competent for regulated exocytosis of glutamate. *Nat Neurosci* 7: 613–620.

Bezzi P, Carmignoto G, Pasti L, Vesce S, Rossi D, Rizzini BL, Pozzan T, Volterra A. 1998. Prostaglandins stimulate calcium-dependent glutamate release in astrocytes. *Nature* 391: 281–285.

Blackburn D, Sargsyan S, Monk PN, Shaw PJ. 2009. Astrocyte function and role in motor neuron disease: a future therapeutic target? *Glia* 57: 1251–1264.

Boison D. 2005. Adenosine and epilepsy: from therapeutic rationale to new therapeutic strategies. *Neuroscientist* 11: 25–36.

Boison D. 2008. The adenosine kinase hypothesis of epileptogenesis. *Prog Neurobiol* 84: 249–262.

Bowser DN, Khakh BS. 2004. ATP excites interneurons and astrocytes to increase synaptic inhibition in neuronal networks. *J Neurosci* 24: 8606–8620.

Bowser DN, Khakh BS. 2007. Vesicular ATP is the predominant cause of intercellular calcium waves in astrocytes. *J Gen Physiol* 129: 485–491.

Brockhaus J, Deitmer JW. 2002. Long-lasting modulation of synaptic input to Purkinje neurons by Bergmann glia stimulation in rat brain slices. *J Physiol* 545: 581–593.

Carmignoto G. 2000. Reciprocal communication systems between astrocytes and neurones. *Prog Neurobiol* 62: 561–581.

Carmignoto G, Gómez-Gonzalo M. 2010. The contribution of astrocyte signalling to neurovascular coupling. *Brain Res Rev* 63: 138–148.

Cauli B, Tong X-K, Rancillac A, Serluca N, Lambolez B, Rossier J, Hamel E. 2004. Cortical GABA interneurons in neurovascular coupling: relays for subcortical vasoactive pathways. *J Neurosci* 24: 8940–8949.

Charles AC, Merrill JE, Dirksen ER, Sanderson MJ. 1991. Intercellular signaling in glial cells: calcium waves and oscillations in response to mechanical stimulation and glutamate. *Neuron* 6: 983–992.

Coco S, Calegari F, Pravettoni E, Pozzi D, Taverna E, Rosa P, Matteoli M, Verderio C. 2003. Storage and release of ATP from astrocytes in culture. *J Biol Chem* 278: 1354–1362.

Cornell-Bell AH, Finkbeiner SM, Cooper MS, Smith SJ. 1990. Glutamate induces calcium waves in cultured astrocytes: long-range glial signaling. *Science* 247: 470–473.

Cotrina ML, Lin JH-C, López-García JC, Naus CCG, Nedergaard M. 2000. ATP-mediated glia signaling. *J Neurosci* 20: 2835–2844.

Cotrina ML, Lin JH-C, Alves-Rodrigues A, Liu S, Li J, Azmi-Ghadimi H, Kang J, Naus CCG, Nedergaard M. 1998. Connexins regulate calcium signaling by controlling ATP release. *Proc Natl Acad Sci USA* 95: 15735–15740.

D'Ambrosio R. 2006. Does glutamate released by astrocytes cause focal epilepsy? *Epilepsy Curr* 6: 173–176.

Duan S, Anderson CM, Keung EC, Chen Y, Swanson RA. 2003. P2X7 receptor-mediated release of excitatory amino acids from astrocytes. *J Neurosci* 23: 1320–1328.

Duffy S, MacVicar BA. 1995. Adrenergic calcium signaling in astrocyte networks within the hippocampal slice. *J Neurosci* 15: 5535–5550.

Dunwiddie TV, Masino SA. 2001. The role and regulation of adenosine in the central nervous system. *Annu Rev Neurosci* 24: 31–55.

Dunwiddie TV, Diao L, Proctor WR. 1997. Adenine nucleotides undergo rapid, quantitative conversion to adenosine in the extracellular space in rat hippocampus. *J Neurosci* 17: 7673–7682.

Evanko DS, Zhang Q, Zorec R, Haydon PG. 2004. Defining pathways of loss and secretion of chemical messengers from astrocytes. *Glia* 47: 233–240.

Fam SR, Gallagher CJ, Salter MW. 2000. P2Y1 purinoceptor-mediated Ca^{2+} signaling and Ca^{2+} wave propagation in dorsal spinal cord astrocytes. *J Neurosci* 20: 2800–2808.

Fellin T, Carmignoto G. 2004. Neurone-to-astrocyte signalling in the brain represents a distinct multifunctional unit. *J Physiol* 559: 3–15.

Fellin T, Haydon PG. 2005. Do astrocytes contribute to excitation underlying seizures? *Trends Mol Med* 11: 530–533.

Fellin T, Gomez-Gonzalo M, Gobbo S, Carmignoto G, Haydon PG. 2006. Astrocytic glutamate is not necessary for the generation of epileptiform neuronal activity in hippocampal slices. *J Neurosci* 26: 9312–9322.

Fellin T, Pascual O, Gobbo S, Pozzan T, Haydon PG, Carmignoto G. 2004. Neuronal synchrony mediated by astrocytic glutamate through activation of extrasynaptic NMDA receptors. *Neuron* 43: 729–743.

Filosa JA, Blanco VM. 2007. Neurovascular coupling in the mammalian brain. *Exp Physiol* 92: 641–646.

Filosa JA, Bonev AD, Nelson MT. 2004. Calcium dynamics in cortical astrocytes and arterioles during neurovascular coupling. *Circ Res* 95: e73–e81.

Finkbeiner S. 1992. Calcium waves in astrocytes—filling in the gaps. *Neuron* 8: 1101–1108.

Gobel W, Kampa BM, Helmchen F. 2007. Imaging cellular network dynamics in three dimensions using fast 3D laser scanning. *Nat Methods* 4: 73–79.

Gomez-Gonzalo M, Losi G, Chiavegato A, Zonta M, Cammarota M, Brondi M, Vetri F, Uva L, Pozzan T, de Curtis M, Ratto GM, Carmignoto G. 2010. An Excitatory Loop with Astrocytes Contributes to Drive Neurons to Seizure Threshold. *PLoS Biology* 8: 1–19.

Gordon GR, Choi HB, Rungta RL, Ellis-Davies GC, MacVicar BA. 2008. Brain metabolism dictates the polarity of astrocyte control over arterioles. *Nature* 456: 745–749.

Guthrie PB, Knappenberger J, Segal M, Bennett MV, Charles AC, Kater SB. 1999. ATP released from astrocytes mediates glial calcium waves. *J Neurosci* 19: 520–528.

Halassa MM, Fellin T, Haydon PG. 2009a. Tripartite synapses: roles for astrocytic purines in the control of synaptic physiology and behavior. *Neuropharmacology* 57: 343–346.

Halassa MM, Florian C, Fellin T, Munoz JR, Lee SY, Abel T, Haydon PG, Frank MG. 2009b. Astrocytic modulation of sleep homeostasis and cognitive consequences of sleep loss. *Neuron* 61: 213–219.

Harder DR, Alkayed NJ, Lange AR, Gebremedhin D, Roman RJ. 1998. Functional hyperemia in the brain: hypothesis for astrocyte-derived vasodilator metabolites. *Stroke* 29: 229–234.

Haydon PG, Carmignoto G. 2006. Astrocyte control of synaptic transmission and neurovascular coupling. *Physiol Rev* 86: 1009–1031.

Iadecola C, Nedergaard M. 2007. Glial regulation of the cerebral microvasculature. *Nat Neurosci* 10: 1369–1376.

Jaiswal JK, Fix M, Takano T, Nedergaard M, Simon SM. 2007. Resolving vesicle fusion from lysis to monitor calcium-triggered lysosomal exocytosis in astrocytes. *Proc Natl Acad Sci USA* 104: 14151–14156.

Jefferys JG. 1990. Basic mechanisms of focal epilepsies. *Exp Physiol* 75: 127–162.

Jourdain P, Bergersen LH, Bhaukaurally K, Bezzi P, Santello M, Domercq M, Matute C, Tonello F, Gundersen V, Volterra A. 2007. Glutamate exocytosis from astrocytes controls synaptic strength. *Nat Neurosci* 10: 331–339.

Kang J, Jiang L, Goldman SA, Nedergaard M. 1998. Astrocyte-mediated potentiation of inhibitory synaptic transmission. *Nat Neurosci* 1: 683–692.

Khakh BS. 2001. Molecular physiology of P2X receptors and ATP signalling at synapses. *Nat Rev Neurosci* 2: 165–174.

Kimelberg HK, Macvicar BA, Sontheimer H. 2006. Anion channels in astrocytes: biophysics, pharmacology, and function. *Glia* 54: 747–757.

Kimelberg HK, Goderie SK, Higman S, Pang S, Waniewski RA. 1990. Swelling-induced release of glutamate, aspartate, and taurine from astrocyte cultures. *J Neurosci* 10: 1583–1591.

Koehler RC, Roman RJ, Harder DR. 2009. Astrocytes and the regulation of cerebral blood flow. *Trends Neurosci* 32: 160–169.

Kreft M, Stenovec M, Rupnik M, Grilc S, Kržan M, Potokar M, Pangršic T, Haydon PG, Zorec R. 2004. Properties of Ca^{2+}-dependent exocytosis in cultured astrocytes. *Glia* 46: 437–445.

Kržan M, Stenovec M, Kreft M, Pangršic T, Grilc S, Haydon PG, Zorec R. 2003. Calcium-dependent exocytosis of atrial natriuretic peptide from astrocytes. *J Neurosci* 23:1580–1583.

Kulik A, Haentzsch A, Luckermann M, Reichelt W, Ballanyi K. 1999. Neuron-glia signaling via 1 adrenoceptor-mediated Ca^{2+} release in Bergmann glial cells in situ. *J Neurosci* 19: 8401–8408.

Li T, Ren G, Lusardi T, Wilz A, Lan JQ, Iwasato T, Itohara S, Simon RP, Boison D. 2008. Adenosine kinase is a target for the prediction and prevention of epileptogenesis in mice. *J Clin Invest* 118: 571–582.

Lovick TA, Brown LA, Key BJ. 2005. Neuronal activity-related coupling in cortical arterioles: involvement of astrocyte-derived factors. *Exp Physiol* 90: 131–140.

Manzoni OJ, Manabe T, Nicoll RA. 1994. Release of adenosine by activation of NMDA receptors in the hippocampus. *Science* 265: 2098–2101.

Maragakis NJ, Rothstein JD. 2006. Mechanisms of disease: astrocytes in neurodegenerative disease. *Nat Clin Pract Neurol* 2: 679–689.

Metea MR, Newman EA. 2006. Glial cells dilate and constrict blood vessels: a mechanism of neurovascular coupling. *J Neurosci* 26: 2862–2870.

Mosso A. 1880. Sulla circolazione del sangue nel cervello dell'uomo. *Mem Real Acc Lincei* 5: 237–358.

Mothet JP, Pollegioni L, Ouanounou G, Martineau M, Fossier P, Baux G. 2005. Glutamate receptor activation triggers a calcium-dependent and SNARE protein-dependent release of the gliotransmitter D-serine. *Proc Natl Acad Sci USA* 102: 5606–5611.

Mothet JP, Parent AT, Wolosker H, Brady RO, Jr, Linden DJ, Ferris CD, Rogawski MA, Snyder SH. 2000. D-serine is an endogenous ligand for the glycine site of the N-methyl-D-aspartate receptor. *Proc Natl Acad Sci USA* 97: 4926–4931.

Mulligan SJ, MacVicar BA. 2004. Calcium transients in astrocyte endfeet cause cerebrovascular constrictions. *Nature* 431: 195–199.

Navarrete M, Araque A. 2008. Endocannabinoids mediate neuron–astrocyte communication. *Neuron* 57: 883–893.

Nedergaard M. 1994. Direct signaling from astrocytes to neurons in cultures of mammalian brain cells. *Science* 263: 1768–1771.

Nedergaard M, Takano T, Hansen AJ. 2002. Beyond the role of glutamate as a neurotransmitter. *Nat Rev Neurosci* 3: 748–755.

Nimmerjahn A, Mukamel EA, Schnitzer MJ. 2009. Motor behavior activates Bergmann glial networks. *Neuron* 62: 400–412.

North RA, Barnard EA. 1997. Nucleotide receptors. *Curr Opin Neurobiol* 7: 346–357.

Oberheim NA, Wang X, Goldman S, Nedergaard M. 2006. Astrocytic complexity distinguishes the human brain. *Trends Neurosci* 29: 547–553.

Panatier A, Theodosis DT, Mothet J-P, Toquet B, Pollegioni L, Poulain DA, Oliet SHR. 2006. Glia-derived D-serine controls NMDA receptor activity and synaptic memory. *Cell* 125: 775–784.

Parpura V, Basarsky TA, Liu F, Jeftinija K, Jeftinija S, Haydon PG. 1994. Glutamate-mediated astrocyte-neuron signalling. *Nature* 369: 744–747.

Pascual O, Casper KB, Kubera C, Zhang J, Revilla-Sanchez R, Sul JY, Takano H, Moss SJ, McCarthy K, Haydon PG. 2005. Astrocytic purinergic signaling coordinates synaptic networks. *Science* 310: 113–116.

Pasti L, Volterra A, Pozzan T, Carmignoto G. 1997. Intracellular calcium oscillations in astrocytes: a highly plastic, bidirectional form of communication between neurons and astrocytes in situ. *J Neurosci* 17: 7817–7830.

Pasti L, Zonta M, Pozzan T, Vicini S, Carmignoto G. 2001. Cytosolic calcium oscillations in astrocytes may regulate exocytotic release of glutamate. *J Neurosci* 21: 477–484.

Perea G, Araque A. 2007. Astrocytes potentiate transmitter release at single hippocampal synapses. *Science* 317: 1083–1086.

Perea G, Navarrete M, Araque A. 2009. Tripartite synapses: astrocytes process and control synaptic information. *Trends Neurosci* 32: 421–431.

Peters A, Palay SL, Webster HdeF. 1991. *The Fine Structure of the Nervous System: Neurons and Their Supporting Cells*. 3rd edition. New York: Oxford University Press.

Petzold GC, Albeanu DF, Sato TF, Murthy VN. 2008. Coupling of neural activity to blood flow in olfactory glomeruli is mediated by astrocytic pathways. *Neuron* 58: 897–910.

Pinto DJ, Patrick SL, Huang WC, Connors BW. 2005. Initiation, propagation, and termination of epileptiform activity in rodent neocortex in vitro involve distinct mechanisms. *J Neurosci* 25: 8131–8140.

Porter JT, McCarthy KD. 1996. Hippocampal astrocytes in situ respond to glutamate released from synaptic terminals. *J Neurosci* 16: 5073–5081.

Pozzan T, Rizzuto R, Volpe P, Meldolesi J. 1994. Molecular and cellular physiology of intracellular calcium stores. *Physiol Rev* 74: 595–636.

Queiroz G, Meyer DK, Meyer A, Starke K, von Kügelgen I. 1999. A study of the mechanism of the release of ATP from rat cortical astroglial cells evoked by activation of glutamate receptors. *Neuroscience* 91: 1171–1181.

Ransom B, Behar T, Nedergaard M. 2003. New roles for astrocytes (stars at last). *Trends Neurosci* 26: 520–522.

Reyes RC, Parpura V. 2008. Mitochondria modulate Ca2+-dependent glutamate release from rat cortical astrocytes. *J Neurosci* 28: 9682–9691.

Roy CS, Sherrington C. 1890. On the regulation of the blood supply of the brain. *J Physiol* 11:85–108.

Schell MJ, Molliver ME, Snyder SH. 1995. D-serine, an endogenous synaptic modulator: localization to astrocytes and glutamate-stimulated release. *Proc Natl Acad Sci USA* 92: 3948–3952.

Schummers J, Yu H, Sur M. 2008. Tuned responses of astrocytes and their influence on hemodynamic signals in the visual cortex. *Science* 320: 1638–1643.

Seifert G, Schilling K, Steinhauser C. 2006. Astrocyte dysfunction in neurological disorders: a molecular perspective. *Nat Rev Neurosci* 7: 194–206.

Serrano A, Haddjeri N, Lacaille JC, Robitaille R. 2006. GABAergic network activation of glial cells underlies hippocampal heterosynaptic depression. *J Neurosci* 26: 5370–5382.

Shelton MK, McCarthy KD. 2000. Hippocampal astrocytes exhibit Ca^{2+}-elevating muscarinic cholinergic and histaminergic receptors in situ. *J Neurochem* 74: 555–563.

Shigetomi E, Bowser DN, Sofroniew MV, Khakh BS. 2008. Two forms of astrocyte calcium excitabilty have distinct effects on NMDA receptor-mediated slow inward currents in pyramidal neurons. *J Neurosci* 28: 6659–6663.

Szatkowski M, Barbour B, Attwell D. 1990. Non-vesicular release of glutamate from glial cells by reversed electrogenic glutamate uptake. *Nature* 348: 443–446.

Takano T, Tian G-F, Peng W, Lou N, Libionka W, Han X, Nedergaard M. 2006. Astrocyte-mediated control of cerebral blood flow. *Nat Neurosci* 9: 260–267.

Takano T, Kang J, Jaiswal JK, Simon SM, Lin JH, Yu Y, Li Y, Yang J, Dienel G, Zielke HR, Nedergaard M. 2005. Receptor-mediated glutamate release from volume sensitive channels in astrocytes. *Proc Natl Acad Sci USA* 102: 16466–16471.

Tian G-F, Azmi H, Takano T, Xu Q, Peng W, Lin J, Oberheim N, et al. 2005. An astrocytic basis of epilepsy. *Nat Med* 11: 973–981.

Traub RD, Wong RK. 1982. Cellular mechanism of neuronal synchronization in epilepsy. *Science* 216: 745–747.

Trevelyan AJ, Sussillo D, Watson BO, Yuste R. 2006. Modular propagation of epileptiform activity: evidence for an inhibitory veto in neocortex. *J Neurosci* 26: 12447–12455.

Ulas J, Satou T, Ivins KJ, Kesslak JP, Cotman CW, Balazs R. 2000. Expression of metabotropic glutamate receptor 5 is increased in astrocytes after kainate-induced epileptic seizures. *Glia* 30: 352–361.

Ventura R, Harris KM. 1999. Three-dimensional relationships between hippocampal synapses and astrocytes. *J Neurosci* 19: 6897–6906.

Verkhratsky A, Kettenmann H. 1996. Calcium signalling in glial cells. *Trends Neurosci* 19: 346–352.

Verkhratsky A, Orkand RK, Kettenmann H. 1998. Glial calcium: homeostasis and signaling function. *Physiol Rev* 78: 99–141.

Volterra A, Meldolesi J. 2005. Astrocytes, from brain glue to communication elements: the revolution continues. *Nat Rev Neurosci* 6: 626–640.

Wallraff A, Kohling R, Heinemann U, Theis M, Willecke K, Steinhauser C. 2006. The impact of astrocytic gap junctional coupling on potassium buffering in the hippocampus. *J Neurosci* 26: 5438–5447.

Wetherington J, Serrano G, Dingledine R. 2008. Astrocytes in the epileptic brain. *Neuron* 58: 168–178.

Ye Z-C, Wyeth MS, Baltan-Tekkok S, Ransom BR. 2003. Functional hemichannels in astrocytes: a novel mechanism of glutamate release. *J Neurosci* 23: 3588–3596.

Zhang J-M, Wang H-K, Ye C-Q, Ge W, Chen Y, Jiang Z-L, Wu C-P, Poo M-M, Duan S. 2003. ATP released by astrocytes mediates glutamatergic activity-dependent heterosynaptic suppression. *Neuron* 40: 971–982.

Zhang Q, Fukuda M, Van Bockstaele E, Pascual O, Haydon PG. 2004a. Synaptotagmin IV regulates glial glutamate release. *Proc Natl Acad Sci USA* 101: 9441–9446.

Zhang Q, Pangršic T, Kreft M, Kržan M, Li N, Sul J-Y, Halassa M, Van Bockstaele E, Zorec R, Haydon PG. 2004b. Fusion-related release of glutamate from astrocytes. *J Biol Chem* 279: 12724–12733.

Zonta M, Angulo MC, Carmignoto G. 2003a. Response: Astrocyte-mediated control of cerebral microcirculation. *Trends Neurosci* 26: 344–345.

Zonta M, Angulo MC, Gobbo S, Rosengarten B, Hossmann K-A, Pozzan T, Carmignoto G. 2003b. Neuron-to-astrocyte signaling is central to the dynamic control of brain microcirculation. *Nat Neurosci* 6: 43–50.

11 A Thorny Question: The Role of Spine Morphogenesis in Adaptive Plasticity

Andrew Hamilton and Karen Zito

One of the fundamental questions in neuroscience today is also one of the oldest: how does the brain change in response to sensory stimuli? This ability of the central nervous system to adapt in response to experience, known as experience-dependent plasticity, is essential not only for the fine-tuning of developing circuits but also for learning and remembering as adults. Over the past 50 years, there has been an intense search for the cellular basis of experience-dependent plasticity. Evidence has been accumulating that changes in neuronal structure underlie experience-dependent plasticity; one structure that has been the focus of intense investigation is the dendritic spine. Recent experiments have demonstrated that dendritic spines are dynamic structures, that changes in spine morphology reflect changes in spine synapse function, and that spine morphological plasticity accompanies circuit plasticity induced by altered sensory experience. These data strongly support the hypothesis that spine synapse plasticity may be responsible for adaptive plasticity of the brain, although definitive evidence remains elusive. In this chapter, we describe some of the most exciting recent discoveries concerning the mechanisms of spine synapse plasticity and outline what we feel are the most intriguing questions which still loom over these tiny cytoplasmic extrusions.

Do Dendritic Spines Twitch?

It was hypothesized that dendritic spines might be dynamic structures even at the time of their first discovery in the late 1800s (Cajal, 1893), and again in the early 1980s (Crick, 1982), yet it wasn't until the application of time-lapse imaging of fluorescently labeled living neurons in the mid-1990s that it was definitively demonstrated that spines were continuously emerging, retracting, and changing shape (Dailey and Smith, 1996; Ziv and Smith, 1996). These early live imaging studies examined fluorescently labeled neurons in dissociated cultures (Ziv and Smith, 1996) or cultured brain slices (Dailey and Smith, 1996) in order to characterize the short-term (minutes to hours) dynamics of dendritic spines. The authors found that spines grew and retracted, lengthened and shortened, and rapidly changed shape. They proposed that this exuberant dendritic motility reflected an active search for presynaptic partners (Ziv and Smith, 1996) and that the generation of new connections during circuit plasticity in the brain involved the emergence and stabilization of these motile structures. Indeed, the extent of spine dynamics decreased as the slices matured (Dailey and Smith, 1996), a trend similar to the decline of plasticity that is observed in the aging brain.

An extensive actin network is one of the hallmarks of dendritic spines (see figure 11.1), and it is the dynamicity of this network which permits spines to rapidly change shape with time scales on the order of seconds to minutes (Matus, 1999; Star et al., 2002). The spine actin network has recently been shown to contain two distinct pools of actin fibers; a stable, slowly treadmilling pool, which tends to stay constant as long as the spine does not retract entirely, and a quickly cycling pool proposed to be the "enlargement" pool, which allows for fast changes in spine size (Honkura et al., 2008). While actin is the dominant cytoskeletal element within spines, recent work has suggested that microtubule invasion does occur infrequently and in response to elevated synaptic activity (Hu et al., 2008; Jaworski et al., 2009). Although these recent experiments suggest a potential specialized role for microtubules in spine morphogenesis, blocking actin dynamics with cytochalasin D, a drug that inhibits actin polymerization, is sufficient to completely block spine motility (Fischer et al., 1998).

The early studies demonstrating spine dynamics were quite convincing and highly regarded; however, skeptics remained concerned that spine motility was an artifact of in vitro preparations and that it would not be observed in the living animal. These criticisms were soon addressed with advanced in vivo imaging approaches using two-photon microscopy (Denk and Svoboda, 1997), which allowed high-resolution imaging of these tiny structures deep within brain tissue. The first set of in vivo imaging experiments (Lendvai et al., 2000) examined dendrites of neurons in the somatosensory cortex of young rats infected with sindbis virus expressing green fluorescent protein (GFP). The authors demonstrated that spines were indeed actively undergoing morphological plasticity over minutes to hours in the living animal. In addition, spine motility decreased as the animals grew older, corroborating the decline of motility observed as slices matured, and once again in parallel with the decrease in plasticity observed upon aging.

This remarkable finding that spines are moving acutely in the brain inspired further characterization of spine morphological changes over longer time intervals. Chronic imaging approaches were developed that allowed repeated imaging of the same dendrites over the course of days, weeks, and even months (Grutzendler et al., 2002; Trachtenberg et al., 2002). These experiments utilized transgenic animals expressing GFP in a subset of cortical pyramidal neurons (Feng et al., 2000), avoiding negative side effects associated with long-term viral infection of neurons. Remarkably, both studies observed that spines appeared and disappeared throughout the lifetime of the animal. However, there were dramatic differences between the studies concerning the extent of spine motility in vivo. Trachtenberg and colleagues observed that only about 50% of spines persisted for one month in the young adult, whereas the remainder were transient, mostly living less than one day (Trachtenberg et al., 2002). They suggested that persistent spines represent elements of established neural circuitry whereas transient spines represent substrates for new synaptic connections during brain plasticity. In contrast, Grutzendler and colleagues observed that approximately 73% of spines in young animals and approximately 96% of spines

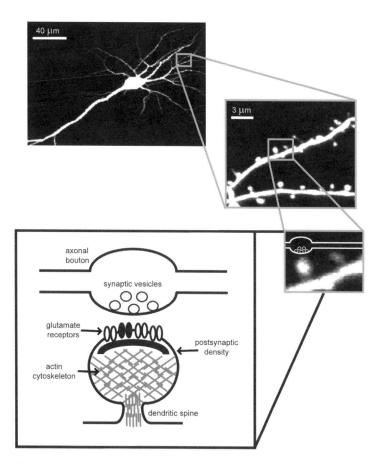

Figure 11.1
Structure of a dendritic spine. Images of dendrites and dendritic spines from a GFP-labeled hippocampal pyramidal neuron and a schematic of a spine synapse. The archetypal dendritic spine is a bulbous extension of the dendritic cytoplasm, with volumes ranging from $0.001–1\ \mu m^3$, connected to the dendrite by a thin neck (diameter $\sim 0.1\ \mu m$), which serves to isolate the spine head from the dendritic shaft. Ultrastructurally, a spine synapse is typically defined by three components: (1) a presynaptic axonal bouton with synaptic vesicles separated by (2) a thin synaptic cleft (~ 20 nm) from (3) a dendritic spine containing an electron dense mass known as the postsynaptic density, or PSD.

in the adult remained stable over a one-month interval (Grutzendler et al., 2002), suggesting a much lower level of plasticity.

The large discrepancy in the spine turnover rates observed by the two studies stirred quite a controversy. However, it is important to note that there were a number of major differences in experimental design between the two initial chronic imaging studies from the Gan and Svoboda labs. First, the laboratories employed different techniques to access the brain for in vivo imaging—the Gan lab used a "thinned-skull" approach, in which a dental drill is used to thin the skull before imaging, while the Svoboda lab replaced a portion of the skull with a glass coverslip, or a "cranial window." Claims were made that use of a cranial window for in vivo imaging is associated with high spine turnover because of activation of microglia after surgery (Xu et al., 2007), although these claims have been disputed (Holtmaat et al., 2009). Second, the Gan lab imaged mainly in the visual cortex, which some studies find to be less plastic than the somatosensory cortex (Holtmaat et al., 2005; Majewska et al., 2006), although other studies find no major differences (Zuo et al., 2005a). Other possible reasons for the discrepancies include different housing environments for the mice, different visibility of spines under the two imaging conditions, and different cell types (layer V versus layer VI pyramidal neurons). Despite all of the controversy, it was an enormous step forward to observe that spines were indeed "twitching" in the adult brain.

Does Sensory Experience Influence Spine Motility?

Changes in dendritic spine densities and morphologies have long been shown to increase or to decrease in response to various environmental stimuli (reviewed by Yuste and Bonhoeffer, 2001). For example, hibernating squirrels lose 40% of their spines, which they regain within a few hours after emerging from hibernation (Popov and Bocharova, 1992). Spine densities are reduced by light deprivation in mice (Valverde, 1967) and increased by visual stimulation (Parnavelas et al., 1973). Most profoundly, animals exposed to enriched environments show altered spine morphologies and, at the same time, these animals are better at solving spatial memory tasks (Greenough and Volkmar, 1973). These studies strongly suggested that sensory experience influences spine motility, yet they were all static snapshots and therefore did not address the acute influence of experience on spine morphogenesis, which requires in vivo imaging of living neurons in behaving animals.

The first thrilling glimpses that sensory experience can influence spine motility in vivo were from the somatosensory cortex of mice. Using in vivo two-photon time-lapse imaging, Lendvai and colleagues demonstrated that spine motility in the somatosensory cortex, but not in neighboring cortical areas, declined in response to sensory deprivation (Lendvai et al., 2000). These studies monitored alterations in spine length over time after clipping all whiskers. Further experiments using a more complex checkerboard whisker clipping pattern (designed to induce maximal plasticity throughout the somatosensory cortex) demonstrated that both growth and retraction, or "turnover," of spines was increased in response to checkerboard whisker clipping, which also induced circuit plasticity as assessed electrophysiologically (Trachtenberg et al., 2002). This adaptive circuit plasticity was accompanied both by increases in the occurrence of new persistent spines, thought to represent new circuit connections, and by loss of preexisting persistent spines, presumed to represent the loss of old circuits (Holtmaat et al., 2006). Finally, Zuo and colleagues examined the effects of trimming all whiskers on spine turnover in vivo (Zuo et al., 2005b). They found that whisker clipping reduced spine loss without affecting spine growth; the reduction in spine loss was abrogated when whiskers were allowed to regrow. Remarkably, a reduction in the rate of spine loss could also be induced simply by infusing drugs that block N-methyl-D-aspartate (NMDA) receptors, and reversed after drug withdrawal, suggesting a role for the NMDA receptor in translating sensory experience into changes in rates of spine morphogenesis.

The visual cortex has also provided a great resource for defining the influence of sensory experience on spine motility in vivo. In a challenging set of experiments designed to link functional plasticity and specific arrangements of dendritic spines, Hofer and colleagues demonstrated that monocular deprivation, which biases electrophysiological responses in the binocular region of the primary visual cortex toward the open eye, increased the rate of spine formation on apical dendrites of layer V cells, leading to an increase in spine density (Hofer et al., 2009). Restoring binocular vision restored the electrophysiological responses and the rate of spine formation to normal levels; however, spine densities remained elevated. Remarkably, spine addition did not increase a second time when the same eye was closed again even though the electrophysiological responses shifted again and even more rapidly. The authors suggested that those spines added during the first monocular deprivation provide a structural basis for subsequent functional shifts (Hofer et al., 2009), a phenomenon resembling that described for axonal growth during auditory map plasticity in the barn owl (Knudsen, 2002).

Another extraordinary set of experiments in the visual cortex helped to define a role for the extracellular matrix (ECM) in regulating the spine structural changes induced by experience. Mataga and colleagues demonstrated that targeted disruption of the tissue-type plasminogen activator (tPA) prevented spine loss on apical dendrites of layer II/III cells induced by monocular deprivation (Mataga et al., 2004). Because proteolysis by tPA increased with monocular deprivation and declined with age (Mataga et al., 2002), this result was interpreted to mean that proteolysis by tPA is permissive for dendritic spine plasticity and that, in the absence of tPA in older animals, the ECM encapsulates the spine and physically blocks plasticity (Berardi et al., 2004; Mataga et al., 2004). Such a model suggested that removing the ECM might lead to increased plasticity. Indeed, in vitro experiments demonstrated that spine motility increased in response to tPA application (Oray et al., 2004). And, in a tour de force set of experiments performed by Maffei and colleagues, in vivo application of chondroitinase ABC, an enzyme that digests the ECM, restored robust visual cortical plasticity to adult animals that would normally exhibit very little plasticity (Pizzorusso et al., 2002). The same authors showed that chondroitinase ABC application, when combined with reverse lid suturing immediately following monocular deprivation, caused a complete recovery of ocular dominance and dendritic spine densities to normal levels (Pizzorusso et al., 2006). These amazing results suggest that targeted degradation of the extracellular matrix might provide a way to restore plasticity in older animals.

What Are the Patterns of Activity That Induce Spine Morphogenesis?

What are the specific patterns of activity that lead to spine morphological plasticity in response to experience? Because experience-dependent plasticity in brain circuitry is thought to occur via associative, synapse-specific changes, a remarkable breakthrough came when spine morphogenesis was shown to be evoked by synaptic activity paradigms that induce associative plasticity. The first of these studies came out in the late 1990s (Engert and Bonhoeffer, 1999; Maletic-Savatic et al., 1999). Despite using very different techniques to locally stimulate dendrites with activity patterns known to induce synaptic strengthening (long-term potentiation, or LTP), both studies observed increased rates of spine outgrowth in stimulated dendritic regions, but not in unstimulated regions on the same neuron. This outgrowth was inhibited by NMDA receptor blockers, which also inhibit synaptic strengthening. In a complementary study, local stimulation in patterns that induce synaptic weakening (long-term depression, or LTD) was shown to decrease synaptic strength and cause spine shrinkage (Zhou et al., 2004), which was inhibited by NMDA receptor blockers. Thus, the NMDA receptor and Hebbian mechanisms of synaptic plasticity appear to play key roles in the induction of spine morphological plasticity.

That spines grew and shrank in response to local stimulation in patterns that induced synaptic strengthening and weakening was indeed remarkable; however, stimulation with local microelectrodes was not restricted to individual spine synapses. Therefore, whether such spine morphological plasticity is input-specific remained unanswered until the development of caged glutamate with a suitable two-photon cross section (Matsuzaki et al., 2001). In a series of elegant experiments using two-photon photolysis of caged glutamate at single spines in patterns that induced synaptic strengthening, Matsuzaki and colleagues demonstrated that individual stimulated spines, and not neighboring unstimulated spines, grew in volume as spine synapses increased in strength (Matsuzaki et al., 2004). This growth in spine volume was dependent on NMDA receptors, calmodulin, and actin polymerization. In a later study, the same authors demonstrated that long-term spine enlargement also depends on protein synthesis and brain-derived neurotrophic factor action (Tanaka et al., 2008). Thus, spine morphological plasticity can be induced in an input-specific manner and shares many molecular mechanisms with LTP and LTD.

Is spine morphological plasticity always input-specific? A series of very challenging experiments demonstrated that there is cross talk between spine synapses. The induction of LTP and spine growth at an individual spine using two-photon glutamate uncaging caused nearby spines (within ten microns) along the dendrite to be more receptive to synaptic strengthening using a normally subthreshold LTP-inducing protocol (Harvey and Svoboda, 2007). In a subsequent study, Harvey and colleagues showed that induction of LTP at a single spine caused the spread of activated Ras, a small GTPase signaling protein, along the dendrite for up to ten microns, and that blocking Ras signaling prevented the reduction in LTP threshold (Harvey et al., 2008), suggesting a critical role for Ras in cross-talk between neighboring synapses. Indeed, in the area surrounding activated spines, the likelihood of new spine appearance is increased (De Roo et al., 2008). These findings suggest that the formation of dendritic spines may be potentiated around sites of high synaptic activity.

Despite all of the success at inducing spine growth and shrinkage in response to glutamate uncaging stimuli, as of yet, de novo spine outgrowth or spine retraction in response to glutamate uncaging has not been reported, and the repertoire of patterns of activity responsible for the de novo gain and complete loss of spines remains somewhat of a mystery.

Do Changes in Spine Shape Reflect Changes in Spine Function?

Spines grow and retract in response to experience, but are these changes in spine morphology functionally relevant? Many neurological diseases resulting in mental retardation have been associated with spine loss or spine morphology changes (Fiala et al., 2002); however, whether these changes are causative or a consequence of the disease is not yet clear. Because almost all spines (approximately 96%) in the adult animal serve as the receiving half of excitatory chemical synapses (Arellano et al., 2007), it is easy to assume that the gain or loss of a spine is associated with the gain or loss of a synapse. However, it could also be that those 4% of spines that were not synapse-associated in the static ultrastructural study are those that are motile in the adult, or, in other words, motile spines don't make synapses and therefore may not have physiological relevance.

One very convincing method to address this question is using in vivo time-lapse two-photon microscopy to identify new spines followed by retrospective serial section electron microscopy (SSEM) to identify whether new spines are synapse associated (Knott et al., 2006; Trachtenberg et al., 2002). Trachtenberg and colleagues reconstructed four spines that were each less than one day old and found that two of the four fulfilled the expectations of a spine synapse; they contacted presynaptic boutons and were apposed to active zones containing clusters of synaptic vesicles. Similar results were obtained in vitro using retrospective SSEM on new spines that grew in response to local high-frequency stimulation (Nagerl et al., 2007). Thus, new spines in the adult brain can form synapses in less than one day from their time of initial emergence. Further studies provided convincing arguments that these new spines were formed de novo and not from preexisting shaft synapses (Knott et al., 2006), thus suggesting that these new spines are integrated into new circuit connections that represent functional circuit plasticity.

New spines can make anatomically mature synapses as assessed by ultrastructural studies, but are newly formed spines functional? Can they receive signals from a presynaptic terminal? Zito and colleagues combined time-lapse imaging to identify spines of different ages with whole-cell recording to measure the responses of new spines and their neighbors to two-photon glutamate uncaging (Zito et al., 2009). They found that new spines expressed glutamate sensitive currents that were indistinguishable from mature spines of comparable volumes. Some spines exhibited negligible AMPA receptor–mediated responses, but the occurrence of these "silent" spines was uncorrelated with spine age. Instead, new spines rapidly accumulated glutamate receptors, within tens of minutes of the time of emergence. In addition, newly emerged spines have been shown to exhibit calcium transients shortly following their appearance (De Roo et al., 2008; Lohmann and Bonhoeffer, 2008). Thus, newly emerged spines rapidly become functional. However, despite these exciting and provocative studies, the time frame within which new spine synapses become functionally relevant for neural circuits remains to be determined.

Experience-dependent spine plasticity can also involve more subtle morphological changes in spine shape. Recent data support that these smaller changes in spine shape could also be functionally relevant. Ultrastructural studies have demonstrated that spine volume, postsynaptic density size, and AMPA receptor content are highly correlated (Harris and Stevens, 1989; Kharazia and Weinberg, 1999; Nusser et al., 1998), suggesting that spine volume should be an accurate indicator of synaptic strength. Indeed, functional studies using two-photon glutamate uncaging demonstrated that the amplitude of excitatory postsynaptic currents at individual spines is proportional to spine volume (Matsuzaki et al., 2001) and that increases in synaptic strength at individual dendritic spines are proportional to spine volume increases (Matsuzaki et al., 2004). Additional studies using local synaptic stimulation found similar results showing that increases and decreases in synaptic strength are associated with increases and decreases in spine volume in the stimulated regions of dendrite and not in unstimulated regions (Bastrikova et al., 2008; Becker et al., 2008; Wang et al., 2007; Yang et al., 2008; Zhou et al., 2004). Finally, even subtle anatomical changes, like increases in spine neck resistance, are likely to have large effects on spine signaling properties and have been shown to be associated with long-term potentiation (Bloodgood and Sabatini, 2005). In sum, even small changes in spine shape are functionally relevant.

Do Spine Morphological Changes Underlie Experience-Dependent Changes in Neuronal Circuits?

The past decade has been a remarkable time for defining the role of dendritic spines in adaptive plasticity in the brain. The experiments described in this chapter demonstrated that spines are motile in vivo, that the rate of spine motility can be modulated by experience, and that changes in spine morphology represent functional changes in synapses. These studies provide strong support for the hypothesis that spine morphological changes underlie experience-dependent changes in neuronal circuits. However, several key questions remain. Are new spine synapses generated in the adult functionally relevant and integrated into neuronal circuits utilized in the intact organism? Is spine motility necessary for circuit plasticity? And finally, will increasing spine motility in adults reactivate plasticity mechanisms that could enable recovery from damage to the central nervous system? These and other key questions related to the molecular mechanisms of spine synapse plasticity will no doubt be the focus of intense investigation in the decade to come.

Acknowledgments

This work was supported by a National Institutes of Health training grant (T32GM007377 to A.H.), a Burroughs Wellcome Fund Career Award in the Biomedical Sciences (K.Z.), and an NSF CAREER Award (K.Z.).

References

Arellano JI, Espinosa A, Fairen A, Yuste R, DeFelipe J. 2007. Non-synaptic dendritic spines in neocortex. *Neuroscience* 145: 464–469.

Bastrikova N, Gardner GA, Reece JM, Jeromin A, Dudek SM. 2008. Synapse elimination accompanies functional plasticity in hippocampal neurons. *Proc Natl Acad Sci USA* 105: 3123–3127.

Becker N, Wierenga CJ, Fonseca R, Bonhoeffer T, Nagerl UV. 2008. LTD induction causes morphological changes of presynaptic boutons and reduces their contacts with spines. *Neuron* 60: 590–597.

Berardi N, Pizzorusso T, Maffei L. 2004. Extracellular matrix and visual cortical plasticity: freeing the synapse. *Neuron* 44: 905–908.

Bloodgood BL, Sabatini BL. 2005. Neuronal activity regulates diffusion across the neck of dendritic spines. *Science* 310: 866–869.

Cajal, S. Ramon Y. (1893). Neue Darstellung vom histologischen Bau des Zentralnervensystem. *Arch Anat Entwick* 319–428.

Crick F. 1982. Do dendritic spines twitch? *Trends Neurosci* 5: 44–46.

Dailey ME, Smith SJ. 1996. The dynamics of dendritic structure in developing hippocampal slices. *J Neurosci* 16: 2983–2994.

De Roo M, Klauser P, Mendez P, Poglia L, Muller D. 2008. Activity-dependent PSD formation and stabilization of newly formed spines in hippocampal slice cultures. *Cereb Cortex* 18: 151–161.

Denk W, Svoboda K. 1997. Photon upmanship: why multiphoton imaging is more than a gimmick. *Neuron* 18: 351–357.

Engert F, Bonhoeffer T. 1999. Dendritic spine changes associated with hippocampal long-term synaptic plasticity. *Nature* 399: 66–70.

Feng G, Mellor RH, Bernstein M, Keller-Peck C, Nguyen QT, Wallace M, Nerbonne JM, Lichtman JW, Sanes JR. 2000. Imaging neuronal subsets in transgenic mice expressing multiple spectral variants of GFP. *Neuron* 28: 41–51.

Fiala JC, Spacek J, Harris KM. 2002. Dendritic spine pathology: cause or consequence of neurological disorders? *Brain Res Brain Res Rev* 39: 29–54.

Fischer M, Kaech S, Knutti D, Matus A. 1998. Rapid actin-based plasticity in dendritic spines. *Neuron* 20: 847–854.

Greenough WT, Volkmar FR. 1973. Pattern of dendritic branching in occipital cortex of rats reared in complex environments. *Exp Neurol* 40: 491–504.

Grutzendler J, Kasthuri N, Gan WB. 2002. Long-term dendritic spine stability in the adult cortex. *Nature* 420: 812–816.

Harris KM, Stevens JK. 1989. Dendritic spines of CA 1 pyramidal cells in the rat hippocampus: serial electron microscopy with reference to their biophysical characteristics. *J Neurosci* 9: 2982–2997.

Harvey CD, Svoboda K. 2007. Locally dynamic synaptic learning rules in pyramidal neuron dendrites. *Nature* 450: 1195–1200.

Harvey CD, Yasuda R, Zhong H, Svoboda K. 2008. The spread of Ras activity triggered by activation of a single dendritic spine. *Science* 321: 136–140.

Hofer SB, Mrsic-Flogel TD, Bonhoeffer T, Hubener M. 2009. Experience leaves a lasting structural trace in cortical circuits. *Nature* 457: 313–317.

Holtmaat A, Bonhoeffer T, Chow DK, Chuckowree J, De Paola V, Hofer SB, Hubener M, et al. 2009. Long-term, high-resolution imaging in the mouse neocortex through a chronic cranial window. *Nat Protoc* 4: 1128–1144.

Holtmaat A, Wilbrecht L, Knott GW, Welker E, Svoboda K. 2006. Experience-dependent and cell-type-specific spine growth in the neocortex. *Nature* 441: 979–983.

Holtmaat AJ, Trachtenberg JT, Wilbrecht L, Shepherd GM, Zhang X, Knott GW, Svoboda K. 2005. Transient and persistent dendritic spines in the neocortex in vivo. *Neuron* 45: 279–291.

Honkura N, Matsuzaki M, Noguchi J, Ellis-Davies GC, Kasai H. 2008. The subspine organization of actin fibers regulates the structure and plasticity of dendritic spines. *Neuron* 57: 719–729.

Hu X, Viesselmann C, Nam S, Merriam E, Dent EW. 2008. Activity-dependent dynamic microtubule invasion of dendritic spines. *J Neurosci* 28: 13094–13105.

Jaworski J, Kapitein LC, Gouveia SM, Dortland BR, Wulf PS, Grigoriev I, Camera P, et al. 2009. Dynamic microtubules regulate dendritic spine morphology and synaptic plasticity. *Neuron* 61: 85–100.

Kharazia VN, Weinberg RJ. 1999. Immunogold localization of AMPA and NMDA receptors in somatic sensory cortex of albino rat. *J Comp Neurol* 412: 292–302.

Knott GW, Holtmaat A, Wilbrecht L, Welker E, Svoboda K. 2006. Spine growth precedes synapse formation in the adult neocortex in vivo. *Nat Neurosci* 9: 1117–1124.

Knudsen EI. 2002. Instructed learning in the auditory localization pathway of the barn owl. *Nature* 417: 322–328.

Lendvai B, Stern EA, Chen B, Svoboda K. 2000. Experience-dependent plasticity of dendritic spines in the developing rat barrel cortex in vivo. *Nature* 404: 876–881.

Lohmann C, Bonhoeffer T. 2008. A role for local calcium signaling in rapid synaptic partner selection by dendritic filopodia. *Neuron* 59: 253–260.

Majewska AK, Newton JR, Sur M. 2006. Remodeling of synaptic structure in sensory cortical areas in vivo. *J Neurosci* 26: 3021–3029.

Maletic-Savatic M, Malinow R, Svoboda K. 1999. Rapid dendritic morphogenesis in CA1 hippocampal dendrites induced by synaptic activity. *Science* 283: 1923–1927.

Mataga N, Mizuguchi Y, Hensch TK. 2004. Experience-dependent pruning of dendritic spines in visual cortex by tissue plasminogen activator. *Neuron* 44: 1031–1041.

Mataga N, Nagai N, Hensch TK. 2002. Permissive proteolytic activity for visual cortical plasticity. *Proc Natl Acad Sci USA* 99: 7717–7721.

Matsuzaki M, Ellis-Davies GC, Nemoto T, Miyashita Y, Iino M, Kasai H. 2001. Dendritic spine geometry is critical for AMPA receptor expression in hippocampal CA1 pyramidal neurons. *Nat Neurosci* 4: 1086–1092.

Matsuzaki M, Honkura N, Ellis-Davies GC, Kasai H. 2004. Structural basis of long-term potentiation in single dendritic spines. *Nature* 429: 761–766.

Matus A. 1999. Postsynaptic actin and neuronal plasticity. *Curr Opin Neurobiol* 9: 561–565.

Nagerl UV, Kostinger G, Anderson JC, Martin KA, Bonhoeffer T. 2007. Protracted synaptogenesis after activity-dependent spinogenesis in hippocampal neurons. *J Neurosci* 27: 8149–8156.

Nusser Z, Lujan R, Laube G, Roberts JD, Molnar E, Somogyi P. 1998. Cell type and pathway dependence of synaptic AMPA receptor number and variability in the hippocampus. *Neuron* 21: 545–559.

Oray S, Majewska A, Sur M. 2004. Dendritic spine dynamics are regulated by monocular deprivation and extracellular matrix degradation. *Neuron* 44: 1021–1030.

Parnavelas JG, Globus A, Kaups P. 1973. Continuous illumination from birth affects spine density of neurons in the visual cortex of the rat. *Exp Neurol* 40: 742–747.

Pizzorusso T, Medini P, Berardi N, Chierzi S, Fawcett JW, Maffei L. 2002. Reactivation of ocular dominance plasticity in the adult visual cortex. *Science* 298: 1248–1251.

Pizzorusso T, Medini P, Landi S, Baldini S, Berardi N, Maffei L. 2006. Structural and functional recovery from early monocular deprivation in adult rats. *Proc Natl Acad Sci USA* 103: 8517–8522.

Popov VI, Bocharova LS. 1992. Hibernation-induced structural changes in synaptic contacts between mossy fibres and hippocampal pyramidal neurons. *Neuroscience* 48: 53–62.

Star EN, Kwiatkowski DJ, Murthy VN. 2002. Rapid turnover of actin in dendritic spines and its regulation by activity. *Nat Neurosci* 5: 239–246.

Tanaka J, Horiike Y, Matsuzaki M, Miyazaki T, Ellis-Davies GC, Kasai H. 2008. Protein synthesis and neurotrophin-dependent structural plasticity of single dendritic spines. *Science* 319: 1683–1687.

Trachtenberg JT, Chen BE, Knott GW, Feng G, Sanes JR, Welker E, Svoboda K. 2002. Long-term in vivo imaging of experience-dependent synaptic plasticity in adult cortex. *Nature* 420: 788–794.

Valverde F. 1967. Apical dendritic spines of the visual cortex and light deprivation in the mouse. *Exp Brain Res* 3: 337–352.

Wang XB, Yang Y, Zhou Q. 2007. Independent expression of synaptic and morphological plasticity associated with long-term depression. *J Neurosci* 27: 12419–12429.

Xu HT, Pan F, Yang G, Gan WB. 2007. Choice of cranial window type for in vivo imaging affects dendritic spine turnover in the cortex. *Nat Neurosci* 10: 549–551.

Yang Y, Wang XB, Frerking M, Zhou Q. 2008. Spine expansion and stabilization associated with long-term potentiation. *J Neurosci* 28: 5740–5751.

Yuste R, Bonhoeffer T. 2001. Morphological changes in dendritic spines associated with long-term synaptic plasticity. *Annu Rev Neurosci* 24: 1071–1089.

Zhou Q, Homma KJ, Poo MM. 2004. Shrinkage of dendritic spines associated with long-term depression of hippocampal synapses. *Neuron* 44: 749–757.

Zito K, Scheuss V, Knott G, Hill T, Svoboda K. 2009. Rapid functional maturation of nascent dendritic spines. *Neuron* 61: 247–258.

Ziv NE, Smith SJ. 1996. Evidence for a role of dendritic filopodia in synaptogenesis and spine formation. *Neuron* 17: 91–102.

Zuo Y, Lin A, Chang P, Gan WB. 2005a. Development of long-term dendritic spine stability in diverse regions of cerebral cortex. *Neuron* 46: 181–189.

Zuo Y, Yang G, Kwon E, Gan WB. 2005b. Long-term sensory deprivation prevents dendritic spine loss in primary somatosensory cortex. *Nature* 436: 261–265.

.

12 The Glutamate Receptor delta2 Subunit in Cerebellar Wiring

Piergiorgio Strata and Georgia Mandolesi

In the mature cerebellar cortex, Purkinje cell (PC) dendrites are characterized by a proximal and a distal domain. The proximal one is innervated by a single climbing fiber (CF), the terminal arbor of inferior olivary neurons. In the rat each CF arbor has about 300 varicosities and each of them makes contact with a cluster of two to six spines. In contrast, the distal domain of the PC dendrites receives about 200,000 parallel fibers (PFs), the axons of the granule cells (Carulli et al., 2004). PFs and CFs compete for PC innervation, and under normal conditions each input is confined to its own dendritic domain where each of them maintains its unique complement of spines. Such heterologous axonal competition is activity dependent (Cesa and Strata, 2009) and represents an excellent model to study structural plasticity events. A molecule involved in such competition is the glutamate receptor delta2 subunit (GluRδ2).

It seems that GluRδ2, during evolution, has lost its channel function to play the role of an adhesion molecule (Yuzaki, 2004; Mandolesi et al., 2009b; see figure 12.1).

Mice carrying spontaneous mutations or a deficiency of the *grid2* gene, coding for the GluRδ2 protein, show cerebellar ataxia due to severe alterations of the cerebellar circuitry. Although no neurological diseases have so far been genetically linked to this locus in humans, it is very likely that at least one of the many human cerebellar ataxias is due to this gene dysfunction. In fact, first, the human GRID2 gene has a 97% identity in amino acid sequence to the mouse gene; second, recently common fragile sites overlapping the mouse *grid2* and its human ortholog have been identified; and finally, in clinical studies antiglutamate receptor delta-2 auto-antibodies have been detected in the serum and cerebrospinal fluid of patients with acute cerebellar ataxia and have been correlated with the time course of the disease (see review, Mandolesi et al., 2009b).

The GluRδ2 Orphan Receptor: A Unique "iGluR" That Does Not Require Channel Activities and Glutamate Analog Ligands

The GluRδ2 subunit is specifically expressed in PC (Lomeli et al., 1993; Mayat et al., 1995). It has never been detected in the rest of the brain except in a few cells of cochlear nucleus (Mayat et al., 1995; Petralia et al., 2004). During postnatal development, it is targeted to both PF and

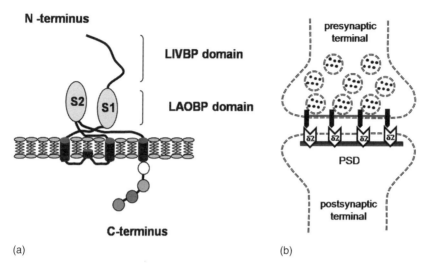

Figure 12.1
Schematic of the glutamate receptor delta2 (GluRδ2) topology and of its role as an adhesion molecule. (a) The GluRδ2 subunit is composed of an N-terminus and a C-terminus domain. The N-terminus contains the LIVBP-like domain and the bipartite LAOBP-like domain, which consists of S1 and S2 regions, the transmembrane TM1, TM3, TM4 domains, and an ion channel forming reentrant loop segment (TM2). The C-terminus domain is divided into four regions (circles). (b) GluRδ2 plays a role in parallel fiber–Purkinje cell synaptogenesis and strengthening. As an adhesion molecule, it may regulate the presynaptic active zone by direct interaction with an active zone component through its N-terminal domain.

CF synapses (Zhao et al., 1998) while in the mature cerebellum it remains only in the distal dendritic compartment of the PC at the PF synapses (Landsend et al., 1997).

The role of the GluRδ2 subunit remains the most puzzling enigma within the ionotropic glutamate receptor family. Despite its high homology with the other iGluR subunits, it is still unclear whether GluRδ2 serves as ion channels *in vivo*. It seems that it does not require ion channel activities or binding to glutamate analogs to achieve its major functions at PF–PC synapses (Yuzaki, 2005). To date, endogenous ligands that modulate the activity of native GluRδ2 in the cerebellum have not been identified. However, taking advantage of the crystallographic structure of GluRδ2 agonist binding domain, two candidate modulators have been recently proposed, D-serine and extracellular calcium (Hansen et al., 2009). Moreover, it has been shown by means of ligand binding domain transplantation that GluRδ2 is capable of gating its intrinsic ion channel (Schmid et al., 2009). Therefore, GluRδ2 function might be controlled by proteins, not yet characterized, that are required to make the GluRδ2 receptor responsive to agonists. On other hand, Torashima et al. (2009) recently produced a GluRδ2 deletion construct that lacks both the ion channel structure and the ligand binding domains and consisted only of the N-terminal domain, one transmembrane domain, and the C-terminus. Such construct is able to rescue the abnormal phenotypes in GluRδ2-deficient mice (Torashima et al., 2009) suggesting ion-channel unrelated functions by which GluRδ2 regulates cerebellar functions. These observations support previous experiments obtained by means of a transgenic rescue approach (Yuzaki, 2005). In conclusion, a debate is still open regarding the ion-channel function of the GluRδ2 subunit.

Finally, the majority of studies on GluRδ2 focused on its metabotropic function; in fact, intracellular signals mediated by the C-terminus are critical to the induction of long-term depression and motor learning (Yuzaki, 2004).

GluRδ2 Is an Adhesion Molecule Involved in Parallel Fiber Synaptogenesis: In Vitro and in Vivo Models

In the last year, several papers have been published almost simultaneously to demonstrate the "adhesive" role of the GluRδ2 subunit by applying different and complementary approaches (Uemura and Mishina, 2008; Kuroyanagi et al., 2009; Mandolesi et al., 2009a; Kakegawa et al., 2009). Observations derived from GluRδ2-null mice (i.e., hotfoot and knockout mice) that show ataxia and impaired motor learning (Kashiwabuchi et al., 1995; Lalouette et al., 1998; Lalouette et al., 2001) had already suggested such a role. In these mutant mice, although the number of distal spines is unchanged, nearly half of them are free of PF innervations (see figure 12.2). In addition, the PF–PC synapses often present a mismatch between the presynaptic and the post-synaptic area (Guastavino et al., 1990; Lalouette et al., 2001). The same phenotype was also observed in conditional GluRδ2 KO mice, in which GluRδ2 is downregulated by inducible and PC-specific gene targeting (Takeuchi et al., 2005); progressive downregulation of GluRδ2 in the adult cerebellum induces a parallel expansion of the postsynaptic density and a reduction of the presynaptic active zone. Therefore, it has been suggested that GluRδ2 is involved in stabilization and strengthening of synaptic connectivity between PFs and PCs.

Coculture of HEK293 Cells and Cerebellar Granule Cells

A first evidence demonstrating the adhesive role of GluRδ2 comes from in vitro culture experiments. Ectopic expression of GluRδ2 in nonneuronal cells, such as HEK293 cells, when cultured in vitro together with cerebellar granule cells, induces granule axons to form junctions that have synapselike properties (Uemura and Mishina, 2008; Kuroyanagi et al., 2009; Mandolesi et al., 2009a). Uemura and Mishina (2008) first observed that the N-terminal domain of GluRδ2 was directly involved in stimulating these effects. Accordingly, Kuroyanagi et al. (2009) demonstrated that GluRδ2 and also its homologue GluRδ1 contribute to establishment of synaptic transmission. In a similar in vitro assay, Mandolesi et al. (2009a) have performed ultrastructural analysis of these contacts by comparing those formed on HEK293 cells expressing GluRδ2 with those on HEK293 cells expressing green fluorescent protein as control (see figure 12.3).

At ultrastructural level the granule axon terminals in culture had two distinct morphological features: first, "round terminals" having the classical profile of presynaptic terminal boutons, with comparable minor and major axes lengths and the absence of cytoskeletal elements, whose density was significantly high in the presence of GluRδ2, and, second, "elongations" that

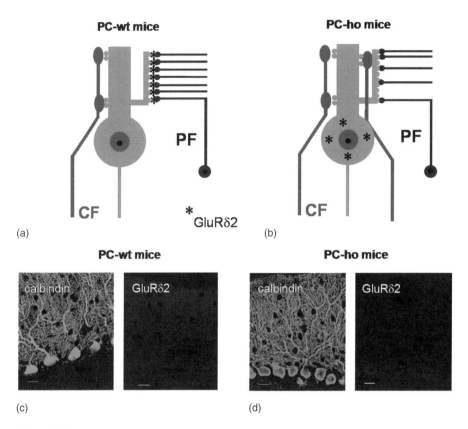

Figure 12.2
A loss of function mutation of the *grid2* gene alters the cerebellar circuitry. (a, b) Schematic representations of Purkinje cell (PC) dendritic compartments and the corresponding glutamatergic inputs in adult wild type (wt, panel a) and hotfoot (ho, panel b) mice. In the wt mice glutamate receptor delta2 (GluRδ2) (*) is targeted to the PC spines of the distal dendritic domain that is innervated by the parallel fiber (PF) input. PCs also receive inputs from climbing fibers (CFs) that abut clusters of spines in the proximal dendritic compartment. In the ho mice, the mutated GluRδ2 protein is retained in the PC soma. PC has free spines in the distal dendritic domain due to a loss of PF innervation, which indicates dysfunctional adhesion. As a consequence, there is a persistence of multiple CF innervation in the mature cerebellum and an extension of the CFs into the distal dendritic compartment. (c, d) Immunostaining of PCs labeled with anti-calbindin (left) and anti-GluRδ2 (right) antibodies in wt mice (c) and ho mice (d). In the ho mice the GluRδ2 truncated protein is retained in the PC soma (d, right panel). Scale bars: c, d = 20 μm. Panels c, d are modified from Mandolesi et al. (2009a).

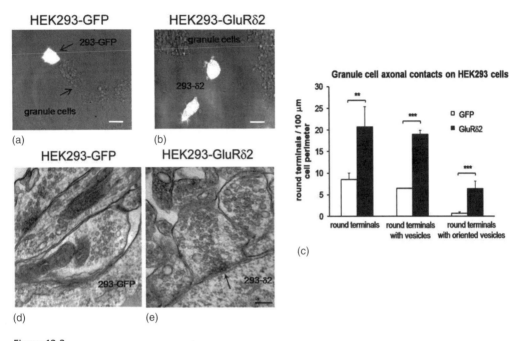

Figure 12.3
Glutamate receptor delta2 (GluRδ2) expressed by HEK293 promotes formation and differentiation of granule cell (GC) axonal contacts. (a, b) Merge of light microphotographs of GCs in coculture with fluorescent 293 cells expressing green fluorescent protein (GFP) alone (a) or GluRδ2 and GFP (b). (c) Electron microscopy (EM) quantitative analysis of the GC axonal contacts on the 293 cell perimeter. The 293-GluRδ2 cells (black bars) are in contact with a higher number of GC round terminals relative to the control (white bars); in both groups, most of the round terminals contained vesicles. In the 293-GluRδ2 cells, more terminals with vesicles oriented toward the postsynaptic membrane were observed. (d, e) EM images of differentiation of the presynaptic GC terminals induced by 293-GluRδ2 cells. (d) Contact between 293-GFP cell and a round GC terminal containing homogeneously distributed vesicles. (e) A 293-GluRδ2 cell contacted by round GC terminal containing oriented vesicles; the arrow indicates the vesicle cluster. Scale bars: a, b = 20 μm; d, e = 0.25 μm. ***p, .001; **p, .01. All panels are modified from Mandolesi et al. (2009a).

are morphologically similar to en passant fibers, whose density was similar in both samples (Mandolesi et al., 2009a). The round terminals have been classified into two types: those with homogeneous vesicle distribution and those that have vesicles oriented toward HEK293 cell membranes. Only the latter type had a higher density in the HEK293–GluRδ2 cells relative to control. In conclusion, GluRδ2 expression in nonneuronal cells not only triggers the formation of contacts with granule cell axons but interactions with an unknown presynaptic protein regulate vesicle clustering.

PF Synaptogenesis in an in Vivo Model: Purkinje Cells and Golgi Cells

With respect to Purkinje cells: the adhesive property of GluRδ2 has also been investigated in vivo. Mandolesi et al. (2009a) found that GluRδ2 alone induces PF synaptic contacts in the distal dendritic compartment of PC-ho mice. In particular, by means of a lentiviral technology, it has been observed that GluRδ2 expression in the distal compartment of the PC dendrite induces the complete recovery of PF contacts in the mature cerebellum of ho-mice (see figure 12.4). Kakegawa et al. (2009) recently supported these in vivo observations by means of electrophysiological and electron microscopy studies.

With respect to Golgi cells: PFs innervate the PC distal dendritic compartments, but they also make contact with stellate, basket, and Golgi interneurons in the molecular layer of the cerebellar cortex. These inhibitory neurons do not express GluRδ2, but their dendrites receive synaptic contacts by PFs on several short neckless spines and on the dendritic shaft (Palay and Chan-Palay, 1974; Castejon and Castejon, 2000; Dieudonne, 1998). Therefore, they represent an ideal recipient cell type to test whether an induced expression of GluRδ2 is able to modify the PF input.

While transfecting PCs of hotfoot mice with a lentivirus carrying the GluRδ2 cDNA under the control of a truncated form of the Pcp2-L7 promoter, Mandolesi et al. (2009a) found serendipitously that Golgi cells also express GluRδ2. This protein was present along the entire Golgi cell dendrite both on spine and on shaft. A location of GluRδ2 in the smooth region of PC dendrites has been recently demonstrated by Cesa et al. (2008) in wild type mice following a prolonged block of electrical activity. GluRδ2 is located in postsynaptic densities together with GluR1 receptors, and these postsynaptic densities are innervated by PFs. By confocal analysis, Mandolesi et al. (2009a) found that GluRδ2 expression in Golgi cells did not increase the number of dendritic spines, but there was a two-fold increase in the number of PF synaptic contacts.

These results strongly suggest that the presence of the GluRδ2 is sufficient to induce the formation of new PF contacts also in cells different from the PCs and further support the concept of a specific interaction between the receptor subunit and the PFs.

GluRδ2 and Heterologous Axonal Competition

Loss of function of the GluRδ2 is accompanied by persistence of multiple CF innervation in the mature cerebellum (Kashiwabuchi et al., 1995; see figure 12.4) and by the extension of the CFs into the distal dendritic compartment (Ichikawa et al., 2002). The same phenotype exists in precerebellin-null mice. Precerebellin is a granule cell-derived secretory factor that has been proposed to regulate PF–PC synaptic formation and heterosynaptic competition in cooperation with GluRδ2 (Yuzaki, 2009). Therefore, in the distal domain, the presence of PF synapses normally limits the CF territory to PC proximal dendrites.

On the other hand, it is known that a lesion to the inferior olive leads to a remarkable increase of spines in the proximal dendritic domain, and the new spines are innervated by the PFs (Sotelo et al., 1975; Rossi et al., 1991). Since, following inactivation or lesion of the inferior olive, PCs become hyperactive for several weeks, this result might seem in line with the main general view that an increase of neuronal activity promotes spinogenesis. However, a similar hyperspiny transformation is present following block of electrical activity by means of an intraparenchymal

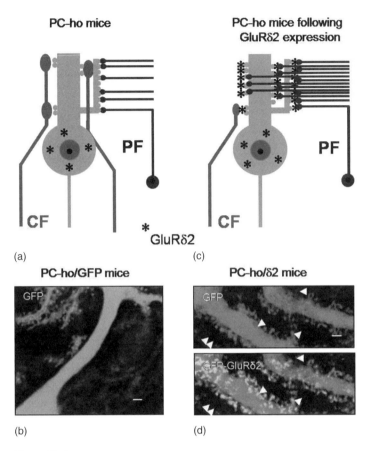

Figure 12.4
Glutamate receptor delta2 (GluRδ2) and cerebellar rewiring. (a) Schematic representation of connection rewiring and Purkinje cell (PC) dendritic changes in ho-mice following lentiviral expression of GluRδ2 (δ2/GFP-ho mice). First, GluRδ2 promotes formation of parallel fiber (PF) contacts in the PC distal domain of δ2/GFP-ho mice. Second, while climbing fiber (CF) terminals undergo marked atrophic changes, numerous new spines appear in the CF compartment and become innervated mainly by PFs; all spines, including those still innervated by the CFs, bear the GluRδ2 subunit. (b–d) Immunostaining of GluRδ2 expression on the PC proximal domain of δ2/GFP-ho mice (d) and GFP-ho mice (b). (d) In the δ2/GFP-ho group, numerous spines (arrowheads) bearing GluRδ2 (white labeling, bottom panel) appear in the proximal domain relative to the control group (b). The PF contacts are more numerous relative to GFP-ho mice (not shown). GFP, green fluorescent protein. Scale bars: b, d = 5 μm. Panels b–d are modified from Mandolesi et al. (2009a).

administration of tetrodotoxin (Bravin et al., 1999), and concomitantly there is a reduction in the number of CF synaptic contacts. Thus, in the absence of activity, the PFs have a competitive advantage. Further, the new proximal spines bear GluRδ2, and, strikingly, this protein appears on the CF synapses and in postsynaptic densities of spines innervated by GABAergic neurons (Morando et al., 2001). Therefore, it has been proposed that GluRδ2 is intrinsically expressed by all PC spines independent of their innervations and that the *active* CFs have a repressive action on PCs spines and on GluRδ2 targeting on their own synapses. Additional experiments have demonstrated that the repressive action is exerted on the postsynaptic dendritic region surrounding their varicosities through ionotropic AMPA receptors thus displacing the PF input (Cesa et al., 2007).

On the whole, in the absence of activity, the PC becomes a uniform territory with a high spine density bearing GluRδ2 subunits and PCs become available to PFs. In the presence of activity, a competition of the two inputs occurs and the *active* CFs are able to acquire and maintain their territory by repressing the PF synapses.

Recently, Mandolesi et al. (2009a) have provided novel evidence that such plastic events occur in mature cerebellar circuitry through changes in GluRδ2 levels in a hotfoot background. In the distal dendritic compartment of ho-PCs, GluRδ2 promotes the recovery of PF contacts, and in the proximal dendritic compartment, spinogenesis develops and the *active* and *intact* CF terminals are displaced. In other words, the pattern of innervations in the PC shifts in favor of the PF input (see figure 12.4).

These experiments suggest that the appearance of GluRδ2 would make CF incompatible with the postsynaptic membrane. This hypothesis is not supported by previous experiments analyzing the distribution of GluRδ2 during the recovery period after removing the electrical block and during the sprouting of the CFs that follows a subtotal lesion of the inferior olive. In these experiments regrowing active CFs are able to establish new synapses with spines bearing GluRδ2 which is later repressed (Cesa et al., 2003).

A second hypothesis that could explain the effects of the GluRδ2 expression is that it interferes with the molecular mechanisms that regulate activity-dependent spines pruning exerted by the CF at the proximal dendrites through ionotropic AMPA/kainate receptors (Cesa et al., 2007). Excess GluRδ2 may shift the generation of tetramer AMPA receptors toward the formation of nonfunctional GluRδ2–AMPA heteromeric channels. This finding is consistent with the observation that GluRδ2, when it assembles in heterologous cells with GluR1 or the kainate receptor GluR6, forms a nonfunctional channel (Kohda et al., 2003). In vivo coimmunoprecipitation experiments demonstrate that endogenous GluRδ2 exists primarily as a homomeric receptor and that at least a portion is closely associated with AMPA or kainate receptors. Similarly, immunogold electron microscopy has revealed that GluRδ2 colocalizes with GluR2/3 in PC spines (Landsend et al., 1997). In conclusion, GluRδ2, by inhibiting the glutamate-induced currents of heteromeric channels (Kohda et al., 2003), may mimic blockage of AMPA receptors (Cesa et al., 2007). As a consequence, the attenuation of CF synapses weakens the repression that they normally exert on the competitor afferent, leading to the emergence of new spines that bear GluRδ2 and the formation of PF synaptic contacts.

Alternatively, GluRδ2 may occupy extrasynaptic regions of CF–PC synapses or the dendritic shaft (Cesa et al., 2008). Because GluRδ2 alone promotes the formation of PF synaptic contacts and PF presynaptic differentiation, we suggest that it generates PF–PC synapses in these compartments. Moreover, GluRδ2 recruits AMPA receptors to the region that faces the active zone by effecting the proper organization of pre- and postsynaptic compartments (Takeuchi et al., 2005). Therefore, in the presence of ectopic PF–PC synapses, competition with the CF inputs is elevated. The PF synapses progressively restrict the surrounding CF territory, and as a consequence, the lateral inhibition that is exerted by the CFs is reduced, intrinsic spinogenesis develops, and new spines that express GluRδ2 result in contact by the PFs.

Conclusion

Regardless of the precise mechanisms by which GluRδ2 exerts its effects, one indisputable role of GluRδ2 is that of an adhesion molecule. By interacting with an unknown ligand, it can induce the formation of PF contacts both in vitro and in vivo independently of its cellular localization. Moreover, GluRδ2 has the potential of inducing plastic events in cerebellar circuitry by promoting heterosynaptic competition in the PC proximal dendritic domain. For this reason, the cerebellar cortex—in particular, the PCs with the PF and CF inputs—tightly regulate GluRδ2 expression and localization to maintain normal architecture under physiological conditions. If its expression is not properly controlled, GluRδ2 effects the formation of excess PF contacts, which is detrimental to cerebellar circuitry.

Dedication

This chapter is dedicated to Lamberto Maffei with whom I (P.S.) shared the best period in the Collegio Medico-Giuridico, now named Collegio Sant'Anna. At that time the College was attached to the Scuola Normale di Pisa, and we were also companions as students in the Medical Faculty of the University. The large community of students made of so many disciplines was astonishingly formative. The rule of the College was to start working in a scientific laboratory from the very beginning. We both were lucky to be admitted in the most prestigious Institute of Physiology under the guidance of Giuseppe Moruzzi, where we stayed together for 20 years. As inexperienced young people, we had to learn a lot of new technologies in electronics and biophysics. After dinner, we often went to the lab to get acclimated to the use of the equipment, discovering how a wave could be modified by passing through a resistance coupled with a capacitance, or assembling single electronic components to generate complex simulation patterns.

I was lucky to share with Lamberto a scientific interest in the activity-dependent plasticity working on two different models, the visual cortex and the cerebellum, an interest supported for many years by European and national grants.

I enjoyed with Lamberto and Giovanni Berlucchi a lot of common activities, a trio tied by a long-lasting friendship. I cannot forget the warm hospitality of his parents in his house in Lucca and the modest quality of our tennis matches without its being possible to tell which of us was better.

The authorship of this chapter is shared with G.M., a former student of Lamberto and at present one of my best collaborators.

Acknowledgments

This work was supported by grants from the Italian Space Agency, the Italian Ministry of Universities and Research, the Ministry of Health, the European Community (contract number 512039), Regione Piemonte, and the Compagnia San Paolo Foundation.

References

Bravin M, Morando L, Vercelli A, Rossi F, Strata P. 1999. Control of spine formation by electrical activity in the adult rat cerebellum. *Proc Natl Acad Sci USA* 96: 1704–1709.

Carulli D, Buffo A, Strata P. 2004. Reparative mechanisms in the cerebellar cortex. *Prog Neurobiol* 72: 373–398.

Castejon OJ, Castejon HV. 2000. Correlative microscopy of cerebellar Golgi cells. *Biocell* 24: 13–30.

Cesa R, Morando L, Strata P. 2003. Glutamate receptor delta2 subunit in activity-dependent heterologous synaptic competition. *J Neurosci* 23: 2363–2370.

Cesa R, Morando L, Strata P. 2008. Transmitter-receptor mismatch in GABAergic synapses in the absence of activity. *Proc Natl Acad Sci USA* 105: 18988–18993.

Cesa R, Scelfo B, Strata P. 2007. Activity-dependent presynaptic and postsynaptic structural plasticity in the mature cerebellum. *J Neurosci* 27: 4603–4611.

Cesa R, Strata P. 2009. Axonal competition in the synaptic wiring of the cerebellar cortex during development and in the mature cerebellum. *Neuroscience* 162: 624–632.

Dieudonne S. 1998. Submillisecond kinetics and low efficacy of parallel fibre-Golgi cell synaptic currents in the rat cerebellum. *J Physiol* 510: 845–866.

Guastavino JM, Sotelo C, Damez-Kinselle I. 1990. Hot-foot murine mutation: behavioral effects and neuroanatomical alterations. *Brain Res* 523: 199–210.

Hansen KB, Naur P, Kurtkaya NL, Kristensen AS, Gajhede M, Kastrup JS, Traynelis SF. 2009. Modulation of the dimer interface at ionotropic glutamate-like receptor delta2 by D-serine and extracellular calcium. *J Neurosci* 29: 907–917.

Ichikawa R, Miyazaki T, Kano M, Hashikawa T, Tatsumi H, Sakimura K, Mishina M, Inoue Y, Watanabe M. 2002. Distal extension of climbing fiber territory and multiple innervation caused by aberrant wiring to adjacent spiny branchlets in cerebellar Purkinje cells lacking glutamate receptor delta 2. *J Neurosci* 22: 8487–8503.

Kakegawa W, Miyazaki T, Kohda K, Matsuda K, Emi K, Motohashi J, Watanabe M, Yuzaki M. 2009. The N-terminal domain of GluD2 (GluRdelta2) recruits presynaptic terminals and regulates synaptogenesis in the cerebellum in vivo. *J Neurosci* 29: 5738–5748.

Kashiwabuchi N, Ikeda K, Araki K, Hirano T, Shibuki K, Takayama C, Inoue Y, et al. 1995. Impairment of motor coordination, Purkinje cell synapse formation, and cerebellar long-term depression in GluR delta 2 mutant mice. *Cell* 81: 245–252.

Kohda K, Kamiya Y, Matsuda S, Kato K, Umemori H, Yuzaki M. 2003. Heteromer formation of delta2 glutamate receptors with AMPA or kainate receptors. *Brain Res Mol Brain Res* 110: 27–37.

Kuroyanagi T, Yokoyama M, Hirano T. 2009. Postsynaptic glutamate receptor delta family contributes to presynaptic terminal differentiation and establishment of synaptic transmission. *Proc Natl Acad Sci USA* 106: 4912–4916.

Lalouette A, Guenet JL, Vriz S. 1998. Hotfoot mouse mutations affect the delta 2 glutamate receptor gene and are allelic to lurcher. *Genomics* 50: 9–13.

Lalouette A, Lohof A, Sotelo C, Guenet J, Mariani J. 2001. Neurobiological effects of a null mutation depend on genetic context: comparison between two hotfoot alleles of the delta-2 ionotropic glutamate receptor. *Neuroscience* 105: 443–455.

Landsend AS, Amiry-Moghaddam M, Matsubara A, Bergersen L, Usami S, Wenthold RJ, Ottersen OP. 1997. Differential localization of delta glutamate receptors in the rat cerebellum: coexpression with AMPA receptors in parallel fiber-spine synapses and absence from climbing fiber-spine synapses. *J Neurosci* 17: 834–842.

Lomeli H, Sprengel R, Laurie DJ, Kohr G, Herb A, Seeburg PH, Wisden W. 1993. The rat delta-1 and delta-2 subunits extend the excitatory amino acid receptor family. *FEBS Lett* 315: 318–322.

Mandolesi G, Autuori E, Cesa R, Premoselli F, Cesare P, Strata P. 2009a. GluRdelta2 expression in the mature cerebellum of hotfoot mice promotes parallel fiber synaptogenesis and axonal competition. *PLoS ONE* 4(4): 1–13.

Mandolesi G, Cesa R, Autuori E, Strata P. 2009b. An orphan ionotropic glutamate receptor: the delta2 subunit. *Neuroscience* 158: 67–77.

Mayat E, Petralia RS, Wang YX, Wenthold RJ. 1995. Immunoprecipitation, immunoblotting, and immunocytochemistry studies suggest that glutamate receptor delta subunits form novel postsynaptic receptor complexes. *J Neurosci* 15: 2533–2546.

Morando L, Cesa R, Rasetti R, Harvey R, Strata P. 2001. Role of glutamate delta-2 receptors in activity-dependent competition between heterologous afferent fibers. *Proc Natl Acad Sci USA* 98: 9954–9959.

Palay SL, Chan-Palay V. 1974. *Cerebellar Cortex: Cytology and Organisation.* Berlin: Springer Verlag.

Petralia RS, Sans N, Wang YX, Vissel B, Chang K, Noben-Trauth K, Heinemann SF, Wenthold RJ. 2004. Loss of GLUR2 alpha-amino-3-hydroxy-5-methyl-4-isoxazoleproprionic acid receptor subunit differentially affects remaining synaptic glutamate receptors in cerebellum and cochlear nuclei. *Eur J Neurosci* 19: 2017–2029.

Rossi F, van der Want JJ, Wiklund L, Strata P. 1991. Reinnervation of cerebellar Purkinje cells by climbing fibres surviving a subtotal lesion of the inferior olive in the adult rat. II. Synaptic organization on reinnervated Purkinje cells. *J Comp Neurol* 308: 536–554.

Schmid SM, Kott S, Sager C, Huelsken T, Hollmann M. 2009. The glutamate receptor subunit delta2 is capable of gating its intrinsic ion channel as revealed by ligand binding domain transplantation. *Proc Natl Acad Sci USA* 106: 10320–10325.

Sotelo C, Hillman DE, Zamora AJ, Llinás R. 1975. Climbing fiber deafferentation: its action on Purkinje cell dendritic spines. *Brain Res* 98: 574–581.

Takeuchi T, Miyazaki T, Watanabe M, Mori H, Sakimura K, Mishina M. 2005. Control of synaptic connection by glutamate receptor delta2 in the adult cerebellum. *J Neurosci* 25: 2146–2156.

Torashima T, Iizuka A, Horiuchi H, Mitsumura K, Yamasaki M, Koyama C, Takayama K, Iino M, Watanabe M, Hirai H. 2009. Rescue of abnormal phenotypes in delta2 glutamate receptor-deficient mice by the extracellular N-terminal and intracellular C-terminal domains of the delta2 glutamate receptor. *Eur J Neurosci* 30: 355–365.

Uemura T, Mishina M. 2008. The amino-terminal domain of glutamate receptor delta2 triggers presynaptic differentiation. *Biochem Biophys Res Commun* 377: 1315–1319.

Yuzaki M. 2004. The delta2 glutamate receptor: a key molecule controlling synaptic plasticity and structure in Purkinje cells. *Cerebellum* 3: 89–93.

Yuzaki M. 2005. Transgenic rescue for characterizing orphan receptors: a review of delta2 glutamate receptor. *Transgenic Res* 14: 117–121.

Yuzaki M. 2009. New (but old) molecules regulating synapse integrity and plasticity: Cbln1 and the delta2 glutamate receptor. *Neuroscience* 162: 633–643.

Zhao HM, Wenthold RJ, Petralia RS. 1998. Glutamate receptor targeting to synaptic populations on Purkinje cells is developmentally regulated. *J Neurosci* 18: 5517–5528.

13 Cortex under Construction: Visual Experience and the Development of Direction Selectivity

Ye Li, Stephen D. Van Hooser, Leonard E. White, and David Fitzpatrick

In order to understand and respond to what we see, the visual system must encode multiple spatial and temporal cues in visual scenes; only then can vision successfully guide motor behavior in a profoundly ambiguous visual environment. The neural representation of such cues arises from the highly selective response properties of neurons in the visual pathway. Especially in the primary visual cortex (V1) where visual signals are first processed by cortical circuits, neurons are tuned to different features of visual stimuli, such as position in visual space, spatial frequency, orientation, and direction of motion. For carnivores and primates, neurons with similar preferences are clustered into radial columns, which are systematically distributed across the cortical surface and organized into functional maps. These maps were first characterized nearly 50 years ago using microelectrode recordings (Hubel and Wiesel, 1962). More recently, the activity of neuronal populations has been assessed with optical imaging methods and, now, two-photon imaging of calcium signals. Based on the results of such imaging studies, numerous functional maps have been characterized for the spatial organization of population activity in V1, including maps of visual space, ocular dominance, orientation, and direction preference (Bonhoeffer and Grinvald, 1991; Shmuel and Grinvald, 1996; Weliky et al., 1996; Issa et al., 2000; Swindale, 2000; Blasdel and Campbell, 2001; Bosking et al., 2002; Ohki et al., 2005; Yu et al., 2005). Although the functional significance of these maps is still in debate (Swindale et al., 2000; Chklovskii and Koulakov, 2004; Horton and Adams, 2005; da Costa and Martin, 2010), they have served as useful models for understanding to what extent these highly organized columnar properties in visual cortex are shaped by vision (experience dependent) and to what extent they are determined by endogenous factors (experience independent).

Our present goal is to take up these themes of brain development in early life by reviewing recent studies of a functional map in the visual cortex that has received far less attention than the more familiar maps of ocular dominance and orientation preference: the map of *direction preference*. Direction preference refers to the differential response of neurons in the visual cortex to motion in one direction across visual space. Neurons are commonly considered direction selective if their responses to the preferred direction are at least twice as great as their responses to the opposite direction. Neurons with such properties are organized into a functional map such that each orientation column or stripe is subdivided into a pair of smaller domains that share the same orientation preference but respond best to opposite directions of motion (Shmuel and Grinvald, 1996; Weliky et al., 1996). Direction preference may be distinguished from more familiar receptive field properties in that it neither reflects the anatomical arrangement of inputs from the peripheral sensory organs (as does ocular dominance), nor is it likely a simple product of the spatial organization of afferent inputs (as orientation preference is commonly conceived). Rather, direction preference must result from neural computations that are sensitive to sequence, that is, the spatial and temporal order of dynamic stimuli in the visual environment. We reasoned that the role of visual experience in the development of direction preference might very well be more formative—and possibly even instructive—than in the development of response properties that more directly reflect peripheral anatomy and the spatial arrangement of afferent input. Our studies of direction selectivity and preference demonstrate the profound influence of early sensory experience over the development of neural circuits in the visual system. In many ways, our studies build on the impressive body of work from Lamberto Maffei and his collaborators, whose creativity and insight continues to emphasize the critical role of experience in brain development (Sale et al., 2009).

The Role of Visual Experience in the Formation of Direction Selectivity

Although unit recordings suggest that at least some cortical neurons may be direction selective near the time of eye opening (Hubel and Wiesel, 1963; Saul and Feidler, 2002), several lines of evidence suggest that the mechanisms by which experience impacts the development of direction selectivity are distinct from those that shape other cortical response properties. Thus, it is well established that both neuronal ocular dominance and orientation selectivity—and the associated maps of ocular dominance and orientation preference—are instantiated in visual cortical circuits without the need for visual experience (Hubel and Wiesel, 1963; Chapman and Stryker, 1993; Horton and Hocking, 1996; Chapman et al., 1996; Crowley and Katz, 2000; White et al., 2001). In contrast, several studies now indicate that the emergence of direction selectivity and the cortical map of direction preference are highly dependent upon visual experience in early life. First, strobe rearing, where kittens were deprived of experience with motion, prevents the development of cortical direction-selective responses (Cynader et al., 1976; Pasternak, 1986; Humphrey and Saul, 1998; Humphrey et al., 1998). The psychophysical measurements of these animals also revealed severe abnormalities in visual discriminations based on differences in motion direction despite the fact that these animals displayed nearly normal spatial vision (Pasternak et al., 1985; Pasternak, 1986; Pasternak and Leinen, 1986). Second, rearing kittens with exposure to a single direction of motion results in a significant increase in the percentage of cortical neurons that respond to the experienced direction; these effects are most prominent during an early period of development that precedes the most sensitive period for ocular dominance plasticity (Daw and Wyatt, 1976; Berman and Daw, 1977; Daw et al., 1978). Importantly, results from both strobe rearing and single-direction rearing show the impact of altered early visual experience on the development of direction selectivity. However, these studies were not designed to indicate whether these changes occurred in a *formative* phase of development, when direction selectivity first emerges, or in the following *plastic* phase, when the established direction selectivity undergoes plasticity by altered experience. Third, and with particular relevance to the formation of direction-selective responses, recent studies in the retinotectal pathway of *Xenopus* tadpoles have shown that the receptive fields of tectal neurons can be "trained" to become direction sensitive within minutes after repetitive exposure to moving bars in a particular direction (Engert et al., 2002; Mu and Poo, 2006). However, retinal ganglion cells that provide input to tectal neurons also display direction selectivity, the emergence of which has been shown to be independent of vision (Niell and Smith, 2005). It is not clear, therefore, whether the formation of direction selectivity in tectal neurons induced by visual training is simply reflecting the neuronal properties that were established in the retina or whether visual training induced changes in retinotectal and intratectal circuits.

We have been using the ferret as a model system to study the development of cortical direction selectivity and the map of direction preference; more generally, our interest has been to understand the role of sensory experience in the construction and maturation of cortical circuits. This species has a visual system that is similar to that of the cat (Linden et al., 1981; Law et al., 1988; Hahm et al., 1991; for a review, see Sengpiel and Kind, 2002), including cortical maps of ocular dominance, orientation, and direction preference. However, ferrets are born with a relatively immature nervous system (roughly three weeks earlier than kittens) and do not open their eyes until about the first month after birth. At the time of eye opening, the lens is clear and cortical cells are visually responsive. Therefore, this species is a satisfying candidate for studying the role of early sensory experience in the *formative* stages of cortical development. Furthermore, there is a substantial body of literature in ferrets on the organization and development of the visual system. Indeed, the ferret may be the species for which we now have the richest knowledge of visual system development, and all of this evidence has served us as the foundation for our studies of cortical direction selectivity (see figure 13.1).

Direction Selectivity Emerges after Eye Opening

Intrinsic signal optical imaging techniques were used to determine when direction selectivity is evident in the population response of early visual cortex (V1 and V2). In the youngest ferrets examined (postnatal days 28–34), there was little or no differential response to opposite directions of motion, despite the presence of columnar patterns of orientation-selective and eye-specific activity (see figure 13.2a, left panels; see Li et al., 2006 for full experimental details and results). In ferrets a few days older (postnatal days 35–37), direction-selective signals could be detected, but they were weak and often localized to restricted portions of visual cortex (see figure 13.2a, second from left), even as orientation selectivity signals became stronger (see figure

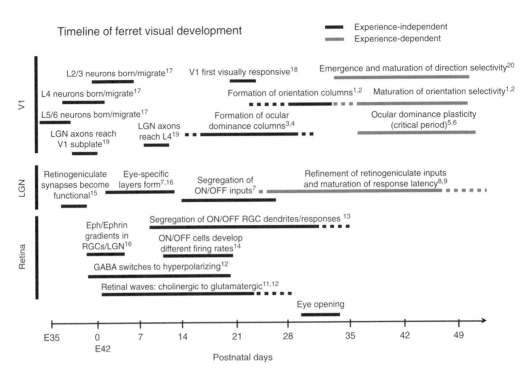

Figure 13.1
Timeline for the development of the ferret visual system. Major events are plotted against embryonic (E) and postnatal age. The maturation of retina is largely completed by the time of eye-opening. However, the development of the lateral geniculate nucleus (LGN) and primary visual cortex (V1) extend beyond the onset of visual experience. These latter events are, therefore, subject to experience-dependent modification. L, layer; RGC, retinal ganglion cell. References: (1) Chapman et al., 1996; (2) White et al., 2001; (3) Crowley and Katz, 2000; (4) Ruthazer et al., 1999; (5) Issa et al., 1999; (6) Liao et al., 2004; (7) Linden et al., 1981; (8) Tavazoie and Reid, 2000; (9) Akerman et al., 2002; (10) Lohmann and Wong, 2001; (11) Wong et al., 1993; (12) Wong et al., 2000; (13) Wang et al., 2001; (14) Wong and Oakley, 1996; (15) Bodnarenko et al., 1999; (16) Huberman et al., 2005; (17) McConnell, 1988; (18) Chapman and Stryker, 1993; (19). Herrmann et al., 1994; (20) Li et al., 2006.

13.2b, second from left). When assessed quantitatively across a large sample of juveniles (n = 45), cortical activity patterns produced by subtracting responses to opposite directions of motion did not differ from nonstimulated background signals until after eye opening (postnatal days 28–33) and did not achieve 50% of mean adult levels until about postnatal day 37, roughly 10 days after the comparable 50% mean adult orientation selectivity index was achieved (about postnatal day 28; see figure 13.2c). Despite this delay, the magnitude of direction selectivity and the distribution of columnar direction-selective signals increased rapidly, such that direction selectivity achieved functional maturity at roughly the same time as orientation selectivity (see figure 13.2c). In sum, these intrinsic signal imaging observations in normal juvenile ferrets showed that direction-selective signals emerged after eye opening and after the establishment of ocular dominance and orientation selectivity.

(a) Light-reared development

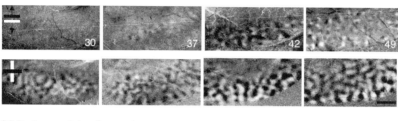

(b) Dark-reared development

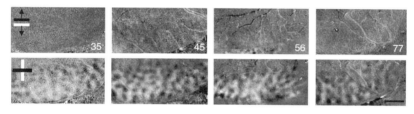

(c) Light-reared   (d) Dark-reared

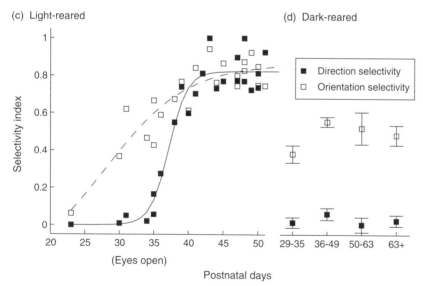

Figure 13.2
Development of direction and orientation selectivity in light-reared and dark-reared ferrets. (a) Difference images showing differential responses to stimulus direction (upper) and orientation (lower) from the same light-reared ferrets; numbers indicate age in postnatal days. Scale bar: 2 mm. (b) Same as (a), but for dark-reared ferrets. (c) Indices of direction (filled squares) and orientation (open squares) selectivity normalized to maximum values. (d) Same as (c), but for dark-reared ferrets with individuals binned.

Dark-Reared Ferrets Lack Direction Selectivity

The emergence of direction-selective responses after eye opening raises the possibility that visual experience is essential for this process. To test this possibility, ferrets were completely deprived of visual experience by absolute dark rearing from postnatal day 17 (before the time of cortical responsiveness to visual stimuli; Chapman and Stryker, 1993) until sedation for terminal experiments. No direction-selective signals were detected by means of intrinsic signal optical imaging in any dark-reared ferret, regardless of age (postnatal days 30–77; see figure 13.2b, d). As these same dark-reared ferrets showed significant orientation selectivity, it was clear that the visual cortex did not simply become unresponsive during dark rearing. Furthermore, no combination of stimulus spatial frequency, temporal frequency, and contrast was found that could elicit direction-selective responses (see Li et al., 2006).

Rapid Emergence of Direction-Selective Responses Driven by Moving Stimuli

Although the deprivation paradigm (i.e., dark rearing) clearly demonstrates the necessity of visual experience for the development of direction selectivity, this approach to understanding the role of experience is indirect and cannot reveal what aspect of vision is required and how these direction-selective domains emerge under the guidance of vision.

To determine whether exposure to a moving visual stimulus was sufficient to induce the emergence of direction-selective responses, animals were exposed to a "training" stimulus (a single sine or square wave grating) that drifted in one of two opposite directions along an axis of motion orthogonal to the grating's orientation (see Li et al., 2008, for experimental details). As illustrated for two example cases (see figure 13.3b, d), no changes were apparent for the first 8–12 hours of stimulation. At later time points, however, direction difference images began to assume a patchy appearance that continued to strengthen in intensity and become more widespread at subsequent time points. The strength of the direction difference signal was quantified by calculating a direction selectivity index (DSI), and there was a notable and progressive increase in DSI that accompanied exposure to the training stimulus (see figure 13.3e).

Compelling evidence that exposure to the training stimulus was responsible for the rapid emergence of direction selectivity came from experiments performed following the training period in which cortical responses to eight directions of motion were examined. Direction-selective responses were evident for stimulus directions that matched that of the training stimulus in 7 of 9 animals but were weak or absent for other directions of motion in all animals that were trained (see figure 13.3f, g). Compared to the initial conditions, the average DSI values after training were significantly increased for responses to stimuli whose properties matched the training stimulus but were not significantly different for responses to stimuli orthogonal to the training stimulus (see figure 13.3g).

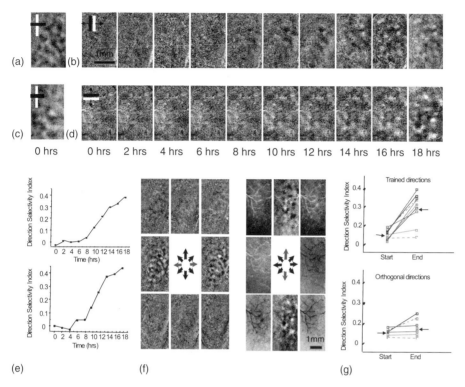

Figure 13.3
Rapid emergence of direction columns with motion training. (a–d) Visually naive animals (postnatal days 34, 35) with orientation columns (a, c) were trained using moving vertical (b) or horizontal (d) gratings. Direction domains emerged after 8 h. (e) Time course of training-induced increases in direction selectivity (top, b; bottom, d). (f) After training, direction domains were present only for the trained directions of motion (arrows; left, b; right, d). (g) Direction selectivity before and after training; each line represents a different animal, and arrows indicate median direction selectivity index, which increased significantly for trained directions (*t* test, p < .001; top) but not orthogonal directions (*t* test, p = 0.12; bottom).

To better understand changes that underlie the emergence of direction columns at the level of individual neurons and local cortical circuits, in vivo 2-photon imaging of calcium signals was employed to explore the direction-selective properties of local populations of layer 2/3 neurons during the rapid emergence of direction columns. In these experiments, the analysis was limited to cells that could be unambiguously identified and whose tuning responses were significant both before and after the training period (see figure 13.4a). Because the calcium-sensitive dye generally fades over time, the training period was shorter (3–6 hours) than that used for intrinsic signal imaging studies. Nevertheless, the distribution of direction index values measured after the training period was significantly higher than the values measured in the same neurons prior to training (see figure 13.4b, c). To test whether motion of the training stimulus was necessary

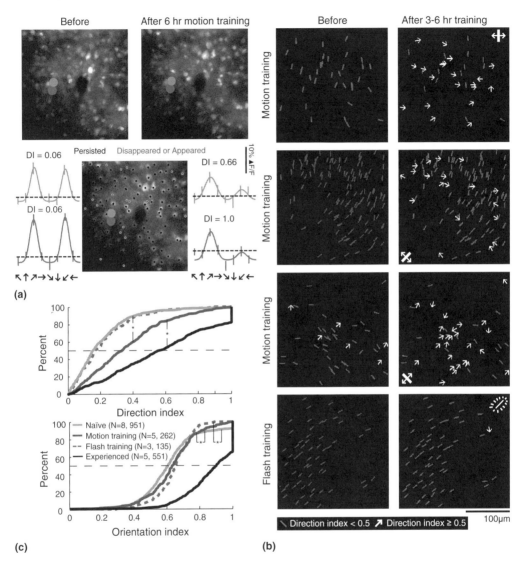

(a)

(b)

(c)

Figure 13.4

Motion training increases direction selectivity in individual cells. (a) Representative 2-photon images (135-μm depth) showing labeled cells evident before (top left) and after training (top right). Cell history over the course of training (persistent, disappeared, appeared) is depicted in the bottom middle. Tuning curves and direction index (DI) values for circled cells are shown at bottom left (before training) and right (after training). (b) Plots of cells from 4 animals before and after motion or flash training; icons indicate training directions or orientation of flashing stimulus. (c) Cumulative histograms of DI and orientation index for naive, motion-trained, flash-trained, and experienced conditions (N = animal, cell number). DI increased significantly following motion training (KW test, p < .01) but not after flash training (KW test, p = .27).

to induce these rapid changes in direction-selective responses, we examined the effects of training with an identical grating stimulus that was flashed. Although this stimulus was effective in driving cortical activity, no significant increase in direction selectivity was found after flash training (see figure 13.4b, c).

Rapid Emergence of Direction Preference during Visual Training

These results provide strong evidence that visual experience increases the magnitude of direction selectivity, and by itself, this could explain the rapid emergence of columnar structure visualized with intrinsic signal imaging (see figure 13.3). But how the directional preferences of motion-sensitive neurons in the visual cortex become specified and organized into a map of direction preference is not yet clear. To address this issue, we also examined the spatial distribution of direction preference by assessing the tuning properties of individual cortical layer 2/3 neurons before and after motion training using 2-photon imaging of calcium signals (see Li et al., 2008, for details on the analysis of neuronal tuning preferences).

At the onset of training, neurons were at best only weakly tuned for direction but nevertheless exhibited significant spatial organization: neighboring neurons tended to have similar direction biases, with this coherence in preference falling off with distance (see figure 13.5a, b). When animals were stimulated with the training stimulus—sinusoidal gratings that drifted in one of two opposite directions in an alternating fashion—cortical neurons acquired a direction preference for one of the two stimulated directions (see figures 13.4b and 13.5c). This finding is especially intriguing given the fact that the information present in the training stimulus is ambiguous: opposite directions of motion were presented and yet neurons rapidly acquired and/or strengthened their preference for a single direction. Evidently, the spatiotemporal cues present in a bidirectional motion training stimulus are sufficient to drive the development of cortical circuits that represent each direction of motion. However, if not by means of biased information present in the training stimulus, what is the source of information that influences neurons to acquire a preference for one direction of motion or another?

A thorough analysis of the spatial distribution of direction preference (i.e., the crude map of direction preference) that was detectable at the start of motion training indicates that the direction preference a neuron acquired during bidirectional training was significantly related to the initial direction biases of its local neighbors. Thus, we found a significant correlation between the likelihood of direction preference reversal and local coherence prior to training (see figure 13.5d) but not with flash training (see figure 13.5e). Neurons that initially had a direction bias that matched their neighbors were likely to maintain their preference following training. However, neurons that initially differed from their neighbors in direction preference were likely to reverse preference by the end of the training period. Consequently, at the conclusion of training, the spatial coherence of direction preference was dramatically increased (see figure 13.5c), consistent with the emergence of a map of direction preference being built up from the weak spatial organization that existed at the onset of training. The relationship between a neuron's acquired

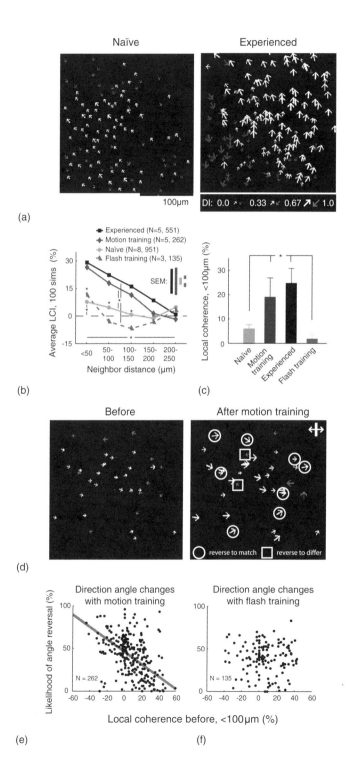

(a)

(b)

(c)

(d)

(e)   (f)

direction preference during bidirectional motion training and the preferences of its neighbors at the start of training raises an obvious question: is a neuron's final direction preference determined by its position in the developing functional map, or can sensory experience dictate the acquired preference? We are now attempting to answer this question by following the emergence of neuronal direction preference under the influence of unidirectional training stimuli. The results to date indicate a clear influence of the vector of motion energy present in the training stimulus on direction preference (Van Hooser et al., 2008). Ongoing experiments are addressing the question of whether this exogenous source of information is capable of changing direction preference, regardless of position in the emerging cortical map.

These findings are shedding light on the neural mechanisms by which structured sensory experience interacts with endogenous mechanisms for symmetry breaking in the functional architecture of developing cortical circuits. It is important to emphasize, however, that our studies of the impact of motion training on neuronal direction selectivity and direction preference have been limited to a few hours of training in acute preparations using anesthetized animals. We do not know whether the experience-dependent advances in visual development would be greater with longer durations of training, with a different regimen of motion training, or if training were performed in awake, behaving animals. Nor do we know—for a given cluster of neurons—if it might be possible to modify one or more of these experimental parameters and completely override the signals derived from local circuits with information present in unidirectional motion stimuli. Nevertheless, the data acquired to date demonstrate the power of motion energy to promote the maturation of neural circuits in the visual cortex and to constrain their emergent tuning preferences.

Lamberto Maffei and his collaborators have broken new ground in the field of experience-dependent brain plasticity by teasing apart the complex and interrelated neuronal and neurohumoral mechanisms by which self-motivated sensorimotor experience shapes the developing brain (see Sale et al., 2009, for a recent review). It is clear from their studies that the impact of experience is mediated by multiple biological mechanisms that act in concert to advance neural development in early life, ameliorate the consequences of sensory deprivation, and enhance neural plasticity in mature nervous systems. Our studies indicate that sensory stimulation structured in both space and time can also have remarkably selective effects in promoting the

Figure 13.5
Impact of normal experience and motion training on direction preference. (a) Plots of direction preference in naive and experienced animals. Arrows indicate preferred direction; length indicates magnitude. Grayscale differentiates cells with opposite preferences ($\pm$ 90 degrees). (b, c) Spatial coherence of direction preference (LCI, local coherence index, the percentage of neighboring cells with similar direction preferences minus the percentage with opposite preferences) increased with experience or motion training but not with flash training (standard error of the mean [SEM] calculated across animals; N = animal, cell number). Significant relations among curves and with distance (analysis of variance), and differences from 0 in naive and flash traces (sign test) indicated by *; sims, simulations. (d) Motion training effects on the direction preference of individual cells. Cells in circles and squares appeared to reverse their preference, coming to prefer rightward (matching their neighbors) and leftward motion (differing from their neighbors), respectively. (e) Influence of initial LCI on motion training effects. Cells whose preferred direction differed from their neighbors were most likely to reverse. (f) No systematic relationship was observed with flash training.

construction of neural circuits that acquire tuning preferences for the pattern of stimulation. The elements of the cortical circuit that are sensitive to the spatiotemporal patterns of stimulation and the cellular and synaptic changes that mediate the rapid emergence of direction-selective responses remain to be determined.

Acknowledgments

The authors thank Mark Mazurek for his contributions to data analysis and interpretation, Maria Christensson for critical discussions, and Prakash Kara, Thomas Mrsic-Flogel, and Aaron Kerlin for help with 2-photon imaging techniques. The work was generously supported by grants from the U.S. National Institutes of Health (D.F. and S.D.V.H.) and the Whitehall Foundation (L.E.W.).

References

Akerman CJ, Smyth D, Thompson ID. 2002. Visual experience before eye-opening and the development of the retino-geniculate pathway. *Neuron* 36: 869–879.

Berman N, Daw NW. 1977. Comparison of the critical periods for monocular and directional deprivation in cats. *J Physiol* 265: 249–259.

Blasdel G, Campbell D. 2001. Functional retinotopy of monkey visual cortex. *J Neurosci* 21: 8286–8301.

Bodnarenko SR, Yeung G, Thomas L, McCarthy M. 1999. The development of retinal ganglion cell dendritic stratification in ferrets. *Neuroreport* 10: 2955–2959.

Bonhoeffer T, Grinvald A. 1991. Iso-orientation domains in cat visual cortex are arranged in pinwheel-like patterns. *Nature* 353: 429–431.

Bosking WH, Crowley JC, Fitzpatrick D. 2002. Spatial coding of position and orientation in primary visual cortex. *Nat Neurosci* 5: 874–882.

Chapman B, Stryker MP. 1993. Development of orientation selectivity in ferret visual cortex and effects of deprivation. *J Neurosci* 13: 5251–5262.

Chapman B, Stryker MP, Bonhoeffer T. 1996. Development of orientation preference maps in ferret primary visual cortex. *J Neurosci* 16: 6443–6453.

Chklovskii DB, Koulakov AA. 2004. Maps in the brain: what can we learn from them? *Annu Rev Neurosci* 27: 369–392.

Crowley JC, Katz LC. 2000. Early development of ocular dominance columns. *Science* 290: 1321–1324.

Cynader M, Berman N, Hein A. 1976. Recovery of function in cat visual cortex following prolonged deprivation. *Exp Brain Res* 25: 139–156.

da Costa NM, Martin KAC. 2010. Whose cortical column would that be? *Front Neuroanat* 4: 1–10.

Daw NW, Berman NE, Ariel M. 1978. Interaction of critical periods in the visual cortex of kittens. *Science* 199: 565–567.

Daw NW, Wyatt HJ. 1976. Kittens reared in a unidirectional environment: evidence for a critical period. *J Physiol* 257: 155–170.

Engert F, Tao HW, Zhang LI, Poo MM. 2002. Moving visual stimuli rapidly induce direction sensitivity of developing tectal neurons. *Nature* 419: 470–475.

Hahm JO, Langdon RB, Sur M. 1991. Disruption of retinogeniculate afferent segregation by antagonists to NMDA receptors. *Nature* 351: 568–570.

Herrmann K, Antonini A, Shatz CJ. 1994. Ultrastructural evidence for synaptic interactions between thalamocortical axons and subplate neurons. *Eur J Neurosci* 6: 1729–1742.

Horton JC, Adams DL. 2005. The cortical column: a structure without a function. *Philos Trans R Soc Lond B Biol Sci* 360: 837–862.

Horton JC, Hocking DR. 1996. An adult-like pattern of ocular dominance columns in striate cortex of newborn monkeys prior to visual experience. *J Neurosci* 16: 1791–1807.

Huberman AD, Murray KD, Warland DK, Feldheim DA, Chapman B. 2005. Ephrin-As mediate targeting of eye-specific projections to the lateral geniculate nucleus. *Nat Neurosci* 8: 1013–1021.

Hubel DH, Wiesel TN. 1962. Receptive fields, binocular interaction and functional architecture in the cat's visual cortex. *J Physiol* 160: 106–154.

Hubel DH, Wiesel TN. 1963. Receptive fields of cells in striate cortex of very young, visually inexperienced kittens. *J Neurophysiol* 26: 994–1002.

Humphrey AL, Saul AB. 1998. Strobe rearing reduces direction selectivity in area 17 by altering spatiotemporal receptive-field structure. *J Neurophysiol* 80: 2991–3004.

Humphrey AL, Saul AB, Feidler JC. 1998. Strobe rearing prevents the convergence of inputs with different response timings onto area 17 simple cells. *J Neurophysiol* 80: 3005–3020.

Issa NP, Trachtenberg JT, Chapman B, Zahs KR, Stryker MP. 1999. The critical period for ocular dominance plasticity in the ferret's visual cortex. *J Neurosci* 19: 6965–6978.

Issa NP, Trepel C, Stryker MP. 2000. Spatial frequency maps in cat visual cortex. *J Neurosci* 20: 8504–8514.

Law MI, Zahs KR, Stryker MP. 1988. Organization of primary visual cortex (area 17) in the ferret. *J Comp Neurol* 278: 157–180.

Li Y, Fitzpatrick D, White LE. 2006. The development of direction selectivity in ferret visual cortex requires early visual experience. *Nat Neurosci* 9: 676–681.

Li Y, Van Hooser SD, Mazurek M, White LE, Fitzpatrick D. 2008. Experience with moving visual stimuli drives the early development of cortical direction selectivity. *Nature* 456: 952–956.

Liao DS, Krahe TE, Prusky GT, Medina AE, Ramoa AS. 2004. Recovery of cortical binocularity and orientation selectivity after the critical period for ocular dominance plasticity. *J Neurophysiol* 92: 2113–2121.

Linden DC, Guillery RW, Cucchiaro J. 1981. The dorsal lateral geniculate nucleus of the normal ferret and its postnatal development. *J Comp Neurol* 203: 189–211.

Lohmann C, Wong RO. 2001. Cell-type specific dendritic contacts between retinal ganglion cells during development. *J Neurobiol* 48: 150–162.

McConnell SK. 1988. Fates of visual cortical neurons in the ferret after isochronic and heterochronic transplantation. *J Neurosci* 8: 945–974.

Mu Y, Poo MM. 2006. Spike timing-dependent LTP/LTD mediates visual experience-dependent plasticity in a developing retinotectal system. *Neuron* 50: 115–125.

Niell CM, Smith SJ. 2005. Functional imaging reveals rapid development of visual response properties in the zebrafish tectum. *Neuron* 45: 941–951.

Ohki K, Chung S, Ch'ng YH, Kara P, Reid RC. 2005. Functional imaging with cellular resolution reveals precise microarchitecture in visual cortex. *Nature* 433: 597–603.

Pasternak T. 1986. The role of cortical directional selectivity in detection of motion and flicker. *Vision Res* 26: 1187–1194.

Pasternak T, Leinen LJ. 1986. Pattern and motion vision in cats with selective loss of cortical directional selectivity. *J Neurosci* 6: 938–945.

Pasternak T, Schumer RA, Gizzi MS, Movshon JA. 1985. Abolition of visual cortical direction selectivity affects visual behavior in cats. *Exp Brain Res* 61: 214–217.

Ruthazer ES, Baker GE, Stryker MP.1999. Development and organization of ocular dominance bands in primary visual cortex of the sable ferret. *J Comp Neurol* 407: 151–165.

Sale A, Berardi N, Maffei L. 2009. Enrich the environment to empower the brain. *Trends Neurosci* 32: 233–239.

Saul AB, Feidler JC. 2002. Development of response timing and direction selectivity in cat visual thalamus and cortex. *J Neurosci* 22: 2945–2955.

Sengpiel F, Kind PC. 2002. The role of activity in development of the visual system. *Curr Biol* 12: R818–R826.

Shmuel A, Grinvald A. 1996. Functional organization for direction of motion and its relationship to orientation maps in cat area 18. *J Neurosci* 16: 6945–6964.

Swindale NV. 2000. Brain development: Lightning is always seen, thunder always heard. *Curr Biol* 10: R569–R571.

Swindale NV, Shoham D, Grinvald A, Bonhoeffer T, Hubener M. 2000. Visual cortex maps are optimized for uniform coverage. *Nat Neurosci* 3: 822–826.

Tavazoie SF, Reid RC. 2000. Diverse receptive fields in the lateral geniculate nucleus during thalamocortical development. *Nat Neurosci* 3: 608–616.

Van Hooser SD, Li Y, Christensson M, White LE, Fitzpatick D. 2008. Emergence and refinement of direction preference in developing visual cortex. Soc Neurosci Abstr 724.5.

Weliky M, Bosking WH, Fitzpatrick D. 1996. A systematic map of direction preference in primary visual cortex. *Nature* 379: 725–728.

White LE, Coppola DM, Fitzpatrick D. 2001. The contribution of sensory experience to the maturation of orientation selectivity in ferret visual cortex. *Nature* 411 1049–1052.

Wang GY, Liets LC, Chalupa LM. 2001. Unique functional properties of on and off pathways in the developing mammalian retina. *J Neurosci* 21: 4310–4317.

Wong RO, Oakley DM. 1996. Changing patterns of spontaneous bursting activity of on and off retinal ganglion cells during development. *Neuron* 16: 1087–1895.

Wong RO, Meister M, Shatz CJ. 1993. Transient period of correlated bursting activity during development of the mammalian retina. *Neuron* 11: 923–938.

Wong WT, Myhr KL, Miller ED, Wong RO. 2000. Developmental changes in the neurotransmitter regulation of correlated spontaneous retinal activity. *J Neurosci* 20: 351–360.

Yu H, Farley BJ, Jin DZ, Sur M. 2005. The coordinated mapping of visual space and response features in visual cortex. *Neuron* 47: 267–280.

14 Neural Plasticity in Humans: Development of Cross-Orientation Contrast Normalization and Cross-Sensory Calibration

M. Concetta Morrone and David C. Burr

Cross-Orientation Inhibition and Gain Control

One of the key mechanisms essential for the versatility of perceptual systems is their capacity to adapt to the prevailing physical conditions. This allows the neural systems to use their full working range, giving an enhanced response to change in average statistics. Searching a cluttered desk for a specific pen would be very difficult if every visual signal were analyzed, encoding all orientated segments in detail. A far more effective strategy is to tune the system to the specific cluttered scene. It seems that the human visual system does this (see, e.g., Morrone, Burr, and Ross, 1983), and one of the main mechanisms it uses is automatic gain control and divisive normalization. (see, e.g., http://www.theswartzfoundation.org/canonical.asp).

As far as orientation is concerned, the normalizing mechanism called "cross-orientation inhibition" or "cross-orientation suppression" was first observed 30 years ago in Pisa while both of us were training with Lamberto. We observed a striking and unexpected effect in simple cells of cat primary visual cortex: although they respond well to stimuli of appropriate orientation, simple cells were absolutely silent when stimulated with two-dimensional random dot patterns even though these patterns have energy at all orientations, including that preferred by the cell (Burr, Morrone, and Maffei, 1981). However, the cell responded well to the same stimulus blurred along the axis of preferred orientation. This surprised us greatly, as the prevailing ideas at the time were that cells in primary visual cortex, particularly simple cells, were essentially linear (Movshon, Thompson, and Tolhurst, 1978; Maffei, Morrone, Pirchio, and Sandini, 1979). Failure to respond to the orientation energy contained within the two-dimensional noise pattern was clear evidence for an essential nonlinearity. We suggested, and demonstrated, that nonlinearity arose from inhibitory mechanisms stimulated from the nonpreferred orientations in the stimulus (Morrone, Burr, and Maffei, 1982).

Together with Lamberto, we quantified what we termed cross-orientation inhibition and showed that the suppression was multiplicative.

Figure 14.1 shows the response of a simple cell to a *test* grating of preferred orientation and variable contrast, with and without a superimposed orthogonal *mask* grating of 18% or 37% contrast. The effect of the orthogonal masks was to reduce considerably responsiveness at high

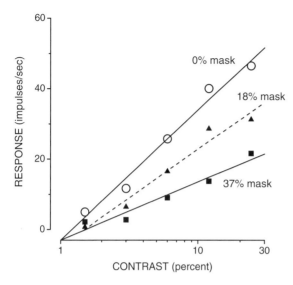

Figure 14.1
Contrast response function for a typical simple cell in cat cortical area V1. The *test* grating was oriented at the cell's preferred orientation and drifted at the preferred speed and direction. The *mask* was orthogonal to the test and drifted at the same speed as the test. The three curves at left show cell response as a function of test contrast (abscissa) for three mask contrasts: 0% (open circles), 18% (filled triangles), and 37% (filled squares). For all masks, cell response increases with test contrast, roughly proportional to log contrast. The masks decreased responsiveness proportionally at all test contrasts, implying a multiplicative suppression, that is, modulation of *response gain*. Reproduced with permission from Morrone, Burr and Maffei (1982).

test contrasts, with little effect at low test contrasts, causing a reduction of the slope (on linear-log scale) in the contrast response plot. In other words, the orthogonal mask decreases the *response gain* without affecting the estimate of threshold (extrapolation to zero response). Parallel masks (not shown) have a different effect, changing the contrast response range over which the cell responds (contrast gain), producing a leftward shift of the curve without changing slope.

More recently, a large body of literature has shown that the effects we observed can best be described as a *divisive normalization* that, depending on the value of the denominator, can simulate both the parallel and the orthogonal behavior. The normalization model of visual cortical responses was introduced in the early 1990s to explain a variety of such suppressive phenomena evident in the response properties of V1 neurons (Burr et al., 1981; Morrone et al., 1982; Bonds, 1989; Carandini and Heeger, 1994; Carandini, Heeger, and Movshon, 1997) and later extended to explain suppression in other visual cortical areas (Heeger, Simoncelli, and Movshon, 1996). The normalization model posits that the stimulus drive is suppressed, effectively normalizing (dividing) the response of each neuron by the sum of the total stimulus drive across a population of neurons.

Normalization is computed by taking the stimulus drive E of each simulated neuron and dividing it by a constant s plus the suppressive drive S. The constant s determines the contrast gain of the neuron's response. The resulting firing rates R of the population of simulated neurons can be expressed as a function of the stimulus drive and suppressive drive:

$$R = \frac{E}{S + s} \tag{14.1}$$

S is pooled across a large sample of neurons of all orientations. What determines whether the normalization results primarily in a shift of the contrast range (contrast gain) or modulation in response (response gain) is the relative size of the pool of neurons contributing to the suppression term S. If this is similar to the pool that contributes to the excitatory response E, the overall effect of the normalization will be a shift in contrast range. However, if the spread of the neuronal population in S is much larger (as happens for gratings of different orientations), the major effect will be a change of the response gain.

The essential feature of this mechanism is the normalization by a nonlinear pool of neurons tuned to different orientations and scales, having the effect of exaggerating the response to an orientation or scale that deviates from the average statistics. Other evidence from our laboratory suggests that cross-orientation suppression is mediated by an inhibitory intracortical GABAergic circuitry (Morrone, Burr, and Speed, 1987).

Interestingly, this type of behavior is not specific to vision and orientation but pervasive in most neuronal circuitry. Both a shift in contrast gain and in response gain can be mediated by GABAergic inhibition, the two mechanisms being determined by different interactions with synaptic depression mechanisms (Rothman, Cathala, Steuber, and Silver, 2009). However, this issue is not completely settled as some evidence suggests that suppression could partly occur at the thalamic stage (Durand, Freeman, and Carandini, 2007). However, there is also good evidence for cross-orientation suppression originating at cortical levels, particularly in the case of eye and orientation specific modulation of the blood-oxygen-level-dependent (BOLD) response (Moradi and Heeger, 2009).

We extended this line of approach to study cross-orientation inhibition in humans by measuring visual evoked potentials (VEPs), a technique pioneered by Lamberto and his friend Fergus Campbell (Campbell and Maffei, 1970). Figure 14.2, taken from Burr and Morrone (Burr and Morrone, 1987), shows in a human subject a set of contrast response curves (VEP amplitude) similar to those of the cat cell of figure 14.1. The paradigm was very similar to that used in the cat, with a vertical *test* and a horizontal *mask*. However, to evoke VEPs, the stimuli were contrast-reversed at a fixed frequency, causing a VEP response at each reversal (twice the frequency of modulation). To separate the response to the test from that to the mask, the test was modulated at 8 Hz and the mask at 7 Hz. The amplitude of the test second-harmonic (16 Hz) response is plotted in figure 14.2a. Like the cell of figure 14.1, the effect of the orthogonal masks is to decrease the response gain, decreasing the slopes of the contrast-amplitude response, without

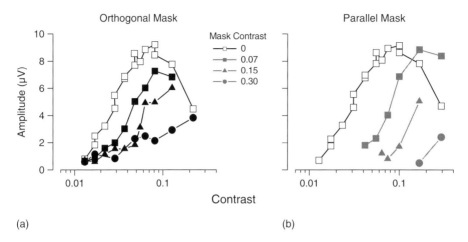

Figure 14.2
Amplitude of visual evoked potentials (VEPs) as a function of test contrast in the presence of orthogonal (A) and parallel (B) masks. The test grating was oriented vertically. The test was contrast-reversed at 8 Hz, and the mask at 7 Hz. The ordinates report the amplitude of the response at 16 Hz, the second harmonic of the test reversal frequency (the second harmonic elicited directly from the mask is at 14 Hz and therefore not analyzed directly. The masks were oriented either orthogonally (a) or parallel (b) to the test of and had 7% (filled squares), 15% (filled triangles), and 30% (filled circles) contrast. The effects of the masks on VEPs are similar to the effects on single cortical cells: the orthogonal masks modulate response gain by changing the slope; parallel masks modulate contrast gain by sliding the curves along the contrast axis. Reproduced with permission from Burr and Morrone (1987).

greatly affecting the extrapolated threshold. Figure 14.2b shows the effect of parallel masks. Similar to the behavior of the single cells (not reported), they do not change the slope of the curves but change the contrast gain, resulting in a rightward shift of the curves.

Cortical inhibition is known to be a key mechanism in modulating the critical period and developmental time course of visual functions (Fagiolini and Hensch, 2000; Fagiolini, Fritschy, Low, Mohler, Rudolph, and Hensch, 2004; Hensch and Fagiolini, 2005). We used the VEP technique described above to study development of orientation-dependent gain control in awake kittens and in infants (Morrone and Burr, 1986; Morrone, Speed, and Burr, 1991b). We measured curves like those of figure 14.2 and characterized them by a change in slope (calculated by regressing the amplitude measured with orthogonal mask against that measured without it). This index of slope change is plotted in figure 14.3a for human infants and figure 14.3b for kittens. For both infants and kittens, the index is constant at 1 (implying that the orthogonal mask caused no change of slope) for quite some time, for 10 months in infants and 40 days in kittens. After this time, inhibition develops quickly, maturing to its asymptotic level of about 0.2 (implying a five-fold change in slope). This shows that this sort of inhibitory process appears late in development, but once it does appear it matures very quickly.

This developmental pattern contrasts sharply with the development of contrast sensitivity, which matures gradually over infancy, to asymptote at about 10 months for infants and 40 days in kittens, more or less the time of onset of cross-orientation inhibition.

The developmental properties of the parallel mask effect are quite different from that of the orthogonal mask. Contrast sensitivity measured with the parallel mask remains roughly constant with age, so its effectiveness (in terms of contrast sensitivity) increases gradually, again saturating at about 10 months for humans and 40 days for infants. The effect of the parallel mask probably reflects the "S-shape" of the neuronal response contrast function, so its slow development suggests the contrast gain mechanisms that generate the S-shape develop slowly. This result has been replicated by Tony Norcia and his group (Skoczenski and Norcia, 1998; Candy, Skoczenski, and Norcia, 2001).

We also studied the plasticity of cross-orientation suppression by rearing monocularly deprived kittens and measuring VEP contrast response curves with and without parallel and orthogonal masks (Speed, Morrone, and Burr, 1991). Even a brief monocular deprivation during the critical period, followed by 4 months of normal binocular vision, produced a very abnormal pattern of results (see figure 14.4b, d): neither parallel nor orthogonal masks affected the response to the test grating, indicating that both response and contrast gain mechanisms, and possibly divisive normalization mechanisms in general, had been severely disrupted by the deprivation.

We also have preliminary data from one amblyopic adult (see figure 14.4a, c). The normal eye has the same pattern of VEP activity observed in normal subjects, while the amblyopic eye shows a much reduced interaction between test and mask. Both parallel and orthogonal masks had some effect on the VEPs, primarily shifting them along the contrast axis (contrast gain), but the pattern is clearly very different from that of the normal eye. These results are in line with very recent studies of the BOLD response in human amblyopes (Jurcoane, Choubey, Mitsieva, Muckli, and Sireteanu, 2009).

Is divisive normalization the inhibition that modulates the critical period? There is ample evidence that inhibitory mechanisms can close the critical period (Fagiolini and Hensch, 2000; Fagiolini et al., 2004) and also that interference with GABAergic inhibition can open the critical period in adults (Maya Vetencourt et al., 2008). It is highly unlikely that all GABAergic inhibition plays the same role. We would like to suggest that the inhibitory mechanisms that subtly change the neuronal working range to adapt it dynamically to the input signals are probably the most important and that divisive normalization may be the key mechanism.

These are key mechanisms during early development, necessary to shape fundamental architecture of the visual system function as we have shown for orientation. However, although visual orientation discrimination is fully mature by 1–2 years in infants, the system still needs to retain a high level of plasticity in order to interact with other less developed systems like the motor system. In the next section we will show how the visual system retains this capability for interactions with other systems.

Plasticity and Multisensory Calibration

Lamberto and his group have recently shown that sensory systems are far more plastic than previously supposed. A fascinating series of experiments shows that rearing animals—

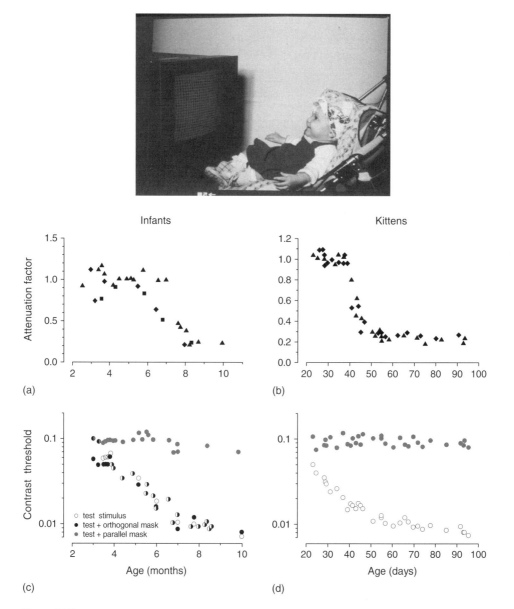

Figure 14.3
Development of inhibitory effects in infants and kittens. (a, b) The effectiveness of orthogonal masks on response gain. For both infants and kittens we recoded contrast response curves like those of figure 14.2a with and without orthogonal masks of 40% contrast and regressed one value against the other. The slope of the regression is taken as an estimate of the multiplicative change in response gain. The value is near unity, implying no change in response slope, for infants until about 7-8 months, for kittens until about 40 days, after which age it decreases dramatically to asymptote near 0.2 (implying a five-fold reduction in response slope). (c, d) Contrast thresholds (calculated from extrapolation of visual

Figure 14.3 (continued)
evoked potential amplitude response curves to zero response) measured with and without a parallel mask of 40% contrast. Thresholds in the presence of the mask (gray symbols) are surprisingly constant, at about 0.1 for both infants and kittens. The thresholds with the parallel mask, however, improve gradually over 8 months in humans and 50 days in kittens. This means that the effect of the mask on threshold, given by the ratio of the masked to unmasked threshold, also develops gradually over the same time span. Reproduced with permission from Morrone and Burr (1986) and Morrone, Speed, and Burr (1991a).

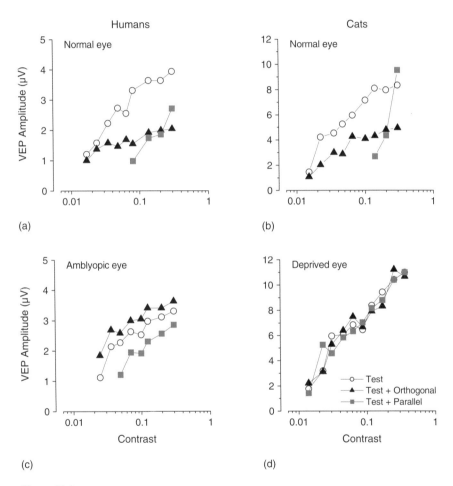

Figure 14.4
Masking in amblyopia. (a, c) Contrast response curves measured with and without parallel and orthogonal masks of 40% contrast. The effect of the masks in the normal eye are similar to those reported in figure 14.2a, while in the amblyopic eye the effect is different: the parallel mask increases slightly the contrast gain (gray symbols), and the orthogonal mask decreases it (black symbols: unpublished observations from our laboratory). (b, d) Same as a and c, except for a cat that had been monocularly deprived for 62 days at day 18, followed by normal vision for 4 months. The pattern of results is similar to the human, except that the three curves for the deprived eye are all identical. VEP, visual evoked potential. Reproduced with permission from Morrone, Speed, and Burr (1991a).

including human infants—in enriched environments can lead to great improvements in sensory sensitivity (see chapter 2, this volume). These studies demonstrate not only the incredible plasticity and capacity for learning of sensory systems but also the multisensory nature of the plasticity: haptic, auditory, and motor enrichment all seem to have an impact on visual development.

We have recently started to study interactions between senses in humans and, in particular, the development of these interactions. A great body of recent work has shown that human adults can fuse signals from different senses in a statistically optimal fashion. Whereas it used to be assumed that one sense—for example, vision—"captures" the other, because it is more "appropriate" for spatial judgments, it is now clear that the brain combines information from the different senses by performing some sort of weighted average, weighting each sense by its *reliability*. The reliability is effectively proportional to the *precision* under the particular conditions. Thus, when visual and auditory stimuli are presented from different sources—for example, from the ventriloquist and his dummy—they seem to emanate from the visual cue, the moving lips of the dummy, because vision is more precise for spatial localization and therefore the more reliable source. The "ventriloquist effect" does not result from vision's being intrinsically more appropriate but from the fact that under most conditions it is more precise. However, when the visual stimulus is blurred, sound can dominate in determining perceived position (Alais and Burr, 2004). The same pattern of results has been demonstrated for the combination of many of sources of information (e.g., Ernst and Banks, 2002; Hillis, Ernst, Banks, and Landy, 2002; Ernst and Bulthoff, 2004; Burr and Alais, 2006).

We recently investigated the combination of visual and tactile signals in young children, using a low-tech child-friendly version of the task used in adults (Gori, Del Viva, Sandini, and Burr, 2008). The results were conclusive but surprising: young children do not integrate haptic and visual information in the way that adults do, but one sense completely dominates the other, even though in the conditions of our experiment it was the least precise. An example of results is shown in figure 14.5 for two representative children, ages 5 and 10. The task involved judging the apparent size of physical blocks that they observed visually and also touched. Although the sizes of the visual and tactile stimuli could be varied independently, there was a strong illusion of continuity making it appear that the two blocks were the same object. The children matched the apparent size of a *standard* stimulus to a *conflict* stimulus, where the height of the visual block was decreased by Δ mm and the haptic block increased by Δ mm ($\Delta = -3$, 0, or +3 mm, plotted in abscissa of figure 14.5). For the 10-year-old the perceived height followed the visual standard (inversely proportional to Δ), but for the 5-year-old it followed the haptic standard (directly proportional to Δ). The dashed line indicates the predictions of an ideal-observer model, based on visual and haptic precision at those ages: the predictions are very similar for the two ages, but while the 10-year-old more or less follows predictions, the results of the 5-year-old go in exactly the opposite direction. It is not optimal integration, nor is it winner-take-all: indeed, it is *loser-take-all* behavior.

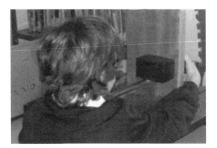

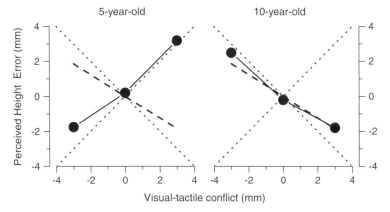

Figure 14.5
Visual–tactile integration in children. Children were asked to compare a *standard* stimulus (average height 50 mm) with a *conflict* stimulus, where the visual block was Δ mm shorter than 50 mm and the haptic stimulus Δ mm taller (Δ reported in abscissa). The dotted lines at +45° show the predictions if the match follows only the haptic standard, the dotted line at –45° the prediction if it follows the visual standard. The dashed lines are the predictions of a maximum-likelihood model, based on visual and haptic discrimination precision at those ages. Although the predictions are similar for both, the 10-year-old follows the predictions closely, while the 5-year-old shows opposite behavior.

We repeated the experiment for another task, orientation discrimination (not shown), and again found domination of one sense rather than integration. However, in this case vision dominated touch rather than the other way around.

Given the overwhelming body of evidence for optimal integration in adults, the result was not to be expected and suggests that multisensory interaction in infants is fundamentally different from that in adults. How could it differ? Although most recent work on multisensory interactions has concentrated on sensory *fusion*, the efficient combination of information from all the senses, an equally important but somewhat neglected potential role is that of *calibration*. In his famous 300-year-old "Essay toward a New Theory of Vision," Bishop George Berkeley (1709) correctly observed that vision has no direct access to attributes such as distance, solidarity, or "bigness." These become tangible only after they have been associated with touch (proposition 45): that is "touch educates vision," perhaps better expressed as "touch *calibrates* vision." Calibration is probably necessary at all ages, but during the early years of life, when children are effectively "learning to see," calibration may be expected to be more important. It is during these years that limbs are growing rapidly, eye length and eye separation are increasing, all necessitating constant recalibration between sight and touch. Indeed, many studies suggest that the first eight years in humans corresponds to the critical period of plasticity for many attributes and properties such as binocular vision (Banks, Aslin, and Letson, 1975) and acquiring accent-free language (Doupe and Kuhl, 1999).

Thus, before eight years of age, calibration may be more important than integration. The advantages of fusing sensory information are probably more than offset by those of keeping the evolving system calibrated: and using one system to calibrate another precludes fusion of the two. So if we accept Berkeley's ideas that vision must be calibrated by touch, that may explain why size discrimination thresholds are dominated by touch, even though touch is less precise than vision. However, why are orientation thresholds dominated by vision? Perhaps Berkeley was not quite right, and touch does not always calibrate vision, but the more robust sense for a particular task is the calibrator. In the same way that the more *precise* sense has the highest weights for sensory fusion, perhaps the more *accurate* sense is used for calibration. And the more accurate need not be the more precise but is probably the more robust. Accuracy is defined in absolute terms, as the distance from physical reality, whereas precision is a relative measure, related to the reliability or repeatability of the results. It is therefore reasonable that for size, touch will be more accurate, as vision cannot code it directly but only by a complex calculation of retinal size and estimate of distance. Orientation, on the other hand, is coded directly by primary visual cortex (Hubel and Wiesel, 1959) and calculated from touch only indirectly via complex coordinate transforms.

If the idea of calibration is correct, then early deficits in one sense should impact on the function of other senses that rely on it for calibration. Specifically, haptic impairment should lead to poor visual discrimination of size and visual impairment to poor haptic discrimination of orientation. We have tested and verified the latter of these predictions (Gori et al, 2010). In 17 congenitally visually impaired children (ages 5–19), we measured haptic discrimination thresholds for both orientation and size and found that orientation, but not size thresholds, were impaired. Figure 14.6 plots size against orientation thresholds, both normalized by age-matched normally sighted children. Orientation discrimination thresholds were all worse than the age-matched controls, on average by more than a factor of two, whereas size discrimination thresholds were generally better than the controls. Interesting, one child with an acquired visual impairment (star symbol) showed a completely different pattern of results, with no orientation deficit. Although we have only one such subject, we presume that his fine orientation thresholds result from the early visual experience (before 2½ years of age) which may have been sufficient for the visual system to calibrate touch.

The suggestion that specific perceptual tasks may require cross-modal calibration during development could have practical implications, possibly leading to improvements in rehabilita-

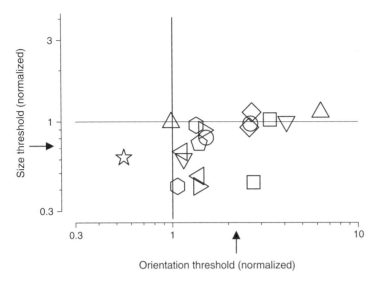

Figure 14.6
Size plotted against orientation discrimination thresholds for 17 congenitally blind and low-vision children (ages 6–20). All thresholds are normalized by the average of the age-matched controls, so values less than unity imply better than age-matched controls, greater than unity imply worse. Most points lie in the lower right quadrant, implying better size and poorer orientation discrimination in the visually impaired children. The arrows refer to group averages, 2.2 ± 0.3 for orientation and 0.8 ± 0.06 for size. The star in the lower left quadrant is the child with acquired low vision.

tion programs. Where cross-sensory calibration has been compromised—for example, by blindness—it may be possible to train people to use some form of "internal" calibration, or to calibrate by another modality such as sound.

Closing Remarks

In this brief chapter we present two lines of research that study plasticity and its development, one looking at inhibitory interactions during early infancy, the other intersensory interactions that take far longer to mature fully, probably because of a continuing need for calibration of sensory systems. Both point to the remarkable plasticity of the human brain, an idea that Lamberto has championed throughout his career. For both of us, this line of research started with Lamberto, in Pisa, some 30 years ago. Since then, our research paths have diverged considerably, so neither of us has since collaborated scientifically with Lamberto. But Lamberto remains a mentor, a colleague, and a close and valued personal friend.

This book is a Festschrift to Lamberto, celebrating an outstandingly creative and fruitful scientific career. The authors of this book know Lamberto well, and we all know he will never give up science. He will simply move into the third stage of his career, one more relaxed, less pressured, and hopefully isolated from the most recent barbarian invasion. We wish him well in his new career!

References

Alais D, Burr D. 2004. The ventriloquist effect results from near-optimal bimodal integration. *Curr Biol* 14(3): 257–262.

Banks MS, Aslin RN, Letson RD. 1975. Sensitive period for the development of human binocular vision. *Science* 190: 675–677.

Berkeley G. 1709/1963. An essay towards a new theory of vision. In: *Works on Vision* (Turbayne CM, ed), pp 19–97. Indianapolis: Bobbs-Merrill.

Bonds, AB. 1989. Role of inhibition in the specification of orientation selectivity of cells in the cat striate cortex. *Vis Neurosci* 2: 41–55.

Burr D, Alais D. 2006. Combining visual and auditory information. *Prog Brain Res* 155: 243–258.

Burr DC, Morrone MC. 1987. Inhibitory interactions in the human visual system revealed in pattern visual evoked potentials. *J Physiol* 389: 1–21.

Burr DC, Morrone MC, Maffei L. 1981. Intracortical inhibition prevents simple cells from responding to textured patterns. *Exp Brain Res* 43: 455–458.

Campbell FW, Maffei L. 1970. Electrophysiological evidence for the existence of orientation and size detectors in the human visual system. *J Physiol* 207: 635–652.

Candy TR, Skoczenski AM, Norcia AM. 2001. Normalization models applied to orientation masking in the human infant. *J Neurosci* 21: 4530–4541.

Carandini M, Heeger D, Movshon A. 1997. Linearity and normalisation in simple cells of the macaque primary visual cortex. *J Neurosci* 17: 8621–8644.

Carandini M, Heeger DJ. 1994. Summation and division by neurons in visual cortex. *Science* 264: 1333–1336.

Doupe AJ, Kuhl PK. 1999. Birdsong and human speech: common themes and mechanisms. *Annu Rev Neurosci* 22: 567–631.

Durand S, Freeman TC, Carandini M. 2007. Temporal properties of surround suppression in cat primary visual cortex. *Vis Neurosci* 24: 679–690.

Ernst MO, Banks MS. 2002. Humans integrate visual and haptic information in a statistically optimal fashion. *Nature* 415: 429–433.

Ernst MO, Bulthoff HH. 2004. Merging the senses into a robust percept. *Trends Cogn Sci* 8(4): 162–169.

Fagiolini M, Fritschy JM, Low K, Mohler H, Rudolph U, Hensch TK. 2004. Specific GABAA circuits for visual cortical plasticity. *Science* 303: 1681–1683.

Fagiolini M, Hensch TK. 2000. Inhibitory threshold for critical-period activation in primary visual cortex. *Nature* 404: 183–186.

Gori M, Del Viva M, Sandini G, Burr DC. 2008. Young children do not integrate visual and haptic form information. *Curr Biol* 18: 694–698.

Gori M, Sandini G, Martinoli C, Burr D. 2010. Poor haptic orientation discrimination in nonsighted children may reflect disruption of cross-sensory calibration. *Curr Biol* 20: 223–225.

Heeger DJ, Simoncelli EP, Movshon JA. 1996. Computational models of cortical visual processing. *Proc Natl Acad Sci USA* 93: 623–627.

Hensch TK, Fagiolini M. 2005. Excitatory–inhibitory balance and critical period plasticity in developing visual cortex. *Prog Brain Res* 147: 115–124.

Hillis JM, Ernst MO, Banks MS, Landy MS. 2002. Combining sensory information: mandatory fusion within, but not between, senses. *Science* 298: 1627–1630.

Hubel DH, Wiesel TN. 1959. Receptive fields of single neurones in the cat's striate cortex. *J Physiol* 148: 574–591.

Jurcoane A, Choubey B, Mitsieva D, Muckli L, Sireteanu R. 2009. Interocular transfer of orientation-specific fMRI adaptation reveals amblyopia-related deficits in humans. *Vision Res* 49: 1681–1692.

Maffei L, Morrone MC, Pirchio M, Sandini G. 1979. Response of visual cortical cells to periodic and non-periodic stimuli. *J Physiol* 296: 27–47.

Maya Vetencourt JF, Sale A, Viegi A, Baroncelli L, De Pasquale R, O'Leary OF, Castren E, Maffei L. 2008. The anti-depressant fluoxetine restores plasticity in the adult visual cortex. *Science* 320: 385–388.

Moradi F, Heeger DJ. 2009. Inter-ocular contrast normalization in human visual cortex. *J Vis* 9(3): 13.1–22.

Morrone MC, Burr DC. 1986. Evidence for the existence and development of visual inhibition in humans. *Nature* 321: 235–237.

Morrone MC, Burr DC, Maffei L. 1982. Functional significance of cross-orientational inhibition. I. Neurophysiological evidence. *Proc R Soc Lond* B216: 335–354.

Morrone MC, Burr DC, Ross J. 1983. Added noise restores recognition of coarse quantised images. *Nature* 305: 226–228.

Morrone MC, Burr DC, Speed HD. 1987. Cross-orientation inhibition in cat is GABA mediated. *Exp Brain Res* 67: 635–644.

Morrone MC, Speed HD, Burr DC. 1991a. Development of inhibitory interactions in kittens. *Vis Neurosci* 7: 321–334.

Morrone MC, Speed HD, Burr DC. 1991b. Development of visual inhibitory interactions in kittens. *Vis Neurosci* 7: 321–334.

Movshon JA, Thompson ID, Tolhurst DJ. 1978. Spatial summation in the receptive fields of simple cells in the cat's striate cortex. *J Physiol* 283: 53–77.

Rothman JS, Cathala L, Steuber V, Silver RA. 2009. Synaptic depression enables neuronal gain control. *Nature* 457: 1015–1018.

Skoczenski AM, Norcia AM. 1998. Neural noise limitations on infant visual sensitivity. *Nature* 391: 697–700.

Speed HD, Morrone MC, Burr DC. 1991. The effects of monocular deprivation on the development of visual inhibitory interactions in kittens. *Vis Neurosci* 7: 335–344.

15 The Developmental Process of Acquiring Multisensory Integration Capabilities

Barry E. Stein, Thomas Perrault, Jr., Terrence R. Stanford, and
Benjamin A. Rowland

Lamberto Maffei has inspired many researchers to examine how the brain develops and crafts its sensory capabilities to adapt to environmental demands. Understanding the inherent plasticity of the developing brain has seemed an obsession with Professor Maffei, on par with his need to swim out of sight into the open ocean. Both endeavors evoke strong reactions from his family and friends.

Professor Maffei has been among the most creative and prolific of researchers in the area of brain plasticity. Although he and most other researchers have concentrated on unisensory processes to understand these remarkable processes of development and plasticity, the ideas they have generated and the insights they have provided are also proving to be extremely helpful in understanding multisensory processes. Somehow the neural mechanisms that process sensory information, regardless of whether they are confined to a single sensory modality or are engaged in integrating information across the senses, must become tuned to the physical properties and statistical likelihoods of the particular environment in which they will function. Thus, the evolutionary strategy has been to ensure that the underlying neural architecture has the flexibility to use sensory experience, most of which must be acquired postnatally, to determine its operational principles. Although we know far less about the maturation of multisensory processes than unisensory processes, and what we do know points to many distinctions between them, they do share this overarching strategy.

Given that multisensory processes are present in all extant organisms that have been examined, and are likely to have predated the evolution of multicellular organisms (see Stein and Meredith, 1993, for a discussion), they, like their unisensory counterparts, have had the benefit of millions of years of selective pressure to achieve their current functional capabilities. The present discussion will use a single model to explore this process: the multisensory neuron in the superior colliculus (SC). The SC is a midbrain structure that plays a primary role in the control of orientation responses, such as gaze shifts (see Stein and Meredith, 1993; Hall and Moschovakis, 2004, for reviews), and has proven to be a highly productive and useful model for understanding multisensory integration at the level of the single neuron. However, before discussing the maturation of multisensory integration, it is useful to examine its general utility, its normal operational principles, and the organization of the model structure.

There Are Many Advantages to Having Multiple Sensory Systems

A driving force in evolution has been to develop systems that facilitate the ability to respond rapidly and appropriately to environmental cues. This includes the creation of storage and retrieval systems that can be used to modify long-term behavior, but it also requires that a broad array of environmental cues can be used to guide that behavior. As a consequence of such evolutionary pressures, brains have access to information from multiple sensory systems, each tuned to a given source of environmental energy. As a result, incomplete information in one sense can be compensated for by additional information in another. Thus, an event that is undetectable along any single sensory dimension may become obvious if simultaneously considered across multiple dimensions. Likewise, an event that cannot be identified along a single dimension (e.g., how it looks, sounds, or feels) may have a unique signature when considered across more than one sensory dimension. Regardless of the problem to be solved, whenever the inputs from different sensory modalities are combined to produce a synthesized product, it is called "multisensory integration" (Stein and Meredith, 1993). This process has been shown to increase the likelihood of detecting and localizing external events, aid in the identification of sensory events, and promote timely and accurate responding. By using such mechanisms, the brain can achieve levels of performance that would not be possible if using the senses independently (Ernst and Banks, 2002, Pouget et al., 2002, etc.)

The Principles of Multisensory Integration

Operationally, multisensory integration enhances (or degrades) the salience of a signal in the brain (Stein and Meredith, 1993), and its functional consequences for perception and behavior have been described in both human and animal subjects (e.g., Busse et al., 2005; Corneil and Munoz, 1996; Frens and Van Opstal, 1995; Ghazanfar and Schroeder, 2006; Grant et al., 2000; Hughes et al., 1994; King and Palmer, 1985; Lakatos et al., 2007; Liotti et al., 1998; Marks, 2004; Newell, 2004; Recanzone, 1998; Sathian, 2000; Sathian, 2005; Sathian and Prather, 2004; Schroeder and Foxe, 2004; Shams et al., 2004; Stein et al., 1989; Talsma et al., 2006a; Talsma et al., 2006b; Wallace et al., 1996; Weisser et al., 2005; Woldorff et al., 2004; Woods and Recanzone, 2004; Zangaladze et al., 1999). Presumably, by enhancing the salience of neuronal responses to cross-modal cues that are derived from the same event, multisensory integration can also aid in the disambiguation of those events. Disambiguation can occur in response to a variety of signals but has been most clearly demonstrated in those involving human speech and animal communication (Bernstein et al., 2004; Ghazanfar et al., 2005; Massaro, 2004; Partan, 2004; Sugihara et al., 2006; Sumby and Pollack, 1954). It also significantly enhances both the speed with which an event is detected and the speed and reliability with which responses can be produced (Corneil and Munoz, 1996; Frens and Van Opstal, 1995; Hughes et al., 1994; Marks, 2004; Newell, 2004; Sathian and Prather, 2004; Shams et al., 2004; Stein et al., 1989; Stein and Meredith, 1993; Stein and Stanford, 2008; Woods and Recanzone, 2004).

Three general operational principles of multisensory integration that have been derived from single-neuron studies of the cat SC that will be discussed below. Two involve space and time and are referred to, respectively, as the "spatial" and "temporal" principles of multisensory integration. In the former case, cross-modal stimuli that are in spatial concordance (as if derived from the same event) enhance neuronal responses, whereas those that are in spatial discordance (as if derived from different events) either fail to be integrated or produce depressed responses. The temporal principle has the same general form, though the depression with temporally discordant stimuli has been less well documented. A third major principle is that of "inverse effectiveness." This principle describes the observation that the proportionate effect of combining cross-modal cues is greater when the effectiveness of the component stimuli is weaker (see Stein and Meredith, 1993, and Stein et al., 2009, for a general discussion of these principles).

Until recently, far less consideration had been given to the developmental prerequisites of multisensory integration or its inherent plasticity than to studies of its general functional organization. Newer studies have shown that its operational principles are very sensitive to experience and are largely or completely instantiated during postnatal life. Nevertheless, some multisensory processes, like cross-modal matching and the recognition of amodal stimulus (e.g., size, intensity, frequency) properties, have been demonstrated in very young children, and the inference is that they may already be present to some degree at birth (e.g., see Bower, 1974; Gibson, 1966; Gibson, 1969; Gibson, 1979; Lewkowicz and Kraebel, 2004; Lickliter and Bahrick, 2004; Marks, 1978; Werner, 1973). Thus, while experiments in animals strongly suggest that "multisensory integration" is acquired postnatally, and only after considerable sensory experience (Wallace et al., 2006; Wallace et al., 1993; Wallace and Stein, 2007; Wallace and Stein, 1997), this should not be taken to mean that there is no communication among the senses at birth. This issue deserves further exploration. However, it appears that regardless of species, multisensory integration develops postnatally, and very recent studies in human subjects, like those in animal subjects, point to the gradual postnatal elaboration of this capability (see Gori et al., 2008; Neil et al., 2006; Putzar et al., 2007).

Collectively, these studies suggest that the neonatal brain must incorporate principles that will guide the integration of inputs from the different senses based on experience. Most of these studies have emphasized multisensory enhancement rather than multisensory depression, and this index of multisensory integration will be emphasized in the following discussion.

Using the Superior Colliculus as a Model of Multisensory Integration

The role of the SC in attentive and orientation behavior has been well documented (Sparks, 1986; Stein and Meredith, 1993). In general, the appearance of a visual, auditory, and/or somatosensory event will activate its topographically organized neurons so that the event is detected, localized, and reacted to with a shift of gaze. Sometimes, the entire body orients to the event, so that the animal is well positioned to respond to it. The neurons activated by these different sensory modalities are located in its deeper aspects where outputs to motor areas of the brainstem and spinal cord originate. Many of these neurons also receive converging inputs from the different senses, rendering them multisensory (it is a primary site of sensory convergence; see Stein and Meredith, 1993; Wallace et al., 1993), and many of them are also output neurons that link multiple sensory inputs to motor behavior (Meredith et al., 1992). These factors make it an excellent model for studying the physiology of multisensory integration and its behavioral consequences. The fact that there is a considerable amount of information concerning the development of the structure, albeit mostly about its unisensory properties (see Stein, 1984), also makes it an ideal model to examine how multisensory integration develops and adapts to the particular environment in which it will function. Indeed, most of what we know about the multisensory properties of single neurons and their ontogeny comes from this model (Peck, 1987; Stein, 1984; Stein and Clamann, 1981; Stein et al., 1973a; Stein et al., 1976; Stein and Meredith, 1993; Stein et al., 1993; Wallace, 2004; but see also Barth and Brett-Green, 2004; Calvert and Lewis, 2004; Groh and Sparks, 1996a; Groh and Sparks, 1996b; Gutfreund and Knudsen, 2004; Jay and Sparks, 1987a; Jay and Sparks, 1987b; King et al., 2004; Lakatos et al., 2007; Sathian and Prather, 2004; Woods and Recanzone, 2004; Zwiers et al., 2003).

One important factor to keep in mind when thinking about SC multisensory integration is that its underlying functional circuits are complex and that the simple fact that afferents from the different senses converge on a common target neuron neither ensures that it will be able to integrate those inputs nor specifies how the inputs would be integrated if the neuron did indeed possess that capability (Jiang et al., 2006; Jiang et al., 2001; Stein and Meredith, 1993; Wallace and Stein, 1997). Experiments have shown that there are several critical factors that must be present, generally during early postnatal life, for this capability to develop, and these factors are discussed below.

Superior Colliculus Organization

Each of the three sensory representations in the multisensory SC (visual, auditory, and somatosensory) is represented in the same topographic fashion. Thus, their maps overlap one another. Neurons in the front of the structure have receptive fields in frontal space or the front portion of the body (e.g., face), those in the rear of the structure are further temporal in visual and auditory space and further back on the body, those medial in the structure have receptive fields in upper space, and those lateral in the structure have receptive fields in lower space (Meredith et al., 1991; Meredith and Stein, 1990; Middlebrooks and Knudsen, 1984; Stein and Gallagher, 1981; Stein et al., 1975; Stein et al., 1993). The overlapping sensory maps are in register with an underlying motor map from which projections to the brainstem and spinal cord translate sensory inputs into motor responses. Thus, a cue in upper space triggers responses from neurons that will produce an upward orientation movement (e.g., gaze shift). This is an elegant and simple way to match sensory input to the output signals that reach the effector organs via the brainstem and spinal cord (Grantyn and Grantyn, 1982; Groh and Sparks, 1996a; Groh and Sparks, 1996b; Guitton and Munoz, 1991; Harris, 1980; Jay and Sparks, 1987a; Jay and Sparks, 1987b; Jay and

Sparks, 1984; Munoz and Wurtz, 1993a; Munoz and Wurtz, 1993b; Peck, 1987; Sparks, 1986; Sparks and Nelson, 1987; Stein and Clamann, 1981; Wurtz and Albano, 1980; Wurtz and Goldberg, 1971).

Because the different sensory maps in the SC overlap one another, so too do the multiple receptive fields of individual multisensory neurons (King et al., 1996; Meredith et al., 1991; Meredith and Stein, 1990; Meredith et al., 1992; see also Brainard and Knudsen, 1998; Gutfreund and Knudsen, 2004; Knudsen and Brainard, 1991; Knudsen et al., 1991; Knudsen and Knudsen, 1989). This is the basis for the spatial principle of multisensory integration (Stein and Meredith, 1993), wherein the magnitude of a neuron's response to a cross-modal stimulus depends on where the component stimuli fall within its receptive fields. As noted earlier, when they fall within its overlapping receptive fields, they generally enhance the neuron's response above that to either stimulus independently, and often above the sum of the responses to each stimulus alone (see figure 15.1).

Although these multisensory properties are most frequently associated with SC neurons in the cat (Meredith and Stein, 1983; Meredith and Stein, 1986a; Meredith and Stein, 1986b; Meredith and Stein, 1996; Stein et al., 1993; Wallace et al., 1993; Wallace and Stein, 1994), they have also been seen in the SC of the hamster (Meredith and Stein, 1983; see also Stein and Dixon, 1979), guinea pig (King and Palmer, 1985), and monkey (Wallace et al., 1996) and also in the cortex of the cat (Wallace et al., 1992), rat (Barth and Brett-Green, 2004; Wallace et al., 2004), monkey (Ghazanfar and Schroeder, 2006; Lakatos et al., 2007; Schroeder and Foxe, 2004; Schroeder and Foxe, 2002; Schroeder et al., 2001), and inferred based on the data acquired in human (Calvert and Lewis, 2004; Fort and Giard, 2004; de Gelder et al., 2004; Hairston et al., 2003; Laurienti et al., 2002; Lovelace et al., 2003; Macaluso and Driver, 2004; Sathian and Prather, 2004; Stein et al., 1996).

Influences from Cortex Are Essential for Multisensory Integration in the Superior Colliculus

Earlier it was noted that multisensory integration is not a simple consequence of the convergence of different sensory inputs onto the same SC neuron. The convergence is a necessary factor but not sufficient for conferring this capacity. This conclusion is based on two sets of studies, the first involving the elimination of selected corticocollicular influences, and the second evaluating the development of multisensory integration.

Studies have shown that reversible deactivation of a region of association cortex (the anterior ectosylvian sulcus, AES; and its neighboring region, the rostral lateral suprasylvian sulcus, rLS) eliminated multisensory integration in SC neurons but didn't preclude their responding to multiple sensory inputs. Thus, a visual–somatosensory neuron remains visual–somatosensory after cortical deactivation but loses the ability to integrate visual and somatosensory information to produce an enhanced response (Jiang et al., 2001; Jiang et al., 2002; Stein et al., 2002; Alvarado et al., 2007a; Alvarado et al., 2007b; Alvarado et al., 2008; see also Burnett et al., 2007). AES appears to be the major cortical contributor to this capacity (Jiang et al., 2001) by virtue of providing converging unisensory inputs to the SC (Wallace et al., 1992, Fuentes-Santamaria

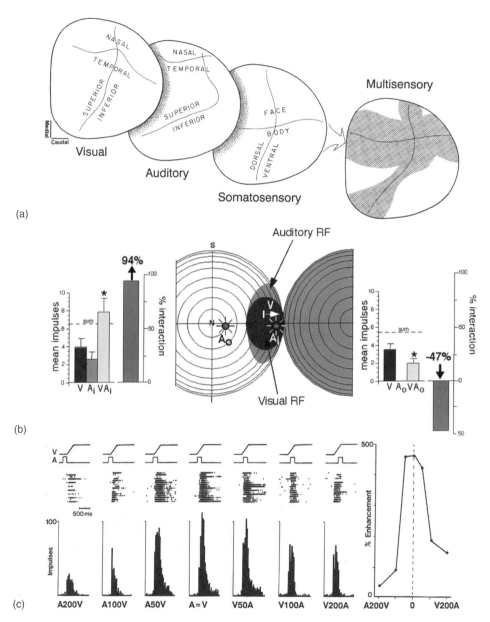

Figure 15.1

Multisensory information converges on individual neurons within the superior colliculus (SC). (a) Visual–auditory–somatosensory maps correspond within the SC creating topographically aligned multisensory representations of the world. (b) Individual neurons within the SC will exhibit response enhancements and depressions depending up on the spatial relationships of unisensory component stimuli. (Center) A visual stimulus (white bar) within the neuron's visual receptive field (RF) and an auditory stimulus (speaker) placed both within and outside the neuron's RF resulted in two different multisensory responses. (Left) When visual and auditory stimuli are placed within the neuron's corresponding et al., 2009); these AES-derived inputs arise from different sensory subdivisions but appear to work synergistically in conferring multisensory integrative capability onto SC neurons (Alvarado et al., 2008). Although AES and rLS can compensate for one another's loss early in life, other brain areas appear to be uninvolved and cannot compensate for the temporary or permanent loss of AES and rLS during neonatal or adult life stages (see figure 15.2; Wilkinson et al., 1996; Jiang et al., 2006: Jiang et al., 2007).

Superior Colliculus Neurons Are Capable of Multisensory Integration Only after a Protracted Period of Postnatal Maturation

The cat is an altricial species, and its comparative immaturity at birth (its eyelids and ear canals are still closed) makes it a good subject for developmental studies. Neither its SC, nor that of its precocial laboratory counterpart, the rhesus monkey, contains neurons capable of integrating inputs from different senses at birth (see figure 15.3; Wallace and Stein, 1997, 2001). A reasonable working assumption is that because the SC develops earlier than does the cerebral cortex (see Stein et al., 1973a; Stein et al., 1973b), there is also little possibility that neurons capable of multisensory integration are present in higher brain areas at this stage of development. This is consistent with recent studies of multisensory development in association cortex (Wallace et al., 2006; Carriere et al., 2007) and is consistent with the gradual elaboration of multisensory perception in humans (Neil et al., 2006; Putzar et al., 2007).

The multisensory layers of the newborn cat's SC are unisensory, and the only sensory-responsive neurons present are somatosensory (Stein et al., 1973a; Stein et al., 1973b). Somatosensory-responsive neurons are already evident in late prenatal stages and are presumably organized prenatally to ensure that the neonate can use perioral tactile cues to find the nipple immediately after birth (Larson and Stein, 1984). The first neurons responsive to auditory stimuli do not appear until several days later, and visual neurons appear last (Stein et al., 1973a; Kao et al., 1994). The maturation of unisensory properties is germane to the maturation of multisensory integration, as the same neurons are often involved. The unisensory information processing of multisensory neurons is very similar to that of their unisensory neighbors. Many of the immature characteristics of these neurons seem independent of modality. Neonatal receptive fields are very large; the neurons respond poorly to stimuli that are highly effective in the adult; they fatigue rapidly and are less selective in their responses to the parameters of the stimulus (e.g., its direction of movement, velocity, size, etc.). As the animal matures, the receptive fields of SC neurons contract and their unisensory selectivities begin to become apparent, but the maturation of multisensory integration lags considerably.

receptive field, the result is response enhancement as depicted by the bar graphs representing mean activity of unisensory and multisensory responses. Right: When visual and auditory stimuli are spatially discordant, response depression is observed. (c) The magnitude of multisensory enhancement is dependent on the temporal relationship component stimuli. Multisensory stimulus presentations were presented at different onset asynchronies. Multisensory stimuli presented simultaneously elicited the greatest response. Modified from Stein and Meredith (1993).

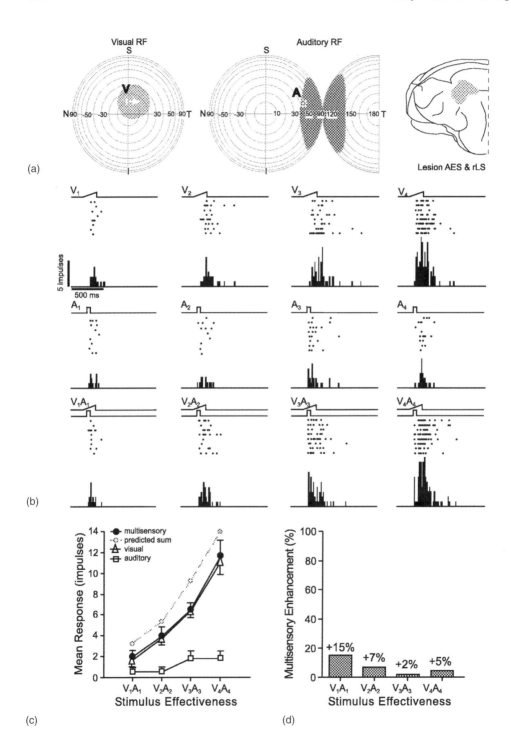

Unisensory Development May Not Readily Be Generalized to Multisensory Development

The different time lines in unisensory and multisensory SC maturation partly reflect the fundamental distinctions between these processes and raise a significant caution. We have to be very
careful when trying to use information about the development of the former to infer something
about the development of the latter. Multisensory integration is a unique process that depends
on the synthesis of information from independent sensory channels (Alvarado et al., 2007a;
Alvarado et al., 2007b; Rowland et al., 2007; Gingras et al., 2006). As noted above, it is possible
to have functional visual and auditory systems yet lack the ability to integrate information across
them. A second distinction is evident in the tendency to specialize (i.e., become specifically
tuned) in one case and to generalize in the other. For example, exposure to all line orientations,
or to complex forms, leads to the maturation of orientation preferences in visual cortical neurons.
Different groups of neurons selectively respond to different line orientations, with all orientations

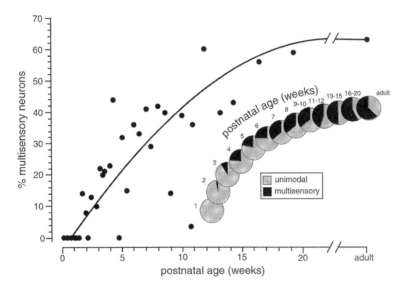

Figure 15.3
The developmental chronology of multisensory neurons. The percentage of multisensory neurons in the deep layer
sensory-responsive population is plotted as a function of postnatal age. Pie charts in the inset show the expansion of
the multisensory population as development progresses.

◀ **Figure 15.2** (opposite)
Neonatal ablation of anterior ectosylvian sulcus (AES) and rostral lateral suprasylvian sulcus (rLS) disrupt the development of superior colliculus (SC) multisensory enhancement. Ablated area of cortex is shown as shading on the schematic
of the brain (top right in a). Characteristically, spatially coincident cross-modal stimuli failed to evoke multisensory
enhancement at any stimulus intensity, and multisensory response was less than response predicted by summing individual unisensory responses (b, c, and d). Multisensory response was nearly identical to the best unisensory response
(visual; taken from Jiang et al., 2001).

being represented among the population of neurons in visual cortex. This represents a process of unisensory specialization. However, multisensory integration appears to have a very different goal. Rather than specializing, multisensory neurons seem to generalize. They are sensitive to the statistical regularities of cross-modal stimuli and use that information to create general principles that guide their integration of information from different sensory sources. Although there is some unisensory selectivity among SC multisensory neurons, as far as we know, they do not group themselves by subpopulations exhibiting different integrative modes based on stimulus properties.

The Developmental Chronology of Multisensory Neurons

Multisensory neurons follow a maturational time course that has the same sequence as their unisensory components, but their initial appearance is somewhat delayed (Stein et al., 1973a). Thus, somatosensory–auditory neurons are the first multisensory neurons to appear. They appear as early as 10 days of age (5 days later than the appearance of auditory neurons). It is not until three weeks later that visually responsive neurons are found in the multisensory layers (their superficial layer counterparts develop much earlier; see Stein et al., 1973a; Stein et al., 1973b; Kao et al., 1994), and visual–somatosensory and visual–auditory neurons are found at about the same time (see figure 15.3). Although these neurons are multisensory, they are not yet capable of integrating their different sensory inputs. This requires 2 to 3 additional months. It is also during this period that corticocollicular projections from association cortex are developing their influence over SC response properties (Stein and Gallagher, 1981; Stein et al., 2002; Wallace and Stein, 2000; Wallace and Stein, 1997).

The Maturation of Multisensory Integration Capabilities

The observation that neonatal multisensory neurons cannot yet integrate their different sensory inputs, and that this capacity requires substantial postnatal development, suggested that this capacity might depend on sensory experience, specifically, experience with cross-modal stimuli. Certainly, early life is a time during which the neonatal brain could learn the statistical regularities of cross-modal stimuli that characterize its environment. It could then use this information to adapt its multisensory integration capabilities to best suit the environment in which they would be used. An underlying assumption here is that multisensory integration is plastic and can, in fact, be crafted to best accommodate the particular stimulus characteristics that are likely to be encountered. However, plasticity is generally associated more with processes in cortex (Buonomano and Merzenich, 1998) than with those in the midbrain (Wickelgren and Sterling, 1969), and, as noted earlier, SC multisensory integration is dependent on influences from association cortex, and these influences develop during the period in which SC multisensory integration develops. In order to explore the possibility that the circuit does adapt to the cross-modal statistics it experiences, and that this process is mostly dependent on cortex, a number of strategies were employed. The first strategy was to examine the effect of eliminating cross-modal experience during early life. If the development of SC multisensory integration was independent of specific experiences, this would not interfere with its normal expression. The easiest way to test this possibility was to use visual–nonvisual integration as a model, not only because of the high incidence of visual multisensory neurons in the normal adult but because such experience can readily be precluded by dark rearing. The second strategy involved altering the cross-modal statistics of the animal's physical world to see if it would affect its multisensory integration in predictable ways. The third strategy was to examine SC multisensory maturation in the absence of the critical cortical inputs, either because they were removed or rendered inoperative.

Rearing Animals without Cross-Modal (i.e., Visual–Nonvisual) Experience

Raising animals in the dark precludes any visual–nonvisual experience and provides a way of testing whether such experience is critical for SC multisensory integration. Using this strategy, cats were raised in the dark until they were 6 months of age (Wallace et al., 2004). The rearing condition did not prevent the maturational appearance of SC sensory neurons with each of the characteristic convergence profiles: unisensory (visual, auditory, somatosensory) and multisensory (visual–auditory, visual–somatosensory, auditory–somatosensory, and trisensory). These neuronal subtypes proved to be in roughly in their normal proportions, but their receptive fields were considerably larger than normal and better approximated those found in much younger animals. Most pertinent in the present context, however, is that they were incapable of multisensory integration. Their general characteristics suggested a failure to mature, as if they were maintained in a neonatal state. The interference with the maturation of multisensory integration might have several possible explanations, but the one that seemed most likely was that, while early visual experience is a key requirement for receptive field contraction, experience with co-occurring cues from different senses (e.g., visual and auditory) is required to later integrate information across them. This was the most attractive possibility because it could also provide a way for the brain to craft multisensory integration capabilities to best fit the particular sensory environment in which this process would operate. If this were the case, one would expect that altering early cross-modal experiences would produce predictable changes in how they would later be integrated.

Rearing Animals with Spatially Disparate Cross-Modal Cues

This strategy here was to examine whether the result predicted above would be induced by rearing animals in an atypical environment in which visual and auditory cues were presented simultaneously but from different locations in space. This was not an ideal circumstance to test this possibility because the stimuli had no intrinsic meaning for the animals and were linked neither to a reward nor to any other event of significance. Therefore, it was not really surprisingly to find that the majority of the SC neurons that were sampled from these animals once they were adults had properties that were very similar to those that characterize neonatal and dark-reared animals. The receptive fields of these neurons were large, and the neurons could not integrate visual–auditory inputs (Wallace and Stein, 2007). These neurons showed no evidence that the cross-modal experience had influenced their development. However, there were many SC neurons that had properties that indicated that their maturation was guided by this cross-modal experience. Their visual and auditory receptive fields had become smaller (albeit not as small as those in normally reared animals), and their spatial register was poor, and some showed no overlap between their visual and auditory receptive fields. The absence of any receptive field overlap was highly unusual. Thus, their organization was such that simultaneous visual and auditory stimuli could fall within their respective receptive fields in a given neuron only if they were disparate in space. When such a stimulus configuration was presented, so that the visual stimulus was within its receptive field and the auditory stimulus was within its receptive field, neurons produced an enhanced response (see figure 15.4). Apparently, the spatial rule of multisensory integration was reversed: now, spatially disparate stimuli produced enhancement rather than depression (see Kadunce et al., 1997; Meredith and Stein, 1996). These observations are highly consistent with the idea that experience with cross-modal cues helps establish the functional features of the circuits underlying multisensory integration. Presumably, much of the impact of this experience is exerted on the cortico–SC projection because of its importance in the normal expression of multisensory integration and because its developmental time course appears to parallel that of multisensory integration (Wallace and Stein, 2000).

Superior Colliculus Maturation after Ablation of Association Cortex

To test the assumption noted above, Jiang et al., (2006) removed AES and/or rLS during early life. As adults, SC neurons in these animals were highly atypical. The different receptive fields of an individual neuron were poorly aligned with each other, and the neurons were unable to engage in multisensory integration. This deficit in multisensory integration was also evident behaviorally (Jiang et al., 2007). Apparently, no other area of the brain could compensate for AES and rLS in this regard. However, it appeared that AES and rLS could compensate for the early loss of one another, because this deficit in multisensory integration was evident only when both areas were removed during neonatal life. In the absence of only one of these areas, SC neurons still developed aligned receptive fields and many still developed the capacity for multisensory integration. Its impact on overt behavior was apparent as well. These results suggest that descending influences from association cortex help ensure that the multisensory processes of SC neurons accurately reflect the statistics of the cross-modal events that have been experienced by the developing brain. Presumably, it doesn't matter whether these statistics are those of "normal" environments or those in which the recurring relationships between visual and auditory events have been varied as long as they are reliable. Without the cortex guiding this development, SC neurons seem to default to the neonatal state where cross-modal cues cannot be used in concert.

Superior Colliculus Development during Long-Term Cortical Deactivation

However, the ablation technique does more than eliminate descending information to the SC. It is a serious insult to the brain that induces a cascade of consequent events in distant areas.

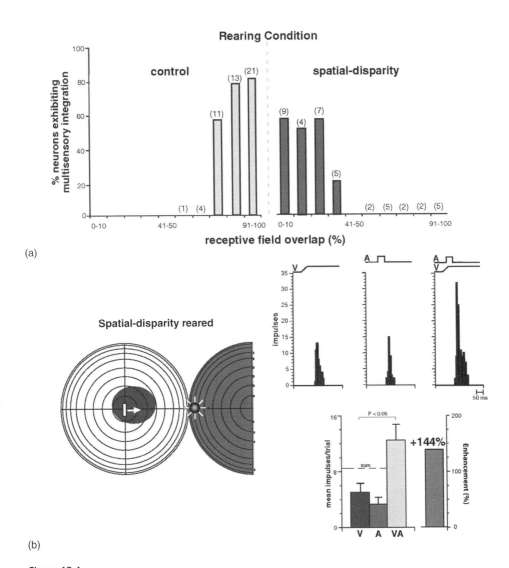

(a)

(b)

Figure 15.4
(a) Receptive field (RF) overlap in normal and spatial-disparity reared animals. The % RF overlap in control animals (light gray) was often 91%–100%, far exceeding that seen in spatial-disparity reared animals (dark gray, often <10%). Modified from Wallace and Stein (2007). (b) Rearing with visual–auditory spatial disparity yields anomalous multisensory integration. When the visual (white bar) and auditory (gray circle) stimuli are spatially disparate and in their respective RFs (left) they produce significant (<.05, t test) enhancement (right bottom)—a striking reversal of the normal condition, but one consistent with the animal's abnormal multisensory experience. Modified from Wallace and Stein (2007).

It also leads to a physical and irreplaceable loss of the cortico–SC synapses, making these sites available to colonization by other afferents. To buttress this observation, ongoing experiments (see Stein et al., 2008; Stein and Rowland, 2007) have been examining the consequences of long-term reversible deactivation of association cortex. This strategy deprives the developing cortex of access to sensory experience but does not remove its projections to the SC and allows it to be reactivated later in life. The deactivation was induced by muscimol that was gradually released over many weeks during the period in which multisensory integration normally develops. The muscimol was infused into chronically implanted pledgets made from the polymer Elvax. Examination of the SC many months later revealed that there were many multisensory neurons. These neurons had developed many of their characteristic unisensory response properties, but even after cortex had been reactivated for many weeks the neurons were still unable to integrate the information derived from cross-modal stimuli and could not enhance SC-mediated behaviors. Once again, the data support the idea that cortex is the portal through which early experiences with cross-modal cues gain access to multisensory SC neurons.

In these experiments, association cortex was unilaterally deactivated and multisensory integration deficits were specific to the ipsilateral SC and to contralateral visual–auditory space. Multisensory responses to stimuli in ipsilateral visual–auditory space were normal and contrasted sharply to those in contralateral space. The deficits appeared to be permanent. However, after four years of normal experience, the animals were retested in a multisensory integration behavioral task and, surprisingly, seemed perfectly normal. All evidence of the prior multisensory integration deficit had disappeared. It seemed that long-term experience, even during adulthood, could compensate for the absence of experiences that are normally acquired during early life. The SC multisensory circuit appeared to be far more flexible than was previously suspected and may be of substantial interest to human subjects with developmental deficits in multisensory integration.

Adult Plasticity

Another ongoing line of research has described how the responses of SC neurons in the adult change or adapt as a consequence of exposure to repeated presentations of cross-modal cues (Yu et al., 2009). These researchers found evidence of short-term plasticity in SC multisensory neurons consistent with the principles of spike-timing-dependent plasticity. When animals were repeatedly presented with sequentially arranged visual–auditory stimuli, the response to the first stimulus increased in magnitude and duration, and the latency of the response to the second stimulus decreased. These findings caused the responses to the sequentially arranged stimuli to appear to "merge," presumably as a consequence of the potentiation of inputs that were previously subthreshold (see figure 15.5). Short-term plasticity of this sort, which reflects the encoding of cross-modal correlations, may provide the basic building blocks on which the "spatial" and "temporal" principles of multisensory integration are founded during long-term development and maturation.

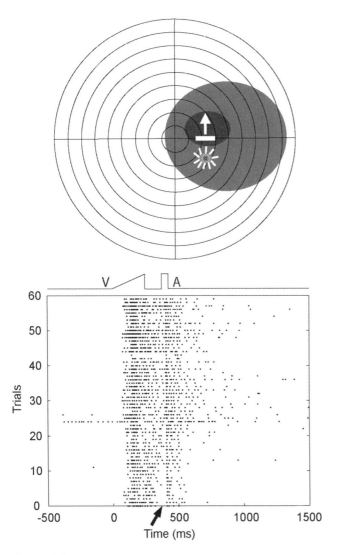

Figure 15.5
Repeated exposure to a sequential auditory–visual stimulus resulted in rapid response changes. (Top) A schematic of visual–auditory space in which concentric circles = 10° of space. A broadband noise burst (shown as a star) and a moving bar of light (shown as a white bar) were within their respective receptive fields (auditory = gray, visual = black). The raster display below the electronic stimulus traces shows the response changes during repeated exposures to the visual stimulus (V) followed 100 milliseconds later by the auditory stimulus (A). This cross-modal stimulus first elicited two distinct unisensory responses, but after several stimulus repetitions, the responses fused into a multisensory response. This was the result of an increase in the amplitude and duration of the first response and a shortening of the latency of the second. The black arrow at the bottom of the raster shows the initial period of silence between the two unisensory responses. Response changes were induced within 2 minutes. Data were taken from ongoing experiments (see Yu et al., 2009).

Recapitulation

Here we have summarized the basic organizational principles of multisensory integration within the SC, its circuitry and experiential antecedents, and evidence for long- and short-term plasticity in these processes. The development of the unisensory systems on which these processes depend provides both a conceptual framework and an interesting foil, as there are clear differences between the development of processing capabilities within a sense and the ability to integrate information across senses. Although we understand that the principles of multisensory integration adapt to the statistics of the cross-modal environment in which the animal functions, we are still in the nascent stages of understanding exactly how the brain determines these statistics and the biological processes by which they are encoded. Future research will expand our focus by studying these adaptive processes and their consequences at different stages of life, from birth to senescence.

Acknowledgments

Portions of the work described here have been supported by National Institutes of Health grants EY016716 and NS036916 and a grant from the Wallace Foundation.

References

Alvarado JC, Stanford TR, Vaughan JW, Stein BE. 2007a. Cortex mediates multisensory but not unisensory integration in superior colliculus. *J Neurosci* 27: 12775–12786.

Alvarado JC, Vaughan JW, Stanford TR, Stein BE. 2007b. Multisensory versus unisensory integration: contrasting modes in the superior colliculus. *J Neurophysiol* 97: 3193–3205.

Alvarado JC, Rowland BA, Stanford TR, Stein BE. 2008. A neural network model of multisensory integration also accounts for unisensory integration in superior colliculus. *Brain Res* 25: 13–23.

Barth DS, Brett-Green B. 2004. Multisensory-evoked potentials in rat cortex. In: *The Handbook of Multisensory Processes* (Calvert GA, Spence C, Stein BE, eds), pp 357–370. Cambridge, MA: MIT Press.

Bernstein LE, Auer ET, Moore JK. 2004. Audiovisual speech binding: convergence or association. In: *The Handbook of Multisensory Processes* (Calvert GA, Spence C, Stein BE, eds), pp 203–224. Cambridge, MA: MIT Press.

Bower TGR. 1974. The evolution of sensory systems. In: *Perception: Essays in Honor of James J. Gibson* (Macleod RGPHL Jr, ed), pp 141–165. Ithaca, NY: Cornell University Press.

Brainard MS, Knudsen EI. 1998. Sensitive periods for visual calibration of the auditory space map in the barn owl optic tectum. *J Neurosci* 18: 3929–3942.

Buonomano DV, Merzenich MM. 1998. Cortical plasticity: from synapses to maps. *Annu Rev Neurosci* 21: 149–186.

Burnett LR, Stein BE, Perrault TJ, Jr., Wallace MT. 2007. Excitotoxic lesions of the superior colliculus preferentially impact multisensory neurons and multisensory integration. *Exp Brain Res* 179: 325–338.

Busse L, Roberts KC, Crist RE, Weissman DH, Woldorff MG. 2005. The spread of attention across modalities and space in a multisensory object. *Proc Natl Acad Sci USA* 102: 18751–18756.

Calvert GA, Lewis JW. 2004. Hemodynamic studies of audiovisual interactions. In: *The Handbook of Multisensory Processes* (Calvert GA, Spence C, Stein BE, eds), pp 483–502. Cambridge, MA: MIT Press.

Carriere B, Royal DW, Perrault TJ, Jr., Morrison SP, Vaughan JW, Stein BE, Wallace MT. 2007. Visual deprivation alters the development of cortical multisensory integration. *J Neurophysiol* 98: 2858–2867.

Corneil BD, Munoz DP. 1996. The influence of auditory and visual distractors on human orienting gaze shifts. *J Neurosci* 16: 8193–8207.

de Gelder B, Vroomen J, Pourtois G. 2004. Multisensory perception of emotion, its time course and its neural basis. In: *The Handbook of Multisensory Processes* (Calvert GA, Spence C, Stein BE, eds), pp 581–596. Cambridge, MA: MIT Press.

Ernst MO, Banks MS. 2002. Humans integrate visual and haptic information in a statistically optimal fashion. *Nature* 415: 429–433.

Fort A, Giard MH. 2004. Multiple electrophysiological mechanisms of audiovisual integration in human perception. In: *The Handbook of Multisensory Processes* (Calvert GA, Spence C, Stein BE, eds), pp 503–514. Cambridge, MA: MIT Press.

Frens MA, Van Opstal AJ. 1995. A quantitative study of auditory-evoked saccadic eye movements in two dimensions. *Exp Brain Res* 107: 103–117.

Fuentes-Santamaria V, Alvarado JC, McHaffie JG, Stein BE. 2009. Axon morphologies and convergence patterns of projections from different sensory-specific cortices of the anterior ectosylvian sulcus onto multisensory neurons in the cat superior colliculus. *Cereb Cortex* 19: 2902–2915.

Ghazanfar AA, Maier JX, Hoffman KL, Logothetis NK. 2005. Multisensory integration of dynamic faces and voices in rhesus monkey auditory cortex. *J Neurosci* 25: 5004–5012.

Ghazanfar AA, Schroeder CE. 2006. Is neocortex essentially multisensory? *Trends Cogn Sci* 10: 278–285.

Gibson JJ. 1966. *The Senses Considered as Perceptual Systems.* Boston, MA: Houghton Mifflin.

Gibson JJ. 1969. *Principles of Perceptual Learning and Development.* Englewood Cliffs, NJ: Prentice Hall.

Gibson JJ. 1979. *An Ecological Approach to Perception.* Boston, MA: Houghton Mifflin.

Gingras G, Rowland BE, Stein BE. 2006. Unisensory versus multisensory integration: computational distinctions in behavior. Program No. 639.9. 2006 Neuroscience Meeting Planner. Atlanta, GA: Society for Neuroscience. Online.

Gori M, Del Viva M, Sandini G, Burr DC. 2008. Young children do not integrate visual and haptic form information. *Curr Biol* 18: 694–698.

Grant AC, Thiagarajah MC, Sathian K. 2000. Tactile perception in blind Braille readers: a psychophysical study of acuity and hyperacuity using gratings and dot patterns. *Percept Psychophys* 62: 301–312.

Grantyn A, Grantyn R. 1982. Axonal patterns and sites of termination of cat superior colliculus neurons projecting in the tecto–bulbo–spinal tract. *Exp Brain Res* 46: 243–256.

Groh JM, Sparks DL. 1996a. Saccades to somatosensory targets. II. Motor convergence in primate superior colliculus. *J Neurophysiol* 75: 428–438.

Groh JM, Sparks DL. 1996b. Saccades to somatosensory targets. III. Eye-position-dependent somatosensory activity in primate superior colliculus. *J Neurophysiol* 75: 439–453.

Guitton D, Munoz DP. 1991. Control of orienting gaze shifts by the tectoreticulospinal system in the head-free cat. I. Identification, localization, and effects of behavior on sensory responses. *J Neurophysiol* 66: 1605–1623.

Gutfreund Y, Knudsen EI. 2004. Visual instruction of the auditory space map in the midbrain. In: *The Handbook of Multisensory Processes* (Calvert GA, Spence C, Stein BE, eds), pp 613–624. Cambridge, MA: MIT Press.

Hairston WD, Wallace MT, Vaughan JW, Stein BE, Schirillo JA. 2003. Visual localization ability influences cross-modal bias. *J Cogn Neurosci* 15: 20–29.

Hall WC, Moschovakis A. 2004. *The Superior Colliculus: New Approaches to Studying Sensorimotor Integration.* Boca Raton: CRC Press.

Harris LR. 1980. The superior colliculus and movements of the head and eyes in cats. *J Physiol* 300: 367–391.

Hughes HC, Reuter-Lorenz PA, Nozawa G, Fendrich R. 1994. Visual–auditory interactions in sensorimotor processing: saccades versus manual responses. *J Exp Psychol Hum Percept Perform* 20: 131–153.

Jay MF, Sparks DL. 1984. Auditory receptive fields in primate superior colliculus shift with changes in eye position. *Nature* 309: 345–347.

Jay MF, Sparks DL. 1987a. Sensorimotor integration in the primate superior colliculus. I. Motor convergence. *J Neurophysiol* 57: 22–34.

Jay MF, Sparks DL. 1987b. Sensorimotor integration in the primate superior colliculus. II. Coordinates of auditory signals. *J Neurophysiol* 57: 35–55.

Jiang W, Jiang H, Rowland BA, Stein BE. 2007. Multisensory orientation behavior is disrupted by neonatal cortical ablation. *J Neurophysiol* 97: 557–562.

Jiang W, Jiang H, Stein BE. 2002. Two corticotectal areas facilitate multisensory orientation behavior. *J Cogn Neurosci* 14: 1240–1255.

Jiang W, Jiang H, Stein BE. 2006. Neonatal cortical ablation disrupts multisensory development in superior colliculus. *J Neurophysiol* 95: 1380–1396.

Jiang W, Wallace MT, Jiang H, Vaughan JW, Stein BE. 2001. Two cortical areas mediate multisensory integration in superior colliculus neurons. *J Neurophysiol* 85: 506–522.

Kadunce DC, Vaughan JW, Wallace MT, Benedek G, Stein BE. 1997. Mechanisms of within- and cross-modality suppression in the superior colliculus. *J Neurophysiol* 78: 2834–2847.

Kao CQ, McHaffie JG, Meredith MA, Stein BE. 1994. Functional development of a central visual map in cat. *J Neurophysiol* 72: 266–272.

King AJ, Doubell TP, Skaliora I. 2004. Epigenetic factors that align visual and auditory maps in the ferret midbrain. In: *The Handbook of Multisensory Processes* (Calvert GA, Spence C, Stein BE, eds), pp 613–624. Cambridge, MA: MIT Press.

King AJ, Palmer AR. 1985. Integration of visual and auditory information in bimodal neurones in the guinea-pig superior colliculus. *Exp Brain Res* 60: 492–500.

King AJ, Schnupp JW, Carlile S, Smith AL, Thompson ID. 1996. The development of topographically-aligned maps of visual and auditory space in the superior colliculus. *Prog Brain Res* 112: 335–350.

Knudsen EI, Brainard MS. 1991. Visual instruction of the neural map of auditory space in the developing optic tectum. *Science* 253: 85–87.

Knudsen EI, Esterly SD, du LS. 1991. Stretched and upside-down maps of auditory space in the optic tectum of blind-reared owls; acoustic basis and behavioral correlates. *J Neurosci* 11: 1727–1747.

Knudsen EI, Knudsen PF. 1989. Vision calibrates sound localization in developing barn owls. *J Neurosci* 9: 3306–3313.

Lakatos P, Chen CM, O'Connell MN, Mills A, Schroeder CE. 2007. Neuronal oscillations and multisensory interaction in primary auditory cortex. *Neuron* 53: 279–292.

Larson MA, Stein BE. 1984. The use of tactile and olfactory cues in neonatal orientation and localization of the nipple. *Dev Psychobiol* 17: 423–436.

Laurienti PJ, Burdette JH, Wallace MT, Yen YF, Field AS, Stein BE. 2002. Deactivation of sensory-specific cortex by cross-modal stimuli. *J Cogn Neurosci* 14: 420–429.

Lewkowicz DJ, Kraebel KS. 2004. The value of multisensory redundancy in the development of intersensory perception. In: *The Handbook of Multisensory Processes* (Calvert GA, Spence C, Stein BE, eds), pp 655–678. Cambridge, MA: MIT Press.

Lickliter R, Bahrick LE. 2004. Perceptual development and the origins of multisensory responsiveness. In: *The Handbook of Multisensory Processes* (Calvert GA, Spence C, Stein BE, eds), pp 643–654. Cambridge, MA: MIT Press.

Liotti M, Ryder K, Woldorff MG. 1998. Auditory attention in the congenitally blind: where, when and what gets reorganized? *Neuroreport* 9: 1007–1012.

Lovelace CT, Stein BE, Wallace MT. 2003. An irrelevant light enhances auditory detection in humans: a psychophysical analysis of multisensory integration in stimulus detection. *Brain Res Cogn Brain Res* 17: 447–453.

Macaluso E, Driver J. 2004. Neuroimaging studies of cross-modal integration for emotion. In: *The Handbook of Multisensory Processes* (Calvert GA, Spence C, Stein BE, eds), pp 529–548. Cambridge, MA: MIT Press.

Marks LE. 1978. *The Unity of the Senses: Interrelations Among the Modalities.* New York: Academic Press.

Marks LE. 2004. Cross-modal interactions in speeded classification. In: *The Handbook of Multisensory Processes* (Calvert GA, Spence C, Stein BE, eds), pp 85–106. Cambridge, MA: MIT Press.

Massaro DW. 2004. From multisensory integration to talking heads and language learning. In: *The Handbook of Multisensory Processes* (Calvert GA, Spence C, Stein BE, eds), pp 153–176. Cambridge, MA: MIT Press.

Meredith MA, Clemo HR, Stein BE. 1991. Somatotopic component of the multisensory map in the deep laminae of the cat superior colliculus. *J Comp Neurol* 312: 353–370.

Meredith MA, Stein BE. 1983. Interactions among converging sensory inputs in the superior colliculus. *Science* 221: 389–391.

Meredith MA, Stein BE. 1986a. Spatial factors determine the activity of multisensory neurons in cat superior colliculus. *Brain Res* 365: 350–354.

Meredith MA, Stein BE. 1986b. Visual, auditory, and somatosensory convergence on cells in superior colliculus results in multisensory integration. *J Neurophysiol* 56: 640–662.

Meredith MA, Stein BE. 1990. The visuotopic component of the multisensory map in the deep laminae of the cat superior colliculus. *J Neurosci* 10: 3727–3742.

Meredith MA, Stein BE. 1996. Spatial determinants of multisensory integration in cat superior colliculus neurons. *J Neurophysiol* 75: 1843–1857.

Meredith MA, Wallace MT, Stein BE. 1992. Visual, auditory and somatosensory convergence in output neurons of the cat superior colliculus: multisensory properties of the tecto–reticulo–spinal projection. *Exp Brain Res* 88: 181–186.

Middlebrooks JC, Knudsen EI. 1984. A neural code for auditory space in the cat's superior colliculus. *J Neurosci* 4: 2621–2634.

Munoz DP, Wurtz RH. 1993a. Fixation cells in monkey superior colliculus. I. Characteristics of cell discharge. *J Neurophysiol* 70: 559–575.

Munoz DP, Wurtz RH. 1993b. Fixation cells in monkey superior colliculus. II. Reversible activation and deactivation. *J Neurophysiol* 70: 576–589.

Neil PA, Chee-Ruiter C, Scheier C, Lewkowicz DJ, Shimojo S. 2006. Development of multisensory spatial integration and perception in humans. *Dev Sci* 9: 454–464.

Newell FN. 2004. Cross-modal object recognition. In: *The Handbook of Multisensory Processes* (Calvert GA, Spence C, Stein BE, eds), pp 123–140. Cambridge, MA: MIT Press.

Partan SR. 2004. Multisensory animal communication. In: *The Handbook of Multisensory Processes* (Calvert GA, Spence C, Stein BE, eds), pp 225–242. Cambridge, MA: MIT Press.

Peck CK. 1987. Visual-auditory interactions in cat superior colliculus: their role in the control of gaze. *Brain Res* 420: 162–166.

Pouget A, Deneve S, Duhamel JR. 2002. A computational perspective on the neural basis of multisensory spatial representations. *Nat Rev Neurosci* 3: 741–747.

Putzar L, Goerendt I, Lange K, Rösler F, Röder B. 2007. Early visual deprivation impairs multisensory interactions in humans. *Nat Neurosci* 10: 1243–1245.

Recanzone GH. 1998. Rapidly induced auditory plasticity: the ventriloquism aftereffect. *Proc Natl Acad Sci USA* 95: 869–875.

Rowland BA, Quessy S, Stanford TR, Stein BE. 2007. Multisensory integration shortens physiological response latencies. *J Neurosci* 27: 5879–5884.

Sathian K. 2000. Practice makes perfect: sharper tactile perception in the blind. *Neurology* 54: 2203–2204.

Sathian K. 2005. Visual cortical activity during tactile perception in the sighted and the visually deprived. *Dev Psychobiol* 46: 279–286.

Sathian K, Prather SCZM. 2004. Visual cortical involvement in normal tactile perception. In: *The Handbook of Multisensory Processes* (Calvert GA, Spence C, Stein BE, eds), pp 703–710. Cambridge, MA: MIT Press.

Schroeder CE, Foxe JJ. 2002. The timing and laminar profile of converging inputs to multisensory areas of the macaque neocortex. *Brain Res Cogn Brain Res* 14: 187–198.

Schroeder CE, Foxe JJ. 2004. Multisensory convergence in early cortical processing. In: *The Handbook of Multisensory Processes* (Calvert GA, Spence C, Stein BE, eds), pp 295–310. Cambridge, MA: MIT Press.

Schroeder CE, Lindsley RW, Specht C, Marcovici A, Smiley JF, Javitt DC. 2001. Somatosensory input to auditory association cortex in the macaque monkey. *J Neurophysiol* 85: 1322–1327.

Shams L, Kamitani Y, Shimojo S. 2004. Modulations of visual perception by sound. In: *The Handbook of Multisensory Processes* (Calvert GA, Spence C, Stein BE, eds), pp 27–34. Cambridge, MA: MIT Press.

Sparks DL. 1986. Translation of sensory signals into commands for control of saccadic eye movements: role of primate superior colliculus. *Physiol Rev* 66: 118–171.

Sparks DL, Nelson JS. 1987. Sensory and motor maps in the mammalian superior colliculus. *Trends Neurosci* 10: 312–317.

Stein BE, Magalhaes-Castro B, Kruger L. 1975. Superior colliculus: visuotopic–somatotopic overlap. *Science* 189: 224–226.

Stein BE. 1984. Development of the superior colliculus. *Ann Rev Neurosci* 7: 95–125.

Stein BE, Labos E, Kruger L. 1973a. Sequence of changes in properties of neurons of superior colliculus of the kitten during maturation. *J Neurophysiol* 36: 667–679.

Stein BE, Labos E, Kruger L. 1973b. Determinants of response latency in neurons of superior colliculus in kittens. *J Neurophysiol* 36: 680–689.

Stein BE, Magalhaes-Castro B, Kruger L. 1976. Relationship between visual and tactile representations in cat superior colliculus. *J Neurophysiol* 39: 401–419.

Stein BE, Dixon JP. 1979. Properties of superior colliculus neurons in the golden hamster. *J Comp Neurol* 183: 269–284.

Stein BE, Gallagher HL. 1981. Maturation of cortical control over superior colliculus cells in cat. *Brain Res* 223: 429–435.

Stein BE, Clamann HP. 1981. Control of pinna movements and sensorimotor register in cat superior colliculus. *Brain Behav Evol* 19: 180–192.

Stein BE, Meredith MA, Huneycutt WS, McDade L. 1989. Behavioral indices of multisensory integration: orientation to visual cues is affected by auditory stimuli. *J Cogn Neurosci* 1: 12–24.

Stein BE, Meredith MA. 1993. *The Merging of the Senses.* Cambridge, MA: MIT Press.

Stein BE, Meredith MA, Wallace MT. 1993. The visually responsive neuron and beyond: multisensory integration in cat and monkey. *Prog Brain Res* 95: 79–90.

Stein BE, London N, Wilkinson LK, Price DD. 1996. Enhancement of perceived visual intensity by auditory stimuli: a psychophysical analysis. *J Cogn Neurosci* 8: 497–506.

Stein BE, Wallace MW, Stanford TR, Jiang W. 2002. Cortex governs multisensory integration in the midbrain. *Neuroscientist* 8: 306–314.

Stein BE, Rowland BA 2007. The critical role of cortico-collicular interactions in the development of multisensory integration. Program No. 614.7. 2007 Neuroscience Meeting Planner. San Diego, CA: Society for Neuroscience, 2007. Online.

Stein BE, Stanford TR. 2008. Multisensory integration: current issues from the perspective of the single neuron. *Nat Rev Neurosci* 9: 255–266.

Stein BE, Perrault TJ, Jr., Vaughan JW, Rowland BA. 2008. Long term plasticity of multisensory neurons in the superior colliculus. Program No. 457.14, 2008 Neuroscience Meeting Planner. Washington, DC: Society for Neuroscience, 2008. Online.

Stein BE, Stanford TR, Ramachandran R, Perrault TJ, Jr., Rowland BA. 2009. Challenges in quantifying multisensory integration: alternative criteria, models, and inverse effectiveness. *Exp Brain Res* 198(2–3): 113–126.

Sugihara T, Diltz MD, Averbeck BB, Romanski LM. 2006. Integration of auditory and visual communication information in the primate ventrolateral prefrontal cortex. *J Neurosci* 26: 11138–11147.

Sumby WH, Pollack I. 1954. Visual contribution to speech intelligibility in noise. *J Acoust Soc Am* 26: 212–215.

Talsma D, Doty TJ, Strowd R, Woldorff MG. 2006a. Attentional capacity for processing concurrent stimuli is larger across sensory modalities than within a modality. *Psychophysiology* 43: 541–549.

Talsma D, Kok A, Ridderinkhof KR. 2006b. Selective attention to spatial and non-spatial visual stimuli is affected differentially by age: effects on event-related brain potentials and performance data. *Int J Psychophysiol* 62: 249–261.

Wallace MT, Meredith MA, Stein BE. 1992. Integration of multiple sensory modalities in cat cortex. *Exp Brain Res* 91: 484–488.

Wallace MT, Meredith MA, Stein BE. 1993. Converging influences from visual, auditory, and somatosensory cortices onto output neurons of the superior colliculus. *J Neurophysiol* 69: 1797–1809.

Wallace MT, Stein BE. 1994. Cross-modal synthesis in the midbrain depends on input from cortex. *J Neurophysiol* 71: 429–432.

Wallace MT, Stein BE. 1997. Development of multisensory neurons and multisensory integration in cat superior colliculus. *J Neurosci* 17: 2429–2444.

Wallace MT, Stein BE. 2000. Onset of cross-modal synthesis in the neonatal superior colliculus is gated by the development of cortical influences. *J Neurophysiol* 83: 3578–3582.

Wallace MT, Stein BE. 2001. Sensory and multisensory responses in the newborn monkey superior colliculus. *J Neurosci* 21: 8886–8894.

Wallace MT. 2004. The development of multisensory integration. In: *The Handbook of Multisensory Processing* (Calvert GA, Spence C, Stein BE, eds), pp 625–642. Cambridge, MA: MIT Press.

Wallace MT, Ramachandran R, Stein BE. 2004. A revised view of sensory cortical parcellation. *Proc Natl Acad Sci USA* 101: 2167–2172.

Wallace MT, Carriere BN, Perrault TJ, Jr., Vaughan JW, Stein BE. 2006. The development of cortical multisensory integration. *J Neurosci* 26: 11844–11849.

Wallace MT, Stein BE. 2007. Early experience determines how the senses will interact. *J Neurophysiol* 97: 921–926.

Wallace MT, Wilkinson LK, Stein BE. 1996. Representation and integration of multiple sensory inputs in primate superior colliculus. *J Neurophysiol* 76: 1246–1266.

Weisser V, Stilla R, Peltier S, Hu X, Sathian K. 2005. Short-term visual deprivation alters neural processing of tactile form. *Exp Brain Res* 166: 572–582.

Werner H. 1973. *Comparative Psychology of Mental Development.* New York: International Universities Press.

Wickelgren BG, Sterling P. 1969. Influence of visual cortex on receptive fields in the superior colliculus of the cat. *J Neurophysiol* 32: 1–15.

Wilkinson LK, Meredith MA, Stein BE. 1996. The role of anterior ectosylvian cortex in cross-modality orientation and approach behavior. *Exp Brain Res* 112: 1–10.

Woldorff MG, Hazlett CJ, Fichtenholtz HM, Weissman DH, Dale AM, Song AW. 2004. Functional parcellation of attentional control regions of the brain. *J Cogn Neurosci* 16: 149–165.

Woods TM, Recanzone GH. 2004. Cross-modal interactions evidenced by the ventriloquism effect in humans and monkeys. In: *The Handbook of Multisensory Processes* (Calvert GA, Spence C, Stein BE, eds), pp 35–48. Cambridge, MA: MIT Press.

Wurtz RH, Albano JE. 1980. Two visual systems: brain mechanisms for localization and discrimination are dissociated by tectal and cortical lesions. *Ann Rev Neurosci* 3: 189–226.

Wurtz RH, Goldberg ME. 1971. Superior colliculus cell responses related to eye movements in awake monkeys. *Science* 171: 82–84.

Yu L, Rowland BA, Stein BE. 2009. Plasticity of multisensory neurons in adult superior colliculus: effects of repeated sequential visual and auditory stimuli. Program No. 847.3. 2009 Neuroscience Meeting Planner. Chicago, IL: Society for Neuroscience, 2009. Online.

Zangaladze A, Epstein CM, Grafton ST, Sathian K. 1999. Involvement of visual cortex in tactile discrimination of orientation. *Nature* 401: 587–590.

Zwiers MP, Van Opstal AJ, Paige GD. 2003. Plasticity in human sound localization induced by compressed spatial vision. *Nat Neurosci* 6: 175–181.

16 Auditory Processing and Plasticity

Josef P. Rauschecker

In an interview with David Burr (Maffei, 2009) for *Current Biology*, Lamberto Maffei fondly refers to the Physiological Laboratory at the University of Cambridge, where he spent several years collaborating with Fergus Campbell, as an "intellectual paradise." Maffei recalls "tea time" at the laboratory with Sir Alan Hodgkin and other giants as "interesting and instructive, and sometimes a sheer joy." Indeed, there is no better way to describe the stimulating and charged atmosphere of the Physiological Laboratory, where I first met Maffei while I was studying under Campbell in 1973 (Rauschecker et al., 1973). The collaboration between Maffei and Campbell led to many seminal publications, not the least of which was a *Scientific American* article (Campbell and Maffei, 1974), certainly read by many students.

The main thrust of the work by Campbell and Maffei, as well as Lamberto's long-time friend and collaborator in Pisa, Adriana Fiorentini (Maffei and Fiorentini, 1973), was the concept that the early visual system served as a spatial frequency analyzer for complex visual scenes and objects. The idea initially came from hearing, in which the inner ear acts as a frequency analyzer that breaks down complex sounds into sinusoidal frequency components (Békésy, 1960; Helmholtz, 1863; Ohm, 1843). The approach of using sinusoidal gratings in visual psychophysics and neurophysiology has continued to be dominant ever since the Cambridge and Pisa studies.

Just as vision scientists have learned from concepts in auditory physiology, auditory neuroscientists are now learning from vision, as this chapter hopes to demonstrate.

Processing of Complex Sounds: Parallels between Vision and Hearing

Georg von Békésy, who won the Nobel Prize in 1961 for his experiments on the mechanics of the inner ear, has often emphasized the "parallelism between vision and hearing" (Békésy, 1971). This parallelism refers to the existence of lateral inhibition at early levels of sensory processing and even more to the increased integration of information from the sensory periphery at higher levels of processing (Rauschecker, 1998b). Just as visual receptive fields get larger and more complex at higher processing levels, the frequency response areas of auditory neurons likewise become broader and more complex at ascending levels of cortical processing (Rauschecker et al., 1995).

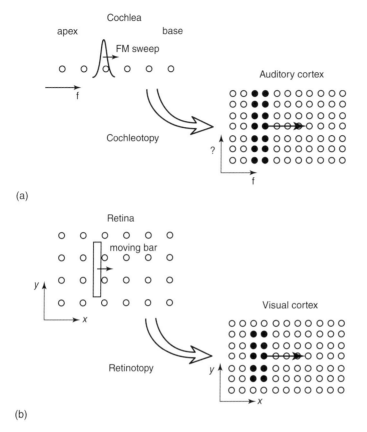

(a)

(b)

Figure 16.1
Equivalence of cortical processing in the auditory (a) and visual (b) systems. Frequency is represented in the tonotopic maps of auditory cortex as compared to two-dimensional retinotopic space in the visual cortex. Accordingly, moving bars or gratings (preferred stimuli in the visual cortex) translate into auditory frequency-modulated (FM) sweeps. Neurons are found in the auditory cortex which respond to FM sweeps in a highly direction-selective manner (Tian and Rauschecker, 2004).

If one equates sensory receptor surfaces (coding of retinal position in the visual system and frequency in the cochlea), direct analogies become immediately obvious: moving bars and gratings—effective stimuli for neurons in the visual cortex—can be equated with the frequency-modulated sweeps that auditory cortical neurons respond to (see figure 16.1). Bandwidth selectivity of neurons in the auditory belt cortex (Rauschecker and Tian, 2004; Rauschecker et al., 1995) can be understood as equivalent to size selectivity in area V4 of the visual cortex (Desimone and Schein, 1987; see figure 16.2). Since size is inversely related to spatial frequency, an analogy can also be drawn between spatial frequency selectivity in the visual cortex and bandwidth selectivity in the auditory cortex.

Auditory Processing Streams

Evidence from Nonhuman Primate Studies

Cortical auditory processing begins with primary auditory cortex (A1), which provides the foundation for many fundamental aspects of hearing. Habituation of neuronal responses in A1, for instance, may form the basis for auditory figure–ground discrimination (Micheyl et al., 2005). However, work in nonhuman primates has also made it abundantly clear that A1 is surrounded by multiple specialized fields processing different aspects of sound (Kaas and Hackett, 2000; Kusmierek and Rauschecker, 2009; Rauschecker et al., 1995; Tian et al., 2001). An anterior stream is devoted to the identification of particular complex sounds; a posterior stream, project-ing to parietal cortex and beyond, is involved in processing spatial aspects of sound (see figure 16.3; Rauschecker and Tian, 2000).

The anterior "what"-stream originates in primary auditory cortex (or area R, the rostral core area) and, via the anterolateral area of the lateral belt cortex, projects to the ventrolateral pre-frontal cortex (Romanski et al., 1999), which has previously been identified as a neural locus for object working memory (Goldman-Rakic, 1996). The what-stream also includes the rostral parabelt and other rostral superior temporal (ST) areas all the way to the rostral pole of ST cortex. Additionally, the what-stream parallels an anteroventral stream in vision, which origi-nates in primary visual cortex (V1) and projects into inferotemporal cortex. The latter includes mechanisms and neurons specific for the processing of complex visual objects, such as faces, hands, houses, or visual scenes in general (Gross, 1992). Similarly, the auditory what-stream is thought to underlie the processing of behaviorally relevant, complex sounds ("auditory objects"), including speech sounds, which are tied to semantic meaning. Auditory and visual what-streams interact throughout the border zone of the superior temporal sulcus (STS). Nonhuman primate studies have demonstrated selective integration of face and voice processing along anterior regions of the STS (Ghazanfar and Logothetis, 2003).

The posterior "where"-stream originates in primary auditory cortex as well but projects pos-teriorly into areas of the caudal belt. These areas contain neurons that are sharply tuned to the spatial location of a sound presented in free field (Recanzone, 2000; Tian et al., 2001). The caudal belt and parabelt project to the ventral inferior parietal area (Lewis and Van Essen, 2000). The caudal belt cortex also projects directly to the dorsolateral prefrontal cortex (Romanski et al., 1999), which is known to play a role in spatial working memory (Goldman-Rakic, 1996).

Evidence from Human Neuroimaging

In addition to nonhuman primate studies, modern neuroimaging techniques, such as positron emission tomography (PET) and functional magnetic resonance imaging (fMRI), have also provided conclusive evidence for a functional parcellation of auditory-responsive brain regions in humans. Anterolateral areas of the superior temporal cortex are activated by intelligible speech or speechlike sounds (Binder et al., 2004; Obleser et al., 2006; Scott et al., 2000) and other auditory objects (Zatorre et al., 2004; Leaver and Rauschecker, 2010). Thus, it has become clear

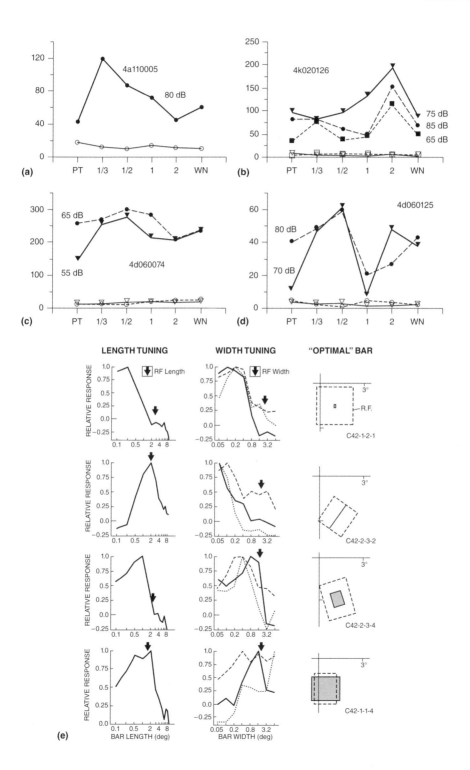

that behaviorally relevant auditory patterns, including speech sounds, are identified and discriminated selectively within an anterior auditory what-stream. Posterior regions in the superior temporal gyrus (STG) and STS of humans, in contrast, are specifically active during spatial tasks, such as auditory spatial discrimination or tasks involving auditory motion in space (Ahveninen et al., 2006; Brunetti et al., 2005; Degerman et al., 2006; Deouell et al., 2007; Jääskeläinen et al., 2004; Krumbholz et al., 2005; Maeder et al., 2001; Tata and Ward, 2005; Warren et al., 2002; Zatorre et al., 2002; Zimmer and Macaluso, 2005).

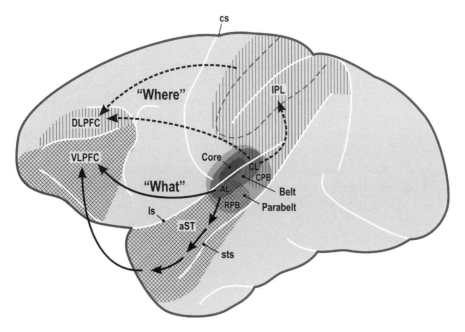

Figure 16.3
Schematic illustration of hierarchical processing in the auditory cortex of the rhesus monkey and processing streams for "what" and "where." Auditory signals arrive first in the core areas (consisting of primary auditory cortex, A1, and two rostral areas) from subcortical inputs in thalamus and brainstem. Activity then propagates to the belt (anterolateral area, AL; caudolateral area, CL, among others) and parabelt areas (rostral and caudal, RPB and CPB, respectively), which give rise to two pathways projecting to two largely segregated regions in the prefrontal cortex (PFC): the ventrolateral and dorsolateral (VLPFC and DLPFC) regions, respectively. The ventral processing stream also includes the anterior superior temporal (aST) cortex, where regions specialized for the processing of communication sounds have been found in both monkeys and humans. The dorsal stream is relayed also through the inferior parietal lobule (IPL) of posterior parietal cortex (PPC; from Rauschecker, 2009). Rich back-projections exist from prefrontal cortex to the PPC as well as to aST (not shown). The significance of these latter projections is discussed in more detail in another recent review (Rauschecker and Scott, 2009). cs, central sulcus.

◀ **Figure 16.2** (opposite)
Equivalence of bandwidth and size tuning in the auditory and visual systems, respectively. a to d show bandwidth tuning curves of single units in the lateral-belt (secondary) auditory cortex in response to band-passed noise bursts (from Rauschecker and Tian, 2004). Illustration of visual size tuning of V4 units in (e) is taken from Desimone and Schein (1987).

In a meta-analysis, Arnott et al. (2004) reviewed evidence from auditory fMRI and PET studies to determine the reliability of the auditory dual-pathway model in humans. Activation coordinates from 11 "spatial" studies and 27 "nonspatial" studies were entered into the analysis. Almost all temporal lobe activity observed during spatial tasks was confined to posterior areas. In addition, all but one of the spatial studies reported activation of the inferior parietal lobule whereas only 41% of the nonspatial studies reported activation in this region. Furthermore, inferior frontal activity (Brodmann's areas 45 and 47) was reported in only 9% of the spatial studies but in 56% of the nonspatial studies. These results support an auditory dual-pathway model in humans in which nonspatial sound information (e.g., sound identity) is processed primarily along an anteroventral stream whereas sound location is processed along a posterodorsal stream, that is, within areas posterior to primary auditory cortex. Interestingly, this dichotomy applies to multisensory integration of auditory and tactile information as well (Renier et al., 2009).

The function of the dorsal stream in all sensory modalities extends beyond the processing of space: it is involved more generally in sensorimotor coupling as relevant to the formation of internal models for behaviors such as reaching and grasping to speech production (Rauschecker and Scott, 2009). Such sensorimotor coupling also includes the learning of sequences—for instance, sequences of sound in speech and music (Leaver et al., 2009). Thus, on a fundamental level, the dorsal processing stream plays a pivotal role in linking perception and action (Fuster, 2008; Goodale and Milner, 1992; Rizzolatti et al., 2006).

Central Auditory Plasticity

Many important functions of the auditory system can only be fully understood with cortical plasticity in mind. For instance, even with an innate capacity for language, normal speech can hardly be acquired without auditory feedback and a capacity for learning. Likewise, a system capable of localizing sound with extraordinary precision, using various sets of cues, cannot accomplish this task without the aid of tuning mechanisms that continuously recalibrate the system, especially during the growth phase of the head and outer ears.

Perception of Speech and Music

As discussed above, functional imaging studies point to an involvement of cortical areas in the anterior STG during the processing of speech and other auditory object information (Binder et al., 2000; Binder et al., 2004; Rauschecker and Tian, 2000; Scott et al., 2000; Zatorre et al., 2004; Leaver and Rauschecker, 2010). Neurophysiologically, one must imagine that neurons specific for certain speech sounds are created by combining input from lower-order neurons, which contain feature detectors for elements of speech, in earlier regions (Rauschecker, 1999; Rauschecker and Scott, 2009). Auditory cortical plasticity enables the formation of such combinations provided the condition of an early phonetic environment. Such self-organization processes ultimately lead to the establishment of phonological representations in higher-order computational maps (Kohonen and Hari, 1999).

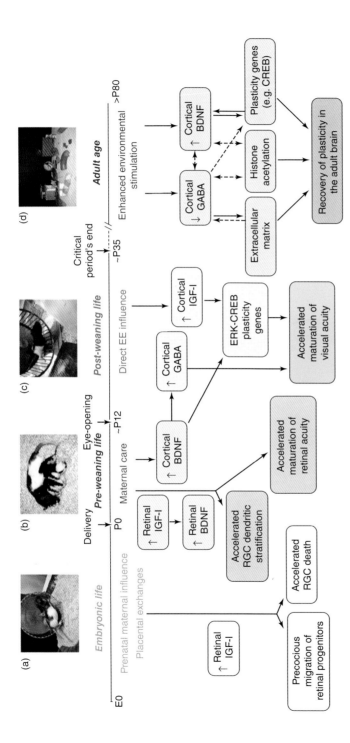

Plate 1 (figure 2.2)

Environmental enrichment (EE) effects on the developing and the adult visual system: an interpretative framework. Three consecutive temporal phases during development are differently controlled by the richness of the environment. (a) The maturation of the nervous system is sensitive to environmental stimulation already during prenatal life, with the mother mediating the influence of the environment through placental exchanges with the fetus. Indeed, exposing pregnant females to EE leads to an acceleration of structural processes critical for retinal maturation in the embryos, an effect mostly due to increased levels of insulin-like growth factor-I (IGF-I). (b) In the early postnatal phase, EE pups receive enhanced maternal care stimulating the expression of experience-dependent factors, such as BDNF, both in the retina and the visual cortex. This drives the accelerated maturation of retinal ganglion cells (RGCs) observed in EE pups and, through an increased GABAergic inhibitory transmission, triggers a faster visual cortex development. (c) Finally, when developing pups are able to autonomously interact with the enriched environment, an increase of cortical IGF-I, which in turn promotes the maturation of the GABAergic system, induces a quite strong acceleration (about one week) in the time course of visual acuity maturation. (d) Recent data have documented a previously unsuspected high potential of neuronal plasticity in the adult visual cortex, with EE in adulthood promoting visual acuity and binocularity recovery from amblyopia. This is due to a decreased intracortical inhibition and to an enhanced BDNF expression. Both the increase in overall cortical activity and BDNF intracellular signaling could in turn induce the activation of other genes promoting plasticity—for instance, through the ERK–CREB pathway. An influence on the epigenetic control of gene transcription has been also suggested for EE. Finally, changes leading to extracellular matrix remodeling may trigger structural modifications at the level of synaptic connectivity. Continuous arrows represent well-documented interactions between boxes; dashed arrows indicate likely interactions in the context of visual cortical plasticity deserving further experimental characterization.

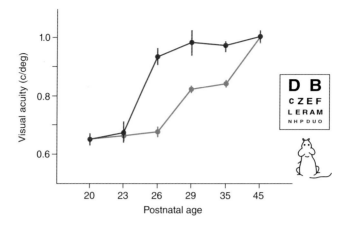

(a)

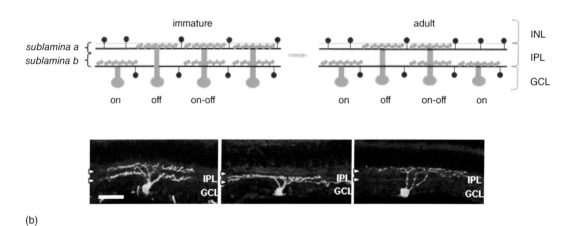

(b)

Plate 2 (figure 2.3)
Acceleration of visual system development by environmental enrichment (EE). (a) Environmental enrichment strongly accelerates visual acuity maturation. Visual acuity measured by visual evoked potentials in non-EE (green) and EE (red) rats during postnatal development is plotted as a function of age to show the leftward shift of the curve for EE animals. (b) Top row: Schematic representation illustrating the passage from immature to adult state during development of retinal ganglion cell (RGC) dendritic stratification (cholinergic amacrine cells in red, RGCs in green). The patterning of cholinergic amacrine cell projections identifies the *a* and *b* sublaminae of the IPL. ON-OFF bistratified RGCs could develop in either ON or OFF RGCs, with dendrites respectively monostratified in the *a* or *b* sublaminae. GCL, ganglion cell layer; IPL, inner plexiform layer; INL, inner nuclear layer. Bottom row: Examples of monostratified or bistratified RGCs. Confocal images are taken from 25-μm vertical retinal sections from P30 transgenic mice expressing the green fluorescent protein. White arrows indicate the sublaminae of the IPL (red bands). Scale bar: 50 μm. Modified from Landi et al. (2007a, 2007b).

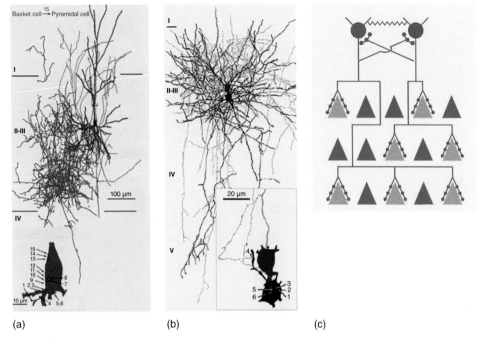

(a)   (b)   (c)

Plate 3 (figure 8.1)
(a) Highly exuberant axonal arborization of a neocortical basket interneuron (blue) and one of its many postsynaptic pyramidal cells (red). Although the basket axon overlaps with a large part of the pyramidal basal dendritic tree, all 15 electron microscopically verified synaptic junctions (bottom panel, right) are clustered around the soma or the most proximal dendrites (bottom left panel) (adapted from Tamas et al., 1997). (b) Reconstructions of the two parvalbumin-containing basket cells connected by both chemical and electrical synapses (presynaptic cell: soma and dendrites, red; axon, green; postsynaptic cell: soma, dendrites, black; axon, blue). Cortical layers (I–V) are indicated on the left. The electron-microscopically identified synaptic junctions (1–4) and gap junctions (5, 6) mediating the interaction between the coupled cells were found nearby on the soma and a proximal dendrite (insert) (adapted from Tamas et al., 2000). (c) A schematic showing prominent features of the innervation pattern of cortical basket interneurons. A single basket cell axon (green) innervating the many pyramidal neurons (red) in its vicinity with clusters of perisomatic synapses (green dots). Basket cells also innervate other basket cells via chemical and electrical (zigzagged lines) synapses. Gray triangles represent pyramidal neurons that are not innervated by these basket cells.

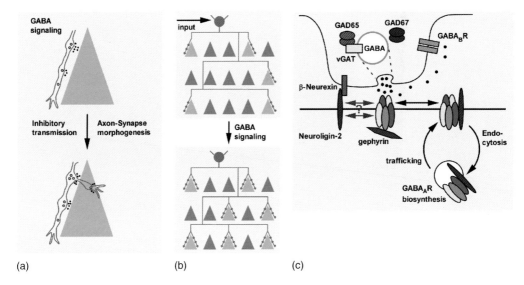

(a)   (b)   (c)

Plate 4 (figure 8.2)

Glutamic acid decaboxylase (GAD) 67 and GABA act beyond inhibitory transmission and regulate inhibitory synapse development and innervation patterns. (a) GABA signaling may regulate the morphogenesis of inhibitory synapses. (b) Since synapse formation is an integral part of axon growth and branching, activity-dependent GABA signaling may further influence the development of GABAergic axon arbor and innervation patterns. (c) A hypothetical model depicting how GABA–GABA receptor signaling and neuroligin–neurexin adhesion may interact and cooperate to regulate the development of inhibitory synapses. Pentameric GABA$_A$ receptors (GABA$_A$Rs) are assembled in the endoplasmic reticulum. Most GABA$_A$Rs are first delivered to extrasynaptic locations; they then either diffuse to and become trapped at postsynaptic sites or undergo endocytosis. Neuroligin 2 (NL2) and synaptic GABA$_A$R stabilize each other, either through intracellular reciprocal interactions aided by scaffolding proteins such as gephyrin or through extracellular cis interaction. In addition, GABA activation of GABA$_A$Rs might further stabilize synaptic GABA$_A$Rs through structural changes or signaling mechanisms. Such activity- and GABA-mediated stabilization of GABA$_A$R might further increase the levels of NL2 at cell–cell contacts and, in turn, stabilize presynaptic terminals through transsynaptic interactions with neurexins.

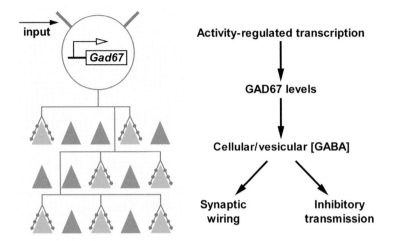

Plate 5 (figure 8.3)
A scheme showing that the level and pattern of neuronal activity may regulate inhibitory synaptic morphogenesis and innervation patterns through glutamic acid decaboxylase (GAD) 67-mediated GABA synthesis and signaling.

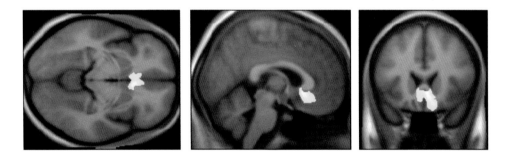

Plate 6 (figure 16.5)
Volume loss in the subcallosal area of tinnitus patients, as shown with voxel-based morphometry (modified from Mühlau et al., 2006). The subcallosal area, which includes medial prefrontal and ventral striatal regions, such as the nucleus accumbens, is thought to participate in the filtering out of unpleasant sounds via serotonergic fibers projecting to the thalamic reticular nucleus. If this region is compromised, as it is here, the "noise cancellation" fails (Rauschecker et al., 2010).

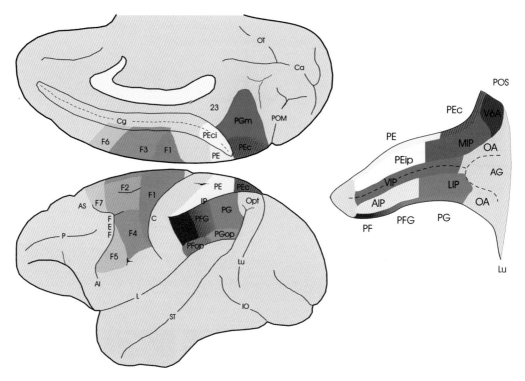

Plate 7 (figure 21.2)
Mesial and lateral views of the macaque brain. Cytoarchitectonic parcellation of the frontal motor cortex (areas indicated with F followed by Arabic numbers) and of the parietal lobe (areas indicated with P and progressive letters). Areas buried within the intraparietal sulcus are shown in an unfolded view of the sulcus (right inset). AIP, anterior intraparietal area; AI, inferior arcuate sulcus; AS, superior arcuate sulcus; C, central sulcus; Ca, calcarine fissure; Cg, cingulate cortex; FEF, frontal eye field; IO, inferior occipital sulcus; IP, intraparietal sulcus; L, lateral sulcus; LIP, lateral intra-parietal area; MIP, medial intraparietal area; Lu, lunate sulcus; OT, occipitotemporal sulcus; P, principal sulcus; PO, parietoccipital sulcus; ST, superior temporal sulcus; VIP, ventral intraparietal area.

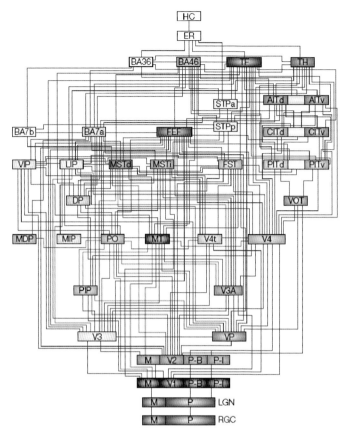

Plate 8 (figure 22.1)
Felleman and Van Essen's (1991) model of the cortical hierarchy.

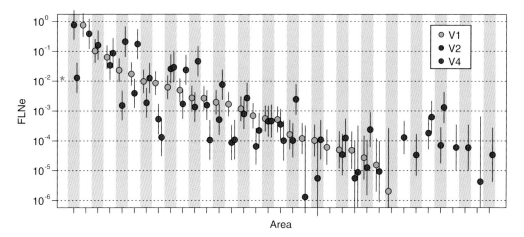

Plate 9 (figure 22.2)
Modeled connectivity profiles of V1, V2, and V4. Cortical areas received repeat injections: V1 (green), V2 (blue), V4 (red). The abscissa represents the source areas ordered according to their fraction of labeled neurons (FLN) when projecting on V1. Green asterisk: FLN value of the lateral geniculate nucleus input to V1. Note the large range (log scale) of FNL. If independently ordered all three profiles show the same envelope distribution that fits with lognormal.

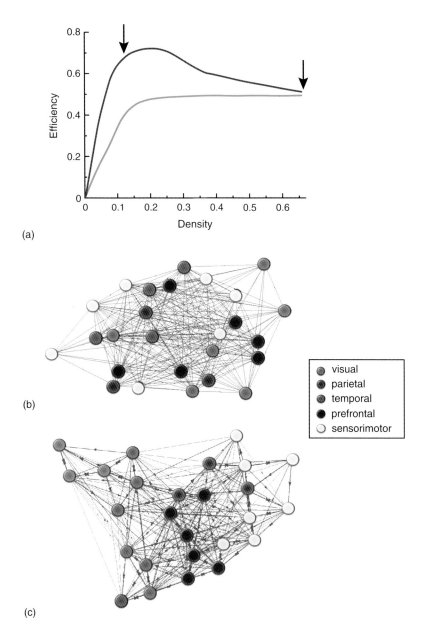

(a)

(b)

(c)

Plate 10 (figure 22.4)
Efficiency and graph topology. (a) illustrates the effect on global and local efficiency of the progressive removal of the weakest connections. Eg (global efficiency): green line; El (local efficiency): blue line. (b) shows the graph topology drawn with the Kamada Kawai algorithm on the unweighted graph, (c) on the weighted.

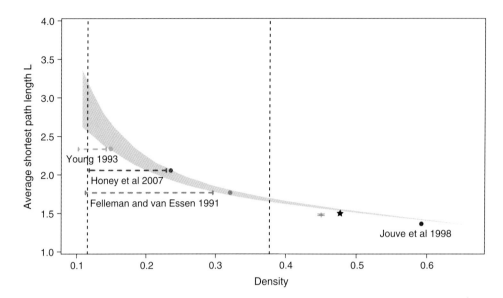

Plate 11 (figure 22.5)
Average shortest path length and graph density and effects of random pathway removal. Gray dot: G_{26x26} (26 nodes, 430 links). Gray area: 95% confidence interval following random removal of connections. Dashed lines 2.5%–97.5% of graphs in the gray zone have infinite *path length* values. Green: Felleman and Van Essen, 1991; purple: Honey et al., 2007 (47 nodes, 505 links); orange: Young 1993 (71 nodes, 746 links). Black star: removal of all new connections in present study. Brown: value predicted by Jouve et al., 1998. This figure shows that while our graph has higher density than previous studies, it is in fact much nearer to the values of Felleman and Van Essen (1991) and the estimated density in Jouve et al. study than of those studies claiming small-world architecture and using a modified database of Felleman and Van Essen.

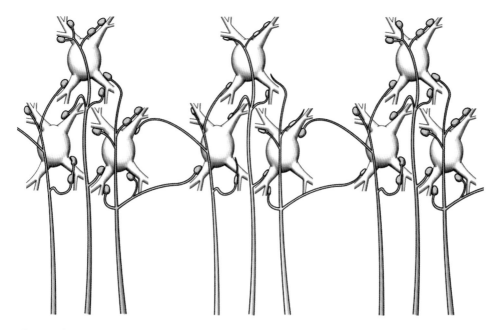

Plate 12 (figure 24.1)

Diagram summarizing the morphological changes of withdrawing lemniscal axons (blue) from the upper limb and upper trunk representations in VPL after transection of the cuneate fasciculus. The same scheme applies to thalamocortical axons withdrawing from the upper limb and upper trunk representation in the somatosensory cortex. The first signs of transneuronal atrophy are a reduction in size and number of synaptic boutons, the presence of incomplete endings, and a loss of short terminal branches. The divergent projections of normal axons (red) from face and lower body representations to the adjacent cuneate representations, normally unable to drive activity, constitute the basis for the expansion of the silenced upper limb/upper trunk representation by adjacent representations of the face and lower body. In the long term, transneuronal atrophy, with shrinkage and loss of deafferented neurons, enhances the expansion of representations with intact innervation. From Graziano and Jones (2009).

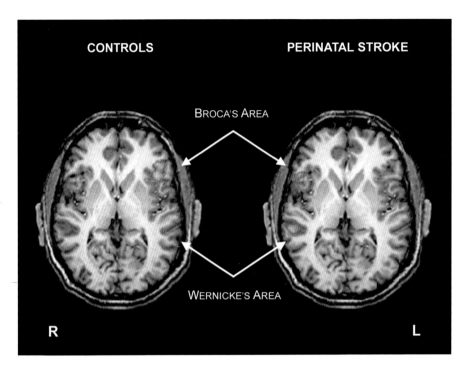

Plate 13 (figure 28.2)
Language representation in patients with left perinatal stroke and right hemispheric reorganization of language. Functional magnetic resonance imaging shows the activation of regions of the right hemisphere which are contralateral and homotopic to the regions of the language circuit activated in normal controls (group analysis performed on 8 patients and 10 normal controls). See Guzzetta et al., 2008.

The same conclusions apply to the acquisition of musical abilities. While there is undoubtedly an inherited component in "musicality," early experience and training has a significant impact on the amount of the brain engaged in music processing. Early musical training in children seems to play an important role in the development of absolute pitch and the concomitant expansion of the auditory cortex (Gaab and Schlaug, 2003; Gaser and Schlaug, 2003; Schlaug et al., 1995).

In the search for a neurophysiological substrate of auditory plasticity, one is again presented with the view that preferences of higher-order neurons for specific types of complex sounds are produced by combining features of lower-order neurons. The binding of lower-order features depends on coincident timing and, thus, coactivation of neurons as postulated originally by Hebb (1949; for a review, see Rauschecker, 1991). Activity-dependent plasticity is also suggested by studies in which monkeys were trained with specific combinations of tones, leading to an over-representation of those frequencies in the auditory cortex (Recanzone et al., 1993).

Cochlear Implants in the Deaf

Profoundly deaf individuals that still have an intact auditory nerve have profited from the dramatic advances made over the past 30 years in the field of cochlear implants (CIs; Loeb, 1985; Rauschecker and Shannon, 2002). Despite the relatively crude CI signal, delivered by a discrete and limited number of stimulating electrodes, most implant listeners are capable of excellent language comprehension. Processing by the auditory cortex fills in much of the missing information, just as the visual cortex fills in the blanks caused by our blind spot or by illusory contours. In other words, by means of its adaptive plasticity, the auditory cortex learns to interpret the impoverished signal, as long as the implant is performed early enough.

Studies in congenitally deaf cats confirm the malleability of the auditory cortex, which is molded by auditory experience from an early age onwards (Klinke et al., 1999). If environmental sounds transmitted via a microphone and CI are used to stimulate the central auditory pathways of young deaf cats, the animals soon begin to respond with appropriate behaviors to these sounds, and their auditory cortex begins to develop normal activation patterns. Much less plasticity is observed in congenitally deaf animals that are exposed to sound at an older age (Klinke et al., 1999). These results are very much in tune with the visual deprivation literature (Rauschecker and Singer, 1981; Wiesel, 1982) and indicate the existence of a sensitive period during early postnatal development of the central auditory system, especially the auditory cortex (Kral et al., 2001; Rauschecker, 1999; Lomber et al., 2010).

Auditory Substitution in the Blind

Cross-modal auditory plasticity has also been demonstrated in blind animals and humans: Auditory spatial tuning of cortical neurons in visually deprived cats is sharper than in normal controls (Rauschecker and Korte, 1993), and normally visual regions are taken over by auditory (and somatosensory) inputs (Rauschecker, 1995). The occipital cortex of congenitally blind humans is likewise activated during sound localization (Weeks et al., 2000). More specifically, it was demonstrated recently that a region in the middle occipital gyrus that participates in visual spatial processing in sighted people is activated during sound localization in the blind (Renier et al., 2010). Accuracy of sound localization correlates with the strength of activation in this region, which suggests direct functional involvement of the reorganized cortex in behavior.

Tinnitus-Related Changes in the Brain

Lesion-Induced Reorganization of Central Auditory Structures

Tinnitus, the hearing of a disturbing tone or noise in the absence of a real sound source, is increasing with old age, although its incidence is also mounting in the younger population (Rauschecker, 1999). One of the most widely held theories on the origin of tinnitus is that it is a form of lesion-induced reorganization of central auditory structures, most likely the auditory cortex (Rauschecker et al., 2010). The assumption that the ultimate cause of tinnitus must be central is based on the fact that tinnitus persists after transection of the auditory nerve, as reported in acoustic neurinoma removal (Matthies and Samii, 1997; Seidman and Jacobson, 1996). Furthermore, studies using 2-deoxyglucose and c-fos autoradiography in gerbils treated with salicylate (which is known to generate tinnitus) demonstrate reduced activity in the inferior colliculus but increased activation in portions of auditory cortex (Wallhäusser-Franke et al., 2003).

According to this cortical hypothesis, the process leading to tinnitus begins with sensorineural hearing loss (usually at high frequencies), which is more common at an older age. While the loss of hair cells corresponding to certain frequencies causes elevated thresholds in that frequency range, adjacent frequency portions may actually be amplified because their central representation expands into the vacated frequency range (see figure 16.4a). Indeed, preliminary evidence from MEG and PET studies indicate an expansion of the frequency representations surrounding the tinnitus frequency in auditory cortex (Lockwood et al., 1998; Mühlnickel et al., 1998). Studies with high-resolution fMRI seem to confirm this conclusion (see figure 16.4b).

Lesions of the cochlea in animals (with loss of hair cells in a specific part of the cochlea) lead to a characteristic cortical reorganization of auditory cortex. Frequency regions neighboring the lesioned part expand into the vacated space and become "overrepresented" compared to other frequency regions. In addition, these regions lose intracortical inhibitory input from the deafferented cortical region, leading to their disinhibition. Cortical neurons with input from frequency ranges next to the cut-off frequency thus display permanently elevated spontaneous activity levels (Rajan and Irvine, 2010).

Increased Gray-Matter Density in Auditory Thalamus

It is possible that the reorganization of the auditory cortex following sensorineural hearing loss is accompanied by changes at the thalamic level. This conclusion derives from high-resolution structural MRI studies using voxel-based morphometry (VBM) that have demonstrated a significant increase in gray-matter density in the auditory thalamus (Mühlau et al., 2006). This result parallels findings in the somatosensory system by Pons and colleagues (Ergenzinger et al., 1998; Pons et al., 1991). Changes in the somatosensory cortex of macaque monkeys after

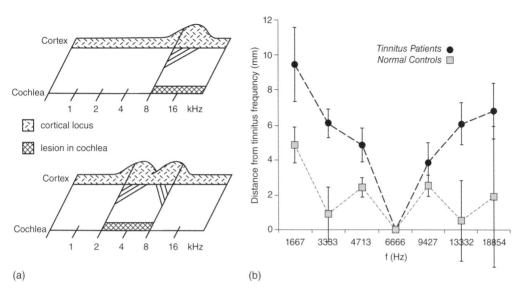

Figure 16.4
Reorganization of auditory cortex in tinnitus. (a) Deafferentation of a particular frequency range in the auditory periphery leads to lesion-induced plasticity and expansion of lesion-edge frequencies into the deafferented region and overrepresentation with a net activity increase of lesion-edge frequencies (modified from Rauschecker, 1999). (b) Distortion of the tonotopic map in primary auditory cortex, as shown with functional magnetic resonance imaging in human tinnitus patients (courtesy of Amber Leaver).

peripheral deafferentation (amputation of an arm) are amplified in the ventromedial nucleus, mediated by N-methyl-D-aspartate-specific corticofugal projections. By analogy, reorganization in the central auditory pathways as a result of noise-induced hearing loss would trigger changes at the thalamic level as well as the auditory cortex (Leaver et al., 2006).

Limbic System Involvement

Although central reorganization of the auditory cortex and thalamus in response to peripheral deafferentation is probably necessary for the generation of tinnitus, it may not be sufficient. Only about one third of patients with noise-induced hearing loss develop tinnitus, and tinnitus strength is modulated significantly by other factors. It seems that, regardless of the changes in the auditory pathways, there exists a switch that can turn the tinnitus sensation on or off.

It has long been assumed that structures in the limbic system associated with the processing of emotions (e.g., the amygdala) must be involved in tinnitus as well, in particular for developing the negative emotions and the suffering associated with tinnitus. Indeed, several imaging studies have pointed to abnormal activation of limbic-related structures in tinnitus patients (Lockwood et al., 1998).

Recently, a potential breakthrough in our understanding of tinnitus came to pass when, in a VBM study, Mühlau et al. (2006) found a highly significant volume loss in the subcallosal area

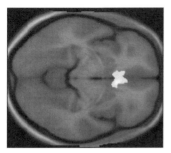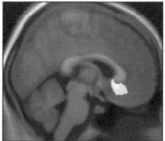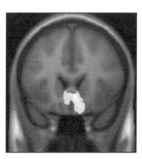

Figure 16.5 (plate 6)
Volume loss in the subcallosal area of tinnitus patients, as shown with voxel-based morphometry (modified from Mühlau et al., 2006). The subcallosal area, which includes medial prefrontal and ventral striatal regions, such as the nucleus accumbens, is thought to participate in the filtering out of unpleasant sounds via serotonergic fibers projecting to the thalamic reticular nucleus. If this region is compromised, as it is here, the "noise cancellation" fails (Rauschecker et al., 2010).

of tinnitus sufferers (see figure 16.5, plate 6). (This was the same group of patients, mentioned above, in which changes in the auditory thalamus were detected.) The subcallosal area includes the limbic-related ventral striatum and the nucleus accumbens (NAc). A volume loss in this region would point to a deterioration of function related to it. One function of the NAc, which receives input from the amygdala and raphe nuclei, seems to be filtering out unpleasant sounds (Blood et al., 1999). The NAc also mediates long-term habituation to repetitive stimulation by the same sounds (McCullough et al., 1993). The latter function may be accomplished via excitatory serotonergic connections from the NAc to the thalamic reticular nucleus (TRN), which in turn inhibit transmission in the medial geniculate, the auditory thalamic relay nucleus (McCormick and Wang, 1991; Sherman and Guillery, 2006; Yu et al., 2009).

Remediation of Tinnitus by Antidepressants?

The comorbidity of tinnitus with depression and insomnia raises the interesting possibility that tinnitus is, in fact, part of a serotonergic deficit syndrome. Serotonergic projections from the NAc to the TRN would normally help to suppress the tinnitus signal, which is generated by lesion-induced reorganization in the central auditory pathways. If the subcallosal area (including the NAc) is compromised, inhibition of the tinnitus signal fails and the signal is relayed to the auditory cortex for conscious perception (Rauschecker, 2008; Rauschecker et al., 2010).

If this serotonin hypothesis of tinnitus is correct, a possible remedy for tinnitus could be antidepressants, which either inhibit the reuptake of serotonin (selective serotonin reuptake inhibitors; SSRIs) or act as indirect agonists of the 5-HT-1A receptor (mirtazapine). Interestingly, a recent study by Maffei and coworkers has shown that the antidepressant fluoxetine, an SSRI, restores plasticity in the adult visual cortex (Maya Vetencourt et al., 2008). As these authors point out, "chronic antidepressant administration promotes neurogenesis and synaptogenesis in the adult hippocampus as well as increased expression of the neurotrophin brain-derived neurotrophic factor (BDNF)" (p. 385). It is possible, therefore, that serotonin plays a role in tinnitus not only by enabling long-term habituation to the tinnitus signal, as postulated above, but also by promoting cortical and thalamic reorganization. Further studies on the general role of serotonin in neural plasticity are clearly needed.

Acknowledgments

The content of this chapter draws substantially from prior reviews by the same author. Grant support for research described here was provided by the National Institutes of Health (grants R01NS052494, RC1DC010720, R01EY018923–01), the Tinnitus Research Consortium (TRC), the National Science Foundation (BCS-0519127, OISE-0730255), the Tinnitus Research Initiative (TRI), and the Skirball Foundation. I would like to thank Marco Piñeyro and Priyanka Chablani for their help with editing this chapter.

References

Ahveninen J, Jääskeläinen IP, Raij T, Bonmassar G, Devore S, Hämäläinen M, Levänen S, et al. 2006. Task-modulated "what" and "where" pathways in human auditory cortex. *Proc Natl Acad Sci USA* 103: 14608–14613.

Arnott SR, Binns MA, Grady CL, Alain C. 2004. Assessing the auditory dual-pathway model in humans. *Neuroimage* 22: 401–408.

Békésy Gv. 1960. *Experiments in Hearing* New York: McGraw-Hill.

Békésy Gv. 1971. Auditory backward inhibition in concert halls. *Science* 171: 529–536.

Binder JR, Frost JA, Hammeke TA, Bellgowan PS, Springer JA, Kaufman JN, Possing ET. 2000. Human temporal lobe activation by speech and nonspeech sounds. *Cereb Cortex* 10: 512–528.

Binder JR, Liebenthal E, Possing ET, Medler DA, Ward BD. 2004. Neural correlates of sensory and decision processes in auditory object identification. *Nat Neurosci* 7: 295–301.

Blood AJ, Zatorre RJ, Bermudez P, Evans AC. 1999. Emotional responses to pleasant and unpleasant music correlate with activity in paralimbic brain regions. *Nat Neurosci* 2: 382–387.

Brunetti M, Belardinelli P, Caulo M, Del Gratta C, Della Penna S, Ferretti A, Lucci G, et al. 2005. Human brain activation during passive listening to sounds from different locations: an fMRI and MEG study. *Hum Brain Mapp* 26: 251–261.

Campbell FW, Maffei L. 1974. Contrast and spatial frequency. *Sci Am* 231: 106–114.

Degerman A, Rinne T, Salmi J, Salonen O, Alho K. 2006. Selective attention to sound location or pitch studied with fMRI. *Brain Res* 1077: 123–134.

Deouell LY, Heller AS, Malach R, D'Esposito M, Knight RT. 2007. Cerebral responses to change in spatial location of unattended sounds. *Neuron* 55: 985–996.

Desimone R, Schein SJ. 1987. Visual properties of neurons in area V4 of the macaque: sensitivity to stimulus form. *J Neurophysiol* 57: 835–868.

Ergenzinger ER, Glasier MM, Hahm JO, Pons TP. 1998. Cortically induced thalamic plasticity in the primate somatosensory system. *Nat Neurosci* 1: 226–229.

Fuster J. 2008. *The Prefrontal Cortex*. Amsterdam: Academic Press/Elsevier.

Gaab N, Schlaug G. 2003. Musicians differ from nonmusicians in brain activation despite performance matching. *Ann N Y Acad Sci* 999: 385–388.

Gaser C, Schlaug G. 2003. Brain structures differ between musicians and non-musicians. *J Neurosci* 23: 9240–9245.

Ghazanfar AA, Logothetis NK. 2003. Neuroperception: facial expressions linked to monkey calls. *Nature* 423: 937–938.

Goldman-Rakic PS. 1996. The prefrontal landscape: implications of functional architecture for understanding human mentation and the central executive. *Philos Trans R Soc Lond B Biol Sci* 351: 1445–1453.

Goodale MA, Milner AD. 1992. Separate visual pathways for perception and action. *Trends Neurosci* 15: 20–25.

Gross CG. 1992. Representation of visual stimuli in inferior temporal cortex. *Philos Trans R Soc Lond B Biol Sci* 335: 3–10.

Hebb DO. 1949. *The Organization of Behavior.* New York: Wiley.

Helmholtz HV. 1863. *Die Lehre von den Tonempfindungen als Physiologische Grundlage für die Theorie der Musik.* Braunschweig: Vieweg.

Jääskeläinen IP, Ahveninen J, Bonmassar G, Dale AM, Ilmoniemi RJLS, Lin FH, May P, Melcher J, Stufflebeam S, Tiitinen H, and Belliveau JW. 2004. Human posterior auditory cortex gates novel sounds to consciousness. *Proc Natl Acad Sci USA* 101: 6809–6814.

Kaas JH, Hackett TA. 2000. Subdivisions of auditory cortex and processing streams in primates. *Proc Natl Acad Sci USA* 97: 11793–11799.

Klinke R, Kral A, Heid S, Tillein J, Hartmann R. 1999. Recruitment of the auditory cortex in congenitally deaf cats by long-term cochlear electrostimulation. *Science* 285: 1729–1733.

Kohonen T, Hari R. 1999. Where the abstract feature maps of the brain might come from. *Trends Neurosci* 22: 135–139.

Kral A, Hartmann R, Tillein J, Heid S, Klinke R. 2001. Delayed maturation and sensitive periods in the auditory cortex. *Audiol Neurootol* 6: 346–362.

Krumbholz K, Schönwiesner M, Rübsamen R, Zilles K, Fink GR, von Cramon DY. 2005. Hierarchical processing of sound location and motion in the human brainstem and planum temporale. *Eur J Neurosci* 21: 230–238.

Kusmierek P, Rauschecker JP. 2009. Functional specialization of medial auditory belt cortex in the alert rhesus monkey. *J Neurophysiol* 102: 1606–1622.

Leaver AM, Rauschecker JP. 2010. Cortical representation of natural complex sounds: Effects of acoustic features and auditory object category. *J Neurosci* 30: 7604–7612.

Leaver AM, Renier L, Purcell J, Costanzo M, Fieger A, Morgan S, Kim HJ, Rauschecker JP. 2006. Auditory cortical map plasticity in tinnitus. *Soc Neurosci Abstracts* 32: 800.802.

Leaver AM, Van Lare J, Zielinski B, Halpern AR, Rauschecker JP. 2009. Brain activation during anticipation of sound sequences. *J Neurosci* 29: 2477–2485.

Lewis JW, Van Essen DC. 2000. Corticocortical connections of visual, sensorimotor, and multimodal processing areas in the parietal lobe of the macaque monkey. *J Comp Neurol* 428: 112–137.

Lockwood AH, Salvi RJ, Coad ML, Towsley ML, Wack DS, Murphy BW. 1998. The functional neuroanatomy of tinnitus: evidence for limbic system links and neural plasticity. *Neurology* 50: 114–120.

Loeb GE. 1985. The functional replacement of the ear. *Sci Am* 252: 104–111.

Lomber SG, Meredith MA, Kral A. 2010. Cross-modal plasticity in specific auditory cortices underlies visual compensations in the deaf. *Nature Neurosci* 13: 1421–1427.

Maeder PP, Meuli RA, Adriani M, Bellmann A, Fornari E, Thiran JP, Pittet A, Clarke S. 2001. Distinct pathways involved in sound recognition and localization: a human fMRI study. *Neuroimage* 14: 802–816.

Maffei L. 2009. Lamberto Maffei [interview by David Burr]. *Curr Biol* 19: R148–R149.

Maffei L, Fiorentini A. 1973. The visual cortex as a spatial frequency analyser. *Vision Res* 13: 1255–1267.

Matthies C, Samii M. 1997. Management of 1000 vestibular schwannomas (acoustic neuromas): clinical presentation. *Neurosurgery* 40: 1–9, discussion 9–10.

Maya Vetencourt JF, Sale A, Viegi A, Baroncelli L, De Pasquale R, O'Leary OF, Castren E, Maffei L. 2008. The antidepressant fluoxetine restores plasticity in the adult visual cortex. *Science* 320: 385–388.

McCormick DA, Wang Z. 1991. Serotonin and noradrenaline excite GABAergic neurones of the guinea-pig and cat nucleus reticularis thalami. *J Physiol* 442: 235–255.

McCullough LD, Sokolowski JD, Salamone JD. 1993. A neurochemical and behavioral investigation of the involvement of nucleus accumbens dopamine in instrumental avoidance. *Neuroscience* 52: 919–925.

Micheyl C, Tian B, Carlyon RP, Rauschecker JP. 2005. Perceptual organization of tone sequences in the auditory cortex of awake macaques. *Neuron* 48: 139–148.

Mühlau M, Rauschecker JP, Oestreicher E, Gaser C, Röttinger M, Wohlschläger AM, Simon F, Etgen T, Conrad B, Sander D. 2006. Structural brain changes in tinnitus. *Cereb Cortex* 16: 1283–1288.

Mühlnickel W, Elbert T, Taub E, Flor H. 1998. Reorganization of auditory cortex in tinnitus. *Proc Natl Acad Sci USA* 95: 10340–10343.

Obleser J, Boecker H, Drzezga A, Haslinger B, Hennenlotter A, Roettinger M, Eulitz C, Rauschecker JP. 2006. Vowel sound extraction in anterior superior temporal cortex. *Hum Brain Mapp* 27: 562–571.

Ohm G. 1843. Ueber die Definition des Tones, nebst daran geknüpfter Theorie der Sirene und ähnlicher tonbildender Vorrichtungen. *Annalen der Physik* 135: 513–565.

Pons TP, Garraghty PE, Ommaya AK, Kaas JH, Taub E, Mishkin M. 1991. Massive cortical reorganization after sensory deafferentation in adult macaques. *Science* 252: 1857–1860.

Rajan R, Irvine DR. 2010. Severe and extensive neonatal hearing loss in cats results in auditory cortex plasticity that differentiates into two regions. *Eur J Neurosci* 31: 1999–2013.

Rauschecker JP. 1991. Mechanisms of visual plasticity: Hebb synapses, NMDA receptors, and beyond. *Physiol Rev* 71: 587–615.

Rauschecker JP. 1995. Compensatory plasticity and sensory substitution in the cerebral cortex. *Trends in Neurosci* 18: 36–43.

Rauschecker JP. 1998a. Cortical control of the thalamus: top-down processing and plasticity. *Nat Neurosci* 1: 179–180.

Rauschecker JP. 1998b. Cortical processing of complex sounds. *Curr Opin Neurobiol* 8: 516–521.

Rauschecker JP. 1999. Auditory cortical plasticity: a comparison with other sensory systems. *Trends Neurosci* 22: 74–80.

Rauschecker JP. 2008. Cortical processing streams and central auditory plasticity. In: *Controversies in Central Auditory Processing Disorder* (Cacace AT, McFarland DJ, eds.). San Diego, CA: Plural Publishing.

Rauschecker JP. 2009. Central auditory processing. In: *Encyclopedia of Perception* (Goldstein B, ed.). Thousand Oaks, CA: SAGE Press.

Rauschecker JP, Campbell FW, Atkinson J. 1973. Colour opponent neurones in the human visual system. *Nature* 245: 42–43.

Rauschecker JP, Korte M. 1993. Auditory compensation for early blindness in cat cerebral cortex. *J Neurosci* 13: 4538–4548.

Rauschecker JP, Leaver AM, Mühlau M. 2010. Tuning out the noise: Limbic-auditory interactions in tinnitus. *Neuron* 66: 819–826.

Rauschecker JP, Scott SK. 2009. Maps and streams in the auditory cortex: nonhuman primates illuminate human speech processing. *Nat Neurosci* 12: 718–724.

Rauschecker JP, Shannon RV. 2002. Sending sound to the brain. *Science* 295: 1025–1029.

Rauschecker JP, Singer W. 1981. The effects of early visual experience on the cat's visual cortex and their possible explanation by Hebb synapses. *J Physiol* 310: 215–239.

Rauschecker JP, Tian B. 2000. Mechanisms and streams for processing of "what" and "where" in auditory cortex. *Proc Natl Acad Sci USA* 97: 11800–11806.

Rauschecker JP, Tian B. 2004. Processing of band-passed noise in the lateral auditory belt cortex of the rhesus monkey. *J Neurophysiol* 91: 2578–2589.

Rauschecker JP, Tian B, Hauser M. 1995. Processing of complex sounds in the macaque nonprimary auditory cortex. *Science* 268: 111–114.

Recanzone GH. 2000. Spatial processing in the auditory cortex of the macaque monkey. *Proc Natl Acad Sci USA* 97: 11829–11835.

Recanzone GH, Schreiner CE, Merzenich MM. 1993. Plasticity in the frequency representation of primary auditory cortex following discrimination training in adult owl monkeys. *J Neurosci* 13: 87–103.

Renier LA, Anurova I, De Volder AG, Carlson S, VanMeter J, Rauschecker JP. 2009. Multisensory integration of sounds and vibrotactile stimuli in processing streams for "what" and "where." *J Neurosci* 29: 10950–10960.

Renier LA, Anurova I, De Volder AG, Carlson S, VanMeter J, Rauschecker JP. 2010. Preserved functional specialization for spatial processing in the occipital cortex of the early blind. *Neuron* 68: 138–148.

Rizzolatti G, Ferrari PF, Rozzi S, Fogassi L. 2006. The inferior parietal lobule: where action becomes perception. Novartis Foundation symposium 270, 129–140; discussion 140–125, 164–129.

Romanski LM, Tian B, Fritz J, Mishkin M, Goldman-Rakic PS, Rauschecker JP. 1999. Dual streams of auditory afferents target multiple domains in the primate prefrontal cortex. *Nat Neurosci* 2: 1131–1136.

Schlaug G, Jancke L, Huang Y, Steinmetz H. 1995. In vivo evidence of structural brain asymmetry in musicians. *Science* 267: 699–701.

Scott SK, Blank CC, Rosen S, Wise RJ. 2000. Identification of a pathway for intelligible speech in the left temporal lobe. *Brain* 123(Pt 12): 2400–2406.

Seidman MD, Jacobson GP. 1996. Update on tinnitus. *Otolaryngol Clin North Am* 29: 455–465.

Sherman SM, Guillery RW. 2006. *Exploring the Thalamus and Its Role in Cortical Function*, 2nd edn. Cambridge, MA: MIT Press.

Tata MS, Ward LM. 2005. Early phase of spatial mismatch negativity is localized to a posterior "where" auditory pathway. *Exp Brain Res* 167: 481–486.

Tian B, Rauschecker JP. 2004. Processing of frequency-modulated sounds in the lateral auditory belt cortex of the rhesus monkey. *J Neurophysiol* 92: 2993–3013.

Tian B, Reser D, Durham A, Kustov A, Rauschecker JP. 2001. Functional specialization in rhesus monkey auditory cortex. *Science* 292: 290–293.

Wallhäusser-Franke E, Mahlke C, Oliva R, Braun S, Wenz G, Langner G. 2003. Expression of c-fos in auditory and non-auditory brain regions of the gerbil after manipulations that induce tinnitus. *Exp Brain Res* 153: 649–654.

Warren JD, Zielinski BA, Green GGR, Rauschecker JP, Griffiths TD. 2002. Analysis of sound source motion by the human brain. *Neuron* 34: 1–20.

Weeks R, Horwitz B, Aziz-Sultan A, Tian B, Wessinger CM, Cohen L, Hallett M, Rauschecker JP. 2000. A positron emission tomographic study of auditory localization in the congenitally blind. *J Neurosci* 20: 2664–2672.

Wiesel TN. 1982. Postnatal development of the visual cortex and the influence of environment. *Nature* 299: 583–591.

Yu XJ, Xu XX, He S, He J. 2009. Change detection by thalamic reticular neurons. *Nat Neurosci* 12: 1165–1170.

Zatorre RJ, Bouffard M, Ahad P, Belin P. 2002. Where is "where" in the human auditory cortex? *Nat Neurosci* 5: 905–909.

Zatorre RJ, Bouffard M, Belin P. 2004. Sensitivity to auditory object features in human temporal neocortex. *J Neurosci* 24: 3637–3642.

Zimmer U, Macaluso E. 2005. High binaural coherence determines successful sound localization and increased activity in posterior auditory areas. *Neuron* 47: 893–905.

17 Functional Plasticity of the Auditory Cortex

Gregg H. Recanzone

One of the most fundamentally important driving forces of normal cortical function is the history of the neuronal activity. As with other sensory systems, normal auditory experience during development is essential for the emergence of normal functional organization of auditory representations within the cortex. These auditory representations are dynamic throughout life and reflect both the ongoing moment-by-moment representational changes and the previous neuronal history of that area. In most cases, a normal, or realistic, environment provides sufficient input for normal functional organization of auditory cortex and, consequently, a normal perception of acoustic events. Under extreme circumstances where normal inputs to the cortex fail to develop or be maintained, the functional organization of auditory cortex can be altered considerably, resulting in abnormal (either better or worse) auditory perception. This plasticity can be the result of changes in anatomical connections, which is more common during development, or from alterations of synaptic strengths, which is common in adult plasticity.

What is the adaptive nature of auditory cortical plasticity? Adult plasticity allows the cerebral cortex to maintain the representations that are used in behaviorally important contexts while having the ability to adapt to ongoing changes in the environment and in the individual. For example, during normal aging, there is a natural growth of the head and ears, as well as a natural decrease in sensitivity to sounds in the cochlea. Thus, the sound localization cues that are dependent on the separation of the two ears will change as the head gets larger. If alterations in the auditory cortex did not adapt to these changes, sound localization ability would be severely disrupted. Auditory cortical plasticity can thus be viewed as a normal process of cortical function that allows for flexibility and for the individual to rapidly adapt to changes in the environment as well as changes in its own physical and neural structure. In this review I will focus on adult plasticity as a consequence of peripheral lesions, experience, and aging and will also discuss the role of the neuromodulator acetylcholine in the plasticity process.

Lesion-Induced Plasticity

A number of early studies in animal models investigated the consequences of cochlear lesions on the functional organization of the auditory cortex. The cochlea is topographically organized sensory epithelium that transduces low frequencies at the apical end with progressively higher frequencies transduced in the basal end. Early experiments examined the effects of a surgical lesion of the high-frequency region of one cochlea on the representation in primary auditory cortex.

Normally, the primary auditory cortex is organized as a series of isofrequency bands that progress from low to high frequency (see figure 17.1a). That is, neurons along one dimension of auditory cortex (the vertical dimension in the schematic of figure 17.1a) respond best to the same restricted frequencies, while in the orthogonal direction neurons respond best to progressively higher (in one direction) or lower (in the opposite direction) frequencies. Several weeks after a partial cochlear lesion, the topography of the isofrequency bands was determined using electrophysiological recording techniques in the guinea pig (Robertson and Irvine, 1989). It was noted that the representation of the frequency that bordered the cochlear lesion was overrepresented in the region of cortex that formerly represented the lesioned frequencies (see figure 17.1b). This finding was later replicated in cats (Rajan et al., 1993), with the addition that the frequency representation was defined for inputs from both the contralateral and ipsilateral ears. In this study it was found that the isofrequency bands were normally organized for the ipsilateral (nonlesioned) ear (see figure 17.1c) while those for the contralateral ear demonstrated abnormal organization as described in guinea pigs. Subsequent experiments in monkeys with bilateral lesions to the cochlea that were induced by ototoxic drugs demonstrated a similar plasticity (Schwaber et al., 1993). In this case, as both cochleas were lesioned, there was an overrepresentation of the frequency that bordered the cochlear lesion in auditory cortex on both sides of the brain. Although the neuromodulator acetylcholine has been demonstrated in previous studies to be an important molecule for cortical plasticity (see below), reducing and/or eliminating the cholinergic input to the cortex does not influence these cortical map changes (Kamke et al., 2005). The site of reorganization has been investigated at subcortical regions of the ascending auditory pathway (Rajan and Irvine, 1998; Irvine et al., 2003; Kamke et al., 2003), and it appears that the thalamus is the first level at which a simple release from inhibition with no change in either anatomical connections or changes in synaptic strengths can account for the result. Thus, the initial site of plasticity is at the thalamic level, but it remains unclear if this plasticity is directed by corticothalamic projections.

Training-Induced Plasticity

In addition to the cortical plasticity that occurs when there is a loss of inputs from the cochlea, several studies have also shown that changes in stimulation history can strongly influence the cortical representation. An important element for this type of plasticity is attention. The individual must actively attend to the new pattern of stimulation and use this information in a behavioral task. In the auditory cortex, studies that have required animals to attend to and discriminate particular acoustic stimuli can result in an expansion of the trained frequencies with a reduction in adjacent frequencies in New World monkeys (Recanzone et al., 1993). In this

(a) Normal

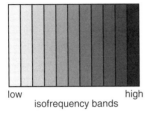

low   high
isofrequency bands

(b) Contralateral ear to cochlear damage

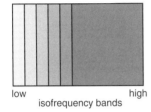

low   high
isofrequency bands

(c) Ipsilateral ear to cochelar damage

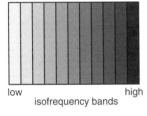

low   high
isofrequency bands

(d) Frequency discrimination training

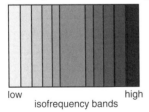

low   high
isofrequency bands

Figure 17.1
Schematic representation of the functional organization of the mammalian primary auditory cortex. (a) The normal A1 is composed of a series of isofrequency bands, where neurons all respond to the same restricted set of frequencies, indicated by shading. (b) Following partial cortical damage, the frequency near the edge of the lesion is overrepresented while the other frequencies are unchanged. (c) Normal organization in the same cortical tissue when stimulated by the nonlesioned ear. (d) Expansion of a restricted frequency range following intense practice and an improvement in performance.

series of experiments, monkeys were trained to discriminate whether two tone pips were the same frequency or the second of the pair was slightly greater than the first. After months of testing, thresholds decreased to well below the initial values. The tuning curves of neurons in the primary auditory cortex were then defined, and the area of cortex where the characteristic frequency of the neurons were within the training stimulus set was greatly expanded compared to those in monkeys that were presented with the same acoustic stimulus set but were performing a tactile discrimination task at the same time (see figure 17.1d). The expanded area of representation was well correlated with the individual monkey's psychophysical performance, suggesting that the population responses across these expanded cortical regions contributed to the improved perceptual abilities.

There are other paradigms that have resulted in changes in the areal extent of a particular frequency representation in auditory cortex. Cortical microstimulation, for example, has been shown to expand the cortical representation of the frequencies represented by the neurons at the stimulation site (Talwar and Gerstein, 2001). This result builds on earlier reports of a similar phenomenon in the motor (Nudo et al., 1990) and somatosensory (Dinse et al., 1993) cortices. Rats tested before and after microstimulation showed no difference in frequency discrimination performance even though the cortical representations had expanded. This is consistent with the idea that attention to the stimulus, and the ability to put the stimulus into a behaviorally relevant context, is necessary for the altered perceptual abilities.

A more recent study in cats, closely following the study of Recanzone et al. (1993), did not reveal a change in the areal extent of the practiced frequencies in A1 (Brown et al., 2004) in spite of the finding that the animals did improve at the task with practice. Several key differences are likely at the heart of this discrepancy. First, the psychophysical performance of the cats was considerably worse than that of the monkeys, even though the paradigms were similar. The best performance achieved by the cats was actually worse than the initial performance of the monkeys, and therefore an expansion of cortical territory may not have been necessary for the perceptual gains. Second, the areal extents of the frequency representations were defined differently. The Recanzone et al. (1993) study used only the frequency range that the monkey was trained on, and it was tailored to the individual animal's performance. The Brown et al. (2004) study used a frequency range that was not as closely matched to the training frequencies. Finally, the Recanzone et al. (1993) study used a frequency range for training that was not initially extensively represented in the cortex, whereas the frequency representation in cortex for the training frequencies was relatively greater in the Brown et al. (2004) study. Thus, there may be some limit in size that a particular cortical representation can achieve using behavioral methods given the wide range of sounds the animal must process in daily life, and this would limit the potential cortical expansion and perceptual gains for any specific task.

A different set of studies has shown that cortical plasticity can occur via normal interactions of the animal with its environment. Such studies usually compare animals raised in enriched environments to those reared in standard laboratory housing. These studies have shown a variety of different changes in different cortical areas (e.g., Diamond et al., 1966, 1972; Volkmar and

Greenough, 1972; Greenough et al., 1973; see van Praag et al., 2000; Godde et al., 2002). Experiments on the physiological response properties in auditory cortex have shown that exposing adult rats to complex environments leads to enhanced responses to acoustic stimuli and an increase in the population of neurons responding to specific stimuli, and these changes occur within two weeks (Engineer et al., 2004). In addition, A1 neurons had shorter response latencies and sharper spectral tuning. These results further indicate that the environment, and specifically the behavioral importance and interactions with the environment, have a strong influence on the functional organization of a cortical field.

Plasticity of Sound Localization

The ability to localize sounds is based on three physical cues: interaural timing differences, interaural intensity differences (binaural cues), and changes in the frequency spectrum (monaural cues). It is known that the auditory cortex is necessary for sound localization ability (Jenkins and Merzenich, 1984; Kavanagh and Kelly, 1987; Heffner and Heffner, 1990), and during normal development and aging these cues will vary. For example, normal growth will result in an increased separation of the two ears, natural aging will result in head and body changes that will influence the monaural cues, and naturally occurring hearing loss will influence all three cues. Sound localization ability is also plastic, and although recent evidence points toward a population code for representing acoustic space in the normal cerebral cortex (Miller and Recanzone, 2009), how this code is altered when these perceptual changes occur has not yet been investigated. Using ferrets as a model, it has been shown that plugging one ear during development results in normal sound localization performance (see King et al., 2001), but there is an immediate deficit in the ability of the animals to localize sounds in ipsilateral space when plugged as an adult (King et al., 2007; see Dahmen and King, 2007). The ability to localize sounds returns over the course of several days, but only if the animal is actively engaged in a sound localization task. This recovery is also dependent on the amount of training that the animal experiences, but not the amount of elapsed time. This is particularly interesting as the ferrets that did not perform the sound localization task were still housed in large environments that would presumably require the animals to localize different sounds. It may be that in these cases the animal depends heavily on visual input for spatial localization and thus does not engage in auditory spatial processing unless specifically tasked to do so. Finally, plasticity in the ability to localize sounds in elevation has been shown in humans by altering the spectral cues in each ear using pinna molds (Hofman et al., 1998). Initially after the spectral cues are altered, the localization ability is dramatically disrupted in elevation but not in azimuth, which relies predominantly on interaural differences in timing, phase, and intensity. The normal localization ability returns over the course of several weeks, and, interestingly, when the molds are removed, the localization behavior is no different than immediately before the molds were inserted weeks before. This indicates that two different representations of acoustic space can coexist.

Normal Aging

Naturally occurring hearing loss as a consequence of aging can be categorized into essentially two types. The first is a sensorineural hearing loss, often of the high frequencies. This type of hearing loss is similar in some respects to the cochlear damage in animal experiments described above. It is currently unclear if the same type of cortical reorganization that occurs in young animals also occurs during normal aging. There is some psychophysical evidence that suggests that it does (see Thai-Van et al., 2007, for a review). For example, the frequency discrimination thresholds for frequencies that border the lost cochlear frequencies is often much better than for lower frequencies, or for the same frequencies in normal-hearing controls.

The second type of age-related hearing deficits is based on poor temporal processing abilities, and this can occur in individuals with normal audiograms. Studies investigating the effects of age on auditory temporal processing have consistently shown that gap detection thresholds increase with age (e.g., Snell, 1997; Snell et al., 2002), but this is not related to audiometric thresholds (e.g., Schneider et al., 1994; Schneider and Hamstra, 1999; Snell and Frisina, 2000). Similar results have been found in speech recognition tasks. Older subjects consistently have more difficulty recognizing normal and altered speech, yet many studies have shown no clear correlation of these deficits with hearing loss (Gordon-Salant and Fitzgibbons, 1993; Strouse et al., 1998; Snell and Frisina, 2000; Snell et al., 2002; Vesfeld and Dreschler, 2002). Thus, normal aging alone can result in deficits in both spectral (e.g., Phillips et al., 2000) and temporal processing abilities (e.g., Gordon-Salant and Fitzgibbons, 2001).

The cortical correlates of these perceptual deficits remain unclear as the age-related effects of normal aging at the cortical level are not well studied. Anatomical changes have been shown to occur in aging rodents, where there is a shrinkage of about half of the cortical thickness and a decrease in NADPH-diaphorase positive neurons, although there is more dendritic branching of NADPH-diaphorase positive neurons (Ouda et al., 2003; Sanchez-Zuriaga et al., 2007). Similar decreases, and in some strains complete loss, of parvalbumin positive neurons have been observed in the auditory cortex of old rats (Ouda et al., 2008). In contrast, in humans it was found that there was no shrinkage of the primary auditory cortex of aged adults, but there was shrinkage of secondary auditory cortical areas (Chance et al., 2006). Electrophysiological experiments in rats suggest that aging results in a shift to more complex receptive field tuning and less reliability in the response to simple stimuli, consistent with a diminished signal-to-noise ratio (e.g., Turner, et al., 2005). Also consistent with the decrease in temporal processing, the responses of neurons in auditory cortex to frequency modulated sweeps in aged animals are diminished at high sweep speeds (Mendelson and Ricketts, 2001). This diminished response is not observed for neurons in the medial geniculate nucleus of the thalamus (Mendelson and Lui, 2004) or inferior colliculus (Lee et al., 2002). Interestingly, these deficits actually begin to emerge in middle age. For example, a magnetoencephalography study showed that the evoked activity in auditory cortex to changes in interaural phase differences decreased partially in middle-aged and more fully in older adults, although discrimination thresholds were only noted in the aged adults (Ross et al., 2007). It may be that these anatomical changes, as well as a host of physiological changes, begin to occur in middle age and a variety of compensatory mechanisms, including cortical plasticity, can maintain perceptual performance for several years or decades before the extent of the loss exceeds the limits of plasticity, at which point the perceptual deficits become measurable.

The Role of Acetylcholine in Cortical Plasticity

Several lines of experiments indicate that different neuromodulators have a strong influence on adult auditory cortical plasticity. The initial studies were performed by pairing electrical stimulation of the basal forebrain with a particular tone stimulus in adult animals over the course of several weeks, with the result that the representation of that tone was increased in the auditory cortex (Kilgard and Merzenich, 1998a; Kilgard et al., 2001). The interpretation of these results is that the basal forebrain stimulation activates cholinergic neurons in the nucleus basalis, and this experimental paradigm in many ways mimics attention to the stimulus. Given that attention is necessary for adult experience-dependent plasticity in the auditory cortex (Recanzone et al., 1993), these results make intuitive sense. In addition, ACH is known to be important in changes of synaptic efficacies under a number of conditions (see Weinberger, 1995). Subsequent experiments showed that this paradigm could also influence temporal response properties (Kilgard and Merzenich, 1998b; Kilgard et al., 2007), single-neuron response thresholds (Chen and Yan, 2007), and responses to frequency-modulated stimuli (Moucha et al., 2005). These effects have also been demonstrated outside of the primary auditory cortex, in the posterior auditory field (Puckett et al., 2007). The reversibility of such pairings has been demonstrated by first pairing stimulation with noise stimuli, which causes a disruption of the tonotopy in A1 and increases spectral bandwidth on cortical neurons. This effect can then be reversed by pairing stimulation with tone stimuli, indicating that the plasticity mechanisms are continuously operating throughout adulthood (Bao et al., 2003a). The role of acetylcholine has also been shown in human subjects, where aversive conditioning paired with a particular tone frequency resulted in a greater blood-oxygen-level-dependent response to the paired tone in subjects given placebo, but not those given the anticholinergic drug scopolamine (Thiel et al., 2002).

While initial observations strongly suggested that acetylcholine was critical for the induction of these plastic changes, a more recent study suggests that this is not entirely the case (Kamke et al., 2005). In these experiments, the cholinergic inputs to the cortex were pharmacologically destroyed prior to mechanical destruction of the high-frequency region of one cochlea. As described above, this type of manipulation leads to a change in the tonotopic organization of the primary auditory cortex that represents the lesioned ear but not the unlesioned ear (see figure 17.1b, c). One would have predicted that ACH-lesioned animals would not show this reorganization, particularly since the equivalent experiment in the somatosensory and motor cortex showed no topographic reorganization (Webster et al., 1991; Juliano et al., 1991; Conner et al., 2005). This was not the case, however, as the usual reorganization did occur. While there were several differences between the Kamke et al. (2005) study and others, particularly the time interval between the deafferentation and the subsequent mapping, it does imply that acetylcholine is only a part of the cortical plasticity mechanisms (see Kilgard, 2005). This is further supported by studies that demonstrate that other neuromodulators, such as norepinephrine and dopamine, can also influence the response properties of auditory cortical neurons (e.g., see Bao et al., 2003b; Manunta and Edeline, 2004; Thiel, 2007).

Summary

In summary, adult auditory cortical plasticity shares many of the features seen in other sensory systems, indicating that plasticity is a general cortical phenomenon. The perceptual consequences are a function of the behavioral importance of the stimuli and the degree of attention that the subject pays to the modifying stimulus. This is consistent with the requirements that an individual's acoustic perception will change over the course of days, weeks, months, and years depending on seasonal changes as well as normal maturation and aging. Neuromodulators, particularly acetylcholine, play a key role in this process.

References

Bao S, Chang EF, Davis JD, Gobeske T, Merzenich MM. 2003a. Progressive degradation and subsequent refinement of acoustic representations in the adult auditory cortex. *J Neurosci* 23: 10765–10775.

Bao S, Chan VT, Zhang LI, Merzenich MM. 2003b. Suppression of cortical representation through backward conditioning. *Proc Natl Acad Sci USA* 100: 1405–1408.

Brown M, Irvine DR, Park VN. 2004. Perceptual learning on an auditory frequency discrimination task by cats: association with changes in primary auditory cortex. *Cereb Cortex* 14: 952–965.

Chance SA, Casanova MF, Switala AE, Crow TJ, Esiri MM. 2006. Minicolumn thinning in temporal lobe association cortex but not primary auditory cortex in normal human ageing. *Acta Neuropathol* 111: 459–464.

Chen G, Yan J. 2007. Cholinergic modulation incorporated with a tone presentation induces frequency-specific threshold decreases in the auditory cortex of the mouse. *Eur J Neurosci* 25: 1793–1803.

Conner JM, Chiba AA, Tuszynski MH. 2005. The basal forebrain cholinergic system is essential for cortical plasticity and functional recovery following brain injury. *Neuron* 46: 173–179.

Dahmen JC, King AJ. 2007. Learning to hear: plasticity of auditory cortical processing. *Curr Opin Neurobiol* 17: 456–464.

Diamond MC, Law F, Rhodes H, Linder B, Rosenzweig MR, Krech D, Bennett EL. 1966. Increases in cortical depth and glia numbers in rats subjected to enriched environment. *J Comp Neurol* 128: 117–126.

Diamond MC, Rosenzweig MR, Bennett EL, Linder B, Lyon L. 1972. Effects of environmental enrichment and impoverishment on rat cerebral cortex. *J Neurobiol* 3: 47–64.

Dinse HR, Recanzone GH, Merzenich MM. 1993. Alterations in correlated activity parallel ICMS-induced representational plasticity. *Neuroreport* 5: 173–176.

Engineer ND, Percaccio CR, Panya PK, Moucha R, Rathbun DL, Kilgard MP. 2004. Environmental enrichment improves response strength, threshold, selectivity, and latency of auditory cortex neurons. *J Neurophysiol* 92: 73–82.

Godde B, Berkefeld T, David-Jurgens M, Dinse HR. 2002. Age-related changes in primary somatosensory cortex of rats: evidence for parallel degenerative and plastic-adaptive processes. *Neurosci Biobehav Rev* 26: 743–752.

Gordon-Salant S, Fitzgibbons PJ. 1993. Temporal factors and speech recognition performance in young and elderly listeners. *J Speech Hear Res* 36: 1276–1285.

Gordon-Salant S, Fitzgibbons PJ. 2001. Sources of age-related recognition difficulty for time-compressed speech. *J Speech Lang Hear Res* 44: 709–719.

Greenough WT, Volkmar FR, Juraska JM. 1973. Effects of rearing complexity on dendritic branching in frontolateral and temporal cortex of the rat. *Exp Neurol* 41: 371–378.

Heffner HE, Heffner RS. 1990. Effect of bilateral auditory cortex lesions on sound localization in Japanese macaques. *J Neurophysiol* 64: 915–931.

Hofman PM, Van Riswick JGA, Van Opstal AJ. 1998. Relearning sound localization with new ears. *Nat Neurosci* 1: 417–421.

Irvine DR, Rajan R, Smith S. 2003. Effects of restricted cochlear lesions in adult cats on the frequency organization of the inferior colliculus. *J Comp Neurol* 467: 354–374.

Jenkins WM, Merzenich MM. 1984. Role of cat primary auditory cortex for sound-localization behavior. *J Neurophysiol* 52: 819–847.

Juliano SL, Ma W, Eslin D. 1991. Cholinergic depletion prevents expansion of topographic maps in somatosensory cortex. *Proc Natl Acad Sci USA* 88: 780–784.

Kamke MR, Brown M, Irvine DR. 2003. Plasticity in the tonotopic organization of the medial geniculate body in adult cats following restricted unilateral cochlear lesions. *J Comp Neurol* 459: 355–367.

Kamke MR, Brown M, Irvine DR. 2005. Basal forebrain cholinergic input is not essential for lesion-induced plasticity in mature auditory cortex. *Neuron* 48: 675–686.

Kavanagh GL, Kelly JB. 1987. Contribution of auditory cortex to sound localization by the ferret (Mustela putorius). *J Neurophysiol* 57: 1746–1766.

Kilgard MP, Merzenich MM. 1998a. Cortical map reorganization enabled by nucleus basalis activity. *Science* 279: 1714–1718.

Kilgard MP, Merzenich MM. 1998b. Plasticity of temporal information processing in the primary auditory cortex. *Nat Neurosci* 1: 727–731.

Kilgard MP, Pandy PK, Vazquez J, Gehi A, Schreiner CE, Merzenich MM. 2001. Sensory input directs spatial and temporal plasticity in primary auditory cortex. *J Neurophysiol* 86: 326–338.

Kilgard MP. 2005. Cortical map reorganization without cholinergic modulation. *Neuron* 48: 529–530.

Kilgard MP, Vazquez JL, Engineer ND, Pandya PK. 2007. Experience dependent plasticity alters cortical synchronization. *Hear Res* 229: 171–179.

King AJ, Kacelnik O, Mrsic-Flogel TD, Schnupp JWH, Parsons CH, Moore DR. 2001. How plastic is spatial hearing? *Audiol Neurootol* 6: 182–186.

King AJ, Bajo VM, Bizley JK, Campbell RAA, Nodal FR, Schultz AL, Schnupp JWH. 2007. Physiological and behavioral studies of spatial coding. *Hear Res* 229: 106–115.

Lee HJ, Wallani T, Mendelson JR. 2002. Temporal processing speed in the inferior colliculus of young and aged rats. *Hear Res* 174: 64–74.

Manunta Y, Edeline JM. 2004. Noradrenergic induction of selective plasticity in the frequency tuning of auditory cortex neurons. *J Neurophysiol* 92: 1445–1463.

Mendelson JR, Ricketts C. 2001. Age-related temporal processing speed deterioration in auditory cortex. *Hear Res* 158: 84–94.

Mendelson JR, Lui B. 2004. The effects of aging in the medial geniculate nucleus: a comparison with the inferior colliculus and auditory cortex. *Hear Res* 191: 21–33.

Miller LM, Recanzone GH. 2009. Populations of auditory cortical neurons can accurately encode acoustic space across stimulus intensity. *Proc Natl Acad Sci USA* 106: 5931–5935.

Moucha R, Pandya PK, Engineer ND, Rathbun DL, Kilgard MP. 2005. Background sounds contribute to spectrotemporal plasticity in primary auditory cortex. *Exp Brain Res* 162: 417–427.

Nudo RJ, Jenkins WM, Merzenich MM. 1990. Repetitive microstimulation alters the cortical representation of movements in adult rats. *Somatosens Mot Res* 7: 463–483.

Ouda L, Nwabueze-Ogbo FC, Druga R, Syka J. 2003. NADPH-diaphorase-positive neurons in the auditory cortex of young and old rats. *Neuroreport* 14: 363–366.

Ouda L, Druga R, Syka J. 2008. Changes in parvalbumin immunoreactivity with aging in the central auditory system of the rat. *Exp Gerontol* 43: 782–789.

Phillips SL, Gordon-Salant S, Fitzgibbons PJ, Yeni-Komshian G. 2000. Frequency and temporal resolution in elderly listeners with good and poor word recognition. *J Speech Lang Hear Res* 43: 217–228.

Puckett AC, Pandya PK, Moucha R, Dai W, Kilgard MP. 2007. Plasticity in the rat posterior auditory field following nucleus basalis stimulation. *J Neurophysiol* 98: 253–265.

Rajan R, Irvine DR. 1998. Absence of plasticity of the frequency map in dorsal cochlear nucleus of adult cats after unilateral partial cochlear lesions. *J Comp Neurol* 399: 35–46.

Rajan R, Irvine DR, Wise LZ, Heil P. 1993. Effect of unilateral partial cochlear lesions in adult cats on the representation of lesioned and unlesioned cochleas in primary auditory cortex. *J Comp Neurol* 338: 17–49.

Recanzone GH, Schreiner CE, Merzenich MM. 1993. Plasticity in the frequency representation of primary auditory cortex following discrimination training in adult owl monkeys. *J Neurosci* 13: 87–103.

Robertson R, Irvine DR. 1989. Plasticity of frequency organization in auditory cortex of guinea pigs with partial unilateral deafness. *J Comp Neurol* 282: 456–471.

Ross B, Fujioka T, Tremblay KL, Picton TW. 2007. Aging in binaural hearing begins in mid-life: evidence from cortical auditory-evoked responses to changes in interaural phase. *J Neurosci* 27: 11172–11178.

Sanchez-Zuriaga D, Marti-Gutierrez N, De La Cruz MAP, Peris-Sanchis MR. 2007. Age-related changes of NADPH-diaphorase-positive neurons in the rat inferior colliculus and auditory cortex. *Microsc Res Tech* 70: 1051–1059.

Schneider BA, Pichora-Fuller MK, Kowalchuk D, Lamb M. 1994. Gap detection and the precedence effect in young and old rats. *J Acoust Soc Am* 95: 980–991.

Schneider BA, Hamstra SJ. 1999. Gap detection thresholds as a function of tonal duration for younger and older listeners. *J Acoust Soc Am* 106: 371–380.

Schwaber MK, Garraghty PE, Kaas JH. 1993. Neuroplasticity of the adult primate auditory cortex following cochlear hearing loss. *Am J Otol* 14: 252–258.

Snell KB. 1997. Age-related changes in temporal gap detection. *J Acoust Soc Am* 101: 2214–2220.

Snell KB, Frisina DR. 2000. Relationships among age-related differences in gap detection and word recognition. *J Acoust Soc Am* 107: 1615–1626.

Snell KB, Mapes FM, Hickman ED, Frisina DR. 2002. Word recognition in competing babble and the effects of age, temporal processing, and absolute sensitivity. *J Acoust Soc Am* 112: 720–727.

Strouse A, Ashmead DH, Ohde RN, Grantham DW. 1998. Temporal processing in the aging auditory system. *J Acoust Soc Am* 104: 2385–2399.

Talwar SK, Gerstein GL. 2001. Reorganization in awake rat auditory cortex by local microstimulation and its effect on frequency-discrimination behavior. *J Neurophysiol* 86: 1555–1572.

Thai-Van H, Micheyl C, Norena A, Veuillet E, Gabriel D, Collet L. 2007. Enhanced frequency discrimination in hearing-impaired individuals: a review of perceptual correlates of central neural plasticity induced by cochlear damage. *Hear Res* 233: 14–22.

Thiel CM. 2007. Pharmacological modulation of learning-induced plasticity in human auditory cortex. *Restor Neurol Neurosci* 25: 435–443.

Thiel CM, Friston KJ, Dolan RJ. 2002. Cholinergic modulation of experience-dependent plasticity in human auditory cortex. *Neuron* 35: 567–574.

Turner JG, Hughes LF, Caspary DM. 2005. Affects of aging on receptive fields in rat primary auditory cortex layer V neurons. *J Neurophysiol* 94: 2738–2747.

van Praag H, Kempermann G, Gage FH. 2000. Neural consequences of environmental enrichment. *Nat Rev Neurosci* 1: 191–198.

Versfeld NJ, Dreschler WA. 2002. The relationship between the intelligibility of time-compressed speech and speech in noise in young and elderly listeners. *J Acoust Soc Am* 111: 401–408.

Volkmar FR, Greenough WT. 1972. Rearing complexity affects branching of dendrites in the visual cortex of the rat. *Science* 176: 1145–1147.

Webster HH, Hanisch UK, Dykes RW, Biesold D. 1991. Basal forebrain lesions with or without reserpine injection inhibit cortical reorganization in rat hindpaw primary somatosensory cortex following sciatic nerve section. *Somatosens Mot Res* 8: 327–346.

Weinberger NM. 1995. Dynamic regulation of receptive fields and maps in the adult sensory cortex. *Annu Rev Neurosci* 18: 129–158.

18 Modulation of Synaptic NMDA Receptors in Striatal Medium Spiny Neurons by Endogenous Dopamine

John G. Partridge and Stefano Vicini

Medium spiny neurons (MSNs) in the striatum integrate converging excitatory glutamatergic inputs from the cortex and thalamus to regulate the smooth execution of movement (Graybiel, 2008). They receive dopamine input from the substantia nigra, the target for degeneration in Parkinson's disease. Based on dopamine (DA) receptor subtype expression patterns, MSNs have been characterized into two major populations whose axons define the direct striatonigral (SN) and the indirect striatopallidal (SP) pathways. These two groups of projection MSNs express dopamine receptors of the D1 and the D2 subtypes, respectively.

Distinct attributes of the two striatal output pathways have recently begun to be elucidated and reviewed (Surmeier et al., 2007; Valjent et al., 2009). Major differences have been identified in morphology and intracellular signaling cascades (Gertler et al., 2008; Bateup et al., 2008). Divergent aspects of inhibitory synaptic input and connectivity have been described as well (Taverna et al., 2008; Janssen et al., 2009). However, it remains to be determined if glutamatergic transmission, particularly that aspect mediated by N-methyl D-aspartate (NMDA) receptors is different in these two populations of MSNs. Furthermore, it is unclear whether the influence of dopamine upon NMDA responses deviates in these neuronal cell types.

Dopaminergic synapses are found in close proximity to the shafts of the dendritic spines (Smith and Bolam, 1990) and are thought to exert a powerful modulatory influence over the excitatory inputs. Dopamine receptor activation affects both pre- and postsynaptic mechanisms to modulate the strength of the excitatory striatal synapse. Postsynaptic action of dopamine on NMDA receptors in both striatal slice preparations and acutely dissociated striatal neurons seems to be mediated mainly by D1 dopamine receptors. Selective D1-like receptor agonists potentiate NMDA receptor currents (Levine et al., 1996) while D2 like agonists are more targeted toward non-NMDA receptors and have generally little effect or cause a reduction of NMDA currents (Cepeda and Levine, 1998). Several pathways have been implicated in the dopamine D1 receptor regulation of striatal NMDA receptors (see Cepeda and Levine, 2006, for a review), including physical interactions and the action of protein kinases, but the molecular mechanism by which D1 activation potentiates NMDA receptor function has not been definitively established.

In this study we have compared the biophysical properties of synaptic NMDA receptors on SN and SP neurons in transgenic mice brain slices. We also addressed the effect of endogenous

DA released with intrastriatal stimulation by comparing the action of DA reuptake inhibition and the antioxidant, ascorbate. We used mice genetically modified by random genomic insertion of a bacterial artificial chromosome (BAC) vector containing the dopamine D2 receptor (*drd2*) promoter driving the expression of the enhanced green fluorescent protein (EGFP) reporter gene (Gong et al., 2003). In a subset of experiments, we also used novel mice lacking the NR2A subunit of NMDA receptors (Sakimura et al., 1995), crossed with BAC-*drd2* mice, obtaining a BAC-*drd2*/NR2A –/– strain. EGFP positive and negative neurons were selected to differentiate SP from SN neurons. Whole-cell voltage clamp recordings in combination with pharmacological isolation of NMDA receptors were used to examine the properties of excitatory postsynaptic currents (NMDA-EPSCs; see Logan et al., 2007, and Partridge et al., 2009, for detailed methods).

We performed whole-cell recordings in initial experiments from 15 EGFP positive SP MSNs and 10 EGFP negative SN MSNs. Prior to recording, we allowed the striatal slice to equilibrate in a recording chamber with constant perfusion of Mg^{2+}-free solution to remove residual Mg^{2+} that block NMDA channels at hyperpolarized membrane potentials. We then adjusted stimulation strength to obtain synaptic responses of 100–400 pA to allow better comparison between neurons. Upon stimulation at 0.1 Hz, we elicited evoked excitatory postsynaptic currents (EPSCs) that, because of the presence of specific AMPA and $GABA_A$ receptor blockers, were identified as NMDA receptor-mediated EPSCs. These currents were characterized by a double exponential decaying current as previously reported (Logan et al., 2007).

Figure 18.1a and b illustrate examples of overlapping NMDA-EPSCs (in gray) derived from an SP and a putative SN MSN together with the average current in black. Shown in the box and whisker summary plot (figure 18.1c) are the weighted time constants (T_ws) of the averaged trace. This parameter did not differ between the two cell types although we observed considerable variability in this measurement. These results show that synaptic NMDA receptors expressed by the two subtypes of MSNs do not differ significantly in deactivation properties. As deactivation has been linked to the presence of distinct NMDA receptor subtypes (Cull-Candy and Leszkiewicz, 2004), this strongly suggests that direct and indirect MSNs respond to glutamate via NMDA receptors similar in composition. These results are comparable to those studied at positive holding potentials (Kreitzer and Malenka, 2007).

With local intrastriatal stimulation, it is quite likely that afferent dopaminergic fibers will also be activated. Current evidence suggests that released dopamine acts in a "volume" transmission fashion from the ubiquitous tyrosine hydroxylase positive nigrostriatal terminals that are present in striatal slices. Thus, we investigated whether dopamine released by local striatal stimulation modulated NMDA receptor mediated transmission.

To this aim, we have used the DA transporter blocker nomifensine (10 µM) and investigated NMDA-EPSC characteristics. As DA may have a differential effect on SP and SN MSNs we compared the action of the DA transporter blocker on both MSN subtypes.

As shown in figure 18.2a and b, local perfusion with 10 µM nomifensine failed to alter on average the amplitude or decay time of the NMDA-EPSCs derived from an SP and an SN MSN.

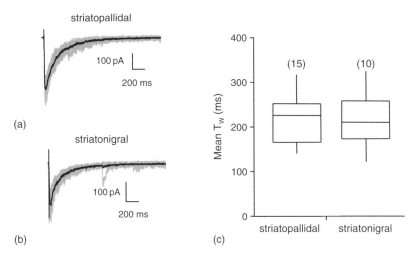

Figure 18.1
NMDA-EPSCs do not differ between MSN subtypes. Superimposed evoked NMDA-EPSCs from a striatopallidal (a) or striatonigral neuron (b). Black trace is mean of ten stimulated responses. (c) Box and whisker plot of decay time constant values from MSN subpopulations. The number of cells examined is shown in parentheses. T_w, weighted time constant.

This is further illustrated by the summary results in figure 18.2c that did not show a significant difference in the action of nomifensine between the two cell types. In eight striatopallidal neurons, 10 μM nomifensine changed the baseline NMDA-EPSC peak amplitude by $98.1 \pm 5.1\%$, while in five striatonigral neurons, this value was $105.5 \pm 5.0\%$. One possible explanation for the lack of action by nomifensine may be due to the rapid oxidation of DA in hyperoxic conditions. Thus, we investigated intrastriatally evoked NMDA-EPSCs in MSNs in the presence of an antioxidant agent, ascorbate.

The use of ascorbate (Vitamin C) in brain slice preparations has been reported to reduce edema and improve the overall health of the acutely prepared tissue sample (Rice, 1999). In addition to its well-known intracellular function as an antioxidant and enzyme cofactor, there is accumulating evidence that it acts extracellularly. Dynamic regulation of ascorbate concentration suggests that the extracellular compartment is an important site of action for ascorbate. Importantly, ascorbate concentrations fluctuate in a circadian fashion and are elevated in the striatum during awake, exploratory behavior in rodents (Rice, 2000). We wanted to determine, in light of the powerful actions of dopamine in basal ganglia physiology, whether ascorbate modulates excitatory synaptic physiology in the striatum either alone or in concert with dopamine.

We found that acute application of 500 μM L-ascorbate had a differential effect upon the amplitude of evoked NMDA-EPSCs. We chose this concentration because active transport mechanisms in the choroid plexus concentrate ascorbate to these levels in cerebrospinal fluid (Spector and Lorenzo, 1973; Rice, 2000). We observed some variability in the effect of acute

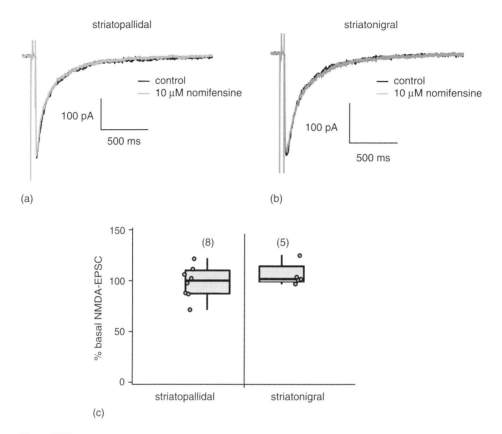

Figure 18.2
Dopamine transport blockade fails to effect synaptic *N*-methyl-D-aspartate (NMDA) responses in the dorsal striatum. Superimposed evoked NMDA-EPSC (excitatory postsynaptic current) averages from a striatopallidal (a) or striatonigral neuron (b) in the presence (black trace) and absence (gray trace) of nomifensine. (c) Box and whisker plot of drug effect on medium spiny neuron subpopulations. The drug effect on single-cell responses is also plotted (gray circles). The number of cells examined is shown in parentheses.

ascorbate upon evoked NMDA-EPSC amplitudes in the striatum. One interpretation of the fluctuations in the effect of ascorbate is in the possibility that the amount of DA release at 0.1 Hz stimulation frequency may be quite variable according to the location of the recorded cell and that of the stimulating electrode. However, when we grouped the cells studied according to their projections being SP or SN MSNs, we observed that ascorbate reduces NMDA-EPSCs selectively in SP neurons. In six SP neurons, the NMDA-EPSC was reduced by ascorbate to $73.0 \pm 7.7\%$ of the baseline amplitude, while in five SN neurons, this value averaged $102.4 \pm 7.6\%$ (see figure 18.3a, b).

It has been previously reported that ascorbate may directly have an effect on NMDA receptors at a "redox" site on several NMDA receptor subunits (Aizenman et al., 1989; Majewska et al.,

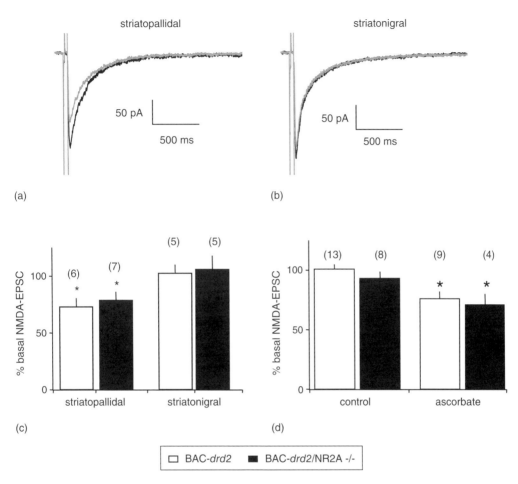

Figure 18.3
Ascorbate reduces NMDA-EPSCs (NMDA, *N*-methyl-D-aspartate; EPSC, excitatory postsynaptic current) selectively in striatopallidal neurons. Superimposed evoked NMDA-EPSCs averages from a striatopallidal (a) or striatonigral neuron (b) in the presence (black trace) and absence (gray trace) of ascorbate. (c) Summary of the effect of ascorbate on NMDA-EPSCs from striatal medium spiny neuron subpopulations investigated in BAC-*drd2* and BAC-*drd2*/NR2A –/– mice (BAC, bacterial artificial chromosome). *p < .05, *t* test comparing medium spiny neuron (MSN) types. (d) Summary of the effect of the combined application of ascorbate and nomifensine on baseline NMDA-EPSC peak amplitude. Data derived from the comparison of pooled MSN subtypes in the two different genotypes investigated. *p < .05, *t* test comparing absence and presence of ascorbate. The number of cells examined is shown in parentheses in both c and d.

1990). Although these effects could mediate a portion of our observed results, we believe that ascorbate modulation of this measurement also involves dopaminergic signaling. The lack of an effect by ascorbate on striatonigral neurons is clear evidence for this hypothesis. As modulation of the NMDA receptor by DA may be influenced by the presence of specific NMDA receptor subunits, we took advantage of the availability of a mouse that lacks the NR2A subunit to extend our study. We crossed NR2A –/– mice to BAC-*drd2* animals to generate a novel strain BAC-*drd2*/NR2A –/–. We found that the average rate of striatal NMDA-EPSC decay in these mice was slower on average (mean T_w: BAC-*drd2*: 213 ± 12 ms; BAC-*drd2*/NR2A –/–: 274 ± 17 ms; p < .01) as reported previously for the background NR2A –/– strain (Logan et al., 2007).

We continued our investigation of acute ascorbate application in the BAC-*drd2*/NR2A –/– animals and found indistinguishable results in comparison to the BAC-*drd2* animals. Again, we observed a depression in SP neurons (78.7 ± 7.5% of baseline, n = 7) with no change in SN neurons (105.7 ± 12.1%, n = 5). These results argue strongly against the "fast" redox site on NR2A subunits contributing to these observations but do not rule out the possibility of an action on the slow redox sites (Köhr et al., 1994).

To extend our investigation, we combined the acute application of ascorbate in combination with nomifensine. As shown in figure 18.3d, pre-incubation of the slice for 5 to 10 minutes with 500 µM ascorbate caused a reduction in the NMDA-EPSC upon application of the DA reuptake blocker. In these data, we did not observe a difference between the MSN types. In six identified SP neurons, nomifensine reduced the peak NMDA-EPSC to 74.5 ± 7.9%, while in three SN neurons, this value averaged 79.3 ± 9.8%. We therefore pooled these data sets across the all MSNs studied. These results were also observed in the BAC-*drd2*/NR2A –/– strain with nomifensine effective in inhibiting NMDA-EPSCs only in the presence of ascorbate.

Together, these data suggest that an interaction is occurring between ascorbate and dopamine. One hypothesis to explain these results could be that rapid oxidation of DA occurs under these recording conditions. DA may be oxidized rather quickly in hyperoxic conditions to an extent where it is difficult to notice an effect of endogenous DA release, even in the presence of the DA reuptake blocker. One possibility is that ascorbate reduces DA oxidation rates, revealing an endogenous modulation of NMDA-EPSCs by DA released by intrastriatal stimulation in SP neurons. As they express D2 dopamine receptors endowed with higher affinity for DA, they are more sensitive to ambient DA produced by the local afferent stimulation. Although other mechanisms to explain these findings cannot be excluded, the data in figure 18.3 show that the selectivity of ascorbate action between D2 and D1 DA receptors expressing MSNs is not lost when the NR2A subunit is absent. This suggests that NMDA receptor composition is not a player in the effect of ascorbate. It is important to note that DA itself does not oxidize rapidly with striatal stimulation in other species (Avshalumov et al., 2003). However, in that study, brain slices were stimulated at 10 Hz for at least three seconds to measure DA release by fast-scan cyclic voltammetry. Our stimulating conditions are quite different, using a single stimulus at 0.1 Hz, 100 µsec in duration.

An alternative hypothesis to explain the extracellular modulation of dopamine action could involve the oxidation state of dopamine receptors—in particular, the D2 receptor and/or the dopamine transporter. Ascorbate has been shown to inhibit dopamine uptake in rat striatal synaptosome preparations (Morel et al., 1998). However, our data show that ascorbate and nomifensine have differential actions on NMDA-EPSCs in the striatum. Still, it may be possible that the mode and degree of inhibition could differ between the two drugs. Finally, the selective actions of ascorbate on MSNs that we observed could be deriving not from its oxidation-reduction capabilities but rather its action as a substrate for the sodium-dependent vitamin C transporter or glutamate-ascorbate heteroexchange mechanisms (Rice, 2000). It remains to be determined if these mechanisms could be contributing to these findings.

Our results imply that ascorbate could facilitate the lifetime of dopamine acting synaptically by altering the oxidation state of DA. If this is the case, one would expect that blockade of the DA transporter would increase these actions of ascorbate. Indeed, we observed that nomifensine in the presence of ascorbate produced a decrease in NMDA-EPSC size in both MSN types profiled.

If DA levels and hence volumetric transmission are increased by these pharmacological manipulations, an intriguing explanation for our results is the possibility of a role for DA-induced endocannabinoid release in MSNs. This would decrease synaptic efficacy as proposed in models of dorsal striatal long-term depression, induced with higher frequency stimulation paradigms (Wang et al., 2006, but see Kreitzer and Malenka, 2007). This hypothesis awaits confirmation with specific blockers of the endocannabinoid pathways. Further work will also be necessary to elucidate a pre- versus postsynaptic expression site of the decrease in NMDA-EPSC we have observed. However, a lack of change in the weighted decay time constant of NMDA-EPSCs points to a presynaptic location. In conclusion, our data reveal a novel regulation of NMDA receptor mediated synaptic responses that may have relevance for neurological diseases of the basal ganglia.

References

Aizenman E, Lipton SA, Loring RH. 1989. Selective modulation of NMDA responses by reduction and oxidation. *Neuron* 2: 1257–1263.

Avshalumov MV, Chen BT, Marshall SP, Peña DM, Rice ME. 2003. Glutamate-dependent inhibition of dopamine release in striatum is mediated by a new diffusible messenger, H2O2. *J Neurosci* 23: 2744–2750.

Bateup HS, Svenningsson P, Kuroiwa M, Gong S, Nishi A, Heintz N, Greengard P. 2008. Cell type-specific regulation of DARPP-32 phosphorylation by psychostimulant and antipsychotic drugs. *Nat Neurosci* 8: 932–939.

Cepeda C, Levine MS. 1998. Dopamine and N-methyl-D-aspartate receptor interactions in the neostriatum. *Dev Neurosci* 20: 1–18.

Cepeda C, Levine MS. 2006. Where do you think you are going? The NMDA-D1 receptor trap. *Sci STKE* 333: pe20.

Cull-Candy SG, Leszkiewicz DN. 2004. Role of distinct NMDA receptor subtypes at central synapses. *Sci STKE* 255: re16.

Gertler TS, Chan CS, Surmeier DJ. 2008. Dichotomous anatomical properties of adult striatal medium spiny neurons. *J Neurosci* 28: 10814–10824.

Graybiel AM. 2008. Habits, rituals, and the evaluative brain. *Annu Rev Neurosci* 31: 359–387.

Gong S, Zheng C, Doughty ML, Losos K, Didkovsky N, Schambra UB, Nowak NJ, Joyner A, Leblanc G, Hatten ME, Heintz N. 2003. A gene expression atlas of the central nervous system based on bacterial artificial chromosomes. *Nature* 425: 917–925.

Janssen MJ, Ade KK, Fu Z, Vicini S. 2009. Dopamine modulation of GABA tonic conductance in striatal output neurons. *J Neurosci* 29: 5116–5126.

Köhr G, Eckardt S, Lüddens H, Monyer H, Seeburg PH. 1994. NMDA receptor channels: subunit-specific potentiation by reducing agents. *Neuron* 12: 1031–1040.

Kreitzer AC, Malenka RC. 2007. Endocannabinoid-mediated rescue of striatal LTD and motor deficits in Parkinson's disease models. *Nature* 445: 643–647.

Levine MS, Li Z, Cepeda C, Cromwell HC, Altemus KL. 1996. Neuromodulatory actions of dopamine on synaptically-evoked neostriatal responses in slices. *Synapse* 1: 65–78.

Logan SM, Partridge JG, Matta JA, Buonanno A, Vicini S. 2007. Long-lasting NMDA receptor-mediated EPSCs in mouse striatal medium spiny neurons. *J Neurophysiol* 98: 2693–2704.

Majewska MD, Bell JA, London ED. 1990. Regulation of the NMDA receptor by redox phenomena: inhibitory role of ascorbate. *Brain Res* 537: 328–332.

Morel P, Fauconneau B, Page G, Mirbeau T, Huguet F. 1998. Inhibitory effects of ascorbic acid on dopamine uptake by rat striatal synaptosomes: relationship to lipid peroxidation and oxidation of protein sulfhydryl groups. *Neurosci Res* 32: 171–179.

Partridge JG, Janssen MJ, Chou DY, Abe K, Zukowska Z, Vicini S. 2009. Excitatory and inhibitory synapses in neuropeptide Y-expressing striatal interneurons. *J Neurophysiol* 102: 3038–3045.

Rice ME. 1999. Use of ascorbate in the preparation and maintenance of brain slices. *Methods* 18: 144–149.

Rice ME. 2000. Ascorbate regulation and its neuroprotective role in the brain. *Trends Neurosci* 23: 209–216.

Sakimura K, Kutsuwada T, Ito I, Manabe T, Takayama C, Kushiya E, Yagi T, Aizawa S, Inoue Y, Sugiyama H, Mishina M. 1995. Reduced hippocampal LTP and spatial learning in mice lacking NMDA receptor epsilon 1 subunit. *Nature* 373: 151–155.

Smith AD, Bolam JP. 1990. The neural network of the basal ganglia as revealed by the study of synaptic connections of identified neurons. *Trends Neurosci* 7: 259–265.

Spector R, Lorenzo AV. 1973. Ascorbic acid homeostasis in the central nervous system. *Am J Physiol* 225: 757–763.

Surmeier DJ, Ding J, Day M, Wang Z, Shen W. 2007. D1 and D2 dopamine-receptor modulation of striatal glutamatergic signaling in striatal medium spiny neurons. *Trends Neurosci* 30: 228–235.

Taverna S, Ilijic E, Surmeier DJ. 2008. Recurrent collateral connections of striatal medium spiny neurons are disrupted in models of Parkinson's disease. *J Neurosci* 28: 5504–5512.

Valjent E, Bertran-Gonzalez J, Hervé D, Fisone G, Girault JA. 2009. Looking BAC at striatal signaling: cell-specific analysis in new transgenic mice. *Trends Neurosci* 32: 538–547.

Wang Z, Kai L, Day M, Ronesi J, Yin HH, Ding J, Tkatch T, Lovinger DM, Surmeier DJ. 2006. Dopaminergic control of corticostriatal long-term synaptic depression in medium spiny neurons is mediated by cholinergic interneurons. *Neuron* 50: 443–452.

19 What Is Callosal Plasticity?

Giovanni Berlucchi

The term plasticity has been in use in brain science for well over a century to refer to multiple changes in neural organization, either ascertained or simply suspected, which may account for various forms of short-lasting or enduring behavioral modifiability, including maturation, adaptation to a mutable environment, specific and unspecific kinds of learning, and compensatory adjustments in response to functional losses from aging or brain damage (Berlucchi and Buchtel, 2009). This heterogeneous, unfocused, and ambiguous use of the general term neural plasticity does not spare the subject of this chapter, the specific plasticity of the corpus callosum.

The corpus callosum is the largest and one of the most important connection systems of the brain because it provides the main link between the neocortical areas of the two cerebral hemispheres. It is an evolutionary innovation restricted to placental mammals because it is absent in the brain of nonmammalian vertebrates as well as of nonplacental mammals, the monotremes and marsupials, whose interhemispheric neocortical connections are carried solely by the anterior commissure (Aboitiz and Montiel, 2003; Mihrshahi, 2006). The afferent and efferent projections to and from the central nervous system are such that each cerebral hemisphere is in receipt of information from the opposite half of the sensory spaces and in control of the contralateral half of the musculature. The corpus callosum provides the anatomical and functional continuity between the sensory and motor half maps on the two sides of the midline. The interhemispheric disconnection syndrome following a surgical section of the corpus callosum in humans and experimental animals (split-brain syndrome) proves beyond doubt that callosal connections are indispensable for integrating and unifying the activities of the right and left cerebral hemispheres in behavioral control and conscious awareness. The split-brain syndrome consists in a disruption of the interhemispheric cooperation required for bilateral sensorimotor integration, bilateral motor coordination, transfer of training, and exchanging of cognitive experiences between the hemispheres. In the normal human brain, all experiences and performances generated within one hemisphere are eventually shared with the other hemisphere via the corpus callosum, whereas each hemisphere of patients submitted to callosotomy for therapeutic reasons seems to be restricted to experiencing its own private perceptions, thoughts, and memories (Sperry, 1961, 1982; Gazzaniga, 2000, 2005).

Early Formation of Callosal Connections

In general, plastic callosal phenomena may refer to modifications of the organization of the callosal system caused by organismic or environmental factors or to modifications induced in other parts of the nervous system by the callosal system itself. Like any other brain system, the callosal system can undergo plastic changes during its early formation and maturation as well as as a result of physiological and pathological experiences during an entire life. A multiplicity of genetic and epigenetic factors are involved in the formation and maturation of the corpus callosum as made clear by the many known causes of developmental aberrations resulting in partial or complete callosal agenesis. Callosal connections may fail to develop because callosally projecting neurons are absent or incorrectly placed in the cortex, or because the midline structures which normally constitute the bridge for the crossing of the callosal fibers are absent or abnormal, or because pathological structures occupying the midline, such as a cyst or tumor, block the transhemispheric growth of callosal axons (Paul et al., 2007). Genetic factors are essential for specifying which cortical neurons are destined to project to the corpus callosum and which are not. In mice, the promotion of the identity of callosally projecting neurons is under the control of two zinc-finger transcription factors, Fezf2 and Ctip2, and a DNA binding protein, Satb2, which is repressed by Fezf2 and in turn represses Ctip2. Cortical neurons expressing Satb2 project to the corpus callosum, and cortical neurons expressing Ctip2 project subcortically. In the absence of Satb2, axons of neurons that should have projected to the corpus callosum fail to extend across the midline and are misrouted to ipsilateral subcortical centers (Leone et al., 2008).

The population of cortical neurons projecting to the corpus callosum (less than 10% of all cortical neurons) has been characterized genetically, biochemically, morphologically, and electrophysiologically and can be distinguished on several counts from populations of cortical neurons not projecting to the corpus callosum (e.g., Hübener and Bolz, 1988; Christophe et al., 2005; Le Bé et al., 2007; Ramos et al., 2008). Most callosally projecting neurons can be classified as pyramidal neurons, though their phenotypic variability is considerable (e.g., Vercelli and Innocenti, 1993; Martinez-Garcia et al., 1994). The few nonpyramidal neurons which project to the corpus callosum in adult animals include aspiny stellate neurons which use the synaptic transmitter gamma-aminobutyric acid (GABA) and are presumably inhibitory to their targets. Reported percentages of GABAergic neurons in total populations of callosally projecting neurons vary from 3% to 5% in rats, according to Gonchar et al. (1995), to 0.7% in rats and 0.8% in cats (Fabri and Manzoni, 2004). Of interest to the subject of callosal plasticity is the finding of a transient contingent (up to 21%–57%) of GABA-containing callosal fibers in fetal or neonatal rats, probably responsible for monosynaptic inhibition of contralateral cortical neurons (Kimura and Baughman, 1997). GABA is one of the earliest neurotransmitters expressed in the immature brain, where its synaptic action is, at least in some cases, facilitatory (depolarizing) rather than inhibitory (hyperpolarizing) as in the mature brain. The early excitatory action of GABA is supposed to influence immature cortical neurons and to play an important role in promoting cortical development (Cancedda et al., 2007; Wang and Kriegstein, 2009). Transient GABAergic callosal connections may take part in driving the activity of immature cortical areas and in shaping their organization (see below), although their specific importance for the formation of cortical networks is largely unknown.

Once cortical neurons have been specified to project to the corpus callosum, a variety of anatomical structures and molecules are required for directing the growth of their axons, their migration toward and across the midline, and then the formation of functioning synaptic relations with the appropriate target neurons in the contralateral cortex. Essential for this highly complex process are midline structures such as the midline zipper, wedge, and indusium griseum, along with numerous molecules including trophic factors, hormones, guidance molecules, and cell-adhesion molecules (Lindwall et al., 2007). Further, in accord with the developmental exuberance of other peripheral and central neuronal populations, a physiological prenatal overproduction of callosal neurons and axons calls for a robust peri- and postnatal elimination of the many elements produced in excess (Innocenti, 1986; LaMantia and Rakic, 1990; Innocenti and Price, 2005).

Some Exogenous and Endogenous Factors of Callosal Plasticity

The more or less definitive organization of the callosal system, from its macrostructure to the fine tuning of the synaptic connections between presynaptic axonal terminals and postsynaptic receptorial sites, is left to functional dynamic interactions between neuronal organization and endogenous or environment-dependent factors. Among the latter factors, one has to consider prenatal intrauterine agents leading to callosal malformations, such as alcohol and other drugs, as well as some so far unknown causes of normal callosal variability. Indeed, normal differences in the morphology of the corpus callosum are greater in pairs of human monozygotic twins with dichorionic placentas than in pairs of monochorionic monozygotic twins (Reed et al., 2002).

In humans, a further possible mechanism of callosal plasticity is a protracted process of callosal axon myelination which continues to operate well into adulthood (Pujol et al., 1993; Giedd et al., 1999) and can be affected by practice and training. The corpus callosum is larger in adult professional musicians than in nonmusicians (Schlaug et al., 1995), and 29 months of intensive practice of playing the piano or string instruments has been shown to increase the size of the anterior midbody of the corpus callosum in prepubertal children. Since postnatal genesis of callosal neurons is not known to occur, the effect is best attributed to an increased myelination of callosal axons linking the cortical areas which project through the anterior midbody of the corpus callosum and are involved in the musical practice, that is, the premotor and supplemental motor areas (Schlaug et al., 2009).

In experimental animals, the plasticity of the callosal system has been the object of many studies with special regard for the visual cortex, where the formation of callosal connections has been shown to be significantly influenced by manipulations of the visual input, ranging from eye enucleation to monocular or binocular visual deprivation and experimental strabismus (e.g.,

Stryker and Antonini, 2001; Milleret et al., 2005; Innocenti, 2007). Among other conditions, and according to the so-called Hebbian rule (Cooper, 2005), the congruence and synchrony between the visual input conveyed by the corpus callosum to a cortical neuron and that directly conveyed to the same neuron by the optic pathways can influence the formation and maintenance of callosal synapses in the visual cortex. The long known existence of binocular receptive fields matched for orientation in split-chiasm cats (Berlucchi and Rizzolatti, 1968; Milleret and Buser, 1993) is consistent with an orderly convergence of congruent optic and callosal visual inputs onto single cortical neurons, which has recently been directly demonstrated with optical imaging of cortical activity and histological visualization of callosal axons in orientation columns of the cat visual cortex (Rochefort et al., 2007, 2009).

In addition to exogenously evoked activity, the spontaneous or endogenous activity of neurons can contribute to a significant degree to the formation, maintenance, and refinement of cortical and subcortical connections. There is recent evidence that the development and the plasticity of the callosal connections of the visual cortex in immature rats depend on the spontaneous activity of callosal neurons no less than on the early action of structural and molecular guidance cues and the influence of visual experience (Mizuno et al., 2007; Tagawa et al., 2008). The three factors operate in part sequentially, with guidance cues coming first, spontaneous activity second, and visual experience third, in part in an overlapping fashion (Tagawa et al., 2008). In one experiment, a significantly decreased number of terminal callosal axons in the visual cortex of neonatal mice before eye opening was observed after blocking the spontaneous activity of callosal neurons by the induced expression of Kir2.1, an inward rectifying potassium channel (Mizuno et al., 2007). Endogenous neuronal activity can act on cortical organization not only by promoting the formation of selective synapses between presynaptic callosal axons and post-synaptic neurons based on the Hebbian rule but also by stimulating the secretion of trophic factors and axon guidance and cell adhesion molecules in an unspecific manner (Tagawa et al., 2008). By their endogenous activity, immature callosal neurons can also modulate the development of their own dendritic arbors (Cancedda et al., 2007). Working on the immature mouse somatosensory cortex, Wang et al. (2007) have confirmed the importance of endogenous callosal activity for cortical maturation, with an additional tentative differentiation between the effect of the reduction of callosal neuronal activity by the expression of Kir2.1 and that of the blockade of callosal synaptic activity by a tetanus toxin. The two effects have proven to be additive, and the authors believe that they are brought about by partly different mechanisms.

Chemical blockade of synaptic transmission in the immature cortex has also been used by Maffei and coworkers (Caleo et al., 2007), providing an interesting different view on the influence of endogenous activity of callosal axons and synapses on the development and plasticity of the visual cortex. Spontaneous and visually evoked neuronal activity was reversibly blocked in the primary visual cortex of one side in rat pups at the time of eye opening, that is, when the cortex is still immature and modifiable. The blockade was obtained by a local injection of the bacterial enzyme botulinum neurotoxin, which silences synapses by interfering with transmitter release. When neuronal activity returned, neurons in the injected cortex displayed a subnormal

visual acuity, consistent with a parallel behavioral deficit, and an abnormally protracted susceptibility to monocular deprivation. The finding relevant to callosal plasticity is that the contralateral visual cortex, whose spontaneous and visually evoked activity was not directly affected by
the neurotoxin, nevertheless suffered the same changes in acuity and susceptibility to monocular
deprivation as the injected cortex. This effect is attributable to toxin-induced absence of electrical
activity of callosal axons, or to the consequent absence of release of callosal synaptic transmitters in the treated cortex, or to both factors. According to Caleo et al. (2007), explanations for
this effect may implicate the lack of a sustaining callosal input to the untreated visual cortex
during the silencing of the contralateral cortex, as well as an equalizing effect of the callosal
connections on cortical activities on the two sides after the recovery from the effects of the
neurotoxin.

Formation of Memory Traces by the Corpus Callosum

A major function of the corpus callosum has been discovered in classical experiments which
involve the learning of a performance with a sensory input or motor output restricted to one
cerebral hemiphere, the trained hemisphere, and then the testing of the performance after the
relevant input or output is switched to the other, untrained hemisphere. An intact corpus callosum
allows an immediate interhemispheric transfer of the performance, whereas if the corpus callosum has been sectioned before training, there is no transfer and the performance must be
learned anew through the untrained hemisphere (Sperry, 1961, 1982; Gazzaniga, 2000, 2005;
Glickstein and Berlucchi, 2008). There has been much discussion as to whether interhemispheric
transfer occurs because the corpus callosum allows the formation of an online memory trace in
the untrained hemisphere, in parallel and simultaneously with that formed in the trained hemisphere, or because the corpus callosum makes available to the untrained hemisphere, when
necessary, a unilateral memory trace restricted to the trained hemisphere. Probably both possibilities exist, but while the formation of concurrent bilateral memories, one direct and the other
through the corpus callosum, has been ascertained as a fact, the hypothesis of a callosal transfer
of unilateral memory traces on demand is not supported by a comparable degree of cogent and
direct evidence (Lepore et al., 1982; Berlucchi, 1990; Doty et al., 1994).

By transferring both environmental and endogenous information between sensory, motor, and
all other cortical areas of the two hemispheres, callosal connections can take part in the formation of memory traces based on such information. Plasticity in the form of short- or long-term
potentiation (LTP) or depression (LTD) of synaptic transmission is generally assumed to be the
main, if not the sole, basis for the laying down of memory traces in neuronal circuits. Before
discussing the potential for callosal connections to undergo and generate plastic synaptic changes,
it is necessary to consider the basic synaptic actions, either facilitatory or inhibitory, of callosal
fibers on their neuronal targets. In behavioral studies of hemispheric interactions, the terms
facilitation and inhibition are often used in a loose sense, simply to mean that a particular
behavioral performance, presumably controlled by one hemisphere, appears to be, respectively,

worsened or improved when that hemisphere is freed from interhemispheric influences (Bloom and Hynd, 2005). While behavioral performance undoubtedly appears to benefit from hemispheric cooperation in certain tasks and from hemispheric dissociation in other tasks (e.g., Banich and Belger, 1990), the attribution of the cooperation to physiological excitation and the dissociation to physiological inhibition of the cortex by the corpus callosum is empirically and logically unwarranted. The phrenological concept that the entirety of neurons of a cortical area can be simultaneously excited or inhibited by the callosal input or any other natural input makes no sense in the light of orthodox cortical physiology. Granted that the action of the callosal input on the total output of a given cortical area can never be purely excitatory or purely inhibitory, electrophysiological evidence in experimental animals indicates that barring some dubious exceptions, all callosal fibers are excitatory to their direct target neurons in the cortex (e.g., Matsunami and Hamada, 1984; Karayannis et al., 2007). Callosal fibers can directly (monosynaptically) activate corticofugal pyramidal neurons, mostly through axospinous synaptic contacts, as well as local nonpyramidal neurons, including spiny excitatory and aspiny inhibitory interneurons. Through the latter inhibitory, GABAergic interneurons, the callosal input can inhibit corticofugal pyramidal neurons (Carr and Sesack, 1998; Karayannis et al., 2007). Callosal fibers use the glutamate transmitter for monosynaptic excitation (e.g., Cissé et al., 2004; Ziskin et al., 2007), while the disynaptic inhibition from callosal inputs uses both $GABA_A$ and $GABA_B$ receptors (Kawaguchi, 1992; Chowdhury et al., 1996; Chowdhury and Matsunami, 2002). Because of its multiple neuronal targets, the basic physiological action of the callosal input to a given cortical area is an obligatory mix of a monosynaptic and di- or polysynaptic excitation, and a di- or polysynaptic inhibition, such that the main functional significance of the callosal input can hardly be that of upregulating or downregulating the total output of a given cortical area. Indeed, in a classical experiment, Asanuma and Okuda (1962) found that electrical stimulation of the corpus callosum generates in discrete cortical regions, such as the motor cortex, a pattern of pyramidal cell activity spatially organized in a concentric fashion, with focal excitation surrounded by inhibition. A possible functional significance of a similar spatial organization of excitation and inhibition generated by callosal inputs has recently been suggested by an experiment on bats. The auditory cortex of bats contains neurons tuned to the combination of the emitted biosonar pulse and its echo with a specific echo delay. The activity of these neurons is modulated by the corpus callosum according to a pattern of a focused facilitation mixed with a widespread lateral inhibition, which according to the authors must represent the most fundamental mechanism for bilateral cortical interactions. In the case of bats, such bilateral cortical interactions are necessary for balancing the delay maps of the two hemispheres in the analysis of orientating echo sounds (Tang et al., 2007).

In relation to neural plasticity, there is ample evidence that repetitive callosal activity can by itself cause effects of LTP and LTD of synaptic transmission which display the canonical properties of cooperativity and heterosynaptic associativity. Such effects have been demonstrated with repetitive callosal stimulation both in slice preparations (e.g., Sah and Nicoll, 1991; Hedberg and Stanton, 1995) and in long-term experiments on freely moving animals (e.g., Teskey and Valentine, 1998; Ivanco et al., 2000; Werk and Chapman 2003; Werk et al., 2006).

Glutamatergic excitatory synapses made by callosal fibers act through both AMPA and *N*-methyl-D-aspartate (NMDA) receptors (e.g., Kawaguchi, 1992: Kumar and Huguenard 2001). NMDA receptors are important for modification of synaptic transmission, and Cissé et al. (2004) have shown that a pharmacological blockade of such receptors suppresses the synaptic enhancement induced through callosal pathways in single neurons of the cat cortex.

Experimentally induced cortical plasticity can also be studied in humans using transcranial magnetic stimulation (Thickbroom, 2007). Appropriately timed bilateral hemispheric stimulation can bring about behavioral effects attributable to a plasticity of the callosal system, as shown, for example, by recent findings of Koganemaru et al. (2009).

Callosal Plasticity: Compensatory Effects in Partial and Total Callosal Agenesis

The deficits in interhemispheric communication caused by a total section of the corpus callosum in adulthood are usually much more severe than those exhibited by subjects who have always lacked the corpus callosum because of an abnormal brain development. In the absence of associated brain abnormalities, the behavior of subjects with agenesis of the corpus callosum may look at first sight entirely normal, even though appropriate tests can disclose some relatively minor deficits in performances requiring the high speed of interhemispheric communication which only the corpus callosum can ensure (Berlucchi et al., 1995). The more efficient functional compensation seen in callosal agenesis than after a callosotomy performed in adulthood is very likely to depend on a greater functional plasticity of the immature compared to the mature brain. In support of this possibility, Lassonde et al. (1990, 1995) have shown that the syndrome of interhemispheric disconnection following callosotomy is considerably less severe if the callosal section is performed in infancy rather than in adulthood, both in cats and in humans. The good functional compensation observed in acallosal and early callosotomized subjects is obviously attributable to a plasticity of noncallosal mechanisms for interhemispheric interaction, which most probably involve the superior colliculi and their cross-midline connections (e.g., Corballis, 1998; Savazzi et al., 2007).

Therefore the term "plasticity of the callosal system" used by Lassonde et al. (1990, 1995) in this connection may not seem entirely appropriate. Nevertheless, it can be argued that the callosal system is involved in these plastic phenomena to the extent that the presence of the corpus callosum appears to repress the potentialities of noncallosal mechanisms to ensure compensatory functional interactions between the hemispheres. Such a repressive influence of the corpus callosum is supported by some evidence that interhemispheric communication may be paradoxically worse in partial than total callosal agenesis (Dennis, 1976; Aglioti et al., 1998). Even disorders which are not regarded as typical of the interhemispheric disconnection syndrome, such as sleep problems, general motor clumsiness, and the delayed attainment of developmental milestones, have recently been reported to be slightly more prevalent in individuals with partial than complete callosal agenesis (Moes et al., 2009). Reasons for this adverse influence of extant callosal connections on the compensatory potentialities of noncallosal hemispheric interactions have been suggested by recent studies using the technique called diffusion tensor imaging (DTI) tractography. DTI tractography is based on the detection of the preferential (anisotropic) diffusion of water molecules along the main direction of parallel bundles of axons and their myelin sheaths. It allows one to measure the location, orientation, and anisotropy of particular tracts within the white matter, in particular the in vivo visualization of pathways within the normal and abnormal corpus callosum. Tovar-Moll et al. (2007) found in subjects with partial callosal agenesis that in addition to a seemingly normal connectivity of part of the existing callosal connections crossing the midline, other connections related to the corpus callosum had formed grossly abnormal white matter tracts. One of these was the long known Probst bundle, containing callosal fibers which fail to cross the midline and establish topographically organized intrahemispheric connections. The other aberrant tract, a long sigmoid asymmetrical connection between the frontal lobe and the contralateral occipitoparietal cortex, was seen in 4 partially acallosal individuals who were neurologically more impaired than 7 other partially acallosal individual without the crossed aberrant tract. Tovar-Moll et al. (2007) postulate that the Probst tract may participate in some kind of advantageous compensatory activity, as an example of good plasticity, whereas the aberrant crossed bundle may exemplify a disadvantageous form of plasticity interfering with normal function and causing pathological disabilities. Wahl et al. (2009) have recently confirmed the presence of frankly aberrant forms of cross-midline connectivity, including the above sigmoid aberrant bundle, in cases of partial callosal agenesis.

Conclusion

The mammalian neocortex is considered by most to be the part of the brain with the greatest potential for plasticity. Although such potential is especially manifested during the early stages of life, effective cognition and behavioral control throughout an entire life depend crucially on an orderly cerebral organization in which an adaptive cortical connectivity plays perhaps the most important role. Cortical connectivity is partly predetermined by genetic and developmental factors and partly continuously adjusted by endogenously driven and environment-dependent adaptations. Being the largest neocortical connection system, the corpus callosum offers a powerful model for understanding various features of the exquisitely malleable organization of cortical connectivity in embryogenesis, development, maturation, learning, and functional recovery after brain damage. In spite of being far from exhaustive, this review of empirical and theoretical knowledge about callosal plasticity in the broadest sense can hopefully illustrate some aspects of the achievements and potentialities of the use of the callosal model as a general model for cortical function.

Dedication

Lamberto Maffei and I first met in the Institute of Physiology of the University of Pisa half a century ago when, as fledgling neurophysiologists, we were being introduced to the mysteries of the brain by the masterly teaching of Giuseppe Moruzzi. As one of Lamberto's oldest friends and colleagues, I am happy to dedicate this chapter to him on the occasion of the felicitous coincidence between his retirement from the university and his election to president of the oldest and most important cultural institution of Italy, the Accademia Nazionale dei Lincei.

References

Aboitiz F, Montiel J. 2003. One hundred million years of interhemispheric communication: the history of the corpus callosum. *Braz J Med Biol Res* 36: 409–420.

Aglioti S, Beltramello A, Tassinari G, Berlucchi G. 1998. Paradoxically greater interhemispheric transfer deficits in partial than complete callosal agenesis. *Neuropsychologia* 36: 1015–1024.

Asanuma H, Okuda O. 1962. Effects of transcallosal volleys on pyramidal tract cell activity of cats. *J Neurophysiol* 25: 198–208.

Banich MT, Belger A. 1990. Interhemispheric interaction: how do the hemispheres divide and conquer a task? *Cortex* 26: 77–94.

Berlucchi G. 1990. Commissurotomy studies in animals. In: *Handbook of Neuropsychology*. Vol. 4 (Boller F, Grafman J, eds.), pp 9–47. Amsterdam: Elsevier.

Berlucchi G, Aglioti S, Marzi CA, Tassinari G. 1995. Corpus callosum and simple visuomotor integration. *Neuropsychologia* 33: 923–936.

Berlucchi G, Buchtel HA. 2009. Neuronal plasticity: historical roots and evolution of meaning. *Exp Brain Res* 192: 307–319.

Berlucchi G, Rizzolatti G. 1968. Binocularly driven neurons in visual cortex of split-chiasm cats. *Science* 159: 308–310.

Bloom JS, Hynd GW. 2005. The role of the corpus callosum in interhemispheric transfer of information: Excitation or inhibition? *Neuropsychol Rev* 15: 59–71.

Caleo M, Restani L, Gianfranceschi L, Costantin L, Rossi C, Rossetto O, Montecucco C, Maffei L. 2007. Transient synaptic silencing of developing striate cortex has persistent effects on visual function and plasticity. *J Neurosci* 27: 4530–4540.

Cancedda L, Fiumelli H, Chen K, Poo M. 2007. Excitatory GABA action is essential for morphological maturation of cortical neurons in vivo. *J Neurosci* 27: 5224–5235.

Carr DB, Sesack SR. 1998. Callosal terminals in the rat prefrontal cortex: synaptic targets and association with GABA-immunoreactive structures. *Synapse* 29: 193–205.

Chowdhury SA, Kawashima T, Konishi T, Niwa M, Matsunami K. 1996. Study of paired-pulse inhibition of transcallosal response in the pyramidal tract neuron in vivo. *Eur J Pharmacol* 314: 313–317.

Chowdhury SA, Matsunami KI. 2002. GABA-B-related activity in processing of transcallosal response in cat motor cortex. *J Neurosci Res* 68: 489–495.

Christophe E, Doerflinger N, Lavery DJ, Molnár Z, Charpak S, Audinat E. 2005. Two populations of layer V pyramidal cells of the mouse neocortex: development and sensitivity to anesthetics. *J Neurophysiol* 94: 3357–3367.

Cissé Y, Crochet S, Timofeev I, Steriade M. 2004. Synaptic enhancement induced through callosal pathways in cat association cortex. *J Neurophysiol* 92: 3221–3232.

Cooper SJ. 2005. Donald O. Hebb's synapse and learning rule: a history and commentary. *Neurosci Biobehav Rev* 28: 851–874.

Corballis MC. 1998. Interhemispheric neural summation in the absence of the corpus callosum. *Brain* 121: 1795–1807.

Dennis M. 1976. Impaired sensory and motor differentiation with corpus callosum agenesis: a lack of callosal inhibition during ontogeny? *Neuropsychologia* 14: 455–469.

Doty RW, Ringo JL, Lewine JD. 1994. Interhemispheric sharing of visual memory in macaques. *Behav Brain Res* 64: 79–84.

Fabri M, Manzoni T. 2004. Glutamic acid decarboxylase immunoreactivity in callosal projecting neurons of cat and rat somatic sensory areas. *Neuroscience* 123: 557–566.

Gazzaniga MS. 2000. Cerebral specialization and interhemispheric communication: does the corpus callosum enable the human condition? *Brain* 123: 1293–1326.

Gazzaniga MS. 2005. Forty-five years of split-brain research and still going strong. *Nat Rev Neurosci* 6: 653–659.

Giedd JN, Blumenthal J, Jeffries NO, Rajapakse JC, Vaituzis AC, Liu H, Berry YC, Tobin M, Nelson J, Castellanos FX. 1999. Development of the human corpus callosum during childhood and adolescence: a longitudinal MRI study. *Prog Neuropsychopharmacol Biol Psychiatry* 23: 571–588.

Glickstein M, Berlucchi G. 2008. Classical disconnection studies of the corpus callosum. *Cortex* 44: 914–927.

Gonchar YA, Johnson PB, Weinberg RJ. 1995. GABA-immunopositive neurons in rat cortex with contralateral projections to SI. *Brain Res* 697: 27–34.

Hedberg TG, Stanton PK. 1995. Long-term potentiation and depression of synaptic transmission in rat posterior cingulate cortex. *Brain Res* 670: 181–196.

Hübener M, Bolz J. 1988. Morphology of identified projection neurons in layer 5 of rat visual cortex. *Neurosci Lett* 94: 76–81.

Karayannis T, Huerta-Ocampo I, Capogna M. 2007. GABAergic and pyramidal neurons of deep cortical layers directly receive and differently integrate callosal input. *Cereb Cortex* 17: 1213–1226.

Kawaguchi Y. 1992. Receptor subtypes involved in callosally-induced postsynaptic potentials in rat frontal agranular cortex in vitro. *Exp Brain Res* 88: 33–40.

Kimura F, Baughman RW. 1997. GABAergic transcallosal neurons in developing rat cortex. *Eur J Neurosci* 9: 1137–1143.

Koganemaru S, Mima T, Nakatsuka M, Ueki Y, Fukuyama H, Domen K. 2009. Human motor associative plasticity induced by paired bihemispheric stimulation. *J Physiol* 587: 4629–4644.

Kumar SS, Huguenard JR. 2001. Properties of excitatory synaptic connections mediated by the corpus callosum in the developing rat neocortex. *J Neurophysiol* 86: 2973–2985.

Innocenti GM. 1986. General organization of callosal connections in the cerebral cortex. In: *Cerebral Cortex*. Vol. 5 (Jones EG, Peters A, eds.), pp 291–353. New York: Plenum Press.

Innocenti GM. 2007. Subcortical regulation of cortical development: some effects of early, selective deprivations. *Prog Brain Res* 164: 23–37.

Innocenti GM, Price DJ. 2005. Exuberance in the development of cortical networks. *Nat Rev Neurosci* 6: 955–965.

Ivanco TL, Racine RJ, Kolb B. 2000. Morphology of layer III pyramidal neurons is altered following induction of LTP in sensorimotor cortex of the freely moving rat. *Synapse* 37: 16–22.

LaMantia AS, Rakic P. 1990. Cytological and quantitative characteristics of four cerebral commissures in the rhesus monkey. *J Comp Neurol* 291: 520–537.

Lassonde M, Ptito M, Lepore F. 1990. La plasticité du système calleux. *Revue Canadienne de Psychologie* 44: 166–179.

Lassonde M, Sauerwein HC, Lepore F. 1995. Extent and limits of callosal plasticity: presence of disconnection symptoms in callosal agenesis. *Neuropsychologia* 33: 989–1007.

Le Bé JV, Silberberg G, Wang Y, Markram H. 2007. Morphological, electrophysiological, and synaptic properties of corticocallosal pyramidal cells in the neonatal rat neocortex. *Cereb Cortex* 17: 2204–2213.

Leone DP, Srinivasan K, Chen B, Alcamo E, McConnell SK. 2008. The determination of projection neuron identity in the developing cerebral cortex. *Curr Opin Neurobiol* 18: 28–35.

Lepore F, Phaneuf J, Samson A, Guillemot JP. 1982. Interhemispheric transfer of visual pattern discriminations: evidence for a bilateral storage of the engram. *Behav Brain Res* 5: 359–374.

Lindwall C, Fothergill T, Richards LJ. 2007. Commissure formation in the mammalian forebrain. *Curr Opin Neurobiol* 17: 3–14.

Martinez-Garcia F, Gonzalez-Hernandez T, Martinez-Millan L. 1994. Pyramidal and nonpyramidal callosal cells in the striate cortex of the adult rat. *J Comp Neurol* 350: 439–451.

Matsunami K, Hamada I. 1984. Effects of stimulation of corpus callosum on precentral neuron activity in the awake monkey. *J Neurophysiol* 52: 676–691.

Mihrshahi R. 2006. The corpus callosum as an evolutionary innovation [Mol Dev Evol]. *J Exp Zool B* 306: 8–17.

Milleret C, Buser P. 1993. Reorganization processes in the visual cortex also depend on visual experience in the adult cat. *Prog Brain Res* 95: 257–269.

Milleret C, Buser P, Watroba L. 2005. Unilateral paralytic strabismus in the adult cat induces plastic changes in interocular disparity along the visual midline: contribution of the corpus callosum. *Vis Neurosci* 22: 325–343.

Mizuno H, Hirano T, Tagawa Y. 2007. Evidence for activity-dependent cortical wiring: formation of interhemispheric connections in neonatal mouse visual cortex requires projection neuron activity. *J Neurosci* 27: 6760–6770.

Moes P, Schilmoeller K, Schilmoeller G. 2009. Physical, motor, sensory and developmental features associated with agenesis of the corpus callosum. *Child Care Health Dev* 35: 656–672.

Paul LK, Brown WS, Adolphs R, Tyszka JM, Richards LJ, Mukherjee P, Sherr EH. 2007. Agenesis of the corpus callosum: genetic, developmental and functional aspects of connectivity. *Nat Rev Neurosci* 8: 287–299.

Pujol J, Vendrell P, Junque C, Marti-Vilalta JL, Capdevila A. 1993. When does human brain development end? Evidence of corpus callosum growth up to adulthood. *Ann Neurol* 34: 71–75.

Ramos RL, Tam DM, Brumberg JC. 2008. Physiology and morphology of callosal projection neurons in mouse. *Neuroscience* 153: 654–663.

Reed T, Pfefferbaum A, Sullivan EV, Carmelli D. 2002. Influences of chorion type on measurements of the corpus callosum in adult monozygotic male twins? *Am J Hum Biol* 14: 338–346.

Rochefort NL, Buzás P, Kisvárday ZF, Eysel UT, Milleret C. 2007. Layout of transcallosal activity in cat visual cortex revealed by optical imaging. *Neuroimage* 36: 804–821.

Rochefort NL, Buzás P, Quenech'du N, Koza A, Eysel UT, Milleret C, Kisvárday ZF. 2009. Functional selectivity of interhemispheric connections in cat visual cortex. *Cereb Cortex* 19: 2451–2465.

Sah P, Nicoll RA. 1991. Mechanisms underlying potentiation of synaptic transmission in rat anterior cingulate cortex in vitro. *J Physiol* 433: 615–630.

Savazzi S, Fabri M, Rubboli G, Paggi A, Tassinari CA, Marzi CA. 2007. Interhemispheric transfer following callosotomy in humans: role of the superior colliculus. *Neuropsychologia* 45: 2417–2427.

Schlaug G, Forgeard M, Zhu L, Norton A, Norton A, Winner E. 2009. Training-induced neuroplasticity in young children. *Ann N Y Acad Sci* 1169: 205–208.

Schlaug G, Jäncke L, Huang Y, Staiger JF, Steinmetz H. 1995. Increased corpus callosum size in musicians. *Neuropsychologia* 33: 1047–1055.

Sperry RW. 1961. Cerebral organization and behavior. *Science* 133: 1749–1757.

Sperry R. 1982. Some effects of disconnecting the cerebral hemispheres. *Science* 217: 1223–1226.

Stryker MP, Antonini A. 2001. Factors shaping the corpus callosum. *J Comp Neurol* 433: 437–440.

Tagawa Y, Mizuno H, Hirano T. 2008. Activity-dependent development of interhemispheric connections in the visual cortex. *Rev Neurosci* 19: 19–28.

Tang J, Xiao Z, Suga N. 2007. Bilateral cortical interaction: Modulation of delay-tuned neurons in the contralateral auditory cortex. *J Neurosci* 27: 8405–8413.

Teskey GC, Valentine PA. 1998. Post-activation potentiation in the neocortex of awake freely moving rats. *Neurosci Biobehav Rev* 22: 195–207.

Thickbroom GW. 2007. Transcranial magnetic stimulation and synaptic plasticity: experimental framework and human models. *Exp Brain Res* 180: 583–593.

Tovar-Moll F, Moll J, De Oliveira-Souza R, Bramati I, Andreiuolo PA, Lent R. 2007. Neuroplasticity in human callosal dysgenesis: A diffusion tensor imaging study. *Cereb Cortex* 17: 531–541.

Vercelli A, Innocenti GM. 1993. Morphology of visual callosal neurons with different locations, contralateral targets or patterns of development. *Exp Brain Res* 94: 393–404.

Wahl M, Strominger Z, Jeremy RJ, Barkovich AJ, Wakahiro M, Sherr EH, Mukherjee P. 2009. Variability of homotopic and heterotopic callosal connectivity in partial agenesis of the corpus callosum: a 3T diffusion tensor imaging and Q-ball tractography study. *AJNR Am J Neuroradiol* 30: 282–289.

Wang CL, Zhang L, Zhou Y, Zhou J, Yang XJ, Duan SM, Xiong ZQ, Ding YQ. 2007. Activity-dependent development of callosal projections in the somatosensory cortex. *J Neurosci* 27: 11334–11342.

Wang DD, Kriegstein AR. 2009. Defining the role of GABA in cortical development. *J Physiol* 587: 1873–1879.

Werk CM, Chapman CA. 2003. Long-term potentiation of polysynaptic responses in layer V of the sensorimotor cortex induced by theta-patterned tetanization in the awake rat. *Cereb Cortex* 13: 500–507.

Werk CM, Klein HS, Nesbitt CE, Chapman CA. 2006. Long-term depression in the sensorimotor cortex induced by repeated delivery of 10 Hz trains in vivo. *Neuroscience* 140(1): 13–20.

Ziskin JL, Nishiyama A, Rubio M, Fukaya M, Bergles DE. 2007. Vesicular release of glutamate from unmyelinated axons in white matter. *Nat Neurosci* 10: 321–330.

20 Time Matters

Wolf Singer

The Role of Synaptic Plasticity in Development and Learning

It is commonly held that the neuronal mechanisms supporting the formation of memories consist of use-dependent long-term modifications of synaptic transmission. In order to explain the formation of new associations, Donald Hebb had postulated that connections among neurons should strengthen if the coupled neurons are repeatedly active in temporal contiguity (Hebb, 1949). This prediction has been confirmed by the seminal discovery of long-term potentiation (LTP) in the hippocampus by Bliss and Lømo (1973). They had found that tetanic stimulation of excitatory pathways led to a long-lasting enhancement of the efficacy of the synapses between the activated fibers and the respective postsynaptic target cells. Later it was shown that this increase in synaptic efficacy occurred only if the postsynaptic cells were actually responding with action potentials to the tetanic stimuli, thus fulfilling the criterion of contingent pre- and postsynaptic activation. If postsynaptic cells were prevented from responding, modifications either did not occur or had opposite polarity, that is, they consisted of a reduction of synaptic efficacy. This latter phenomenon has become known as long-term depression (LTD). It is now well established that these modifications depend on a surge of calcium in the subsynaptic space of the postsynaptic dendrites and that the polarity of the modifications depends on the rate of rise and the amplitude of this calcium increase (Bröcher et al., 1992a; Hansel et al., 1996, 1997). Accordingly, both modifications can be obtained merely by raising intracellular calcium concentrations through the liberation of caged calcium in a concentration-dependent manner (Neveu and Zucker, 1996). Fast and strong increases lead to LTP while slow and smaller increases trigger LTD. Moreover, the source of the calcium increase is of importance. Calcium entering through N-methyl-D-aspartate (NMDA) receptor-associated channels favors the induction of LTP while calcium entering through voltage-dependent calcium channels is more likely to trigger LTD. A vast number of studies have subsequently been performed in order to elucidate the molecular cascades mediating these use-dependent changes in synaptic transmission. They involve to variable degrees changes of the presynaptic transmitter release mechanisms, of postsynaptic receptors, and of cell excitability. Use-dependent long-term modifications of neuronal connectivity are also a hallmark of the epigenetic shaping of neuronal architectures during development. The selective stabilization and removal of connections that accompanies the maturation of neuronal networks is to a substantial extent guided by patterned neuronal activity, either self-generated activity during embryogenesis or experience-dependent activity after birth. These processes have been investigated as thoroughly as those underlying learning and memory, and this has revealed striking similarities between the two. They seem to follow similar rules with respect to their dependence on patterned activity, and they are mediated by similar synaptic mechanisms. Major differences appear to exist only with respect to the long-term consequences of the changes in coupling efficacy. In the developing but not in the mature system, functional weakening of connections eventually results in their physical removal.

The NMDA Hypothesis

For long it had been held that the polarity of use-dependent synaptic gain changes depended merely on the extent to which pre- and postsynaptic activity was correlated in time as initially proposed by Hebb. The evidence that activation of NMDA receptors was one of the decisive variables in determining the polarity of synaptic gain changes agreed with this notion because these channels open and become permeable for calcium ions only if the excitatory transmitter glutamate is bound to the receptor and if the postsynaptic cell is sufficiently depolarized to remove the magnesium block that makes the channel impermeable at hyperpolarized membrane potential levels (Artola and Singer, 1987; Bear et al., 1990; Kleinschmidt et al., 1987). Thus, LTP would occur when presynaptic afferents release glutamate while the postsynaptic membrane is sufficiently depolarized to remove the magnesium block (Artola et al., 1990). Since the level of depolarization of the postsynaptic neuron does not only depend on the level of activity of the pathways under consideration but also on all the other excitatory and inhibitory inputs, this mechanism can also elegantly account for the cooperativity of synaptic modifications. Even weak inputs can increase their gain if at the same time strong inputs are active to assure sufficient depolarization of the postsynaptic membrane to remove the magnesium block. Likewise, concomitant activation of inhibitory inputs can prevent NMDA receptor activation at levels of presynaptic activity that would normally induce LTP. In this case, the outcome is usually LTD or no change (Artola et al., 1990).

In conclusion, this mechanism is ideally suited to strengthen excitatory interactions among pairs of cells that are frequently activated in temporal contiguity and, due to cooperativity, it strengthens excitatory inputs converging on a common target cell if these inputs are frequently active in temporal contiguity. Conversely, modifications of opposite polarity occur if the respective activation patterns are anticorrelated. In this conceptual framework, the crucial variable that determines the occurrence and the polarity of synaptic gain changes is the discharge rate of the pre- and postsynaptic elements and the temporal coherence of fluctuations in discharge rate. The precise timing of individual spikes appeared irrelevant in this context.

A Role for Precise Timing

This notion has changed considerably over the last years due to three initially independent lines of research that converged in the conclusion that the precise timing of spikes matters both in signal processing and synaptic plasticity (Gray and Singer, 1989; Gray et al., 1989; Markram et al., 1997). In experiments based on paired recordings from coupled neurons in slices, it had been deduced that the polarity of synaptic gain changes depends crucially on the temporal relation between excitatory postsynaptic potentials (EPSPs) and postsynaptic action potentials. It had been discovered that somatic action potentials can propagate backward into the dendrites due to activation of voltage-dependent dendritic sodium channels and electrotonic propagation and that contingency of this back-propagating action potential with a simultaneously generated EPSP can be sufficient to remove the magnesium block of the NMDA channels and, in certain cases, even allow for the generation of a dendritic calcium spike, thus allowing for a sufficient increase of postsynaptic calcium to induce LTP (Stuart and Häusser, 2001). Varying the timing between the EPSP and the back-propagating spike, the latter elicited by somatic current injection, revealed that the timing between individual EPSPs and back-propagating spikes was critical both for the induction of long-term modifications and for the determination of their polarity. No changes occurred when the interval between the EPSP and the back-propagating spike was longer than about 50 milliseconds. When the EPSP preceded the back-propagating action potential, the probability of obtaining LTP increased with decreasing delays and then there was a sharp transition toward LTD as soon as the EPSP occurred after the back-propagating spike. The discovery of spike-timing-dependent plasticity (STDP) had two important implications. First, it showed that the precise timing of spikes matters in determining the occurrence and polarity of synaptic gain changes. Second, it suggests that the mechanism subserving synaptic modifications does not only evaluate covariations between pre- and postsynaptic firing rates but also evaluates causal relations. It increases the gain of excitatory connections whose activity can be causally related to the activation of the postsynaptic neuron, and it weakens connections whose activity could not have contributed to the postsynaptic response (Markram et al., 1997; but see Stiefel et al., 2005).

Precise Timing in Signal Processing

At about the same time, evidence was obtained suggesting that the precise timing of individual spikes is relevant in signal processing. In vivo recordings from higher visual areas and the auditory and the somatosensory cortex revealed that the discharge latencies of individual neurons could signal the temporal structure of stimuli with a precision in the millisecond range, suggesting that precise timing of discharges can be preserved despite numerous intervening synaptic transmission steps (Buracas et al., 1998; Reinagel and Reid, 2002). Simulation studies, partly based on the concept of synfire chains proposed by Moshe Abeles (1991), confirmed that conventional integrate-and-fire neurons are capable of transmitting temporal information with the required precision (Diesmann et al., 1999; Mainen and Sejnowski, 1995).

In parallel to these discoveries, evidence had been obtained in the visual system for the existence of mechanisms capable of adjusting the timing of individual spikes, again with millisecond precision independently of external stimuli (Engel et al., 2001; Fries et al., 2001a; Gray and Singer, 1989; Gray et al., 1989). Applying multielectrode recording techniques, it had been shown that neurons in the visual cortex engage in oscillatory firing patterns in the range of the gamma frequency band and that these periodic discharges are synchronized with a precision in the millisecond range. This synchronization was observed not only between neurons located within the same cortical area but also between cells in different cortical areas and even among cells in corresponding areas of the two hemispheres (Roelfsema et al., 1997; Singer, 1999). While synchronization probability did reflect to some extent the layout of corticocortical association connections (Löwel and Singer, 1992), it soon became apparent that synchronization was the result of a highly dynamic self-organizing process that enables rapid generation and dissolution of synchronized cell assemblies as a function of stimulus configuration, central state, and attentional mechanisms (for a review, see Engel et al., 2001; Singer, 1999). Initially, this precise synchronization of discharges of spatially distributed neurons had been seen mainly in the context of low-level visual processes such as feature binding and figure–background segregation. Later it became clear that it is a ubiquitous phenomenon in most structures of the nervous system (Brecht et al., 1999; Castelo-Branco et al., 1998) and with all likelihood serves a large number of different functions that have to do with the definition of relations in the context of distributed processing (Womelsdorf et al., 2006). Because synchronized discharges have a stronger impact on target neurons than temporally dispersed inputs and because the communication between oscillating cell groups depends critically on the phase relations between the respective oscillations, synchronization serves multiple functions. It can be used interchangeably with rate increases to enhance perceptual saliency (Biederlack et al., 2006), select signals for the control of behavior (Fries et al., 1997), mediate effects of focused attention (Fries et al., 2001b), dynamically adjust coupling among interconnected neuron groups (Womelsdorf et al., 2007), support maintenance of contents in working memory (Buschman and Miller, 2007), and facilitate access of stimuli to consciousness (Gaillard et al., 2009; Melloni et al., 2007).

Oscillations as Timing Mechanism

Extensive experimental and theoretical studies have demonstrated that the oscillatory patterning of neuronal activity is crucial for the adjustment of precise spike timing (König et al., 1995; Volgushev et al., 1998). Due to reciprocal coupling via chemical and electrical synapses, networks of inhibitory interneurons engage in oscillatory activity, the frequency of which is often characteristic for particular networks and conveys periodic inhibition to excitatory neurons, in the case of the neocortex and the hippocampus the pyramidal cells (Whittington et al., 2001).

The effect is that the timing of spikes generated by pyramidal cells does not solely depend on the timing of the arriving EPSPs. During the hyperpolarizing phase of the oscillation cycle, arriving EPSPs have only a small chance to drive action potentials in the postsynaptic neuron because of the initial shunting and then hyperpolarizing effect of the barrages of inhibitory postsynaptic potentials (IPSPs). This limits spiking essentially to the depolarizing phase in the peak of the oscillation cycle, causing synchronization of discharges in cells oscillating in phase. Moreover, the precise timing of spikes generated during the depolarizing cycle does depend on the strength of the excitatory input (Fries et al., 2007). A strong excitatory input will elicit spikes earlier during the depolarizing cycle than a weak input. Thus, the phase relation between the time of occurrence of a spike and the peak of the oscillation cycle does reflect the amplitude of the excitatory drive that generated the spike. Through this mechanism, known as phase precession in the hippocampus, rate coded amplitude values can be converted into a temporal code that is expressed in the timing of spikes relative to the oscillation cycle. As shown in numerous theoretical studies, such temporal codes are advantageous for fast processing because information on spike times can be transmitted and read out much more rapidly than information encoded in discharge rates not requiring temporal integration for transmission or readout (for a review, see Fries et al., 2007).

There is thus a mechanism that can generate the precise temporal relations among individual spikes required for the gating of synaptic plasticity. This very same mechanism adjusts the precise timing of spikes during signal processing and can be used to convert rate coded information into timing relations. Both the classical Hebbian mechanism as well as STDP, which most certainly do coexist, evaluate temporal relationship among activity patterns in order to convert correlations into synaptic gain changes. For these modifications to be meaningful, the signatures of relatedness used for engram formation must be exactly the same as those used for signal processing. Otherwise, correlations occurring spuriously during signal processing would lead to changes in synaptic coupling that are functionally meaningless. Because STDP does depend so critically on the precise timing of spikes and is susceptible to changes in timing relations in the order of milliseconds, relations between the distributed firing of neurons need to be defined and evaluated with similar precision during signal processing. However, this does require that neurons can act as coincidence detectors and distinguish between precisely synchronized and temporally dispersed input activity.

Integrate and Fire or Detect Coincidences

Finally, there is a third line of independent evidence favoring the notion that precise spike timing may play an important role both in neuronal processing and synaptic plasticity. Data are accumulating which indicate that cortical circuits, synaptic properties, and the characteristics of neurons are optimized for the transmission and detection of coincident activity. A prominent feature of cortical connectivity is sparseness, and, as proposed by Abeles and confirmed later in extensive simulation studies (Diesmann et al., 1999; König et al., 1996; Mainen and Sejnowski,

1995), such networks strongly favor transmission of synchronized activity over transmission of temporally dispersed activity. Likewise, the frequency adaptation of transmitter release and the adaptation of postsynaptic receptors attenuate transmission of frequency coded information. These adaptive mechanisms favor transmission of singular synchronized events and tend to filter out discharge sequences occurring at high frequencies. Sensitivity to single but coincident EPSPs is further enhanced by cooperative mechanisms in the postsynaptic dendrites. The existence of voltage-dependent sodium and calcium channels in the dendrites and their ability to convert into regenerative spikes high-amplitude EPSPs, such as result from coincident inputs, greatly enhance the coincidence sensitivity of cortical neurons (Ariav et al., 2003; Stuart and Häusser, 2001). Finally, there is evidence that spike thresholds lower as the depolarizing slope preceding the spike becomes steeper (Azouz and Gray, 2003). This also favors responses to coincident inputs as compared to temporally dispersed inputs. Last, but not least, the membrane time constants of cortical neurons are shorter than previously assumed, especially when the neurons are in the upstate. This is due to the reduced membrane resistance caused by the simultaneous bombardment by EPSPs and IPSPs in the upstate.

Thus, several lines of evidence indicate that cortical networks are capable of exploiting precise temporal relations among the discharges of interconnected neurons both for signal processing and for the induction of use-dependent synaptic gain changes such as support specification of developing nerve networks and the formation of memories.

However, a problem arises if precise timing of discharges is achieved through an oscillatory modulation of neuronal excitability, especially when it comes to the coordination of timing relations over larger distances, and if synaptic gain changes depend essentially on STDP. If coupled neuron groups engage in oscillatory activity in the same frequency range but oscillate 180 degrees out of phase, one can anticipate situations in which EPSPs always arrive in the trough of the oscillation cycle and, hence, at equal distance to the preceding and the following peak of enhanced excitability where spikes tend to occur. Thus, EPSPs are preceded and followed by spikes at the same interval. In this case, different outcomes are predicted by the classical Hebbian correlation rule and STDP. If the pre- and postsynaptic neurons discharge at high frequencies as would be the case, for example, if they are engaged in gamma oscillations, the classical Hebbian rule would predict LTP because of the contingency of high-frequency pre- and postsynaptic activation. The STDP rule cannot make a clear prediction because EPSPs are preceding and following spikes at about the same interval, which should lead to a cancellation of the antagonistic effects. This problem has recently been addressed in an in vitro study on slices of the visual cortex (Wespatat et al., 2004). The results indicated that inputs oscillating at the same frequency as the target cell (20 or 40 Hz) underwent LTP when they were in phase with the depolarizing peak of the oscillation cycle, whereby it was irrelevant whether the EPSPs arrived shortly before or after the action potentials, while the same input underwent LTD when it oscillated 180 degrees out of phase, so that the EPSPs arrived during the hyperpolarizing troughs of the oscillation cycle of the postsynaptic neuron.

Evidence for Relations between Oscillatory Activity and Synaptic Plasticity and Learning

Given that learning mechanisms evaluate temporal correlations among the activity patterns of coupled neurons and that the temporal patterning of neuronal activity is often structured by an oscillatory modulation, one expects to find close relations between synaptic plasticity and oscillatory activity. Although research on this issue is still at its very beginning, such evidence is indeed available.

Indirect evidence for a relationship between synaptic plasticity and oscillatory patterning comes from studies relating oscillatory activity to central states and attentional mechanisms. While synaptic modifications can be induced with artificial stimulation conditions irrespective of the state of neuronal networks and even in fully deafferented slice preparations, there is consensus that under natural conditions, learning-related modifications of synaptic gain do occur only when the brain is in an activated state and when attentional mechanisms are functional. The reason is that synaptic modifications require the presence of an appropriate mix of neuromodulators such as acetylcholine, dopamine, and noradrenaline and that these modulators are available in the required concentrations only when the brain is in an awake and activated state. Another likely reason is that the induction of synaptic modifications requires a minimum of cooperativity—for example, a sufficient amount of synchronized input activity—and that such cooperativity is only achieved in the activated brain. These activated brain states favor the emergence of oscillatory activity in various frequency bands and the synchronization of the oscillations across structures that need to cooperate for memory processes. In this context, the most important frequency bands appear to be the theta, the beta, and the gamma band. Gamma oscillations in the neocortex and the associated precise synchronization of neuronal discharges are greatly facilitated by the presence of acetylcholine and its action on muscarinic receptors (Herculano-Houzel et al., 1999; Munk et al., 1996). Acetylcholine also facilitates use-dependent synaptic modifications, and it is likely that there is a relation between the two phenomena (Bröcher et al., 1992b, Wespatat et al., 2004). Attention facilitates gamma oscillations (Fries et al., 2001b). Preliminary evidence suggests that there may be a causal relation between the occurrence of synchronized oscillatory activity in the gamma-frequency band and the induction of synaptic plasticity. It is possible to modify the receptive fields of neurons in the visual cortex by appropriate visual stimulation even in anaesthetized animals if the brain is concomitantly activated by electrical stimulation of the mesencephalic reticular formation (unpublished observation). This stimulation increases the release of plasticity enhancing neuromodulators and at the same time favors the occurrence of gamma oscillations in response to the applied stimuli. Post hoc analysis of the neuronal responses to the change-inducing light stimuli revealed that lasting changes in receptive field properties occurred only in the trials associated with a strong oscillatory modulation and synchronization of neuronal responses in the gamma-band. A similar relation, albeit in the theta-frequency range, has been found in the hippocampus (Huerta and Lisman, 1995). Here, the so-called beta-burst stimulation that entrains the hippocampus in the characteristic theta rhythm of the structure turned out to be particularly effective for the induction of long-lasting synaptic modifications. Moreover, when the hippocampal circuits were engaged in spontaneous theta oscillations, the effectiveness of the stimuli applied for the induction of synaptic gain changes and the polarity of the resulting synaptic modifications depended critically on the phase relation between the ongoing theta activity and the change-inducing stimuli (Huerta and Lisman, 1995). A similar finding has been obtained in the somatosensory barrel cortex where synchronous oscillatory activity occurs in conjunction with the whisking movements. Again, the efficacy of the change-inducing electrical stimuli depended critically on the timing of the stimuli relative to the whisking cycle. Finally, experiments in which hippocampus theta was recorded while animals were exposed to classical conditioning paradigms show that memory traces could be established only if the conditioning stimuli were given during a particular phase of the theta cycle. While these experiments only showed a relation between the timing of inducing stimuli relative to oscillatory activity, more direct evidence for an instrumental role of long-range synchronization of oscillations in memory processes has been obtained with multielectrode recordings from structures relevant for memory formation (Fell et al., 2001; Tallon-Baudry et al., 2001, 2004). In human subjects implanted with depth electrodes for the localization of epileptic foci, it was found that successful formation of episodic memories was accompanied by transient increases in gamma- and theta-oscillatory synchrony between the hippocampus and neighboring entorhinal cortex, structures known to be involved in memory formation. In trials in which memory formation was not successful, these changes in synchronization were not observed (Fell et al., 2001, 2003). Likewise, simultaneous recordings from limbic structures (amygdala and hippocampus) have shown that fear conditioning is associated with transient synchronization of oscillatory activity between the two structures (Narayanan et al., 2007; Seidenbecher et al., 2003). EEG and magnetoencephalography studies in healthy human subjects revealed that classical Pavlovian conditioning leads to a lasting enhancement of the synchronization of gamma oscillations between cortical areas encoding the conditioned and nonconditioned stimulus, respectively (Miltner et al., 1999).

The recall of memories also appears to be associated with enhanced oscillatory patterning of neuronal responses in the theta, beta, and gamma band (Guderian and Duzel, 2005; Herrmann et al., 2004; Raghavachari et al., 2001; Rizzuto et al., 2003; Sederberg et al., 2003; Tallon-Baudry et al., 2001). Auditory stimuli that matched a previously stored template led to significantly more gamma-band synchrony than those that did not match (Debener et al., 2003). Visual stimuli for which subjects have a long-term memory representation caused significantly greater gamma oscillations in the occipital cortex than similar stimuli that were not stored in long-term memory (Herrmann et al., 2004). A close relation between encoding and retrieval of memory contents and enhanced gamma oscillations has also been found in experiments on working memory (Strüber et al., 2000; Tallon-Baudry et al., 1997, 2001, 2004). Here, the increase of oscillatory activity was particularly pronounced over parietal, central, and frontal regions of the brain. Finally, there appears to be a relation between the access to declarative memory and long-range synchronization of gamma oscillations (Melloni et al., 2007). In humans performing a delayed matching-to-sample task on stimuli that were only perceived in a subset of trials and gained access to consciousness and declarative recall, it was possible to demonstrate that only those stimuli that were consciously perceived and encoded in declarative memory evoked large-scale phase synchronization of gamma oscillations across distributed cortical networks. In addition, only those trials were associated with sustained, enhanced theta activity throughout the hold period. The latter finding agrees well with the growing evidence that large-scale synchronization in the theta-frequency band is closely related to the encoding and recall of stimulus material in declarative memory. Successful recognition of known faces is associated with increased activity in a distributed network that includes prefrontal, mediotemporal, and visual areas in occipital cortex (Guderian and Duzel, 2005). Finally, invasive recordings in patients suggest that theta-band oscillations are implicated in spatial navigation, working memory, and episodic memory (Caplan et al., 2001, 2003; Raghavachari et al., 2001; Rizzuto et al., 2003; Sederberg et al., 2007).

Last, but not least, there is recent evidence from studies in human subjects that consolidation of memories during sleep is closely related to an oscillatory patterning of neuronal activity (Marshall et al., 2006).

Conclusion

So far, most of the evidence suggesting a relation between synchronized oscillatory activity in various frequency bands and synaptic plasticity is correlative in nature and does not allow us to conclude that synchronized oscillatory activity is a necessary prerequisite for the induction of synaptic gain changes. However, the evidence reviewed above concerning the importance of precise temporal relations in synaptic plasticity and the pivotal role of oscillations for the establishment of precise temporal relations between neuronal activity provides strong support for the hypothesis that oscillations and the associated synchronization of spike discharges play a crucial role in the coordination of distributed neuronal processing, on the one hand, and the gating of synaptic plasticity on the other. It has long been suspected that not only stimulus-induced but also self-generated synchronized activity plays a crucial role in the activity-depending shaping of neuronal architectures during development. The evidence that self-generated activity of ganglion cells is synchronized at very early stages in development supports this notion and has initiated a systematic search for relations between synchronized, self-generated activity and the development of ordered neuronal networks (Maffei and Galli-Resta, 1990). Since then, ample evidence has been obtained that temporally structured activity, whether caused by interactions with the environment or by internal mechanisms, plays a pivotal role in the developmental self-organization of the brain. In the last two decades, much progress has been made in the identification of the molecular cascades that translate electrical activity into lasting changes of neuronal architectures, and the pioneering studies of Lamberto Maffei have been and are instrumental for this progress.

References

Abeles M. 1991. *Corticonics*. Cambridge: Cambridge University Press.

Ariav G, Polsky A, Schiller J. 2003. Submillisecond precision of the input–output transformation function mediated by fast sodium dendritic spikes in basal dendrites of CA1 pyramidal neurons. *J Neurosci* 23: 7750–7758.

Artola A, Bröcher S, Singer W. 1990. Different voltage-dependent thresholds for the induction of long-term depression and long-term potentiation in slices of the rat visual cortex. *Nature* 347: 69–72.

Artola A, Singer W. 1987. Long-term potentiation and NMDA receptors in rat visual cortex. *Nature* 330: 649–652.

Azouz R, Gray CM. 2003. Adaptive coincidence detection and dynamic gain control in visual cortical neurons in vivo. *Neuron* 37: 513–523.

Bear MF, Kleinschmidt A, Gu Q, Singer W. 1990. Disruption of experience-dependent synaptic modifications in striate cortex by infusion of an NMDA receptor antagonist. *J Neurosci* 10: 909–925.

Biederlack J, Castelo-Branco M, Neuenschwander S, Wheeler DW, Singer W, Nikolic D. 2006. Brightness induction: rate enhancement and neuronal synchronization as complementary codes. *Neuron* 52: 1073–1083.

Bliss TVP, Lømo T. 1973. Long-lasting potentiation of synaptic transmission in the dentate area of the anaesthetized rabbit following stimulation of the perforant path. *J Physiol* 232: 331–356.

Brecht M, Singer W, Engel AK. 1999. Patterns of synchronization in the superior colliculus of anesthetized cats. *J Neurosci* 19: 3567–3579.

Bröcher S, Artola A, Singer W. 1992a. Intracellular injection of Ca++ chelators blocks induction of long-term depression in rat visual cortex. *Proc Natl Acad Sci USA* 89: 123–127.

Bröcher S, Artola A, Singer W. 1992b. Agonists of cholinergic and noradrenergic receptors facilitate synergistically the induction of long-term potentiation in slices of rat visual cortex. *Brain Res* 573: 27–36.

Buracas G, Zador A, Deweese M, Albright T. 1998. Efficient discrimination of temporal patterns by motion-sensitive neurons in primate visual cortex. *Neuron* 20: 959–969.

Buschman TJ, Miller EK. 2007. Top-down versus bottom-up control of attention in the prefrontal and posterior parietal cortices. *Science* 315: 1860–1862.

Caplan JB, Madsen JR, Raghavachari S, Kahana MJ. 2001. Distinct patterns of brain oscillations underlie two basic parameters of human maze learning. *J Neurophysiol* 86: 368–380.

Caplan JB, Madsen JR, Schulze-Bonhage A, Aschenbrenner-Scheibe R, Newman EL, Kahana MJ. 2003. Human theta oscillations related to sensorimotor integration and spatial learning. *J Neurosci* 23: 4726–4736.

Castelo-Branco M, Neuenschwander S, Singer W. 1998. Synchronization of visual responses between the cortex, lateral geniculate nucleus, and retina in the anesthetized cat. *J Neurosci* 18: 6395–6410.

Debener S, Herrmann CS, Kranczioch C, Gembris D, Engel AK. 2003. Top-down attentional processing enhances auditory evoked gamma band activity. *Neuroreport* 14: 683–686.

Diesmann M, Gewaltig M-O, Aertsen A. 1999. Stable propagation of synchronous spiking in cortical neural networks. *Nature* 402: 529–533.

Engel AK, Fries P, Singer W. 2001. Dynamic predictions: oscillations and synchrony in top-down processing. *Nat Rev Neurosci* 2: 704–716.

Fell J, Klaver P, Elfadil H, Schaller C, Elger CE, Fernández G. 2003. Rhinal–hippocampal theta coherence during declarative memory formation: interaction with gamma synchronization? *Eur J Neurosci* 17: 1082–1088.

Fell J, Klaver P, Lehnertz K, Grunwald T, Schaller C, Elger CE, Fernández G. 2001. Human memory formation is accompanied by rhinal–hippocampal coupling and decoupling. *Nat Neurosci* 4: 1259–1264.

Fries P, Neuenschwander S, Engel AK, Goebel R, Singer W. 2001a. Rapid feature selective neuronal synchronization through correlated latency shifting. *Nat Neurosci* 4: 194–200.

Fries P, Reynolds JH, Rorie AE, Desimone R. 2001b. Modulation of oscillatory neuronal synchronization by selective visual attention. *Science* 291: 1560–1563.

Fries P, Roelfsema PR, Engel AK, König P, Singer W. 1997. Synchronization of oscillatory responses in visual cortex correlates with perception in interocular rivalry. *Proc Natl Acad Sci USA* 94: 12699–12704.

Fries P, Nikolic D, Singer W. 2007. The gamma cycle. *Trends Neurosci* 30: 309–316.

Gaillard R, Dehaene S, Adam C, Clémenceau S, Hasboun D, Baulac M, Cohen L, Naccache L. 2009. Converging intracranial markers of conscious access. *PLoS Biol* 7(3): e1000061.

Gray CM, Singer W. 1989. Stimulus-specific neuronal oscillations in orientation columns of cat visual cortex. *Proc Natl Acad Sci USA* 86: 1698–1702.

Gray CM, König P, Engel AK, Singer W. 1989. Oscillatory responses in cat visual cortex exhibit inter-columnar synchronization which reflects global stimulus properties. *Nature* 338: 334–337.

Guderian S, Duzel E. 2005. Induced theta oscillations mediate large-scale synchrony with mediotemporal areas during recollection in humans. *Hippocampus* 15: 901–912.

Hansel C, Artola A, Singer W. 1996. Different threshold levels of postsynaptic [Ca^{2+}]i have to be reached to induce LTP and LTD in neocortical pyramidal cells. *J Physiol (Paris)* 90: 317–319.

Hansel C, Artola A, Singer W. 1997. Relation between dendritic Ca^{2+} levels and the polarity of synaptic long-term modifications in rat visual cortex neurons. *Eur J Neurosci* 9: 2309–2322.

Hebb DO. 1949. *The Organization of Behavior.* New York: John Wiley and Sons.

Herculano-Houzel S, Munk MHJ, Neuenschwander S, Singer W. 1999. Precisely synchronized oscillatory firing patterns require electroencephalographic activation. *J Neurosci* 19: 3992–4010.

Herrmann CS, Lenz D, Junge S, Busch NA, Maess B. 2004. Memory-matches evoke human gamma-responses. *BMC Neurosci* 5: 13.

Huerta PT, Lisman JE. 1995. Bidirectional synaptic plasticity induced by a single burst during cholinergic theta oscillation in CA1 in vitro. *Neuron* 15: 1053–1063.

Kleinschmidt A, Bear MF, Singer W. 1987. Blockade of "NMDA" receptors disrupts experience-dependent plasticity of kitten striate cortex. *Science* 238: 355–358.

König P, Engel AK, Singer W. 1995. Relation between oscillatory activity and long-range synchronization in cat visual cortex. *Proc Natl Acad Sci USA* 92: 290–294.

König P, Engel AK, Singer W. 1996. Integrator or coincidence detector? The role of the cortical neuron revisited. *Trends Neurosci* 19(4): 130–137.

Löwel S, Singer W. 1992. Selection of intrinsic horizontal connections in the visual cortex by correlated neuronal activity. *Science* 255: 209–212.

Maffei L, Galli-Resta L. 1990. Correlation in the discharges of neighboring rat retinal ganglion cells during prenatal life. *Proc Natl Acad Sci USA* 87: 2861–2864.

Mainen ZF, Sejnowski TJ. 1995. Reliability of spike timing in neocortical neurons. *Science* 268: 1503–1506.

Markram H, Lübke J, Frotscher M, Sakmann B. 1997. Regulation of synaptic efficacy by coincidence of postsynaptic APs and EPSPs. *Science* 275: 213–215.

Marshall L, Helgadóttir H, Mölle M, Born J. 2006. Boosting slow oscillations during sleep potentiates memory. *Nature* 44: 610–613.

Melloni L, Molina C, Pena M, Torres D, Singer W, Rodriguez E. 2007. Synchronization of neural activity across cortical areas correlates with conscious perception. *J Neurosci* 27: 2858–2865.

Miltner WHR, Braun C, Arnold M, Witte H, Taub E. 1999. Coherence of gamma-band EEG activity as a basis for associative learning. *Nature* 397: 434–436.

Munk MHJ, Roelfsema PR, König P, Engel AK, Singer W. 1996. Role of reticular activation in the modulation of intracortical synchronization. *Science* 272: 271–274.

Narayanan RT, Seidenbecher T, Kluge C, Bergado J, Stork O, Pape H-C. 2007. Dissociated theta synchronization in amygdalo–hippocampal circuits during various stages of fear memory. *Eur J Neurosci* 25: 1823–1831.

Neveu D, Zucker RS. 1996. Postsynaptic levels of [Ca^{2+}]i needed to trigger LTD and LTP. *Neuron* 16: 619–629.

Raghavachari S, Kahana MJ, Rizzuto DS, Caplan JB, Kirschen MP, Bourgeois B, Madsen JR, Lisman JE. 2001. Gating of human theta oscillations by a working memory task. *J Neurosci* 21: 3175–3183.

Reinagel P, Reid RC. 2002. Precise firing events are conserved across neurons. *J Neurosci* 22: 6837–6841.

Rizzuto DS, Madsen JR, Bromfield EB, Schulze-Bonhage A, Seelig D, Aschenbrenner-Scheibe R, Kahana MJ. 2003. Reset of human neocortical oscillations during a working memory task. *Proc Natl Acad Sci USA* 100: 7931–7936.

Roelfsema PR, Engel AK, König P, Singer W. 1997. Visuomotor integration is associated with zero time-lag synchronization among cortical areas. *Nature* 385: 157–161.

Sederberg PB, Kahana MJ, Howard MW, Donner EJ, Madsen JR. 2003. Theta and gamma oscillations during encoding predict subsequent recall. *J Neurosci* 23: 10809–10814.

Sederberg PB, Schulze-Bonhage A, Madsen JR, Bromfield EB, McCarthy DC, Brandt A, Tully MS, Kahana MJ. 2007. Hippocampal and neocortical gamma oscillations predict memory formation in humans. *Cereb Cortex* 17: 1190–1196.

Seidenbecher T, Laxmi TR, Stork O, Pape H-C. 2003. Amygdala and hippocampal theta rhythm synchronization during fear memory retrieval. *Science* 301: 846–850.

Singer W. 1999. Neuronal synchrony: a versatile code for the definition of relations? *Neuron* 24: 49–65.

Stiefel KM, Tennigkeit F, Singer W. 2005. Synaptic plasticity in the absence of backpropagating spikes of layer II inputs to layer V pyramidal cells in rat visual cortex. *Eur J Neurosci* 21: 2605–2610.

Strüber D, Basar-Eroglu C, Hoff E, Stadler M. 2000. Reversal-rate dependent differences in the EEG gamma-band during multistable visual perception. *Int J Psychophysiol* 38: 243–252.

Stuart GJ, Häusser M. 2001. Dendritic coincidence detection of EPSPs and action potentials. *Nat Neurosci* 4: 63–71.

Tallon-Baudry C, Bertrand O, Delpuech C, Permier J. 1997. Oscillatory gamma-band (30–70 Hz) activity induced by a visual search task in humans. *J Neurosci* 17: 722–734.

Tallon-Baudry C, Bertrand O, Fischer C. 2001. Oscillatory synchrony between human extrastriate areas during visual short-term memory maintenance. *J Neurosci* 21: RC177.

Tallon-Baudry C, Mandon S, Freiwald WA, Kreiter AK. 2004. Oscillatory synchrony in the monkey temporal lobe correlates with performance in a visual short-term memory task. *Cereb Cortex* 14: 713–720.

Volgushev M, Chistiakova M, Singer W. 1998. Modification of discharge patterns of neocortical neurons by induced oscillations of the membrane potential. *Neuroscience* 83(1): 15–25.

Wespatat V, Tennigkeit F, Singer W. 2004. Phase sensitivity of synaptic modifications in oscillating cells of rat visual cortex. *J Neurosci* 24: 9067–9075.

Whittington MA, Doheny HC, Traub RD, LeBeau FEN, Buhl EH. 2001. Differential expression of synaptic and nonsynaptic mechanisms underlying stimulus-induced gamma oscillations in vitro. *J Neurosci* 21: 1727–1738.

Womelsdorf T, Fries P, Mitra PP, Desimone R. 2006. Gamma-band synchronization in visual cortex predicts speed of change detection. *Nature* 439: 733–736.

Womelsdorf T, Schoffelen J-M, Oostenveld R, Singer W, Desimone R, Engel AK, Fries P. 2007. Modulation of neuronal interactions through neuronal synchronization. *Science* 316: 1609–1612.

21 The Two Dorsal Visual Streams and Their Role in Perception

Giacomo Rizzolatti, Leonardo Fogassi, and Giuseppe Luppino

Unlike most chapters in this book, this chapter does not deal with plasticity. Its aim is different: to give a new account of functions of the dorsal stream and to discuss the possible origin of conscious perception. To this purpose, we review first, adopting an evolutionary perspective, how visual information is transformed into motor acts. We then analyze the concept of two visual systems and, on the basis of recent anatomical and functional evidence, show that the dorsal stream is actually formed by two basically independent pathways. Finally, we address the issue of the role of different visual streams in perception. This essay is dedicated to Lamberto Maffei with whom one of us (G.R.) worked in the past and from whom he learned a great deal on how to carry out neurophysiological experiments and, most importantly, how to address fundamental problems in neuroscience. We hope that this essay would reflect this lesson for which we all are grateful to Lamberto.

Visuomotor Transformations in Amphibians and Rodents

One of the aspects that characterize animals' behavior is their capacity to navigate in space and reach specific objects. A prerequisite for both these capacities is the ability to have an internal representation of space (space perception). Without it, neither action nor object perception is possible.

The traditional view on space perception derives from clinical and psychological studies. It assumes that inside our brain there is a kind of general map where objects are located. This map is unitary, independent of motor activity, and used for organizing all types of actions (see De Renzi, 1982; Heilman et al., 1993; Ungerleider and Mishkin, 1982).

A series of experiments carried out in amphibians and rodents started to challenge this view (see, for review, Milner and Goodale, 1995). Particularly influential was a series of studies of Ingle (1973, 1975) on the frog's visuomotor behavior. He examined two behaviors: turning and snapping at small preylike objects and jumping away from large looming discs. The study of these two behaviors was carried out before and following removal of the optic tectum, the most important visuomotor integration center in amphibians. Note that in amphibians the projections from the retina to the brain regrow following transection.

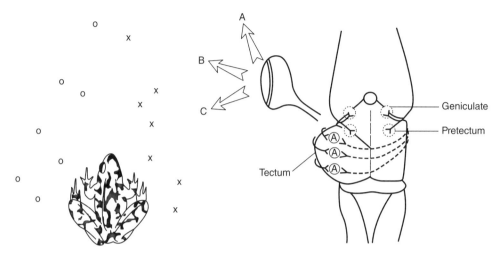

Figure 21.1
Responses and anatomical organization of visuomotor circuits in a "rewired" frog. (Left) Circles represent the location of prey objects and the crosses the corresponding, mirror position frog's snaps in the opposite visual field. (Right) Diagram of the "rewired" projections (interrupted lines) from the retina of the remaining eye to the ipsilateral tectum. Besides the right eye, also the contralateral tectum has been ablated. Inputs from loci A, B, and C on the retina now cross the contralateral tectum, their target in normal nonrewired frog, and project to sites in the ipsilateral tectum that would normally receive input from corresponding points in the retina of the right eye. When these tectal sites are activated by stimulation of the left eye, they direct responses to contralateral locations, as if those sites were activated by the right eye. (Modified from Ingle, 1973.)

Immediately following unilateral removal of the optic tectum, frogs totally ignored stimuli presented in the field contralateral to the ablated tectum. However, over the next month vision recovered, but the observed responses were bizarre. When presented with prey stimuli in the formerly blind contralateral field, the frogs, instead of turning and snapping toward them, directed their responses toward a location roughly symmetrical to the position of the stimulus, located in the ipsilateral field. Similarly, when a large threatening disc was suddenly introduced into the field opposite to the lesion, instead of jumping away from the disc, they jumped toward it (see figure 21.1).

What occurred? Histological analysis revealed that the transected optic tract regenerated and innervated the tectum opposite to the lesion. With this in mind, the explanation is simple. When prey objects or looming discs were shown to the eye *ipsilateral* to the intact tectum, they elicited the behavior proper to this tectum, that is, a response to stimuli within the visual field of the eye *contralateral* to the tectum. It was as if the stimulus was presented to this eye—hence, the paradoxical responses.

It is important to note that not the entire visual space of the rewired frog was a mirror image of what it had been before. In fact, not all visuomotor behaviors were reversed in these animals. The same rewired frog, which jumped against a suddenly presented "threatening" disc, avoided obstacles placed in front of it when its movements were elicited by a touch applied on the rear.

This capacity of circumventing barriers was preserved because this behavior was not mediated by retinal projections to the tectum, but by projections to the pretectum, another visual structure. This pathway was not destroyed by the lesion.

These findings illustrate that what counts in the organization of the visuomotor response is the *activation of the motor centers*. Furthermore, most importantly, it shows that in the frog there is no such a thing as a unified representation of the external world. The frogs possess a parallel set of *independent visuomotor* circuits, each of which has a space representation. These circuits are activated by specific stimuli present in the environment and determine the appropriate responses.

A similar organization of the visual system in parallel visuomotor circuits is also present in rodents (Goodale and Milner, 1982). As in amphibians, a projection from the retina to the superior colliculus—the mammalian homolog of the optic tectum—mediates eye, head, and body orienting movements to stimuli presented in their visual field. A second retinal projection to the superior colliculus mediates, in a manner very similar to that described in the frog, escape reactions. Finally, there is evidence that a visual projection from the retina to the pretectum mediates barrier avoidance much as in the frog. This striking homology in neural machinery underlying visuomotor behavior in amphibians and rodents indicates that a separate control of visuomotor behavior rather than a unified representation of the visual space was the solution that evolution chose for providing individuals with an efficient way to interact with the external environment.

Visuomotor Organization in Primates

In primates, the organization of movements in space is controlled, besides by the same subcortical structures as in other animals, also by cortical areas and, in particular, by those of the parietal lobe. The parietal lobe was classically viewed as an association region that "puts together" (associates) different sensory modalities (Denny-Brown and Chambers, 1958; De Renzi, 1982). Space perception is the result of this association process. A series of anatomical and functional studies, starting from the early work of Hyvarinen (1982) and Mountcastle et al. (1975), showed that the organization of this region is very similar to that present in the subcortical structures. There is no such a thing as a dedicated space area, but rather a series of areas that transform sensory information into action.

For example, a recent study that assessed the neural properties of the convexity of the inferior parietal lobule (IPL) showed that actions done with different effectors are represented in different cytoarchitectonic areas. The rostral part of IPL (areas PF and PFG) encodes mouth and hand actions; the central part of it (PG) mediates reaching arm movements; finally, the caudal part encodes eye movements (Rozzi et al., 2008).

These findings clearly show that the traditional notion that the parietal lobe is the region responsible for space perception, independent of motor system and preceding motor activity, does not capture the essence of the parietal lobe function. The parietal lobe is formed by a series

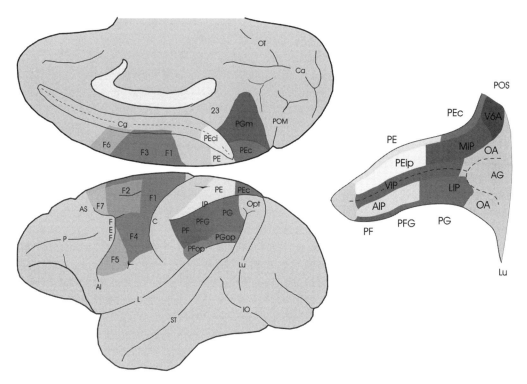

Figure 21.2 (plate 7)
Mesial and lateral views of the macaque brain. Cytoarchitectonic parcellation of the frontal motor cortex (areas indicated with F followed by Arabic numbers) and of the parietal lobe (areas indicated with P and progressive letters). Areas buried within the intraparietal sulcus are shown in an unfolded view of the sulcus (right inset). AIP, anterior intraparietal area; AI, inferior arcuate sulcus; AS, superior arcuate sulcus; C, central sulcus; Ca, calcarine fissure; Cg, cingulate cortex; FEF, frontal eye field; IO, inferior occipital sulcus; IP, intraparietal sulcus; L, lateral sulcus; LIP, lateral intraparietal area; MIP, medial intraparietal area; Lu, lunate sulcus; OT, occipitotemporal sulcus; P, principal sulcus; PO, parietoccipital sulcus; ST, superior temporal sulcus; VIP, ventral intraparietal area.

of distinct cytoarchitectonic areas specifically linked with areas located in the premotor cortex (see figure 21.2, plate 7). Together these areas form a series of visuomotor circuits coding different types of motor behavior among which are hand grasping, arm reaching, mouth movements, and different types of eye movements. These circuits are activated by specific sets of sensory inputs that are conveyed to the parietal lobe from other somatosensory, visual, and auditory areas (see Rizzolatti et al., 1998; Rizzolatti and Luppino, 2001).

The New Demands to Visual System in Primates

Up to now we have stressed the basic similarities of the organization of visuomotor behavior in lower animals and primates. However, if the basic evolutionary functional skeleton is similar, evolution provided primates with some new fundamental capacities poorly developed in lower animals. One is the amazing capacity to discriminate and code visual stimuli; the other is the appearance of a prehensile hand.

The evolution of rich visual discrimination capacities had profound consequences on brain organization. For a frog, a stimulus has a *double* function: it says *what* the stimulus is and specifies *how* to interact with it. A thin rectangular piece of paper moved horizontally means prey, and, simultaneously, provides information necessary to act upon it. In primates, these two stimulus aspects are separate. It is not sufficient to have a round object for determining a grasping movement in a hungry person. This could occur if the round object is an orange, but not if it is a tennis ball.

Similarly, the evolution of a prehensile hand and the associated manual dexterity radically changed the way in which primates relate themselves to the external world. While, in rodents, motor behavior consists mostly of the control of navigation, prey catching, obstacle avoidance, escape from predators, and some very limited manual capacities, the prehensile hand allowed primates to interact in a sophisticated way with objects. Thus, coming back to the previous example, regardless of whether the round object is an orange or a tennis ball, when an individual wants to grasp it, he or she will use the same circuit that transforms spherical objects into a particular hand shaping. Thus, while the visual information is unitary in frogs, it "doubled" in primates.

These new evolutionary acquisitions led to an enormous increase in the neural space devoted to vision. The necessity to encode a large variety of visual objects determined the enlargement of the temporal lobe with appearance of a large ventral sector in this structure, the "inferotemporal cortex." This was accompanied by the appearance of visual areas that finely analyze the details of visual stimuli and send their information to the temporal lobe. These areas form a specific functional stream: the "ventral visual stream" (Ungerleider and Mishkin, 1982; see figure 21.3).

At the same time, the increased capacity to interact with objects also had important consequences on the sensorimotor system transforming visual objects into actions. First, reaching an object requires a space computation different from that for directing the gaze on it. This new requirement determined most likely the evolution of areas encoding the "peripersonal space," that is, the space around the body where objects are reachable (see Rizzolatti et al., 2000). Second, grasping requires a particular description of objects in terms of their affordances, a description different from that necessary for coding their figural aspects (Jeannerod et al., 1995). Third, the "reaching-to-grasp" action required a sophisticated control system to correctly perform the desired movements.

These new functions, computationally akin to those necessary for other types of visuomotor transformations, were allocated in the parietal lobe and, similarly to what occurred to the ventral system, required specific areas mostly devoted to these new functions. These areas formed a second visual stream, referred to as the "dorsal visual stream" (see Milner and Goodale, 1995).

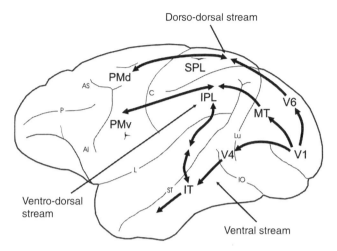

Figure 21.3
Schematic view of the cortical visual streams. Arrows indicate the main pathways of the ventral stream, of the two subdivisions of the dorsal stream and their premotor target areas. The reciprocal connection between the ventrodorsal and ventral stream is also indicated. IPL, inferior parietal lobule; MT, middle temporal area; PMd, dorsal premotor cortex; PMv, ventral premotor cortex; SPL, superior parietal lobule. Other conventions as in figure 21.2.

An Analysis of the Dorsal Stream

Whereas there is a general agreement that the ventral stream mediates a pictorial description of objects and biological motions, there are divergent views on the functional role of the dorsal stream. We will address this issue at the end of this chapter after reviewing the organization of this stream.

Recently, Rizzolatti and Matelli (2003), on the basis of the connectivity patterns of the parietal visuomotor areas, have proposed that the various parietofrontal circuits can be grouped into two anatomically and functionally distinct main components, the dorsodorsal (d-d) stream, formed by circuits involving the superior parietal lobule (SPL) and dorsal premotor cortex (PMd) areas and the ventrodorsal (v-d) stream, formed by circuits involving the IPL and, mostly, ventral premotor cortex (PMv) areas and the frontal eye field (FEF; see figure 21.3).

Besides the anatomical differences in the parietal regions involved in the d-d and in the v-d streams (SPL vs. IPL, respectively) and the markedly different roles in motor control played by their final target areas in the agranular frontal cortex (PMd vs. PMv and FEF), one major argument in favor of this subdivision is represented by the marked difference in the sources of visual information feeding the two streams.

Both dorsal visual streams are mostly under the influence of the so-called "magnocellular" pathway, which, at the cortical level, originates from layer IV B of V1. In its original definition, the nodal point of this pathway was the extrastriate area MT/V5. This area directly, or through the neighboring area MST, is the major source of visual inputs to the caudal IPL, considered the final target of this pathway. The discovery that the caudal SPL (e.g., Caminiti et al., 1996; Galletti et al., 2003) is also involved in visuomotor processing raised the question of which is the source of visual inputs to this parietal sector.

Recent evidence showed that another extrastriate area—V6, placed at the same level as MT/V5 in the hierarchy of visual extrastriate areas—is a further main nodal point of the magnocellular pathway and represents the major source of visual information to the caudal SPL (Galletti et al., 2001). Thus, at the origin of the d-d and the v-d streams, there are two distinct extrastriate areas, V6 and V5/MT, respectively.

Second, another major difference between the d-d and the v-d streams is that the visuomotor areas of IPL, but not those of SPL, are connected to the temporal lobe (Baizer et al., 1991; Rozzi et al., 2006; Borra et al., 2008). Accordingly, the v-d stream operates under the influence not only of the magnocellular pathway but also of the ventral visual stream and of higher order polysensory areas of the superior temporal gyrus.

The Dorsodorsal Stream

As noted above, at the origin of the d-d stream is area V6, an area located deeply in the anterior wall of the parieto-occipital sulcus. This region, classically considered part of the occipital cytoarchitectonic cortex, consists of two architectonically and functionally distinct areas (see Galletti et al., 2003; Luppino et al., 2005): a ventral smaller one, V6, showing architectonic features typical of the occipital cortex, and a more dorsal and larger one, V6A, showing architectonic features typical of the parietal cortex.

V6 is a pure visual area. It is retinotopically organized, with a complete representation of the contralateral visual hemifield. Unlike what is observed in other extrastriate areas, the representation of the central visual field is not so emphasized in V6 (Galletti et al., 1999a). In contrast to V6, in V6A only about 60% of the neurons are responsive to visual stimuli. Their receptive fields are typically large, and there is no clear topographic organization in the representation of the visual field. Nonvisual neurons in V6A are sensitive to gaze direction and/or saccadic eye movements, some to somatosensory stimulation, and others discharge in association to arm movements (Galletti et al., 1999b).

V6 is the target of strong projections from V1 and is connected to several other occipital areas, including V2, V3, V3A, V4T, and V5/MT (Galletti et al., 2001). V6 is not connected with the frontal lobe, and its parietal connections are almost completely limited to the caudalmost part of SPL, in particular to V6A and medial intraparietal area (MIP), an area involved in the organization of reaching movements (Colby and Duhamel, 1996; Andersen and Buneo, 2002). Area V6A is not connected with extrastriate areas except to V6 and is the source of strong projections to PMd (Matelli et al., 1998; Marconi et al., 2001; Gamberini et al., 2009), mainly with the ventral and rostral part of area F2, which contains a representation of proximal and distal arm movements. V6A is also strongly connected with two neighboring SPL areas, MIP and PGm, that, in turn, are the sources of strong projections to different PMd sectors (Matelli et al., 1998).

Specifically, MIP mostly projects to ventrolateral F2 whereas PGm projects to the rostral PMd (area F7).

Altogether, these data strongly support the notion that V6 is an extrastriate area at the origin of a relatively direct ("fast") visuomotor pathway (the d-d stream), which, in few steps, conveys visual information to caudal SPL areas, which are the source of parieto-frontal projections to arm-related fields of PMd.

The Ventrodorsal Stream

The major source of visual inputs to the v-d stream is MT/V5, in part through the neighboring area MST. IPL targets of MT/V5 and MST are two areas located in the intraparietal sulcus, the oculomotor area lateral intraparietal area (LIP) and ventral intraparietal area (VIP), involved in peripersonal space coding for arm and face movements (Colby et al., 1993), and the caudal part of the IPL convexity (Boussaoud et al., 1990).

Recent evidence showed that the IPL consists of a multiplicity of distinct visuomotor areas. More specifically, in the lateral bank of the IPS, an area rostral to LIP—anterior intraparietal area (AIP)—plays a crucial role in visuomotor control of hand actions (Sakata et al., 1995). Furthermore, the IPL convexity cortex can be subdivided into four architectonically distinct areas, designated, from the rostral to the caudal end, as PF, PFG, PG, and Opt (Gregoriou et al., 2006). All of them are involved in visuomotor control of different types of actions (Rozzi et al., 2008). Connection studies in which neural tracers were injected in these newly defined IPL areas showed that, in addition to LIP and VIP, AIP and the three caudal IPL convexity areas PFG, PG, and Opt are the targets of projections from MT and/or MST (Rozzi et al., 2006; Borra et al., 2008). Accordingly, all these areas can be considered to be located along the main pathway of the v-d stream.

A further finding of these connection studies, very important for functionally characterizing the v-d stream with respect to the d-d stream, has been that all these MST-recipient areas of IPL are robustly and reciprocally connected with the temporal cortex. These connections involve two temporal regions, the rostral two-thirds of the dorsal bank of the superior temporal sulcus (STS) and the areas of the lower bank of the STS (TEa/m) and of the middle temporal gyrus (TEa and TEp). Both these temporal regions are potential sources of different types of high-order visual information. Specifically, while the three caudal IPL convexity areas (PFG, PG, and Opt) are predominantly and extensively connected to the upper bank of the STS, AIP is very robustly and exclusively connected with the different subdivisions of inferotemporal area TE.

The rostral sector of the dorsal bank of the STS is generally referred to as the "superior polysensory area" (STP; Bruce et al., 1981). STP is a site of convergence of projections from somatosensory, auditory, and visual areas of both the dorsal and the ventral visual stream. Functional findings are in accord with this pattern of afferent projections showing that neurons in this area often have somatosensory, auditory, and visual receptive fields (Bruce et al., 1981; Bayliss et al., 1987). Visually responsive neurons in STP may have very complex properties as shown by Perrett and coworkers (Perrett et al., 1989; Carey et al., 1997). In contrast, the rostral inferotemporal areas connected to area AIP are located at the highest hierarchical levels of the ventral visual stream. Neurons in this area have complex visual responses related to recognition and discrimination of objects and actions (Gross et al., 1972; Tanaka, 1996).

Functional Hypotheses on the Role of the Ventrodorsal and Dorsodorsal Streams

The data reviewed above suggest the two dorsal streams play a differential role in the organization of visuomotor behavior. As far as the d-d is concerned, there are three important aspects worth stressing. First, this stream represents a shorter pathway than both v-d and ventral stream for conveying visual information to the premotor cortex. Second, in contrast to the organization of most visual areas, the periphery of visual field is richly represented in this stream. Third, there are no connections with the areas of the temporal cortex, and therefore the d-d stream does not receive higher order visual information.

Considering these properties, the organization of the d-d stream appears to be similar to that of the evolutionarily oldest visuomotor circuits present in amphibians and rodents. There is, however, a noticeable difference. D-d stream is endowed with neurons related to arm reaching movements and, to some extent, even to hand grasping movements, suggesting an evolutionary new function of this stream: that of a forelimb movement control (see also below).

A completely different picture emerges from the anatomy and functional properties of the v-d stream. This stream conveys magnocellular visual information to the motor system but, in addition, integrates this information with that coming from inferotemporal cortex and the polysensory areas of STS. This indicates the this stream may organize object-directed movements according to the semantic properties of objects in addition to that based on intrinsic (physical) object properties (see Jeannerod, 1997).

Most interestingly, the areas of this stream represent a node where motor action representations, present in IPL, integrate with the description of objects and biological movements coming from the temporal lobe. In virtue of this fact, areas of v-d stream have been found to play an important role in cognitive motor functions, such as space perception and action understanding (see Rizzolatti and Matelli, 2003; Rizzolatti et al., 2004).

An additional cognitive function mediated by the connections between v-d and ventral stream is the possibility to give a full semantic description of objects, based not only on the object visual aspect but also on its common use. Finally, the same circuit might play a role in cross-modal transfer from somatosensory and motor knowledge of a given object to its visual and semantic representation.

Syndromes Resulting from Damage to the Superior Parietal and Inferior Parietal Lobule

The data reviewed in the previous sections (based mostly on monkey data) indicate a marked difference in the anatomical connections and functional properties of the d-d and v-d streams.

Are these differences also present in humans? In the past, there has been marked disagreement concerning the homology between the monkey and human posterior parietal cortex. Some authors—for example, Brodmann (1909)—considered IPL as an evolutionary new lobule present only in humans. Today, however, there is convincing evidence coming from brain imaging studies that show that the areas located inside the intraparietal sulcus have similar functional properties in the two species (Simon et al., 2002; Grefkes and Fink, 2005). This finding, together to the fact that the intraparietal sulcus is a very ancient sulcus, already present in prosimians, strongly suggests that this sulcus is an ancient divide between two different anatomical and functional streams. With this in mind, it is interesting to examine whether the different properties of SPL and IPL fit and possibly explain the clinical deficits observed in humans following damage to SPL and IPL, respectively.

A relatively common syndrome following damage to SPL is *optic ataxia*. Optic ataxia is a disorder of arm visually guided movements toward a target. The affected arm gropes for the target, making errors in both frontal and sagittal planes, until it runs, almost by chance, into the object. The deficit is particularly severe when the target is located in the peripheral part of the visual field, decreases when the target is in parafoveal vision, and often completely disappears when the patient fixates the target. Interestingly enough, most patients, albeit not all of them, are able to point correctly to targets on their own body (see De Renzi, 1982; Perenin and Vighetto, 1988).

From this brief description of the basic features of optic ataxia it is obvious that the core deficit in the syndrome is a deficit in sensorimotor control. There is no hint of perceptual deficits. The patients know where the objects are. Their difficulty is to reach them, especially when the visual information is limited to peripheral vision.

The most common clinical syndrome following damage to the IPL (typically to the right IPL) is spatial neglect. When neglect is full-fledged, patients show a deviation of the head and eyes toward the side of the lesion. If addressed by the the left (contralesional) side, they may fail to respond or look for the examiner in the opposite (ipsilesional) side of the room. Frequently, patients with neglect do not take food from the left half of the dish and, when asked to make a drawing, draw only the right side of it (see Bisiach and Vallar, 2000).

Neglect affects typically both the space near to and far from the body. Dissociations, however, have been described first in the monkey (Rizzolatti et al., 1983) and then in humans (e.g., Halligan and Marshall, 1991; Cowey et al., 1994; see Berti and Rizzolatti, 2002). Thus, near (peripersonal) space or far space can be affected, either independently or in prevalent form. In the first case, neglect patients respond normally to visual stimuli presented far from them but are unable to respond to near stimuli ("peripersonal neglect"). Vice versa, in the second case, they respond well to near visual stimuli but ignore those located far away ("extrapersonal neglect").

In addition to these disturbances, neglect may affect the patient's body ("personal neglect"). Patients with personal neglect become untidy in their personal appearance, not caring about the part of their body contralateral to the lesion. Neurological examination shows that patients with personal neglect fail to respond to tactile stimuli delivered on the body side contralateral to the lesion (see Bisiach and Vallar, 2000).

It is obvious that, unlike in optic ataxia, the dominant aspect of neglect is a deficit in perception. However, a series of motor deficits are also present, especially in the severe forms and in its early phases.

The third major syndrome following posterior parietal lesion is apraxia. Apraxia is an impaired ability to perform gestures that is not caused by weakness, sensory loss, abnormality of tone or movements, intellectual deterioration, or poor comprehension (Geschwind, 1965; De Renzi and Faglioni, 1999). Apraxia takes two major forms: ideational apraxia and ideomotor apraxia. In the first form, the patients have difficulties in retrieving motor ideas on how to use objects, especially when more than one object is involved (e.g., lighting a candle). In the second, they fail to implement the internal representation of a motor act or a gesture into the appropriate motor action.

Of the two major apraxic syndromes, of interest here is the ideomotor apraxia. Classically, this syndrome was conceived as a motor syndrome, characterized by an automatic–voluntary dissociation. This term indicates that the same gesture that fails on the examiner's request is well executed in the presence of an appropriate context. For example, the same patient that in front of an object is perfectly able to grasp it is unable to replicate the same gesture following a verbal command or on imitation in the absence of the object. In this description of ideomotor apraxia, perception is not involved. There is evidence, however, that the situation may be more complex. Heilman and his colleagues (Heilman et al., 1982; Rothi et al., 1985) demonstrated that apraxic patients with posterior parietal lesions might show inability to distinguish well-performed from poorly performed actions. There was also a trend to confound different gestures, but this deficit was rare. More recently, Pazzaglia et al. (2008) studied patients with limb and/or buccofacial ideomotor apraxia. The patients were asked to match sounds evoking human-related actions or nonhuman action sounds with specific visual pictures. They found that hand and mouth action-related sound recognition was specifically impaired in limb and buccofacial apraxia patients, respectively. Most interestingly, the localization of the damage revealed that the left frontoparietal cortex is crucial for recognizing the sound of limb movements, while the left inferior frontal gyrus and adjacent insular cortex were associated with recognition of buccofacial-related action sounds. These behavioral and neural double dissociations indicate that a left-lateralized multimodal network (mirror network) is actively involved in the body-part-specific motor mapping of limb and mouth action-related sounds, as well as in the execution of the very same actions.

Summing up, the three syndromes described above have three different anatomical locations. Lesions centered to SPL determine optical ataxia (Ratcliff and Davies-Jones, 1972; Perenin and Vighetto, 1988). Lesions of the right IPL, especially its lower part, produce neglect (Vallar and Perani, 1987; Perenin and Vighetto, 1988). Damage to a parietofrontal circuit that includes the rostral part of the left IPL causes ideomotor apraxia (De Renzi and Faglioni, 1999).

Conclusions

In recent times, it became fashionable to freely use mental terms like perception or consciousness in discussing neurophysiological findings. Perception, however, is a concept referring to an individual's personal experience of a perceived item. It does not seem to us that, at present, there is any satisfactory neurophysiological explanation of *how* this experience may occur and which are the neural mechanisms responsible. Therefore, the use of these terms within the context of neuroscience is premature and probably can even be misleading.

Nonetheless, the term perception may be operationally useful, especially in clinical neurology, to describe syndromes where patients are unable to recognize certain items (visual agnosia) or are unaware of their presence (spatial neglect). As far as the visual system is concerned, these deficits may occur following damage to the ventral or the dorsal visual system, respectively.

Damage to the *ventral visual stream* may selectively impair the recognition of certain categories of visual stimuli like objects, faces, written words, or colors while leaving others intact (Farah, 1990). The occurrence of visual deficits selectively impairing the perception of certain categories of stimuli is in agreement with neuroimaging data showing that separate, discrete areas of the ventral visual stream are dedicated to the analysis and storage of objects, faces, or colors (Kanwisher et al., 1997; Downing et al., 2001). There is no reason, however, to think that a patient with one of these deficits (visual *agnosia* or specific forms of it) does not perceive these stimuli because of damage to a mechanism devoted to perception in the proper sense. It is much more plausible that, the damage being localized to specific visual areas, the processing of some types of visual information is lost and therefore not available to the complex network of areas and centers that, in a manner that we do not yet understand, determine perception.

Damage to the v-d stream, besides deficits concerning action organization and action execution, yields deficits in space perception and action understanding. Neglect is the most convincing case of a syndrome in which patients *are not conscious,* in the proper sense, of aspects of the external world. The arguments in favor of this conclusion are the following. First, it is difficult to conceive of object representation without space representation. Second, in spite of the integrity of the ventral visual system and evidence that this system is active in patients with neglect, these patients do not perceive objects in the contralateral space (Volpe et al., 1979; Marshall and Halligan, 1988; Berti and Rizzolatti, 1992). Third, in anaesthetized individuals, who are unconscious by definition, the ventral system is active and its neurons respond to appropriate visual stimuli, while the dorsal visual system is unresponsive. Fourth, patients with visual agnosia are often able to recognize and name objects presented in tactile modality (Farah, 1990). Thus, the dorsal visual stream (more than the ventral one) appears to be the neural substrate on which perception in the proper sense is built.

In conclusion, the types of deficit occurring following damage of the visuomotor circuits responsible for actions suggest that actions and space organization are the building blocks on which perception is built. These evolutionarily old visuomotor circuits thus appear to represent the neural basis from which, starting from a mere elaboration of visual information, the first person knowledge of the external world emerged.

References

Andersen RA, Buneo CA. 2002. Intentional maps in posterior parietal cortex. *Annu Rev Neurosci* 25: 189–220.

Baizer JS, Ungerleider LG, Desimone R. 1991. Organization of visual inputs to the inferior temporal and posterior parietal cortex in macaques. *J Neurosci* 11: 168–190.

Bayliss GC, Rolls ET, Leonard CM. 1987. Functional subdivisions of the temporal lobe neocortex. *J Neurosci* 7: 330–342.

Berti A, Rizzolatti G. 1992. Visual processing without awareness: evidence from unilateral neglect. *J Cogn Neurosci* 4: 345–351.

Berti A, Rizzolatti G. 2002. Coding far and near space. In: *The Cognitive and Neural Bases of Spatial Neglect* (Karnath H-O, Milner D, Vallar G, eds), pp 313–326. Oxford, UK: Oxford University Press.

Bisiach E, Vallar G. 2000. Unilateral neglect in humans. In: *Handbook of Neuropsychology*, 2nd edition (Boller F, Grafman J, eds), pp 459–502. Amsterdam: Elsevier.

Borra E, Belmalih A, Calzavara R, Gerbella M, Murata A, Rozzi S, Luppino G. 2008. Cortical connections of the macaque anterior intraparietal (AIP) area. *Cereb Cortex* 18: 1094–1111.

Boussaoud D, Ungerleider L, Desimone R. 1990. Pathways for motion analysis: cortical connections of the medial superior temporal and fundus of the superior temporal visual areas in the macaque. *J Comp Neurol* 296: 462–495.

Brodmann K. 1909. Vergleichende Lokalisationslehre der Groshirnrinde. Leipzig (Reprinted 1925): Barth.

Bruce C, Desimone R, Gross CG. 1981. Visual properties of neurons in a polysensory area in superior temporal sulcus of the macaque. *J Neurophysiol* 46: 369–384.

Caminiti R, Ferraina S, Johnson PB. 1996. The sources of visual information to the primate frontal lobe: a novel role for the superior parietal lobule. *Cereb Cortex* 6: 319–328.

Carey DP, Perrett DI, Oram MW. 1997. Recognizing, understanding and reproducing actions. In: *Handbook of Neuropsychology* (Boller F, Grafman J, eds), pp 111–129. Amsterdam: Elsevier.

Colby CL, Duhamel J-R, Goldberg ME. 1993. Ventral intraparietal area of the macaque: anatomic location and visual response properties. *J Neurophysiol* 69: 902–914.

Colby CL, Duhamel JR. 1996. Spatial representations for action in parietal cortex. *Brain Res Cogn Brain Res* 5: 105–115.

Cowey A, Small M, Ellis S. 1994. Left visuo-spatial neglect can be worse in far than near space. *Neuropsychologia* 32: 1059–1066.

Denny-Brown D, Chambers RA. 1958. The parietal lobe and behavior. *Res Publ Assoc Res Nerv Ment Dis* 36: 35–117.

De Renzi E. 1982. *Disorders of Space Exploration and Cognition.* New York: Wiley.

De Renzi E, Faglioni P. 1999. Apraxia. In: *Clinical and Experimental Neuropsychology* (Denes G, Pizzamiglio L, eds), pp 421–440. East Sussex, UK: Psychology Press.

Downing PE, Jiang J, Shuman M, Kanwisher N. 2001. Cortical area selective for visual processing of the human body. *Science* 293: 2470–2473.

Farah M. 1990. *Visual Agnosia: Disorders of Object Recognition and What They Tell Us About Normal Vision.* Cambridge, MA: MIT Press.

Galletti C, Fattori P, Gamberini M, Kutz DF. 1999a. The cortical visual area V6: brain location and visual topography. *Eur J Neurosci* 11: 3922–3936.

Galletti C, Fattori P, Kutz DF, Gamberini M. 1999b. Brain location and visual topography of cortical area V6A in the macaque monkey. *Eur J Neurosci* 11: 575–582.

Galletti C, Gamberini M, Kutz DF, Fattori P, Luppino G, Matelli M. 2001. The cortical connections of area V6: an occipito–parietal network processing visual information. *Eur J Neurosci* 13: 1572–1588.

Galletti C, Kutz DF, Gamberini M, Breveglieri R, Fattori P. 2003. Role of the medial parieto–occipital cortex in the control of reaching and grasping movements. *Exp Brain Res* 153: 158–170.

Gamberini M, Passarelli M, Fattori P, Zucchelli M, Bakola S, Luppino G, Galletti C. 2009. Cortical connections of the visuomotor parietooccipital area V6Ad of the macaque monkey. *J Comp Neurol* 513: 622–642.

Geschwind N. 1965. Disconnexion syndromes in animals and man. *Brain* 88: 237–294.

Goodale MA, Milner AD. 1982. Fractionating orienting behavior in rodents. In: *Analysis of Visual Behavior* (Ingle DJ, Goodale MA, Mansfield RJW, eds), pp 549–586. Cambridge, MA: MIT Press.

Grefkes C, Fink GR. 2005. The functional organization of the intraparietal sulcus in humans and monkeys. *J Anat* 207: 3–17.

Gregoriou GG, Borra E, Matelli M, Luppino G. 2006. Architectonic organization of the inferior parietal convexity of the macaque monkey. *J Comp Neurol* 496: 422–451.

Gross CG, Rocha-Miranda CE, Bender DB. 1972. Visual properties of neurons in inferotemporal cortex of the macaque. *J Neurophysiol* 35: 96–111.

Halligan PW, Marshall JC. 1991. Left neglect for near but not far space in man. *Nature* 350: 498–500.

Heilman KM, Rothi LJ, Valenstein E. 1982. Two forms of ideomotor apraxia. *Neurology* 32: 342–346.

Heilman KM, Watson RT, Valenstein E. 1993. Neglect and related disorders. In: *Clinical Neuropsychology*, 3rd ed. (Heilman KM, Valenstein E, eds), pp 279–336. London: Oxford University Press.

Hyvarinen J. 1982. Posterior parietal lobe of the primate brain. *Physiol Rev* 62: 1060–1129.

Ingle DJ. 1973. Two visual systems in the frog. *Science* 181: 1053–1055.

Ingle DJ. 1975. Selective visual attention in frogs. *Science* 188: 1033–1035.

Jeannerod M, Arbib MA, Rizzolatti G, Sakata H. 1995. Grasping objects: the cortical mechanisms of visuomotor transformation. *Trends Neurosci* 18: 314–320.

Jeannerod M. 1997. *The Cognitive Neuroscience of Action.* Oxford, UK: Blackwell.

Kanwisher N, Mc Dermott J, Chun MM. 1997. The fusiform face area: A module in human extrastriate cortex specialized for face perception. *J Neurosci* 17: 4302–4311.

Luppino G, Ben Hamed S, Gamberini M, Matelli M, Galletti C. 2005. Occipital (V6) and parietal (V6A) areas in the anterior wall of the parieto-occipital sulcus of the macaque: a cytoarchitectonic study. *Eur J Neurosci* 21: 3056–3076.

Marconi B, Genovesio A, Battaglia Mayer A, Ferraina S, Squatrito S, Molinari M, Lacquaniti F, Caminiti R. 2001. Eye–hand coordination during reaching. I. Anatomical relationships between parietal and frontal cortex. *Cereb Cortex* 11: 513–527.

Marshall JF, Halligan PW. 1988. Blindsight and insight in visuo-spatial neglect. *Nature* 336: 766–767.

Matelli M, Govoni P, Galletti C, Kutz DF, Luppino G. 1998. Superior area 6 afferents from the superior parietal lobule in the macaque monkey. *J Comp Neurol* 402: 327–352.

Milner D, Goodale MA. 1995. *The Visual Brain in Action.* Oxford, UK: Oxford University Press.

Mountcastle VB, Lynch JC, Georgopoulos A, Sakata H, Acuna C. 1975. Posterior parietal association cortex of the monkey: command functions for operations within extrapersonal space. *J Neurophysiol* 38: 871–908.

Pazzaglia M, Pizzamiglio L, Pes E, Aglioti SM. 2008. The sound of actions in apraxia. *Curr Biol* 18: 1766–1772.

Perenin MT, Vighetto A. 1988. Optic ataxia: a specific disruption in visuomotor mechanisms. I. Different aspects of the deficit in reaching for objects. *Brain* 111: 643–674.

Perrett DI, Harries MH, Bevan R, Thomas S, Benson PJ, Mistlin AJ, Chitty AK, Hietanen JK, Ortega JE. 1989. Frameworks of analysis for the neural representation of animate objects and actions. *J Exp Biol* 146: 87–113.

Ratcliff G, Davies-Jones GA. 1972. Defective visual localization in focal brain wounds. *Brain* 95: 49–60.

Rizzolatti G, Luppino G. 2001. The cortical motor system. *Neuron* 31: 889–901.

Rizzolatti G, Matelli M. 2003. Two different streams form the dorsal visual system: anatomy and functions. *Exp Brain Res* 153: 146–157.

Rizzolatti G, Berti A, Gallese V. 2000. Spatial neglect: neurophysiological bases, cortical circuits and theories. In: *Handbook of Neuropsychology* 2nd Ed., Vol. I (Boller F, Grafman J, Rizzolatti G, eds), pp 503–537. Amsterdam: Elsevier.

Rizzolatti G, Fogassi L, Gallese V. 2004. Cortical mechanism subserving object grasping, action understanding and imitation. In: *The Cognitive Neuroscience*, Third Ed. (Gazzaniga MS, ed), pp 427–440. Cambridge, MA: MIT Press.

Rizzolatti G, Luppino G, Matelli M. 1998. The organization of the cortical motor system: new concepts. *Electroencephalogr Clin Neurophysiol* 106: 283–296.

Rizzolatti G, Matelli M, Pavesi G. 1983. Deficits in attention and movement following the removal of postarcuate (area 6) and prearcuate (area 8) cortex in macaque monkeys. *Brain* 106: 655–673.

Rothi LJ, Heilman KM, Watson RT. 1985. Pantomime comprehension and ideomotor apraxia. *J Neurol Neurosurg Psychiatry* 48: 451–454.

Rozzi S, Calzavara R, Belmalih A, Borra E, Gregoriou GG, Matelli M, Luppino G. 2006. Cortical connections of the inferior parietal cortical convexity of the macaque monkey. *Cereb Cortex* 16: 1389–1417.

Rozzi S, Ferrari P, Bonini L, Rizzolatti G, Fogassi L. 2008. Functional organization of inferior parietal lobule convexity in the macaque monkey: electrophysiological characterization of motor, sensory and mirror responses and their correlation with cytoarchitectonic areas. *Eur J Neurosci* 28: 1569–1588.

Sakata H, Taira M, Murata A, Mine S. 1995. Neural mechanisms of visual guidance of hand action in the parietal cortex of the monkey. *Cereb Cortex* 5: 429–438.

Simon O, Mangin JF, Cohen L, Le Bihan D, Dehaene S. 2002. Topographical layout of hand, eye, calculation, and language-related areas in the human parietal lobe. *Neuron* 33: 475–487.

Tanaka K. 1996. Inferotemporal cortex and object vision. *Annu Rev Neurosci* 19: 109–139.

Ungerleider LG, Mishkin M. 1982. Two cortical visual systems. In: *Analysis of Visual Behavior* (Ingle DJ, Goodale MA, Mansfield RJW, eds), pp 549–586. Cambridge, MA: MIT Press.

Vallar G, Perani D. 1987. The anatomy of spatial neglect in humans. In: *Neurophysiological and Neuropsychological Aspects of Spatial Neglect* (Jeannerod M, ed), pp 235–258. Amsterdam: North-Holland Co. Elsevier Science Publishers.

Volpe BT, Ledoux JE, Gazzaniga MS. 1979. Information processing of visual stimuli in an "extinguished" field. *Nature* 282: 722–724.

22 The Tribal Networks of the Cerebral Cortex

Nikola T. Markov, Maria-Magdolina Ercsey-Ravasz, Marie-Alice Gariel,
Colette Dehay, Kenneth Knoblauch, Zoltán Toroczkai, and Henry Kennedy

Overview

This chapter is an effort to remedy the lack of data on the interareal network of the cortex. Our exploration reveals that, contrary to what has been previously thought, the cortical network is dense. We show the crucial importance of weight and distance information in order to understand this embedded network. An exponential distance rule is found to govern and organize the global and local properties of the network. The network is small-scale, and this, along with its density and the distance rule, impacts the algorithms that it can implement. We propose that tribal is a better adapted descriptor for the cortical network than the famous small world.

There is a long history of attempts at understanding how information flow through the cortex is shaped by the organizational principles of cortical connectivity. The work of Hubel and Wiesel was greatly inspired by the structure/function relations in the visual system, and their formulation of the functional architecture of the visual cortex is a monument in favor of this approach to understanding mechanisms underlying perception and development (Hubel, 1995). Using both single-unit recording and transsynaptic labeling of thalamic terminals in area V1, they were able to describe the ocular dominance and orientation columns. They extended this approach to tackle the issue of interareal connectivity from a functional perspective. Their insight into the anatomy of the cortex coupled with single-unit recording suggested that simple, complex, and hypercomplex receptive fields reflected stages of information processing in successive and distinct levels of the system. However, strange as it may seem, in the 1970s anatomy and physiology were considered as two distinct disciplines, and while bridging the gap was permissible at Harvard, it was more questionable in the conservative atmosphere of Lyon, France. This was the point I (H.K.) was bitterly complaining about to Lamberto Maffei over an andouillette and a pot of dry white Macon wine in a Lyonnais bouchon on a foggy November night in the early 1970s.

In the decade that followed my encounter with Lamberto, tract tracing became increasingly accessible and anatomy and physiology became progressively more combined. However, as tracers' sensitivity increased, the number of connections made by a cortical area became larger, and, paradoxically, anatomy was perceived to play only a minor role in explaining function. This has led to the present demise of anatomy, when anatomists are becoming a rare and endangered species. Of course, there are some rare and therefore brave exceptions. For instance, Christof Koch has recently argued that a neurobiological approach to the question of consciousness must be firmly anchored in an understanding of structure (Koch, 2004). However, generally, it is as if there has been a collective amnesia for the fact that it was first the structure of DNA that allowed the code to be deciphered, thereby providing the basis of all modern molecular biology. Out of structure comes forth strength!

With the discovery of increasing numbers of connections, the more interesting approaches to the issue of cortical connectivity have looked at general principles rather than the detailed connectivity of a single area. Probably one of the most influential publications in this direction is that of the investigation of the hierarchy of the cortex conducted by Felleman and Van Essen (Felleman and Van Essen, 1991). Their study employed concepts of cortical organization developed earlier by Pandya and Rockland (Rockland and Pandya, 1979). In their pioneering work, Rockland and Pandya had noted that the laminar organization of interareal connections shows strong regularities. Projections from the primary sensory areas to subsequent levels of cortical processing (associated with the increase of both size and complexity of the receptive field) predominantly stem from supragranular layers, whereas projections from higher to lower areas originate mostly from infragranular layers. This and the analogy with cortical projections to subcortical structures led to the suggestion that these two sets of projections constitute bottom-up (feedforward) and top-down (feedback) pathways of a sequential processing of information.

In their meta-analysis of the connections linking cortical areas, obtained from numerous tract-tracing experiments in different laboratories, Felleman and Van Essen presented a model in which their 32 cortical areas are distributed over 10 hierarchical levels (see figure 22.1, plate 8). In this layout, virtually all known feedforward projections link a source area to a target higher up in the hierarchy, and these feedforward projections are reciprocated by feedback ones. They had been able to find a hierarchical ordering of the cortical areas with almost no exceptions to these simple topological rules, which were subsequently shown to be a consistent feature of sensory cortex (Felleman and Van Essen, 1991; Kaas and Collins, 2001). In many ways, the famous Felleman and Van Essen model of the cortical hierarchy is the best map we have of the cortex. It captures many features of the cortex, it reveals a clearly hierarchical structure with numerous parallel pathways including the main trunks of the ventral and dorsal streams, and it shows that feedforward information can only go from lower to higher levels whereas feedback information travels in the opposite direction. In their study, Young and colleagues showed that nonmetric multidimensional scaling of an adjacency matrix (a matrix containing the binary connection information within a set of areas) obtained from the database compiled by Felleman and Van Essen confirmed a hierarchical organization of the major cortical pathways as well as their levels of convergence (Young, 1992). However, because of the numerous parallel pathways and given the arbitrary number and positions of levels used in the Felleman and Van Essen model, the analysis of Young's group showed that there were 150,000 equally plausible solutions to the

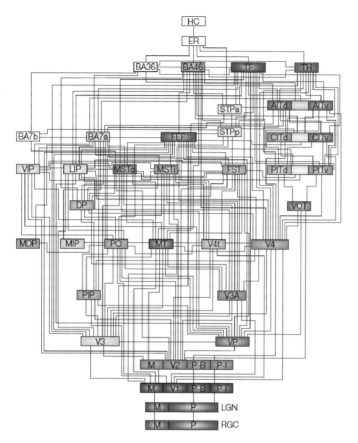

Figure 22.1 (plate 8)
Felleman and Van Essen's (1991) model of the cortical hierarchy.

model (Hilgetag et al., 1996). One way to resolve this ambiguity is to use a hierarchical distance measure that holds the promise of allowing a definitive solution to the hierarchy (Barone et al., 2000).

While the Felleman and Van Essen map reveals important unifying features of the cortex, it remains conceptually frustrating. Its construction depends entirely on the notion that there are feedforward, ascending pathways versus feedback or descending pathways. The common assumption is that feedforward pathways contribute to determining the receptive field features in their target areas while feedback projections have a modulatory role. At the systems level, there are few experimental verifications of these notions (Ekstrom et al., 2008; Hupé et al., 1998), and there are none at the cellular level. This is in large part due to the fact that interareal corticocortical projection cells are hard to identify, for they are only a minute fraction of cortical cells, and the molecular markers for this cellular type are still to be found.

Recently, an alternative approach to understanding cortical pathways appeals to graph theoretic analysis of cortical networks. Since the early 1990s, there has been an increasing focus on network representations of complex systems with the goal of gaining an insight into the functional processes supported by these networks (Barabasi and Albert, 1999; Newman, 2003). Among the major discoveries coming out of this approach was the recognition that many real-world networks, on the binary connectivity level, share small-world (Watts and Strogatz, 1998) and scale-free properties (Barabasi and Albert, 1999). The description of the small-world and scale-free phenomena seemed to be particularly relevant to understanding the brain (Watts, 1999). In particular, small-world networks are characterized by short path lengths between nodes, coupled with high levels of clustering, and ensure maximum integration with minimum wire length. Translated into anatomical terms, nodes are areas, and a small-world network would imply that the average number of areas (hops or steps) crossed in the path between any two areas would be small even though areas are mostly linked to a few other areas, forming a densely clustered neighborhood. Minimum wire would mean that there would be multiple interconnections within a set of areas but only some of these areas will have extensive connections that form long-distance pathways to other tightly grouped areas. These would effectively provide the shortcuts necessary to keep average path lengths optimally short. Small-world networks were initially used for describing social networks, where it has been claimed that no two individuals on the planet are more than six handshakes from each other—truly a small world, made possible because although most of your friends know each other (clustering), some of them plug into other social groups (and provide the shortcuts across the graph). These features provide the integrative function typical of modern society, and it is easy to imagine that they are important in cortical function (Bassett and Bullmore, 2006). Inspired from these early studies on small worlds, and using the compilation of Felleman and Van Essen (Felleman and Van Essen, 1991), several studies have confirmed the clustering of functionally related areas and found evidence of short average path lengths suggestive of small-world architecture (Hilgetag et al., 2000; Sporns et al., 2000).

Previous graph theory studies of the cortex have largely described cortical topology obtained from binary data (i.e., describing areas as being connected or not connected; Hilgetag et al., 2000; Sporns et al., 2000). Modeling studies of the cortex have used published databases compiled from numerous studies, many using antiquated techniques and variable definitions of a cortical area and restricting their investigations to limited regions of the cortex, so that the present day cortical graph is predicted to be incomplete. Further, it is increasingly recognized that new and fundamental insight into the functional organization of real-world systems requires the use of *weighted* networks (i.e., the strength of connections), possibly incorporating spatial distance (Boccaletti et al., 2006). In cortex, however, the study of spatial, weighted networks is hindered by the absence of reliable published data concerning the distance and numbers of neurons involved in the links between cortical areas (Scannell et al., 2000). We have therefore undertaken a detailed anatomical investigation of the macaque cortex using stereotyped protocols. This has amounted to a huge work effort (on the order of 70 person years). It has enabled us to compile a consistent and extensive database of the weight and distance of interareal connections, which we have analyzed using graph theoretic procedures. To achieve this goal, we used retrograde fluorescent tracers, which, as we have previously demonstrated (Falchier et al., 2002), have maximum sensitivity. These tracers are picked up by axon terminals at the injection site and retrogradely transported back to the cell bodies of the neurons projecting to the injected area. Previously, we have also shown that folding of the cortex makes it necessary to have high-frequency sampling of the projection zone in each area (Vezoli et al., 2004). Many previous studies have suffered from the "looking under the street lamp" bias, restricting their observations to those areas which are known to project to the injected area. Here we show that the optimization of tracer sensitivity coupled with brainwide examination reveals many (in the range of 30%) pathways that have not been previously reported. We have made retrograde tracer injections in 26 target areas distributed across occipital, temporal, parietal, frontal, and prefrontal lobes. The number of labeled neurons in a given source structure (cortical area or subcortical nuclei) over the total number of labeled neurons in the brain defines the fraction of labeled neurons (FLN) of that structure.

We believe that the effort has been fully rewarded. It shows that contrary to what has been claimed, interareal connectivity of the cortex does not exhibit small-world features and instead conforms to what could be thought of as a system of tribal networks, suggesting very different constraints on network dynamics from what has previously been considered (Gariel et al., 2009; Knoblauch et al., 2009; Markov et al., 2010).

Cortical Connectivity Profiles

If connectivity weight does play a role in shaping the network properties of the cortex, then we predict that cortical areas would exhibit weight-specific connectivity profiles. That is to say, we would predict that if area X, Y, and Z have, respectively, strong, medium, or weak projections to area W, this will be consistent across animals. There have been very few studies that have attempted to test this possibility. The few quantitative studies that have been reported claim that there is a 100-fold, interindividual variation in the density of connections of a given cortical pathway (MacNeil et al., 1997; Musil and Olson, 1988a, 1988b; Olson and Musil, 1992; Scannell et al., 2000). We have therefore examined this issue in visual areas V1, V2, and V4. Here the advantage is that the areal boundaries of these large areas are well established as are the retinotopic maps, making it possible to make large, stereotypic injections of retrograde tracers in similar retinotopic positions across animals. By employing standardized methods to define areal boundaries within the whole cortical sheet, we obtained a range of variations for FLN values with median and means less than a factor of two. Thus, while the observed values are overdispersed with respect to a Poisson distribution, importantly they are systematically less than that predicted by a geometric distribution. The negative binomial distribution has proven valuable in the analysis of overdispersed count data (Hilbe, 2007; Lindsey, 1999; Venables and Ripley, 2002) and provides a reasonable prediction of the relationship between the mean and

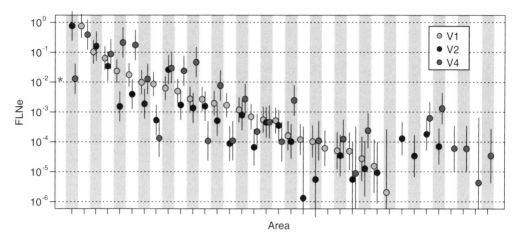

Figure 22.2 (plate 9)
Modeled connectivity profiles of V1, V2, and V4. Cortical areas received repeat injections: V1 (green), V2 (blue), V4 (red). The abscissa represents the source areas ordered according to their fraction of labeled neurons (FLN) when projecting on V1. Green asterisk: FLN value of the lateral geniculate nucleus input to V1. Note the large range (log scale) of FNL. If independently ordered all three profiles show the same envelope distribution that fits with lognormal.

the standard deviation of FLN values. For repeated injections in the same site (V1, V2, or V4), the model that best predicts without overparametrization includes no main effect of the factor "injection CASE" and therefore each area exhibits a connectivity profile (see figure 22.2, plate 9). These results show that there is a connectivity profile despite large intercase variation, and the observed consistency is possible because the connection weights span nearly 7 orders of magnitude. The FLN distribution is heavy-tailed and resembles a lognormal distribution. Globally, the connectivity profile is expressed as follows. The mean intrinsic connectivity FLN percentage was nearly 80% (68%–89%) of the total connectivity and is highly local, occurring within 1.2 to 1.9 mm from the injection site. The next largest contribution is from the neighboring cortical areas (14%). The remaining connectivity is shared between 3.3% long-range corticocortical connections and 1.3% subcortical connections. This pattern of high local connectivity coupled with very small subcortical input and weak long distance connectivity is consistent across the cortex.

Effects of Distance on Connectivity Weight

The lognormal distribution of the FLN is the expression of a distance rule, which has a profound effect on the organization of the cortex. The pathways linking cortical areas were measured through the white matter and their distribution estimated by determining the fraction of labeled neurons extending to a given distance. This showed that in all injections there is an exponential decay in the density of connections with distance. This distance information enabled us to show that the strength of interconnections follows an exponential distance rule (EDR; i.e., strength of

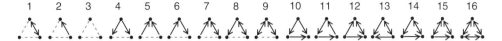

Figure 22.3
Graph motifs. Visualization of the 16 possible motifs of triadic subgraphs. An arrow indicates the existence and direction of a projection between two nodes. A dashed line means that there is no direct projection between the two nodes.

connections decays exponentially with increasing projection distance). We examined how distance and strength of connections shape cortical connectivity by building random models of connectivity based on the same number of pathways and areas as in the data and complying to the EDR, and we compared this to the properties of networks generated using a constant distance rule (CDR).

We then examined the capacity of the two models (the EDR and the CDR) to capture the measured features of the data, the rational being that if the EDR is an important principle governing cortical connectivity, then it will show an enhanced capacity compared to the CDR to capture the characteristic features.

The average number of unidirectional and bidirectional (reciprocated) connections (as area pairs) measured on 1,000 random graphs based on the EDR gives an almost perfect match to the experimental data while that for CDR differs considerably. One characteristic binary feature of a network is the relative frequency distribution of directed triads (see figure 22.3). Any three areas are taken and the connections examined, giving a total of 16 possible motifs. Studies looking at motifs' distribution frequencies have reported that specific types of network (signal transduction, gene transcription, social, etc.) have characteristic motif distributions, which are thought to constrain the function of the network (Milo et al., 2004). We were able to show that random models of cortical connectivity constructed with CDR failed to capture the motifs and bidirectionality of the data. This contrasted with the EDR model, which leads to excellent estimations of these binary features.

Graph Density and Efficiency

Global efficiency reflects the average bandwidth for information flow through the weighted graph (see figure 22.4A, plate 10; Latora and Marchiori, 2003). Here we have sought to determine the pathways that ensure the global efficiency of the graph. The global efficiency is the sum of the conductance between all pairs of areas, where the maximum resistance comes from the weakest links. We tested the effect of attacking the graph by removing connections in order of strength, starting with the weakest ones. This does not show an effect on global efficiency until 81% of pathways (containing 7% of total neurons) have been removed. Hence, the efficiency of the network is ensured by the remaining 19% of pathways exhibiting the highest weights (93% of the cortical projection neurons). These pathways with the highest FLN that ensure the global efficiency have a mean projection distance of 14 mm, considerably shorter than the 38 mm of the connections that do not contribute to global efficiency. The network

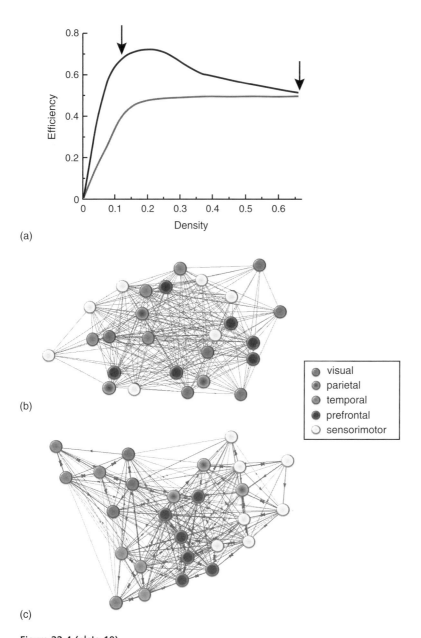

(a)

(b)

(c)

Figure 22.4 (plate 10)
Efficiency and graph topology. (a) illustrates the effect on global and local efficiency of the progressive removal of the weakest connections. Eg (global efficiency): green line; El (local efficiency): blue line. (b) shows the graph topology drawn with the Kamada Kawai algorithm on the unweighted graph, (c) on the weighted.

formed by the 19% of pathways that confer efficiency constitute a backbone of the graph. It is the minimal set of connections that provide unaffected global efficiency. Interestingly, given the large average path length (3.7 steps) and the diameter of the graph (9 steps), the efficiency backbone does not seem to correspond to a small-world architecture.

A complementary measure of efficiency is the local efficiency (Vragovic et al., 2005), which is the summed conductance between all the areas connected to an area X after removal of area X. It is like assessing how easily you can travel between the satellites of a town, without using routes passing through the town. Again, this is averaged across the entire graph. Local efficiency evolves differently with weak link removal (see figure 22.4a). Whereas global efficiency shows a very modest decline with weak link removal, local efficiency shows a gradual increase, peaking in the region just prior to the breakdown of the global backbone.

The differential responses of the local and global efficiencies are predicted by the EDR and not the CDR, showing that the geometry and weight configuration has a particular significance in the efficiency configuration of the network. Further, the differential response of the local and global efficiencies suggests interesting dynamics of the system. The effect of weak pathway removal is one way of examining how threshold changes in the network will influence information flow. High activity levels in the network could raise neuron response threshold (Azouz and Gray, 2003; Braitenberg and Schüz, 1998; Destexhe and Pare, 1999). This suggests that activity-dependent increases in threshold (Braitenberg and Schüz, 1998) could lead to a small decrease in global efficiency that is offset by a large increase in local efficiencies, as has been suggested in the local microcircuit (Binzegger et al., 2004). In this way the control of assembly dynamics in the cortex will have a spatial component in large part due to the spatial and weight characteristics of the cortical network described here. A simple way to illustrate the role of connection weight and distance is to plot the graph either using a binary or weighted, adjacency matrix. When weights are not taken into account, the algorithm converges to a layout where there is no biologically relevant node clustering (see figure 22.4b). Remarkably, when the weighted matrix is provided to the algorithm, it converges to groupings that strongly reflect the functional lobes (see figure 22.4c). This is highly illustrative of the link between connection weight and distance that we reveal in the EDR.

Discussion

The small FLN of the thalamic input to the cortex, coupled with the high FLN values of intrinsic connectivity, fits with the evidence that local recurrent excitatory networks amplify a numerically sparse thalamic input (Douglas et al., 1995). For instance, we find that the FLN of the lateral geniculate nucleus projection onto area V1 is 0.16% (Markov et al., 2010). This result is consistent with the fact that less than 10% of all synapses found in area V1 arise from the lateral geniculate nucleus (da Costa and Martin, 2009; Peters et al., 1994). The intrinsic FLN is around 80% and reveals the high investment of the cortex in local processing, which is thought to be largely responsible for generating receptive field properties (Douglas et al., 1995; Somers et al., 1995). The massive allocation of the neuronal resources of the cortex to local processing and its ongoing patterned activity likewise account for much of the brain's energy consumption (Kenet et al., 2003; Raichle and Mintun, 2006; Tsodyks et al., 1999). This view of the brain insists on the importance of intrinsic operations, so that the input to a given level interacts with ongoing activity.

Short-distance interareal connections from neighboring areas could be envisaged to provide input that interacts with the recurrent local connectivity very much in the same way as the feedforward input from the thalamus to cortex as described above. However, the long-range interareal connectivity has FLN values up to 4 orders of magnitude weaker than the FLN of the lateral geniculate and does not contribute to the global efficiency of the network. The surprisingly weak corticocortical connections are employed for long-range coordination of neuronal assemblies, possibly required for high-level representations (Buzsaki, 2007; Buzsaki and Draguhn, 2004; Lakatos et al., 2008). Importantly, long-range connections are not randomly organized, as thought by numerous authors, but instead link specific sets of cortical areas and have very precisely determined strengths.

Previous studies were performed on a binary level of cortical connectivity matrices (connected or not) lacking information on the strength and spatial distance of the connections. Collecting all the connections found and their FLN values, we obtained a *weighted* and *spatially embedded directed network* of 26 nodes (each node representing an area). By using this 26×26 matrix, we are excluding areas in which no injections were made. In this way, the subset contains the complete information of both in- and outlinks (and their weights) and is a subgraph of the full cortical network of approximately 83 source areas projecting into the 26 target areas. While lognormal distributions have been reported for a number of biological phenomena, importantly they are found for the distributions of synaptic strengths of single neurons (Song et al., 2005). The observation of lognormal distributions of strength of interaction at both the cell and areal levels suggests that an identical logical principle might be functioning over multiple scales.

Spatial information is a crucial feature of the cortical network. The EDR, coupled with interareal distances, generates the lognormal distribution of connection strengths as well as the basic binary connectivity properties of the interareal network. It is interesting that binary network properties are recovered from a distance rule, which is a continuous spatial property of the system. Because the EDR strongly shapes the cortical network structure, it is to be expected that it is a selector for the types of information theoretic algorithms implemented by the cortex.

The novel anatomical connectivity data, including the strengths of connections and spatial information, suggest a revision of the cortical network given by previous studies. In particular, the newly uncovered anatomical connections lead to a very strongly connected interareal network (over 66% of the possible connections exist). In the light of such high density, the small-world-like properties of the graph (average directed path length = 1.34 steps and diameter = 2 steps are not significant. Neither can the network be described as scale free in terms of its binary connectivity, given that the number of nodes is small and given their non-power-law degree distributions.

With a density of over 66%, binary features of the cortex, such as small-world properties and hubs, provide little functional insight, given that nonsparse graphs can hardly be rewired in a manner not to express short path and high clustering. Instead, the range of weights of connection and distance must be examined. Doing so reveals a strong regularity of the cortex, where each area has strong connections with its neighbors, and where weights of connections fall off exponentially with distance to give place to weak, mid-to-long-distance projections. These latter connections greatly contribute to linking areas standing on very distant levels of the cortical hierarchy and yet appear to make only a poor contribution to the global efficiency of the cortex. We see a dichotomy between the circuit of few very strong connections and the myriad of weak links that do not provide channels broad enough to transfer detailed, extensive fine-grain information.

The outstanding reason why interareal connectivity does not correspond to a small-world network is that the density of the graph is way too high. Lock 100 people in a room, and shortly they will all know each other, leading to a social graph of 100% density, with path length of 1 hop and a single large cluster. Small-world properties only become interesting when the number of nodes is large and the number of links is small. In other words, short path lengths and clustering can be identified at various densities; however, for a dense graph they are uninformative about any architectural specificity. In figure 22.5 (plate 11) we show how average shortest path length relates to graph density. At 66% (that is, with all observed connections included) we have a path length of 1.34, and, as connections are randomly removed, there is a progressive increase of the average path length. This allows us to compare our graph density to those of earlier studies, some of which have claimed small-world architectures in cortical interareal connectivity. The Felleman and Van Essen (1991) study provided a compilation of data taken from over 300 anatomical studies. Felleman and Van Essen cautiously questioned their network and found it to have a density of 30%. They distinguished three possible states: documented (existing), not found (explored but reported absent), and unknown (nonexplored connections). By taking into account the unknown connections, they predicted that the real density of cortex would be round 45%. Later Jouve et al. (1998) first updated the database of Felleman and Van Essen and then implemented an algorithm that uses the properties of the network to predict whether there are projections within the unknown category that are very likely to exist (Jouve et al., 1998). This led to a density prediction of 50%. All subsequent studies examining the small-world properties of the cortex have used the database of Felleman and Van Essen. However, these studies firstly considered the unknown connections as if they were nonexistent, and secondly, they increased the number of areas by referring to publicly available databases where the unknown category is actually higher than that in the Felleman and Van Essen database. This automatically increased the sparseness of their graphs (15%–20%; Sporns et al., 2007; Sporns et al., 2000; Young, 1993).

The interareal network is actually a dense network, and it does not correspond to a small world. One of the fascinating aspects of network science is that basic properties of networks are found across many widely different physical systems. If the binary properties of interareal

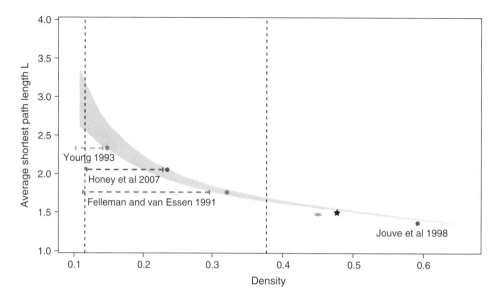

Figure 22.5 (plate 11)
Average shortest path length and graph density and effects of random pathway removal. Gray dot: G_{26x26} (26 nodes, 430 links). Gray area: 95% confidence interval following random removal of connections. Dashed lines 2.5%–97.5% of graphs in the gray zone have infinite *path length* values. Green: Felleman and Van Essen, 1991; orange: Honey et al., 2007 (47 nodes, 505 links); purple: Young 1993 (71 nodes, 746 links). Black star: removal of all new connections in present study. Brown: value predicted by Jouve et al., 1998. This figure shows that while our graph has higher density than previous studies, it is in fact much nearer to the values of Felleman and Van Essen (1991) and the estimated density in Jouve et al. study than of those studies claiming small-world architecture and using a modified database of Felleman and Van Essen.

cortical connectivity do not constitute a small world, what type of social network does it resemble?

An analogy can be found in another class of social networks. Human societies are evolving systems, and small-world networks have been identified in modern urban society. An early societal structure is the tribe, which can be composed of 100 to 200 individuals, unified by common language and culture. The characteristic feature of the tribe is that the majority of individuals are directly related to each other (high density). The increase in scale (size) of human societies first led to the imperial structure where the network of interactions is centralized around a principal node, "the emperor," and the density of the network is reduced compared to tribal society. This intermediate structure has given rise to modern society, retaining the sparse structure of the imperial network, but at the same time it has also been decentralized. The major difference between the tribal and modern world is in the density and scale of the connected network.

Up to the 1960s, anthropology largely focused on the social structure of tribes in different parts of the globe, employing largely empirical methodology, without the use of graph theoretical methods. Later, when studies focused on modern society, the graph theoretical methods became an increasingly attractive method of investigation. Milgram's famous chain-letter experiment (Milgram, 1967) emphasized the surprisingly small diameter of the large-scale modern society and introduced the concept of the small world.

Hence, the notion of small world is very descriptive and useful in the framework of modern society, as it gives insight in to the role of social dynamics in shortening the diameter of an otherwise very large graph. However, the small-world graph is irrelevant to the tribal societal structure. The anthropologists who have explored the tribal network have rightly paid little attention to the small-world concept. On the contrary, they claim that the high density and small scale of the tribal network are the major elements underlying its functionality.

Conclusion

Our proposition of a tribal cortical network has profound implications for understanding cortical function. Coming back to Felleman and Van Essen's model, a small-world network would envisage connections spanning multiple levels like so many information highways, providing numerous shortcuts across the graph. In such a network, one would envisage the long-distance connections of the cortex providing an integrated circuit, allowing messages to shuttle back and forth in the cortical loom across multiple levels. We would expect to find hubs, perhaps in the posterior parietal cortex or in the prefrontal cortex. One might expect to see some sort of essential feature attached to such a hub, perhaps a sense of self, crouching like a homunculus in the middle of the web of connections, directing all. Instead, what one has in the tribal networks are strong "driving" connections, mostly between neighboring areas on the same hierarchical level and adjacent levels, no centers, no hubs, no information highways but instead, distributed processing dependant on myriad trickle down and trickle up effects from a sea of weak connections, acting upon and coordinating the neuronal assemblies of synchronized, reverberating activity.

We need to ponder the advantages of such dense tribal networks, envisage the high density not as a constraint but as a necessary advantage. This type of network offers the synchronization properties that are thought to play a major role in cortical operations and relates the wide range of strength of projections (a newly documented fact) to spatial distance in the brain. The high density constrains the functional algorithms that can be implemented within such a network, bridging the gap between local and global processing. It hints that brain connectivity could be governed by such rules as the EDR both at the area and cell levels.

The notion that the cortex is a small world and scale free, thus echoing the planetary society and the World Wide Web (among many others), has an enormous appeal. The fact that the principles of cortical organization may have far more in common with small-scale, high-density tribal networks may, to some, come as a disappointment. However, let us remember, it is the dense social network that saw the emergence of man. It could be the large-scale, sparse network that sees civilization's demise.

Acknowledgments

We thank D. Autran, J. Beneyton, A. Batardiere, P. Barone, S. Clavagnier, A. Falchier, P. Giroud, C. Huissoud, A. Kennedy, C. Lamy, P. Misery, R. Quilodran, J. Sallet, J. Vezoli, and S. Zouaoui, for histological assistance and data collection, N. Kolomitre, M. Seon, and M. Valdebenito for animal husbandry, V. Vezoli for administrative assistance, and Louis-Jan Pilaz for software development. This work was supported by DAISY FP6–2005 IST-1583 (H.K.); ANR-05-NEUR-088 (H.K.), SECO FP7–2007-ICT-216593 (H.K.), and in part by HDTRA 201473–35045 (Z.T., M.M.E.R.) and the Hungarian Bioinformatics MTKD-CT-2006–042794, Marie Curie Host Fellowships for Transfer of Knowledge program (Z.T.).

References

Azouz R, Gray CM. 2003. Adaptive coincidence detection and dynamic gain control in visual cortical neurons in vivo. *Neuron* 37: 513–523.

Barabasi AL, Albert R. 1999. Emergence of scaling in random networks. *Science* 286: 509–512.

Barone P, Batardiere A, Knoblauch K, Kennedy H. 2000. Laminar distribution of neurons in extrastriate areas projecting to visual areas V1 and V4 correlates with the hierarchical rank and indicates the operation of a distance rule. *J Neurosci* 20: 3263–3281.

Bassett DS, Bullmore E. 2006. Small-world brain networks. *Neuroscientist* 12: 512–523.

Binzegger T, Douglas RJ, Martin KA. 2004. A quantitative map of the circuit of cat primary visual cortex. *J Neurosci* 24: 8441–8453.

Boccaletti S, Latora V, Moreno Y, Chavez M, Hwang DU. 2006. Complex networks: structure and dynamics. *Phys Rep* 424: 175–308.

Braitenberg V, Schüz A. 1998. *Cortex: Statistics and Geometry of Neuronal Connectivity*, 2nd edn. Berlin: Springer-Verlag.

Buzsaki G. 2007. The structure of consciousness. *Nature* 446: 267.

Buzsaki G, Draguhn A. 2004. Neuronal oscillations in cortical networks. *Science* 304: 1926–1929.

da Costa NM, Martin KA. 2009. The proportion of synapses formed by the axons of the lateral geniculate nucleus in layer 4 of area 17 of the cat. *J Comp Neurol* 516: 264–276.

Destexhe A, Pare D. 1999. Impact of network activity on the integrative properties of neocortical pyramidal neurons in vivo. *J Neurophysiol* 81: 1531–1547.

Douglas RJ, Koch C, Mahowald M, Martin KA, Suarez HH. 1995. Recurrent excitation in neocortical circuits. *Science* 269: 981–985.

Ekstrom LB, Roelfsema PR, Arsenault JT, Bonmassar G, Vanduffel W. 2008. Bottom-up dependent gating of frontal signals in early visual cortex. *Science* 321: 414–417.

Falchier A, Clavagnier S, Barone P, Kennedy H. 2002. Anatomical evidence of multimodal integration in primate striate cortex. *J Neurosci* 22: 5749–5759.

Felleman DJ, Van Essen DC. 1991. Distributed hierarchical processing in the primate cerebral cortex. *Cereb Cortex* 1: 1–47.

Gariel MA, Vezoli J, Markov NT, Douglas RJ, Knoblauch K, Kennedy H. 2009. Weak connections, economy and antihierarchy in the cortex. In 2009 Neuroscience Meeting Planner (Chicago, Society for Neuroscience).

Hilbe JM. 2007. *Negative Binomial Regression*. Cambridge: Cambridge University Press.

Hilgetag CC, Burns GA, O'Neill MA, Scannell JW, Young MP. 2000. Anatomical connectivity defines the organization of clusters of cortical areas in the macaque monkey and the cat. *Philos Trans R Soc Lond B Biol Sci* 355: 91–110.

Hilgetag CC, O'Neill MA, Young MP. 1996. Indeterminate organization of the visual system. *Science* 271: 776–777.

Hubel D. 1995. *Eye, Brain and Vision.* New York: Freeman and Co.

Hupé JM, James AC, Payne BR, Lomber SG, Girard P, Bullier J. 1998. Cortical feedback improves discrimination between figure and background by V1, V2 and V3 neurons. *Nature* 394: 784–787.

Jouve B, Rosenstiehl P, Imbert M. 1998. A mathematical approach to the connectivity between the cortical visual areas of the macaque monkey. *Cereb Cortex* 8: 28–39.

Kaas JH, Collins CE. 2001. The organization of sensory cortex. *Curr Opin Neurobiol* 11: 498–504.

Kenet T, Bibitchkov D, Tsodyks M, Grinvald A, Arieli A. 2003. Spontaneously emerging cortical representations of visual attributes. *Nature* 425: 954–956.

Knoblauch K, Ercsey-Ravasz MM, Markov NT, Vezoli J, Gariel MA, Barone P, Dehay C, Toroczkai Z, Kennedy H. 2009. Distance rules in the cortex. In 2009 Neuroscience Meeting Planner (Chicago, Society for Neuroscience).

Koch C. 2004. *The Quest for Consciousness A Neurobiological Appraoch.* Englewood, CO: Roberts and Company.

Lakatos P, Karmos G, Mehta AD, Ulbert I, Schroeder CE. 2008. Entrainment of neuronal oscillations as a mechanism of attentional selection. *Science* 320: 110–113.

Latora V, Marchiori M. 2003. Economic small-world behavior in weighted networks. *Eur Phys J B* 32: 249–263.

Lindsey JK. 1999. *Models Repeated Measurements,* 2nd edn. Oxford: Oxford University Press.

MacNeil MA, Lomber SG, Payne BR. 1997. Thalamic and cortical projections to middle suprasylvian cortex of cats: constancy and variation. *Exp Brain Res* 114: 24–32.

Markov NT, Misery P, Falchier A, Lamy C, Vezoli J, Quilodran R, Gariel MA, et al. 2010. Weight Consistence Specifies Regularities of Macaque Cortical Networks. *Cereb Cortex,* Nov 2, Epub ahead of print.

Milgram S. 1967. The small world problem. *Psychol Today* 1: 60–67.

Milo R, Itzkovitz S, Kashtan N, Levitt R, Shen-Orr S, Ayzenshtat I, Sheffer M, Alon U. 2004. Superfamilies of evolved and designed networks. *Science* 303: 1538–1542.

Musil SY, Olson CR. 1988a. Organization of cortical and subcortical projections to anterior cingulate cortex in the cat. *J Comp Neurol* 272: 203–218.

Musil SY, Olson CR. 1988b. Organization of cortical and subcortical projections to medial prefrontal cortex in the cat. *J Comp Neurol* 272: 219–241.

Newman MEJ. 2003. The structure and function of complex networks. *SIAM Rev* 45: 167–256.

Olson CR, Musil SY. 1992. Topographic organization of cortical and subcortical projections to posterior cingulate cortex in the cat: evidence for somatic, ocular, and complex subregions. *J Comp Neurol* 324: 237–260.

Peters A, Payne BR, Budd J. 1994. A numerical analysis of the geniculocortical input to striate cortex in the monkey. *Cereb Cortex* 4: 215–229.

Raichle ME, Mintun MA. 2006. Brain work and brain imaging. *Annu Rev Neurosci* 29: 449–476.

Rockland KS, Pandya DN. 1979. Laminar origins and terminations of cortical connections of the occipital lobe in the rhesus monkey. *Brain Res* 179: 3–20.

Scannell JW, Grant S, Payne BR, Baddeley R. 2000. On variability in the density of corticocortical and thalamocortical connections. *Philos Trans R Soc Lond B Biol Sci* 355: 21–35.

Somers DC, Nelson SB, Sur M. 1995. An emergent model of orientation selectivity in cat visual cortical simple cells. *J Neurosci* 15: 5448–5465.

Song S, Sjostrom PJ, Reigl M, Nelson S, Chklovskii DB. 2005. Highly nonrandom features of synaptic connectivity in local cortical circuits. *PLoS Biol* 3: e68.

Sporns O, Honey CJ, Kotter R. 2007. Identification and classification of hubs in brain networks. *PLoS ONE* 2: e1049.

Sporns O, Tononi G, Edelman GM. 2000. Theoretical neuroanatomy: relating anatomical and functional connectivity in graphs and cortical connection matrices. *Cereb Cortex* 10: 127–141.

Tsodyks M, Kenet T, Grinvald A, Arieli A. 1999. Linking spontaneous activity of single cortical neurons and the underlying functional architecture. *Science* 286: 1943–1946.

Venables WN, Ripley BD. 2002. *Modern Applied Statistics with S,* 4th edn. New York: Springer.

Vezoli J, Falchier A, Jouve B, Knoblauch K, Young M, Kennedy H. 2004. Quantitative analysis of connectivity in the visual cortex: extracting function from structure. *Neuroscientist* 10: 476–482.

Vragovic I, Louis E, Diaz-Guilera A. 2005. Efficiency of informational transfer in regular and complex networks. *Phys Rev E Stat Nonlin Soft Matter Phys* 71: 036122.

Watts DJ. 1999. Networks, dynamics, and the small-world phenomenon. *Am J Sociol* 105: 493–527.

Watts DJ, Strogatz SH. 1998. Collective dynamics of "small-world" networks. *Nature* 393: 440–442.

Young MP. 1992. Objective analysis of the topological organization of the primate cortical visual system. *Nature* 358: 152–155.

Young MP. 1993. The organization of neural systems in the primate cerebral cortex. *Proc R Soc Lond B Biol Sci* 252: 13–18.

23 Neurophysiological Correlates of Cortical Plasticity in the Normal and Diseased Human Brain

Paolo Maria Rossini and Jean-Marc Melgari

Plasticity as an Inner Property of the Nervous System ... The Potential for Change of Everybody ... Yes, We Can!

The term *plasticity* describes the capacity for pliancy and malleability. When applied to a dynamic system, such as the brain, the concept of plasticity usually includes the *potential for change* as well as all the mechanisms of self-repair and/or of reorganization.

The study of neuroplasticity has clearly shown that the developing brain, the adult brain, and the aging brain are shaped by environmental inputs both under normal conditions (i.e., learning) and after a lesion. Plastic phenomena are at the basis of learning as well as of damage repair; cortical maps can be modified by sensory input, experience, and learning. Indeed, cortical maps undergo continuous transient changes during life experiences, in response to repeated sensory experience, practice of motor patterns, and cognitive tasks as well as in response to their deprivation. The nervous system is a continuously changing structure, basically due to its plastic properties.

Neuroimaging techniques (electrophysiological, flow/metabolic) are suitable to investigate structural and functional changes subtending neuronal plasticity in humans (Rossini et al., 2003; Rossini and Dal Forno 2004; Rossini and Rossi 2007). The review presented in this chapter is mainly focused on the results of studies performed with neurophysiological techniques; their integration with flow/metabolic methods constitutes, at present, the best way to assess plasticity in the normal and abnormal brain as represented by three paradigmatic conditions: healthy aging, neurodegeneration, and ischemic stroke.

Noninvasive Neuromagnetic Methods for Functional Neuroimaging

Nowadays, many neuroimaging techniques (electrophysiological, flow/metabolic) are suitable to investigate structural and functional changes subtending neuronal plasticity (Rossini et al., 2003, 2007; Rossini and Dal Forno, 2004; Rossini and Rossi, 2007). Some techniques measure regional blood flow and metabolic modifications linked with function-related changes in neuronal firing level, such as positron emission tomography (PET) and functional magnetic resonance imaging (fMRI), while others, namely, high resolution electroencephalography (EEG), magne-toencephalography (MEG), and transcranial magnetic stimulation (TMS), analyze the electro-magnetic properties of neuronal activation. None of them individually has a temporal and spatial resolution accurate enough to exhaustively follow up neuroplastic mechanisms; therefore, mul-timodal integration constitutes the best way to describe and understand plastic phenomena.

Since the present review is focused on neurophysiological correlates of cortical plasticity, presently available neurophysiological methods need a brief description.

Electroencephalography

Since its introduction, the electroencephalogram was viewed with a great enthusiasm as the only methodology allowing a direct and online view of the "brain at work." The traditional EEG method has been recently enriched by a number of modern approaches able to analyze and localize in three dimensions the signal's generator sources as well as to track hierarchical con-nectivity characterizing electromagnetic brain activity linked with a given cerebral function. When this is integrated with PET and fMRI structural and functional imaging, the result is a tool theoretically able to discern—with a time resolution which follows "brain time," which is on the order of milliseconds—the sequential recruitment of different neural centers within a putative network underlying the task under investigation. Advanced EEG analysis can identify changes in specific cerebral rhythms oscillating at different frequencies over time and provide quantitative and individual measurements of them (Babiloni et al., 2001). EEG coherence or synchronicity of rhythmic signals recorded from individual scalp electrodes in various frequency bands from different cortical areas can also be measured. Moreover, spectral coherence analysis indexes the temporal synchronization of two EEG time series among electrodes in the frequency domain and permits characterization of linear functional corticocortical connectivity. Decreased coherence reflects reduced linear functional connections and information transfer (i.e., functional uncoupling) among cortical areas or modulation of common areas by a third region while coher-ence increase reflects augmented linear functional connections and information transfer (i.e., functional coupling), which reflects the interaction of different cortical structures for a given task. Finally, the direction of the information flow within the coupled EEG rhythms can be estimated by a direct transfer function (Babiloni et al., 2004a, 2004b).

Magnetoencephalography

MEG represents a noninvasive technique for recording neuronal electromagnetic fields, able to spatially identify the synchronous firing of neurons—either spontaneous or in response to a stimulus—from specific cortical areas. The MEG signal is not influenced by extracerebral tissue layers overlying the brain, therefore allowing for easier and more faithful head–brain modeling. It does not require any "reference," and therefore it allows localization and measurement of the intracellular currents in a shallow brain region exactly below the recording sensor, without any contributions from volume currents. Signals originate from current flow of tangential dipoles as created by parallel pyramidal cells in cortical gyri and sulci (Romani et al., 1982) and reflect the spatial and temporal production of a dipolar source modeled as an equivalent current dipole (ECD) and its three-dimensional localization with a time resolution of milliseconds (Williamson and Kaufman, 1990). ECD spatial properties indicate not only location of neural sources but also their orientation and strength. A decrease or increase in the responsive area caused by recruitment or loss of neurons surrounding the central core causes a corresponding increase or decrease in the dipole strength (roughly reflecting the number of neurons firing synchronously). A decrease or increase of dipole strength can be due to restriction or enlargement of the responsive area studied, possibly because of recruitment of a fringe of neurons surrounding those usually firing in response to the incoming stimulus. ECD orientation can be measured; response morphology provides indirect information on the underlying neural circuitries. These variations can be secondary to dynamic phenomena, such as use-dependent modulation of synaptic efficacy, changes of excitatory–inhibitory input from adjacent or remote damaged brain areas (diaschisis), or changes in the amount of sensory information (Rossini et al., 1994a, 1994b, 2003, 2007; Tecchio et al., 2000).

Both EEG and MEG signals mainly originate from postsynaptic currents associated with synchronous neuronal firing. EEG detects the electric potential difference measured from the scalp, that is, it is a reference-dependent measure. It requires contact between the recording electrodes and the scalp. MEG detects magnetic fields at the cranial surface, giving an absolute measure at each point without any direct sensor–scalp contact. EEG is equally sensitive to radially and tangentially oriented cerebral sources; MEG is almost selectively sensitive to the latter. The EEG signal is perturbed in its space and time properties by the passage through the extracerebral layers (cerebrospinal fluid, meninges, skull, and scalp) while the MEG signal is transparent to them.

Transcranial Magnetic Stimulation

TMS was introduced by Barker et al. (1985) and is a safe, painless, and noninvasive technique increasingly employed in brain functions studies (Kobayashi and Pascual Leone, 2003; Rossini and Rossi, 2007, for a review).

When applied over the scalp regions corresponding to the motor strip, TMS triggers a transient electromyographic response (motor evoked potentials; MEPs) in the connected "target" muscles.

Cortical mapping procedures with single TMS pulses focally applied on several scalp positions overlying the motor cortex take into account the number of cortical sites eliciting MEPs and its "center of gravity" (Rossini et al., 1994a, 1994b). They are useful to track plastic changes originating from physiological manipulations—that is, changing the sensory feedback or during motor learning or secondary to a disease process involving the motor system. Use-dependent changes—or changes secondary to a lesion—have been shown in cortical maps, with or without variations in the amplitude-weighted center of gravity, probably owing to the recruitment or inhibition of adjacent neurons at the periphery of the map (Rossini et al., 2003). The area of maximal excitability, also called the "hot spot," can migrate outside the usual boundaries (Rossini et al., 2003; Ferreri et al., 2003) either because of the activation of a secondary hot spot previously hidden by the predominant one or due to the recruitment of silent but already existing synapses or even the creation of new synaptic connections and neural networks.

Paired-pulse TMS (pp-TMS) protocols are a powerful tool for studying mechanisms of intra-cortical inhibition and excitation. Typically, intracortical inhibitory and excitatory mechanisms can be tested by pp-TMS in which a conditioning subthreshold TMS stimulus precedes a supra-threshold test stimulus by a programmable interstimulus interval (ISI), typically between 1 and 15 milliseconds. The amplitude modulation of the test MEP provides a direct measure of intracortical inhibitory (ISIs 1–4 ms = intracortical inhibition; ICI) and facilitatory (at longer ISIs = intracortical facilitation; ICF) phenomena, which are likely mediated by GABAa and glutamate, respectively (Kujirai et al., 1993; Ziemann, 2004).

Single TMS pulses delivered in trains with a constant frequency and intensity for a given time is the principle of repetitive TMS (rTMS), which can produce changes—outlasting the period of stimulation—in cortical excitability via a transient potentiation or decrement of the underlying brain area activity (i.e., making a "virtual lesion"). The net result of rTMS is highly dependent on the stimulus rate, which is the basis for the reported clinical benefits in diseases linked with brain excitability dysfunctions (Rossini and Rossi, 2007).

Neurophysiological Correlates of Cortical Plasticity

Neurophysiological techniques had a major impact in the study of neuroplasticity, particularly in cognitive neuroscience and in the presence of localized brain damage. For this reason, three main clinical settings have been selected as prototypical models of neuroplasticity for the present review:

- Normal brain and normal brain aging
- Mild cognitive impairment and Alzheimer's disease (AD): a model of neurodegenerative disease
- Monohemispheric stroke: a model of localized brain lesion

Normal Brain and Normal Brain Aging

In 1894, Cajal, speaking about the plasticity of cellular processes, claimed that it was a dynamic process varying throughout different ages, being maximum in young people, lower in adults, and nearly disappearing in the aged (DeFelipe, 2006). Today, we know from neurobiological, neuroradiological, and neurophysiological studies that the aging brain maintains properties for regional plastic reorganization.

The normal aged brain undergoes many neurofunctional changes as revealed by neurophy-siological studies. The resting EEG of an healthy aging brain shows a global "slowing" of its background activity paired with ongoing modifications in its spectral power profile consistent with a marked amplitude decrease of alpha (8–13 Hz) and increases in power and topographic location in the slower delta (2–4 Hz) and theta (4–8 Hz) frequency ranges (Rossini et al., 2007).

The age-dependent power decrement of low-frequency alpha rhythms (8–10.5 Hz) is recorded in parietal, occipital, and temporal regions, as is a decrease of delta rhythms in occipital regions (Babiloni et al., 2006a). Alpha oscillations reflect the activity of a dominant oscillatory neural network in the resting awake brain that is modulated by thalamocortical and corticocortical interactions facilitating–inhibiting the transmission of sensorimotor information and the retrieval of semantic information from cortical storage. The age-dependent alpha power reduction might be associated with changes in cholinergic system functionality.

An interferential TMS study showed that rTMS applied in young subjects on the right dorsolateral prefrontal cortex (DLPFC) simultaneously with the presentation of memoranda during a visuospatial recognition memory task interfered with retrieval more than left DLPFC stimulation. The asymmetry of the effect progressively vanished with aging, suggesting that the bilateral engagement of the DLPFC has a compensatory role in episodic memory performance across the age span (Rossi et al., 2001, 2004).

Moreover, analyzing EEG recordings during a memory task, it was found that EEG spatial distribution displays an increasing uniformity with age. This effect can be attributed to an increased number of coupling interactions among cortical areas, which may reflect loss of lateralized (right–left hemisphere) and localized abilities such that progressively more distributed networks are engaged for performing relatively simple tasks (i.e., index finger movement) as the brain gets older, at the same level as for complex tasks (i.e., sequential movements of all fingers) in younger subjects (Babiloni et al., 2000; for a review on this subject, see Rossini et al., 2007).

As a general consideration, findings from neurophysiological (as well as neuroradiological) studies in normal aging suggest compensatory mechanisms as well as nonselective recruitment of disinhibited regions or dedifferentiation of cerebral cortex.

Since plasticity can be considered as an inner property of the nervous system, a large bulk of literature has addressed the issue of plasticity in the normal brain. Apart from normal aging, the study of short-term plastic events in sensorimotor cortical areas is intriguing for its translational perspectives in brain injuries (i.e., stroke). Short-term plastic effects following changes of the sensory input on cortical sensorimotor organization have been documented by our group. It has been observed that cortical activity accompanying voluntary movements is strongly modified by an induced loss of the cutaneous feedback from the moving hand and that fingers anesthesia induces short-term enlargement and lateral or medial shifts of the parietal cortical representation of the unanesthetized finger (Rossini et al., 1994a) as well as transient and rapid modifications in the cortical motor maps of muscles surrounded by anesthetized skin, reducing the cortical somatotopical representation of the muscle area deprived of its natural sensory feedback without modifying (or even enhancing) the one of neural pools controlling the adjacent muscles (Rossini et al., 1996; Rossi et al., 1998). It is to be noted that all the mentioned human studies (like the animal studies) involve the use of nonphysiological experimental stimulation profoundly different from everyday experience. On the contrary, a recent TMS study carried out via simultaneous mapping of 12 upper limb muscles of healthy subjects in "physiological" experimental conditions (Melgari et al., 2008) was performed in order to disentangle functional topography (i.e., dynamic associations) by measuring cortical overlapping and correlation (standardized covariation). Interhemispheric differences and the short-term influence of posture were evaluated as well. Findings demonstrate significant difference between muscles' pairs in cortical overlapping (high for hand–forearm muscles, very low for arm vs. hand–forearm) and higher overlapping in the left hemisphere. This interhemispheric difference could be due to long-term plastic changes in the left (dominant) hemisphere related to its lifetime higher training with respect to the right hemisphere. Moreover, the arm–hand posture transiently influenced both measures of association resulting in a higher overlapping with the prone versus supine hand, but only for the muscles subjected to the proprioceptive change. Those last findings suggest that a sort of "short-term" plasticity can take place in primary motor area induced by a simple change of posture.

A Model of Neurodegenerative Disease: Mild Cognitive Impairment and Alzheimer's Disease

Dementia is one of the most frequent diseases in the elderly (Vicioso, 2002). From a neuro-pathological perspective, AD is characterized by macroscopic hallmarks such as cortical atrophy and ventricular enlargements, mainly due to temporal and parietal neuronal loss, and by microscopic hallmarks including neurofibrillary tangles and amyloid plaques, mostly concentrated in the hippocampus, parahippocampal structures, entorhinal cortex, and postcentral parietal neocortex. Typically, heralding symptoms are represented by mild memory difficulties after the sixth decade of life, slowly affecting also executive functions, visuospatial abilities, language, and other cognitive and behavioral domains, finally leading to loss of independency in daily life activities. Many neurophysiological studies have faced the question of disease-related cortical reorganizations in the demented brain both in the resting state and in poststimulus conditions. In the resting state, AD patients, compared to healthy normal elderly subjects, show a higher EEG power for delta and theta and lower power for posterior alpha (8–12 Hz) and/or beta (13–30 Hz) frequencies (Babiloni et al., 2004c; Rossini et al., 2007).

MEG findings confirmed an enhancing of parietotemporal delta and theta power sources in AD compared to normal controls paired with hippocampal atrophy and a decrease of parieto-occipital alpha sources power possibly compensated by an increase of temporal alpha sources (Osipova et al., 2005). In line with neuroradiological results, in AD patients spectral EEG coherence showed an impairment of functional connectivity with abnormal linear coupling of EEG rhythms among cortical regions, suggesting a linear temporal synchronicity of coupled EEG rhythms from simultaneously engaged neural sources (Rossini et al., 2008). Linear and nonlinear EEG nalysis, as well as supervised artificial neural networks, improves classification accuracy of AD compared to unaffected controls and gives indications about disease severity (Babiloni et al., 2004d, 2006b; Rossini et al., 2008; Rossini et al., 2007). TMS can be used within this clinical frame in order to assess cortical excitability, intracortical facilitatory and inhibitory mechanisms resulting from the balance among neurotransmitters, and dynamic synaptic adaptations to progressive neuronal loss. Even if the findings do not always converge, the majority of TMS studies indicate that the AD cortex is hyperexcitable. An interesting result has been obtained by TMS-mapping studies of representational plasticity of motor maps in AD patients: it has been demonstrated that motor maps of hand muscles are early modified in AD despite the lack of clinically evident motor deficits (Ferreri et al., 2003). Mapping of motor output in mild AD patients, asymptomatic for motor deficits, has revealed frontal and medial shift of the cortical motor maps for hand muscles as well as an increased (with respect to healthy subjects) "cortical distance" between the hot spot (point with MEP having maximal amplitude and minimal latency) and the center of the map in terms of center of gravity (Ferreri et al., 2003). Those studies seem to confirm that plastic brain reorganization is a widespread phenomenon in AD even in the preclinical stage; in fact, the reorganization is not selective only for memory circuits. An altered synaptic plasticity in AD has also been demonstrated by high-frequency (facilitatory) rTMS, which induces an increase in MEP size in normal age-matched controls but produces opposite changes in patients with AD (Inghilleri et al., 2006). This finding could be interpreted as an altered short-term synaptic enhancement in excitatory circuits of the motor cortex.

A Model of Localized Brain Damage: Monohemispheric Stroke

Functional recovery from an ischemic stroke relies mainly on restorative brain plasticity. Post-stroke brain reorganization of hand sensorimotor function has been extensively studied through neurophysiological and neurometabolic methods.

In healthy humans, the organization of the sensorimotor areas for hand–finger control is rather symmetrical between the two hemispheres (Rossini et al., 2003; Rossini and Dal Forno, 2004; Rossini and Rossi, 2007). Therefore, the comparison of the affected (ipsilesional; ILH) hemisphere to the unaffected (contralesional; CLH) hemisphere in a monohemispheric lesion is a sensitive procedure to follow up reorganization phenomena.

From a methodological point of view, MEG has an optimal capability to identify cerebral regions devoted to hand control, and sensory stimulation seems to be more appropriate and more standardized in order to detect interhemispheric asymmetries of homologous areas, with respect to active motor tasks, where the functional demand to control the paretic hand versus the nonparetic one cannot be met. For this reason, studies with active motor tasks suffer from recruitment bias since patients with severe motor deficits are generally excluded.

About a decade ago, our group introduced and validated (Tecchio et al., 1997) an ad hoc procedure with galvanic median nerve (or finger) stimulation in patients with monohemispheric stroke in the middle cerebral artery territory since it equals the input to the two hemispheres. It was shown that the ipsilesional hand sensory area undergoes a significant reorganization; specifically, an excessive asymmetry of spatial parameters and response morphology was identified when localizing the generator source of short-latency somatosensory evoked field (Tecchio et al., 2000). Sensory hand cortical topography was larger on ILH than CLH, suggesting that brain areas outside the normal boundaries and usually not reached by a dense sensory input from the opposite hand and fingers may act as somatosensory hand centers. A reduction of afferent signal in ILH was observed to be inversely correlated with the clinical outcome (Rossini et al., 1998). With a prognostic perspective MEG parameters were recorded at rest and after median nerve stimulation in acute stroke (T0 = within 10 days from symptom onset) and in a chronic phase (T1 = an average of 8 months after symptom onset) to correlate with neuroradiological and clinical outcomes. The lesion volume showed the strongest ability to prognosticate the clinical outcome at T1, but ILH gamma and CLH delta band powers were predictive factors and CLH delta added prognostic indication to lesion volume (Tecchio et al., 2007).

There is evidence showing that overall reduction of interhemispheric responsiveness asymmetry seen in acute state is accompanying clinical amelioration during follow-up.

MEG findings, in subacute and chronic stroke patients, show a clear positive correlation linking a better clinical outcome to a higher interhemispheric asymmetry of cortical neuronal sources recruited by a sensory stimulus from the hand in those patients unable to reach a complete recovery (Rossini et al., 1998; Rossini, 2001). On this basis, there are indications that different cerebral mechanisms sustain complete and partial healing.

Also TMS has been used to investigate residual motor function in stroke because the size of map and amplitude of the MEP depend on the stimulus intensity, the excitability and number of cortical neurons, and the number and integrity of the corticospinal tract fibers. Poststroke TMS studies of ILH and/or CLH have been used to investigate neuroplastic mechanisms promoting functional recovery and to assess the efficacy of rehabilitative strategies. During the acute stage, presence and amplitude of MEPs, and delayed central motor conduction time from ILH, had a positive correlation with clinical presentation and long-term outcome (Cicinelli et al., 1997; Traversa et al., 2000; Rossini et al., 2003). Other typical abnormalities are an excessive asymmetry of the hand muscle motor maps between the ILH and CLH and the migration of the excitable area of ILH outside the usual boundaries (Cicinelli et al., 1997). These changes tend to occur to a maximum degree within the three months poststroke and become stable in the chronic stages of recovery. In general, the electrophysiological behavior of the CLH and contralesional corticospinal tract is within normal limits in both acute and chronic stages (Shimizu et al., 2002), but sometimes the amplitude of MEPs elicited from the CLH may be enhanced in the first 24 hours after stroke. This interhemispheric asymmetry can decrease in the chronic stage, possibly reflecting a progressive "balancing" of interhemispheric transcallosal modulation, and is more prominent in patients with subcortical strokes. TMS, in addition, is a powerful tool for studying mechanisms of intracortical inhibition and excitation (Shimizu et al., 2002), which cannot be addressed with neuroimaging methods based on blood flow because it is not possible to distinguish whether activation of a certain brain area corresponds to the activity of excitatory or inhibitory neuronal networks. Particularly, the study of short-latency intracortical inhibition (SICI) and facilitation (ICF) via pp-TMS early after stroke sheds light on some plasticity mechanisms. SICI is suppressed in the ILH in the first weeks whereas ICF is consistently normal. Along this vein, an enhanced pattern of imagery-induced facilitation in the affected hemisphere has been reported in stroke (Cicinelli et al., 2006), and it has been suggested that the rapid clinical improvement of some patients might be induced by motor cortical disinhibition, secondary to the remote effects of structurally intact areas ("diaschisis"), and/or to the preexisting organization of the motor areas (i.e., the number of ipsilateral uncrossed corticospinal fibers; Rossini et al., 2003). An intriguing perspective is the possible application of rTMS as a potential therapy to promote reorganization and improve response to conventional treatments. Particularly, preliminary studies demonstrated that rTMS results in improvement in motor function, upregulating excitability within M1 of the ILH (Khedr et al., 2005) or downregulating excitability in the CLH. This proposal is consistent with the finding that downregulation of excitability in CLH may correct abnormally high interhemispheric transcallosal inhibition to ILH and cause an indirect functional facilitation of the affected hand. Even though the possible application of rTMS in therapy and for rehabilitation is exciting, further research is needed before proceeding toward a therapeutic application in stroke patients: for example, high-frequency rTMS reduces cerebral vasomotor reactivity, a possibly dangerous impact on cerebral hemodynamics (Vernieri et al., 2009; Rossini and Johnston, 2005).

Conclusion and Take-Home Message

As mentioned above, an integrated approach with technologies able to investigate functional brain imaging is of considerable value in providing information on the excitability, extension, localization, and functional hierarchy of cortical brain areas. Since, both in healthy aging and in different models of disease, neuroplasticity is an efficient way to maintain brain function despite progressive loss of its resources, deepening our knowledge on the mechanisms regulating cerebral function and plastic phenomena might prompt newer and more efficacious therapeutic and rehabilitative strategies for neurologic diseases.

Integration of different imaging technologies is just one of the possible applications of a more general multidisciplinary approach that should always lead the activity of clinicians and researchers.

Dedication

I (P.M.R.) was working in Lamberto's lab located in Via S. Zeno in Pisa between 1975 and 1977. At that time, I was a young MD, specializing in neurology and full of enthusiasm for clinical applications of evoked potentials (mainly visual evoked potentials) and for the use of HRP in studying thalamocortical connectivity under the guidance of Giorgio Macchi. Even though all my work there was on animal models, Lamberto always encouraged my tendency to translate into a clinical context the experimental methods and technologies. The atmosphere of the lab was extremely exciting and had a strong international character for those times (at least for Italy). Every week there was a lecture from someone coming from abroad, and most of the lecturers were the very top names in neurophysiology and the neurosciences. Going to the library was also an experience because it was actually the study of Giuseppe Moruzzi (a living monument of the Italian neurosciences), and we entered this area as if going to church.

Lamberto was—and he probably still is—a tennis player. There were at that time two main problems: first, he wanted to play in the very early morning hours (like at 6 a.m.) in order to have time for the next experiment; second, he couldn't bear to lose; in other words, if defeated, he was then like a lion in a cage for the following hours and, in fact, sometimes for the whole day. In those years, the designated victim or "sparring partner" was Giulio Sandini (who often slept in my apartment when he came from Genoa to stay overnight). I remember the whole staff of the lab encouraging Giulio to set his sights on an honorable defeat in order to make Lamberto happy and to make our life with him easier!

For the young visitors of the lab, Lamberto was a model for his geniality, enthusiasm, rigorous approach to the experimental data, open mind to suggestions and even criticisms, for not being intrusive and invasive in excess with respect to others' research but always being ready to listen and suggest, to drive toward the right type of analysis. I have taken all these "gifts" with me for more than 30 years, trying to transfer his style and philosophy in my everyday fight against patients' troubles and in my clinical research. I am deeply in debt to him and the whole staff of the Via S. Zeno Lab (Adriana, Silvia, Mario, and Nicoletta, among others), and I feel really honored to celebrate Lamberto's career with this contribution.

References

Babiloni C, Babiloni F, Carducci F, Cincotti F, Del Percio C, De Pino G, Maestrini S, et al. 2000. Movement-related electroencephalographic reactivity in Alzheimer disease. *Neuroimage* 12: 139–146.

Babiloni C, Vecchio F, Babiloni F, Brunelli GA, Carducci F, Cincotti F, Pizzella V, et al. 2004a. Coupling between "hand" primary sensorimotor cortex and lower limb muscles after ulnar nerve surgical transfer in paraplegia. *Behav Neurosci* 118: 214–222.

Babiloni, C, Babiloni F, Carducci F, Cincotti F, Vecchio F, Cola B, Rossi S, et al. 2004b. Functional frontoparietal connectivity during short-term memory as revealed by high-resolution EEG coherence analysis. *Behav Neurosci* 118: 687–697.

Babiloni C, Binetti G, Cassetta E, Cerboneschi D, Dal Forno G, Del Percio C, Ferreri, F, et al. 2004c. Mapping distributed sources of cortical rhythms in mild Alzheimer's disease: A multicentric EEG study. *Neuroimage* 22: 57–67.

Babiloni C, Ferri R, Moretti DV, Strambi A, Binetti G, Dal Forno G, Ferreri F, et al. 2004d. Abnormal frontoparietal coupling of brain rhythms in mild Alzheimer's disease: a multicentric EEG study. *Eur J Neurosci* 19: 2583–2590.

Babiloni C, Frisoni G, Steriade M, Bresciani L, Binetti G, Del Percio C, Geroldi C, et al. 2006a. Frontal white matter volume and delta EEG sources negatively correlate in awake subjects with mild cognitive impairment and Alzheimer's disease. *Clin Neurophysiol* 117: 1113–1129.

Babiloni C, Ferri R, Binetti G, Cassarino A, Forno GD, Ercolani M, Ferreri F, et al. 2006b. Fronto-parietal coupling of brain rhythms in mild cognitive impairment: a multicentric EEG study. *Brain Res Bull* 69: 63–73.

Babiloni F, Carducci F, Cincotti., Del Gratta C, Pizzella V, Romani GL, Rossini PM, et al. 2001. Linear inverse source estimate of combined EEG and MEG data related to voluntary movements. *Hum Brain Mapp* 14: 197–209.

Barker AT, Jalinous R, Freeston IL. 1985. Non-invasive magnetic stimulation of the human motor cortex. Lancet 1: 1106–1107.

Cicinelli P, Marconi B, Zaccagnini M, Pasqualetti P, Filippi MM, Rossini PM. 2006. Imagery-induced cortical excitability changes in stroke: a transcranial magnetic stimulation study. *Cereb Cortex* 16: 247–253.

Cicinelli P, Traversa R, Rossini PM. 1997. Post-stroke reorganization of brain motor output to the hand: a 2–4 month follow-up with focal magnetic transcranial stimulation. *Electroencephalogr Clin Neurophysiol* 105: 438–450.

DeFelipe J. 2006. Brain plasticity and mental processes: Cajal again. *Nat Rev Neurosci* 7: 811–817.

Ferreri F, Pauri F, Pasqualetti P, Fini R, Dal Forno G, Rossini PM. 2003. Motor cortex excitability in Alzheimer's disease: a transcranial magnetic stimulation study. *Ann Neurol* 53: 102–108.

Inghilleri M, Conte A, Frasca V, Scaldaferri N, Gilio F, Santini M, Fabbrini G, et al. 2006. Altered response to rTMS in patients with Alzheimer's disease. *Clin Neurophysiol* 117: 103–109.

Khedr EM, Ahmed MA, Fathy N, Rothwell JC. 2005. Therapeutic trial of repetitive transcranial magnetic stimulation after acute ischemic stroke. *Neurology* 65: 466–468.

Kobayashi M, Pascual Leone A. 2003. Transcranial magnetic stimulation in neurology. *Lancet Neurol* 2: 145–156.

Kujirai T, Caramia MD, Rothwell JC, Day BL, Thompson PD, Ferbert A, Wrose S, et al. 1993. Corticocortical inhibition in human motor cortex. *J Physiol* 471: 501–519.

Melgari JM, Pasqualetti P, Pauri F, Rossini PM. 2008. Muscles in "concert": study of primary motor cortex upper limb functional topography. *PLoS ONE* 3: e3069.

Osipova D, Ahveninen J, Jensen O, Ylikoski A, Pekkonen E. 2005. Altered generation of spontaneous oscillations in Alzheimer's disease. *Neuroimage* 27: 835–841.

Romani GL, Williamson SJ, Kaufman L. 1982. Tonotopic organization of the human auditory cortex. *Science* 216: 1339–1340.

Rossi S, Pasqualetti P, Tecchio F, Sabato A, Rossini PM. 1998. Modulation of corticospinal output to human hand muscles following deprivation of sensory feedback. *Neuroimage* 8: 163–175.

Rossi S, Cappa SF, Babiloni C, Pasqualetti P, Miniussi C, Carducci F, Babiloni F, Rossini PM. 2001. Prefrontal [correction of Prefontal] cortex in long-term memory: an "interference" approach using magnetic stimulation. *Nat Neurosci* 4: 948–952.

Rossi S, Miniussi C, Pasqualetti P, Babiloni C, Rossini PM, Cappa SF. 2004. Age-related functional changes of prefrontal cortex in long-term memory. A repetitive transcranial magnetic stimulation (rTMS) study. *J Neurosci* 24: 7939–7944.

Rossini PM, Martino G, Narici L, Pasquarelli A, Peresson M, Pizzella V, Tecchio F, et al. 1994a. Short-term brain "plasticity" in humans: transient finger representation changes in sensory cortex somatotopy following ischemic anesthesia. *Brain Res* 642: 169–177.

Rossini PM, Barker AT, Berardelli A, Caramia MD, Caruso G, Cracco RQ, Dimitrijevic MR, et al. 1994b. Non-invasive electrical and magnetic stimulation of the brain, spinal cord and roots: basic principles and procedures for routine clinical application. Report of an IFCN committee. *Electroencephalogr Clin Neurophysiol* 91: 79–92.

Rossini PM, Rossi S, Tecchio F, Pasqualetti P, Finazzi-Agrò A, Sabato A. 1996. Focal brain stimulation in healthy humans: motor maps changes following partial hand sensory deprivation. *Neurosci Lett* 214: 191–195.

Rossini PM, Caltagirone C, Castriota-Scanderbeg A, Cicinelli P, Del Gratta C, Demartin M, Pizzella V, et al. 1998. Hand motor cortical area reorganization in stroke: a study with fMRI, MEG and TCS maps. *Neuroreport* 9: 2141–2146.

Rossini PM. 2001. Tracking post-stroke recovery with magnetoencephalography. *Ann Neurol* 49: 136.

Rossini PM, Calautti C, Pauri F, Baron JC. 2003. Post-stroke plastic reorganisation in the adult brain. *Lancet Neurol* 2: 493–502.

Rossini PM, Dal Forno G. 2004. Neuronal post-stroke plasticity in the adult. *Restor Neurol Neurosci* 22: 193–206.

Rossini PM, Johnston CS. 2005. Facilitating acute stroke recovery with magnetic fields? *Neurology* 65: 353–354.

Rossini PM, Rossi S. 2007. Transcranial magnetic stimulation: diagnostic, therapeutic and research potential. *Neurology* 68: 484–488.

Rossini PM, Rossi S, Babiloni C, Polich J. 2007. Clinical neurophysiology of aging brain: from normal aging to neurodegeneration. *Prog Neurobiol* 83: 375–400.

Rossini PM, Buscema M, Capriotti M, Grossi E, Rodriguez G, Del Percio C, Babiloni C. 2008. Is it possible to automatically distinguish resting EEG data of normal elderly vs. mild cognitive impairment subjects with high degree of accuracy? *Clin Neurophysiol* 119: 1534–1545.

Shimizu T, Hosaki A, Hino T, Sato M, Komori T, Hirai S, Rossini PM. 2002. Motor cortical disinhibition in the unaffected hemisphere after unilateral cortical stroke. *Brain* 125: 1896–1907.

Tecchio F, Rossini PM, Pizzella V, Cassetta E, Romani GL. 1997. Spatial properties and interhemispheric differences of the sensory hand cortical representation: a neuromagnetic study. *Brain Res* 767: 100–108.

Tecchio F, Pasqualetti P, Pizzella V, Romani G, Rossini PM. 2000. Morphology of somatosensory evoked fields: inter-hemispheric similarity as a parameter for physiological and pathological neural connectivity. *Neurosci Lett* 287: 203–206.

Tecchio F, Pasqualetti P, Zappasodi F, Tombini M, Lupoi D, Vernieri F, Rossini PM. 2007. Outcome prediction in acute monohemispheric stroke via magnetoencephalography. *J Neurol* 254: 296–305.

Traversa R, Cicinelli P, Oliveri M, Palmieri M, Filippi MM, Pasqualetti P, & Rossini PM. 2000. Neurophysiological follow-up of motor cortical output in stroke patients. *Clin Neurophysiol* 111: 1695–1703.

Vernieri F, Maggio P, Tibuzzi F, Filippi MM, Pasqualetti P, Melgari JM, Altamura C, Palazzo P, Di Giorgio M, Rossini PM. 2009. High frequency repetitive transcranial magnetic stimulation decreases cerebral vasomotor reactivity. *Clin Neurophysiol* 120: 1188–1194.

Vicioso BA. 2002. Dementia: when is it not Alzheimer disease? *Am J Med Sci* 324(2): 84–95.

Williamson SJ, Kaufman L. 1990. Evolution of neuromagnetic topographic mapping. *Brain Topogr* 3: 113–127.

Ziemann U. 2004. TMS and drugs. *Clin Neurophysiol* 115: 1717–1729.

Subcortical Contributions to Cortical Reorganization after Massive
Somatosensory Deafferentation

Alessandro Graziano and Edward G. Jones

The primary somatosensory cortex (SI) of primates contains a finely detailed, topographically organized representation of cutaneous and deep receptors on the contralateral side of the body (Penfield and Rasmussen, 1950). In the adult brain, somatosensory maps are relatively stable (Dreyer et al., 1975), but events that disrupt the normal sensory input from the periphery cause changes in their topographic organization. For example, silencing afferent input from one or two digits, by amputation, peripheral nerve transection, or spinal cord lesion, will at first cause silencing of the cortical representation of those digits, followed by expansion of the cortical representations of adjacent digits with intact input into the silenced region of cortex (Kaas et al., 1983; Merzenich et al., 1983; Merzenich et al., 1984). The inverse holds for increased input activity, by which the overuse of a digit causes its cortical representation to expand at the expense of adjacent representations (Allard et al., 1991; Jenkins et al., 1990; Recanzone et al., 1990; Recanzone et al., 1992a; Recanzone et al., 1992b; Recanzone et al., 1992c). These shifts can be very large; after amputation of the upper limb, or its complete sensory deafferentation by dorsal root transections or lesions of the dorsal columns of the spinal cord, the face representation in SI, which lies lateral to the upper limb representation, expands medially up to 14 mm in macaque monkeys (Pons et al., 1991) or 20 mm in humans (Elbert et al., 1994), and in the long term, the face representation may completely replace the silenced representation of the deafferented arm.

Plasticity of somatosensory cortical and subcortical neurons after limited denervation has been extensively studied, and some of its mechanisms are relatively well understood. Very rapid changes depend on uncovering of silent synapses and release of GABA-mediated inhibition, followed in the short tem by modulation of synaptic efficacy (Buonomano and Merzenich, 1998; Calford, 2002; Cowan et al., 2003; Wall, 1977). These synaptic mechanisms will not be discussed here. By contrast, mechanisms underlying the extensive plasticity that follows long-term massive deafferentation (Jones and Pons, 1998; Pons et al., 1991) are less well understood. This is very unfortunate, because cortical reorganization may form the physiological substrate of phantom sensations in amputees and in patients with spinal cord injuries. Deafferentation pain, for example, is invariably associated with significant reorganization of cortical somatosensory maps (Flor et al., 1995). There are three lines of evidence that support this association. First, procedures that temporarily control pain cause immediate and reversible normalization of the reorganized cortical maps (Birbaumer et al., 1997; Huse et al., 2001). Second, pathological conditions causing chronic pain of peripheral origin—for example, chronic back pain or complex regional pain syndrome—are accompanied by cortical map reorganization (Flor et al., 1997; Pleger et al., 2004). Finally, in conditions of intensive use of a body part, such as a hand in professional musicians, dystonia is a common occurrence, a condition characterized by intense pain in the affected hand and large expansion of its cortical sensorimotor representation (Candia et al., 2003). It is clear, therefore, that understanding the mechanisms leading to long-term cortical reorganization represents a fundamental step toward unveiling the central mechanisms of pain and controlling its most debilitating manifestations, such as chronic and central pain.

Two major hypotheses have been advanced in order to explain the mechanisms underlying massive long-term expansions of cortical maps: either sprouting of axons of nondeafferented central neurons with the formation of synapses on deafferented neurons (Kaas et al., 2008) or withdrawal of overlapping inputs from atrophying deafferented neurons to reveal hitherto silent inputs from body parts with intact innervation (Jones, 2000). In this chapter, we will first discuss the sprouting hypothesis, underlining its inadequacy in the face of experimental and clinical evidence. Secondly, we will present the atrophy view and show its potential for explaining both short- and long-term cortical plasticity after central and peripheral denervation.

The Case for New Axon Growth

A number of studies have shown that peripheral deafferentation can induce new axon growth from spared portions of the periphery to innervate deafferented regions in the CNS. For example, Jain et al. (2000) reported that, after cutting the cuneate fasciculus at cervical levels in New World monkeys, and later injecting an anterograde axonal tracer in the skin of the chin and lower face, terminal labeling could be found in the ipsilateral cuneate nucleus on the side of the spinal lesion. By using a similar technique, the same group also reported new growth of cortical axons from neurons in area 3b of SI, innervating larger-than-normal portions of area 1 in monkeys with disrupted somatosensory input (Florence et al., 1998). In both studies, the tracing experiments were accompanied by extensive mapping of the cortical body representation, and the authors proposed that new axonal growth at cortical or subcortical levels is necessary and sufficient for large-scale cortical map plasticity after massive deafferentation. For a number of reasons, such evidence, and the conclusions derived from it, should be interpreted carefully, especially in regard to a causal role of sprouting in cortical reorganization.

First, more parsimonious explanations can account for the presence of anterogradely labeled axons from the skin of the chin in the cuneate nucleus. Jain et al.'s (2000) interpretation that their results indicated sprouting of trigeminal axons into the cuneate nucleus is open to question. In primates, the transverse cutaneous nerve of the neck, whose axons enter the spinal cord at C2–C3 level and terminate in the cuneate nucleus, extends its innervation field from the neck as far as the chin, overlapping the field innervated by the mandibular branch of the trigeminal nerve (Carpenter and Sutin, 1983; Sherrington, 1939). It is not surprising, therefore, to find anterogradely labeled axons in the cuneate nucleus after tracer injections in the chin area. To draw conclusions on the causal role of brainstem sprouting in cortical reorganization (Jain et al., 2000), it would be necessary to closely control the amount of tracer and the extent of the area injected, in conjunction with a detailed evaluation of cortical map reorganization, and this has yet to be done. The significance of this observation becomes all the more evident by considering that the region of periphery where trigeminal and cuneate projecting nerves overlap corresponds to the same portions of cortical and thalamic face representations which expand into those of a deafferented hand (Jones and Pons, 1998; Pons et al., 1991); these cortical and thalamic representations are characterized by dense reciprocal connectivity (Manger et al., 1997). The evidence for sprouting of cortical axons after disruption of somatosensory input (Florence et al., 1998) suffers from a similar shortcoming, in that it may depend on the amount and extent of tracer injected, a possibility that needs to be convincingly ruled out. In an attempt to clarify the results of tracer injections from which intracortical sprouting was inferred (Florence et al., 1998), we compared in the illustrations of the authors the ratio between the spread of tracer at the injection sites in area 1 and the extent of the distribution of retrogradely labeled cells in area 3b (see figure 2 of reference Florence et al., 1998) obtaining results virtually identical in normal monkeys and in monkeys with disrupted somatosensory input from the hand (for extensive studies of corticocortical connectivity between SI fields, see Burton and Fabri, 1995; DeFelipe et al., 1986; Jones et al., 1978). Even assuming that growth of new long-range axons does occur in significant amounts after massive deafferentation, the sprouting hypothesis remains unconvincing on physiological grounds as well. The trigeminal axons reported to sprout into the cuneate nucleus are those normally ending in the adjacent spinal trigeminal nucleus (Jain et al., 2000). These are slow-conducting A-delta and C fibers, known to carry information from pain and temperature receptors (Willis and Westlund, 1997), clearly different from those mediating the fast, low-threshold responses evoked in the reorganized SI by light tactile stimulation (Pons et al., 1991). Moreover, trigemino- and spinothalamic projections have no role in maintaining activity of the somatosensory cortex after lesion (Jain et al., 1997). It should also be added that newly formed dorsal column axons reaching the cuneate nucleus after spinal cord lesion are chronically demyelinated and remain in a pathophysiological state (Tan et al., 2007). Thus, many lines of evidence demand reconsideration of the significance of sprouting in cortical reorganization.

Lane et al. (2008) showed that the reorganization of cortical maps after forepaw amputation in rats does not depend on the sprouting of gracile axons into the denervated cuneate nucleus, an observation in line with recent results from Jain et al. (2008), who, two years after lesioning the cuneate fasciculus at C5–C7 in adult monkeys, observed massive reorganization in SI, finding neurons with face-receptive fields as far medially as the representation of the foot. The foot area receives input from the gracile nucleus via the ventral posterior lateral nucleus of the thalamus (VPL). Based on the sprouting hypothesis, one would expect to find new trigeminal axons terminating in the gracile nucleus. It is significant that, at comparable postlesion times, sprouting of spinal trigeminal axons after more massive deafferentations, produced by lesioning both cuneate and gracile fasciculi at higher cervical levels (C3–C5), was limited to the cuneate nucleus (Jain et al., 2000), making it unlikely that cortical reorganization depends solely, or to any significant extent, upon axonal sprouting in the brainstem.

Clinical evidence also does not support sprouting as a leading mechanism of cortical reorganization . In amputees suffering from phantom pain, peripherally or centrally induced analgesia can cause immediate and temporary normalization of cortical maps, with concomitant release from phantom pain (Birbaumer et al., 1997; Huse et al., 2001). Moreover, one patient reported precise, topographically organized phantom sensations after stimulation of the face as early as 24 hours after arm amputation (Borsook et al., 1998). These clinical observations, while not dismissing the possibility of sprouting phenomena occurring at different levels of the somatosensory pathways after deafferentation, question a causal role for newly formed long-range projections in cortical reorganization (Knecht et al., 1998).

If Not Sprouting, Then …

The rapid emergence of phantom sensations and the long-term cortical reorganization occurring after massive deafferentation can be explained by the joint action of two mechanisms: divergence of the normal somatosensory ascending projections and activity-dependent transneuronal atrophy of neurons along the somatosensory pathway from periphery to cortex, with progressive axon withdrawal from deafferented thalamus and cortex.

Divergence in Ascending Somatosensory Projections

At all levels of the somatosensory pathway, the divergence of ascending projections is remarkable. In the medulla oblongata, primary sensory axons from one digit terminate in an elongated field, extending throughout the rostrocaudal extent of the pars rotunda of the cuneate or gracile nucleus, corresponding to a column of approximately 3×0.2 mm (Culberson and Brushart, 1989; Florence et al., 1989; Nyberg and Blomqvist, 1982; Rasmusson, 1988). This means that, despite the limited extension of single axonal arborizations, the cumulative input to the cuneate nucleus from a single body part involves thousands of cells, and in any given position approximately 300 peripheral afferents overlap (Weinberg et al., 1990). Such extensive divergence and convergence can readily explain the immediate reorganization of cuneate receptive fields after limited denervation. Divergence of ascending projections is even more dramatic in the thalamus, where a single body part is represented in a lamellar volume of approximately $3 \times 3.5 \times 0.1$ mm and increases exponentially in the thalamocortical projections, where 0.1 mm^3 of VPL can project to a cortical area as wide as 20 mm^2 (Rausell et al., 1998). This organization implies that the cortical area influenced by a single body part is much larger than that revealed by extracellular multiunit mapping. Thalamic projections to cortical representations of adjacent body parts significantly overlap, providing input to an appropriate cortical representation but overlapping into adjacent representations (Snow et al., 1988). Under the conditions of extracellular multiunit mapping, these divergent projections are not seen to drive postsynaptic cells in the inappropriate representation; however, excitatory postsynaptic potentials have been recorded intracellularly from inappropriate cortical neurons after stimulation of adjacent digits (Smits et al., 1991; Zarzecki et al., 1993). Loss of input activity from one digit will unmask these "silent" projections, and stimulation of an adjacent digit with preserved input to the cortex will become effective in driving activity in neurons that have lost peripheral input from an amputated or deafferented digit. By the divergence at each step of the ascending somatosensory pathway, small changes in the input to the brainstem are magnified along their way to the thalamus and cortex and can support large expansions of cortical representations with intact input into regions of SI cortex that have lost input. The underlying anatomical organization provides a basis for the adult CNS to be intrinsically capable of large, activity-dependent changes in the short term. It also explains the observation that a few spared projections, after otherwise massive deafferenting lesions, can maintain a full cortical representation of the deafferented body part (Jain et al., 1997). Divergence also allows for more than 35% of a thalamic representation of a single digit to be destroyed before the cortical representation of that digit begins to shrink (Jones et al., 1997).

There are, however, limitations to divergence-mediated map reorganization. Massive deafferentations, such as amputations or complete dorsal columns lesions, or thalamic lesions involving over 40% of the thalamic volume cause silencing of the SI cortex that lasts for months or years (Jones et al., 1997). This implies that mechanisms other than divergence are needed to account for the emergence of new responses in the deafferented cortex long after massive loss of somatosensory input.

Long-Term Transneuronal Atrophy

An important clue in the search for mechanisms of long-term plasticity in response to massive peripheral or spinal deafferentation comes from studies of the long-term effects of large-scale somatosensory deafferentation in the thalamus of monkeys. Twenty years after cutting spinal dorsal roots C2–T4, the deafferented VPL of the thalamus displays dramatic atrophic changes compared to the normal thalamus, with cells more densely packed, reflecting reduced neuropil mass and loss of lemniscal axons; neuronal somata are shrunken and stain more darkly in Nissl preparations, and there is gliosis (Woods et al., 2000). Such changes are well documented at earlier times in the deafferented cuneate nucleus (Loewy, 1973), but until relatively recently there was no documentation of similar changes in the thalamus. On a larger scale, these changes are reflected in a conspicuous volume reduction of the deafferented VPL. Such physical rearrangement causes the face representation, normally contained within the boundaries of the ventral posterior medial nucleus, to collapse into the deafferented hand representation in VPL, so that cells with receptive fields on the face lie adjacent to cells with receptive fields on the foot (Jones and Pons, 1998), a proximity never observed in the normal thalamus, where face and foot representations are separated by the large representation of the hand (Jones, 2007).

Two aspects of the transneuronal atrophic process are especially important in relation to long-term cortical reorganization. First, both in brainstem and thalamus, actual cell loss by death of neurons is small, not more than 15% of the cells in the cuneate nucleus and even fewer in the thalamus disappearing 20 years after deafferentation (Woods et al., 2000).Thus, the majority of the cells undergoing primary (in the cuneate nucleus) and secondary (in the thalamus) transneuronal atrophy do survive and may be able to drive postsynaptic activity in the reorganized cortex, because in patients with long-standing amputations who underwent neurosurgery, electrical stimulation of the deafferented thalamus elicited clear sensations in the missing limb (Davis et al., 1998). Second, the process leading to secondary transneuronal atrophy in the thalamus is progressive and extremely slow. It begins to become identifiable 10 years after deafferentation, and more than 10 years is necessary for cellular changes to reach their fullest observed extent (Woods et al., 2000). The slow, progressive but inexorable shrinkage of neurons and withdrawal of their axons from thalamus and cortex may represent a powerful stimulus to reorganization under conditions of long-term deafferentations, and the physical proximity of face and foot representations in the deafferented thalamus should facilitate the synaptic rearrangement of intact divergent projections mediating the expansion of the cortical face representation into the neighboring silenced cortex. This has profound clinical implications. In amputees and patients with spinal cord lesions, phantom sensations and central pain can emerge years after the deafferenting injury (Hill, 1999; Störmer et al., 1997), and an atrophic process unfolding at such a slow pace is the only plausible mechanism that can explain the late appearance of signs of deafferentation-induced thalamic and cortical reorganization.

Transneuronal Atrophy in the Short Term

While the slow progression of transneuronal atrophy represents an important potential mechanism of long-term cortical plasticity and its clinical manifestations, it has not been without its detractors. They have sought to minimize the role of transneuronal atrophy in cortical plasticity, reasoning that clinical symptoms associated with massive deafferentations usually take much shorter than 10 years to emerge and, in many cases, cortical reorganization takes place in the absence of any microscopic sign of atrophy at any level of the central somatosensory pathways (Kaas and Florence, 2001; Kaas et al., 2008; Merzenich, 1998). These arguments, however, fail to recognize the progressive nature of activity-dependent transneuronal atrophy and do not take into account the likelihood that the axon of a deafferented cuneate or thalamic neuron may be undergoing changes long before shrinkage of its cell body becomes microscopically visible. The inexorable progression of transneuronal atrophy in the years after cell body atrophy becomes identifiable strongly suggests that its action is already affecting the deafferented neurons along the somatosensory pathway well before. In order to verify this, it was essential to look at the axons themselves of deafferented neurons to determine whether they were in fact withdrawing from higher centers before the detection of shrinkage of their parent somata.

We investigated this issue (Graziano and Jones, 2009) by using a quantitative approach. We studied morphological changes in a large population of lemniscal and thalamocortical axons two years after complete transection of the cuneate fasciculus at the level of the first cervical segment in adult monkeys. Two years is almost a decade before cell body shrinkage and gliosis can be identified in the thalamus (Woods et al., 2000). We examined the morphology of axons of cuneate neurons terminating in the thalamus and of thalamic axons terminating in the cortex by injection of anterograde tracers in the cuneate nucleus or thalamus and collected data from more than 15 miles of axon reconstructions in physiologically identified regions of thalamus and cortex, obtaining two important results.

Two years after complete cuneate fasciculotomy, the deafferented regions in the brainstem, thalamus, and cortex were virtually silent, with no detectable expansion of the adjacent face representation. The lack of frank expansion of the face representation in our experiments suggests that early cortical map reorganization, reported by other studies after lesion of the dorsal columns at levels varying from C3 to C7 (Jain et al., 1997; Jain et al., 2008), may depend on preserved input from upper cervical segments. Because of the overlap of cuneate and trigeminal innervation of the neck and the chin (see above), lesions at or below the C3 level will preserve input from this part of the face in the cuneate nucleus. By interrupting the cuneate fasciculus at C1, we effectively removed all input to the cuneate nucleus, resembling the massive denervation performed by cutting the dorsal roots from C2 to T4 (Pons et al., 1991). After deafferentation of this extent, the area of cortex receiving cuneate input is completely silenced (Bioulac and Lamarre, 1979), with the exception of a small region receiving head input behind the arm representation, present in normal monkeys (Dreyer et al., 1975; Ullrich and Woosley, 1954). Unfortunately, the only available data on cortical reorganization from 6 to 8 months to 2 years and thus relevant to our discussion were obtained after lesions at levels ranging from C3 to C7, so they do not shed light on this issue. It must be noted that even after more restricted deafferentations of single digits, areas of silenced cortex persist for as long as 32 weeks, and the extent of cortical reactivation at this time depends on the size of the deafferenting lesion (Darian-Smith and Ciferri, 2006). These observations suggest that after complete cuneate deafferentation, thalamic and cortical hand representations may remain silent for years before becoming occupied by inputs from the face.

The second, more important result of our study is that transneuronal atrophy affected the morphology of second-order lemniscal and third-order thalamocortical axons long before overt shrinkage of their deafferented parent cells could be identified in dorsal column nuclei or thalamus (Graziano and Jones, 2009). The effects of the two-year-long deafferentation on the terminal arbors of axons in thalamus and cortex were similar, consisting primarily of a considerable reduction in size and number of synaptic boutons (see figure 24.1, plate 12).

The inability to detect transneuronal atrophy in earlier studies of peripheral deafferentation is the consequence of focusing only on somal morphology. Our results demonstrate that even at relatively early postlesional stages, transneuronal atrophy has affected lemniscal and

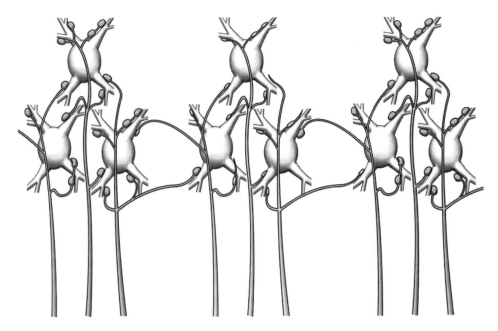

Figure 24.1 (plate 12)
Diagram summarizing the morphological changes of withdrawing lemniscal axons (blue) from the upper limb and upper trunk representations in VPL after transection of the cuneate fasciculus. The same scheme applies to thalamocortical axons withdrawing from the upper limb and upper trunk representation in the somatosensory cortex. The first signs of transneuronal atrophy are a reduction in size and number of synaptic boutons, the presence of incomplete endings, and a loss of short terminal branches. The divergent projections of normal axons (red) from face and lower body representations to the adjacent cuneate representations, normally unable to drive activity, constitute the basis for the expansion of the silenced upper limb/upper trunk representation by adjacent representations of the face and lower body. In the long term, transneuronal atrophy, with shrinkage and loss of deafferented neurons, enhances the expansion of representations with intact innervation. From Graziano and Jones (2009).

thalamocortical axon terminations, suggesting that transneuronal atrophy and withdrawal of the axons of deafferented neurons from centers higher in the somatosensory pathway is likely to contribute to cortical reorganization. Even in the short term, and even after deafferenting peripheral injuries that are not commonly thought to induce loss of dorsal root ganglion cells (Kaas and Florence, 2001), there may be withdrawal of primary afferents from the dorsal column nuclei. Indeed, limb amputations or transections of nerves which sever the peripheral axons of dorsal root ganglion cells do cause extensive loss of dorsal root ganglion cells and of sensory axons entering the brainstem and spinal cord (Csillik et al., 1982; Knyihar-Csillik et al., 1987; Liss et al., 1996; Liss and Wiberg, 1997a; 1997b). Moreover, this is accompanied by transneuronal atrophy of neuronal somata in the cuneate nucleus and thalamus (Florence and Kaas, 1995; Jones and Pons, 1998; Woods et al., 2000), and in humans there is a decrease in thalamic gray matter demonstrable by magnetic resonance imaging (Draganski et al., 2006). The atrophy of cuneate cell bodies will be accompanied by changes of the type we have described in their axons terminating in the thalamus and transynaptically in the axons of deafferented thalamic relay neurons in the cortex. Thus, peripheral and central deafferentation may act through the same mechanisms.

Transneuronal Atrophy Commences Very Early

Mechanisms of central plasticity that depend upon transneuronal effects upon the axonal terminations of deafferented neurons may come into play even before morphological changes become evident in the axonal terminations. Two months after unilateral cuneate fasciculotomies in adult monkeys, we studied differential gene expression in the deafferented regions of brainstem, thalamus, and cortex (Graziano and Jones, 2006). Analysis of the biological functions associated with up- or downregulated genes showed a clear overrepresentation of genes associated with neuronal atrophy, neurodegeneration, and neuroinflammation. In adjacent regions, in which representations receiving inputs from the face and lower limb were located and which expand to occupy the deafferented regions, we also found upregulated genes associated with positive plasticity, such as neurogenesis, synaptogenesis, and short- and long-term synaptic plasticity. These findings imply that, even at very early stages after denervation, activity-dependent transneuronal changes are already affecting neurons and their terminations along the somatosensory pathway. The many intracellular metabolic pathways that are up- or downregulated under these conditions may lead not only to axon withdrawal and cell atrophy in the short and long term but also to the synaptic plasticity necessary to mediate the early and late changes in the receptive field properties of cells that lead to cortical map reorganization.

The evidence that somatosensory denervation induces early regulation of genes related to neuronal atrophy, together with progressive atrophic changes, first involving axon terminals and synapses, and later causing axon withdrawal and cell body atrophy and death in thalamus and cortex, suggests that a neurodegenerative process leading to anatomical and functional reorganization of thalamus and cortex at all stages of peripheral and central deafferentations likely to be a powerful inducement of representational plasticity.

Acknowledgments

We thank Phong Nguyen for technical support and Prabhakara Choudary and Karl Murray for advice. This work was supported by grant number NS21377 from the National Institutes of Health, United States Public Health Service.

References

Allard T, Clark SA, Jenkins WM, Merzenich MM. 1991. Reorganization of somatosensory area 3b representations in adult owl monkeys after digital syndactyly. *J Neurophysiol* 66: 1048–1058.

Bioulac B, Lamarre Y. 1979. Activity of postcentral cortical neurons of the monkey during conditioned movements of a deafferented limb. *Brain Res* 172: 427–437.

Birbaumer N, Lutzenberger W, Montoya P, Larbig W, Unertl K, et al. 1997. Effects of regional anesthesia on phantom limb pain are mirrored in changes in cortical reorganization. *J Neurosci* 17: 5503–5508.

Borsook D, Becerra L, Fishman S, Edwards A, Jennings CL, et al. 1998. Acute plasticity in the human somatosensory cortex following amputation. *Neuroreport* 9: 1013–1017.

Buonomano DV, Merzenich MM. 1998. Cortical plasticity: from synapses to maps. *Annu Rev Neurosci* 21: 149–186.

Burton H, Fabri M. 1995. Ipsilateral intracortical connections of physiologically defined cutaneous representations in areas 3b and 1 of macaque monkeys: projections in the vicinity of the central sulcus. *J Comp Neurol* 355: 508–538.

Calford MB. 2002. Dynamic representational plasticity in sensory cortex. *Neuroscience* 111: 709–738.

Candia V, Wienbruch C, Elbert T, Rockstroh B, Ray W. 2003. Effective behavioral treatment of focal hand dystonia in musicians alters somatosensory cortical organization 1. *Proc Natl Acad Sci USA* 100: 7942–7946.

Carpenter MB, Sutin J. 1983. *Human Neuroanatomy.* Baltimore: Williams and Wilkins.

Cowan WM, Südhof TC, Stevens CF. 2003. *Synapses.* Baltimore: Johns Hopkins University Press.

Csillik B, Knyihar E, Rakic P. 1982. Transganglionic degenerative atrophy and regenerative proliferation in the Rolando substance of the primate spinal cord: discoupling and restoration of synaptic connectivity in the central nervous system after peripheral nerve lesions. *Folia Morphol (Praha)* 30: 189–191.

Culberson JL, Brushart TM. 1989. Somatotopy of digital nerve projections to the cuneate nucleus in the monkey. *Somatosens Mot Res* 6: 319–330.

Darian-Smith C, Ciferri M. 2006. Cuneate nucleus reorganization following cervical dorsal rhizotomy in the macaque monkey: its role in the recovery of manual dexterity. *J Comp Neurol* 498: 552–565.

Davis KD, Kiss ZH, Luo L, Tasker RR, Lozano AM, Dostrovsky JO. 1998. Phantom sensations generated by thalamic microstimulation. *Nature* 391: 385–387.

DeFelipe J, Conley M, Jones EG. 1986. Long-range focal collateralization of axons arising from corticocortical cells in monkey sensory-motor cortex. *J Neurosci* 6: 3749–3766.

Draganski B, Moser T, Lummel N, Ganssbauer S, Bogdahn U, et al. 2006. Decrease of thalamic gray matter following limb amputation. *Neuroimage* 31: 951–957.

Dreyer DA, Loe PR, Metz CB, Whitsel BL. 1975. Representation of head and face in postcentral gyrus of the macaque. *J Neurophysiol* 38: 714–733.

Elbert T, Flor H, Birbaumer N, Knecht S, Hampson S, et al. 1994. Extensive reorganization of the somatosensory cortex in adult humans after nervous system injury. *Neuroreport* 5: 2593–2597.

Flor H, Braun C, Elbert T, Birbaumer N. 1997. Extensive reorganization of primary somatosensory cortex in chronic back pain patients. *Neurosci Lett* 224: 5–8.

Flor H, Elbert T, Knecht S, Wienbruch C, Pantev C, et al. 1995. Phantom-limb pain as a perceptual correlate of cortical reorganization following arm amputation. *Nature* 375: 482–484.

Florence SL, Kaas JH. 1995. Large-scale reorganization at multiple levels of the somatosensory pathway follows therapeutic amputation of the hand in monkeys. *J Neurosci* 15: 8083–8095.

Florence SL, Taub HB, Kaas JH. 1998. Large-scale sprouting of cortical connections after peripheral injury in adult macaque monkeys. *Science* 282: 1117–1121.

Florence SL, Wall JT, Kaas JH. 1989. Somatotopic organization of inputs from the hand to the spinal gray and cuneate nucleus of monkeys with observations on the cuneate nucleus of humans. *J Comp Neurol* 286: 48–70.

Graziano A, Jones EG. 2006. Changes in gene expression accompanying somatosensory plasticity in adult monkeys. Program No: 212.8. 2006 Neuroscience Meeting Planner. Atlanta, GA. Society for Neuroscience. Online.

Graziano A, Jones EG. 2009. Early withdrawal of axons from higher centers in response to peripheral somatosensory denervation. *J Neurosci* 29: 3738–3748.

Hill A. 1999. Phantom limb pain: a review of the literature on attributes and potential mechanisms. *J Pain Symptom Manage* 17: 125–142.

Huse E, Larbig W, Flor H, Birbaumer N. 2001. The effect of opioids on phantom limb pain and cortical reorganization. *Pain* 90: 47–55.

Jain N, Catania KC, Kaas JH. 1997. Deactivation and reactivation of somatosensory cortex after dorsal spinal cord injury. *Nature* 386: 495–498.

Jain N, Florence SL, Qi HX, Kaas JH. 2000. Growth of new brainstem connections in adult monkeys with massive sensory loss. *Proc Natl Acad Sci USA* 97: 5546–5550.

Jain N, Qi HX, Collins CE, Kaas JH. 2008. Large-scale reorganization in the somatosensory cortex and thalamus after sensory loss in macaque monkeys. *J Neurosci* 28: 11042–11060.

Jenkins WM, Merzenich MM, Ochs MT, Allard T, Guic-Robles E. 1990. Functional reorganization of primary somatosensory cortex in adult owl monkeys after behaviorally controlled tactile stimulation. *J Neurophysiol* 63: 82–104.

Jones EG. 2000. Cortical and subcortical contributions to activity-dependent plasticity in primate somatosensory cortex. *Annu Rev Neurosci* 23: 1–37.

Jones EG. 2007. *The Thalamus*, second edition. Cambridge, UK: Cambridge University Press.

Jones EG, Coulter JD, Hendry SH. 1978. Intracortical connectivity of architectonic fields in the somatic sensory, motor and parietal cortex of monkeys. *J Comp Neurol* 181: 291–347.

Jones EG, Manger PR, Woods TM. 1997. Maintenance of a somatotopic cortical map in the face of diminishing thalamocortical inputs. *Proc Natl Acad Sci USA* 94: 11003–11007.

Jones EG, Pons TP. 1998. Thalamic and brainstem contributions to large-scale plasticity of primate somatosensory cortex. *Science* 282: 1121–1125.

Kaas JH, Florence SL. 2001. Reorganization of sensory and motor systems in adult mammals after injury. In The Mutable Brain: Dynamic and Plastic Features of the Developing and Mature Brain (Kaas JH ed.), pp 165–242. Amsterdam: Harwood Academic Publishers.

Kaas JH, Merzenich MM, Killackey HP. 1983. The reorganization of somatosensory cortex following peripheral nerve damage in adult and developing mammals. *Annu Rev Neurosci* 6: 325–356.

Kaas JH, Qi HX, Burish MJ, Gharbawie OA, Onifer SM, Massey JM. 2008. Cortical and subcortical plasticity in the brains of humans, primates, and rats after damage to sensory afferents in the dorsal columns of the spinal cord. *Exp Neur* 209: 407–416.

Knecht S, Henningsen H, Hohling C, Elbert T, Flor H, et al. 1998. Plasticity of plasticity? Changes in the pattern of perceptual correlates of reorganization after amputation. *Brain* 121(Pt 4): 717–724.

Knyihar-Csillik E, Rakic P, Csillik B. 1987. Transganglionic degenerative atrophy in the substantia gelatinosa of the spinal cord after peripheral nerve transection in rhesus monkeys. *Cell Tissue Res* 247: 599–604.

Lane RD, Pluto CP, Kenmuir CL, Chiaia NL, Mooney RD. 2008. Does reorganization in the cuneate nucleus following neonatal forelimb amputation influence development of anomalous circuits within the somatosensory cortex? *J Neurophysiol* 99: 866–875.

Liss AG, af Ekenstam FW, Wiberg M. 1996. Loss of neurons in the dorsal root ganglia after transection of a peripheral sensory nerve: an anatomical study in monkeys. *Scand J Plast Reconstr Surg Hand Surg* 30: 1–6.

Liss AG, Wiberg M. 1997a. Loss of nerve endings in the spinal dorsal horn after a peripheral nerve injury: an anatomical study in Macaca fascicularis monkeys. *Eur J Neurosci* 9: 2187–2192.

Liss AG, Wiberg M. 1997b. Loss of primary afferent nerve terminals in the brainstem after peripheral nerve transection: an anatomical study in monkeys. *Anat Embryol (Berl)* 196: 279–289.

Loewy AD. 1973. Transneuronal changes in the gracile nucleus. *J Comp Neurol* 147: 497–510.

Manger PR, Woods TM, Munoz A, Jones EG. 1997. Hand/face border as a limiting boundary in the body representation in monkey somatosensory cortex. *J Neurosci* 17: 6338–6351.

Merzenich M. 1998. Long-term change of mind. *Science* 282: 1062–1063.

Merzenich MM, Kaas JH, Wall J, Nelson RJ, Sur M, Felleman D. 1983. Topographic reorganization of somatosensory cortical areas 3b and 1 in adult monkeys following restricted deafferentation. *Neuroscience* 8: 33–55.

Merzenich MM, Nelson RJ, Stryker MP, Cynader MS, Schoppmann A, Zook JM. 1984. Somatosensory cortical map changes following digit amputation in adult monkeys. *J Comp Neurol* 224: 591–605.

Nyberg G, Blomqvist A. 1982. The termination of forelimb nerves in the feline cuneate nucleus demonstrated by the transganglionic transport method. *Brain Res* 248: 209–222.

Penfield W, Rasmussen T. 1950. *The Cerebral Cortex of Man*. New York: Macmillan.

Pleger B, Tegenthoff M, Schwenkreis P, Janssen F, Ragert P, et al. 2004. Mean sustained pain levels are linked to hemispherical side-to-side differences of primary somatosensory cortex in the complex regional pain syndrome I. *Exp Brain Res* 155: 115–119.

Pons TP, Garraghty PE, Ommaya AK, Kaas JH, Taub E, Mishkin M. 1991. Massive cortical reorganization after sensory deafferentation in adult macaques. *Science* 252: 1857–1860.

Rasmusson DD. 1988. Projections of digit afferents to the cuneate nucleus in the raccoon before and after partial deafferentation. *J Comp Neurol* 277: 549–556.

Rausell E, Bickford L, Manger PR, Woods TM, Jones EG. 1998. Extensive divergence and convergence in the thalamocortical projection to monkey somatosensory cortex. *J Neurosci* 18: 4216–4232.

Recanzone GH, Allard TT, Jenkins WM, Merzenich MM. 1990. Receptive-field changes induced by peripheral nerve stimulation in SI of adult cats. *J Neurophysiol* 63: 1213–1225.

Recanzone GH, Jenkins WM, Hradek GT, Merzenich MM. 1992a. Progressive improvement in discriminative abilities in adult owl monkeys performing a tactile frequency discrimination task. *J Neurophysiol* 67: 1015–1030.

Recanzone GH, Merzenich MM, Dinse HR. 1992b. Expansion of the cortical representation of a specific skin field in primary somatosensory cortex by intracortical microstimulation. *Cereb Cortex* 2: 181–196.

Recanzone GH, Merzenich MM, Jenkins WM, Grajski KA, Dinse HR. 1992c. Topographic reorganization of the hand representation in cortical area 3b owl monkeys trained in a frequency-discrimination task. *J Neurophysiol* 67: 1031–1056.

Sherrington CS. 1939. On the distribution of sensory nerve roots. In Selected Writings of Sir Charles Sherrington (Denny-Brown D, ed), pp 31–93. London: Hamish Hamilton.

Smits E, Gordon DC, Witte S, Rasmusson DD, Zarzecki P. 1991. Synaptic potentials evoked by convergent somatosensory and corticocortical inputs in raccoon somatosensory cortex: substrates for plasticity. *J Neurophysiol* 66: 688–695.

Snow PJ, Nudo RJ, Rivers W, Jenkins WM, Merzenich MM. 1988. Somatotopically inappropriate projections from thalamocortical neurons to the SI cortex of the cat demonstrated by the use of intracortical microstimulation. *Somatosens Res* 5: 349–372.

Störmer S, Gerner HJ, Gruninger W, Metzmacher K, Follinger S, et al. 1997. Chronic pain/dysaesthesiae in spinal cord injury patients: results of a multicentre study. *Spinal Cord* 35: 446–455.

Tan AM, Petruska JC, Mendell LM, Levine JM. 2007. Sensory afferents regenerated into dorsal columns after spinal cord injury remain in a chronic pathophysiological state. *Exp Neurol* 206: 257–268.

Ullrich DP, Woosley CN. 1954. Trigeminal nerve representation in the upper head area of the postcentral gyrus of Macaca mulatta. *Trans Am Neurol Assoc* 13: 23–28.

Wall PD. 1977. The presence of ineffective synapses and the circumstances which unmask them. *Philos Trans R Soc Lond B Biol Sci* 278: 361–372.

Weinberg RJ, Pierce JP, Rustioni A. 1990. Single fiber studies of ascending input to the cuneate nucleus of cats. I. Morphometry of primary afferent fibers. *J Comp Neurol* 300: 113–133.

Willis WD, Westlund KN. 1997. Neuroanatomy of the pain system and of the pathways that modulate pain. *J Clin Neurophysiol* 14: 2–31.

Woods TM, Cusick CG, Pons TP, Taub E, Jones EG. 2000. Progressive transneuronal changes in the brainstem and thalamus after long-term dorsal rhizotomies in adult macaque monkeys. *J Neurosci* 20: 3884–3899.

Zarzecki P, Witte S, Smits E, Gordon DC, Kirchberger P, Rasmusson DD. 1993. Synaptic mechanisms of cortical representational plasticity: somatosensory and corticocortical EPSPs in reorganized raccoon SI cortex. *J Neurophysiol* 69: 1422–1432.

25 Environmental Influences on Neurodegenerative Disease: The Impact of Systemic Inflammation

V. Hugh Perry

As the human population lives longer, so diseases of the elderly and aging are thrown into sharp focus. Chronic progressive degenerative diseases of the central nervous system (CNS) are an enormous social and economic burden: it is estimated that neurological disease accounts for a highly significant proportion of the global health burden (Menken et al., 2000). Globally, approximately 24 million persons suffer from dementia, the most common form being Alzheimer's disease (AD), and this number is predicted to rise to 80 million persons by the year 2040 (Ferri et al., 2005). It is believed that the causes of the most common chronic neurodegenerative diseases are the result of complex interactions between the genetics of a given individual and multiple environmental factors. In AD, three genes have been identified that lead to rare familial forms of the disease, amyloid precursor protein (APP), presenilins-1 and 2 (PSN-1, PSN-2), and a further gene, apolipoprotein-4 (ApoE4), has been identified that confers increased susceptibility (Blennow et al., 2006). With the application of powerful new methodologies and techniques (Hardy and Singleton, 2009), there is a rapidly growing list of loci that will lead to the identification of genes that either increase susceptibility to disease or are protective. Testing how each of these genes, or interactions between these genes, contributes to disease progression will be a formidable challenge. Identification of the environmental factors that impact a particular disease has depended on epidemiology studies, and again a diverse list of factors has been identified including smoking, obesity, and diabetes among others (Blennow et al., 2006). Of interest is that these risk factors are typically associated with low-grade systemic inflammation.

Inflammation in Alzheimer's Disease: Consequence or Contributor?

Evidence that inflammation might contribute to the onset or progression of AD has arisen from the observations on postmortem material from AD patients. The classical hallmarks of AD neuropathology are the deposition of amyloid in plaques, and neurofibrillary tangles, which are in turn associated with massive neuronal loss and brain atrophy. In addition, the pathology is associated with changes in the resident macrophage population of the brain, the microglia (Akiyama et al., 2000). In the normal brain, the microglia are a quiescent or downregulated population of macrophages (Ransohoff and Perry, 2009) that have a very slow turnover when compared to other tissue macrophages (Lawson et al., 1992) and are involved in the surveillance of their local microenvironment (Nimmerjahn et al., 2005). In the AD brain, and in other chronic neurodegenerative diseases of the CNS, the microglia change their morphology and increase the level of expression of a number of cell surface and intracellular proteins and are typically referred to as "activated microglia." The presence of activated microglia in the brains of AD patients can also be imaged in life using positron emission tomography (PET) scanning and the ligand PK11195 (Edison et al., 2008). The significance of microglia activation is by no means obvious; it could simply be a consequence of the deposition of amyloid and the degeneration of neurons, or microglia may be a contributor to disease progression. Furthermore, as is discussed below, the change in morphology of the microglia and upregulation of several surface antigens such as major histocompatibility antigens, the complement type 3 receptor, or binding of a particular lectin are not related in any simple way to the other aspects of the phenotype. Macrophages can adopt diverse activation states depending on the local microenvironment (Mosser and Edwards, 2008). A particular phenotypic state associated with the production of a spectrum of cytokines is not, however, fixed but may be rapidly changed by external factors such as cytokines or pathogen derived products (Stout et al., 2005). We also need to bear in mind, of course, that the innate inflammatory response is not only essential for host protection in the presence of a pathogen or tissue injury but plays a role in tissue repair (Mosser and Edwards, 2008).

Evidence that the innate inflammatory response in the AD brain is not simply a consequence of the neurodegeneration but can contribute to disease pathogenesis has come from epidemiology studies on patient populations taking nonsteroidal anti-inflammatory drugs (NSAIDs) over long periods. Not all studies have shown protection from the onset or progression of AD, but a meta-analysis of some nine studies shows that overall there is some modest protection (Etminan et al., 2003). However, studies in animal models of AD have demonstrated that NSAIDs may have important effects other than inhibiting cyclooxygenase activity: some NSAIDs reduce production of the Aβ peptides (Gasparini et al., 2004), a major component of amyloid in plaques and around cerebral blood vessels. A recent study examined the influence of long-term use of NSAIDs that were shown to influence Aβ1–42 production and those that did not (Vlad et al., 2008). The study showed that NSAID use was effective in protecting against AD, but there was no difference between NSAIDs that did or did not alter Aβ1–42 production. Despite these positive findings in epidemiology studies, the impact of NSAIDs has not yet translated into clinical efficacy in a number of clinical trials. The reasons for this are at present unclear but may include the class of NSAID used, the time of initiation of the trial, the length of the trial, and other as yet uncontrolled for variables.

While these epidemiology data suggest that inflammation may contribute to AD progression, precisely how is much less clear; if we are to understand mechanisms, we need to study animal models. These models are commonly carried out in well-defined environmental conditions that then allow the experimenter to address which of the myriad of environmental factors may influence disease progression in AD.

Inflammation in Models of Alzheimer's Disease

It is well recognized that no single animal model can recapitulate all aspects of a human disease, and choice of a particular model will much depend on the particular question that is being asked. There are now many animal models that mimic different aspects of AD pathology in genetically modified mice. Several mouse lines carry transgenes leading to overexpression of human APP and deposition of Aβ1–40/42 in amyloid plaques within the brain parenchyma (McGowan et al., 2006). Although these mice show memory deficits with advancing age and increasing deposition of amyloid, there is little evidence of the catastrophic widespread neurodegeneration that is typical of the AD brain. The generation of genetically modified mice with multiple trans-genes has to date failed to generate a model with a robust progressive neurodegenerative disease. The triple transgenic mice carrying three mutated human genes (APP, PS-1, and tau) show the hallmarks of human AD with both amyloid deposits and intracellular tangles, but again there are no reports of widespread extensive neurodegeneration typical of AD pathology.

In the light of the potential role of inflammation in AD, my colleagues and I were interested in understanding how microglia would respond to the presence of both slowly accumulating misfolded protein or amyloid and chronic slowly evolving degeneration of neurons and their processes. Mouse models of prion disease have been studied for many years, and the selection of mouse strain and prion agent permits the experimenter to chose a combination that will target a particular brain region and disease that will evolve over varying periods of time (Bruce, 1993). Murine prion disease is also a valuable model since it is readily inducible in strains of geneti-cally modified mice, which in turn allows dissection of the role of selected molecules or molecu-lar pathways in influencing disease progression.

Microglia Response to Chronic Neurodegenerative Disease

The ME7 prion agent, when injected into C57BL mice, leads to pathology in the hippocampus, other regions of the limbic system, thalamus, and cortex. In this model the overt behavioral changes commonly used to classify disease onset appear at about 140 days, and terminal disease is at 165 days. To understand the contribution of inflammation to disease progression, we wanted to identify the earliest components of the disease since simply extending the terminal phases of disease would be of little benefit if translated to a clinical setting. We developed a battery of behavioral tasks that have largely relied on species-specific spontaneous behaviors that previous work suggested may be of value (see Guenther et al., 2001, for references). These tasks detect deficits in rewarding behaviors such as glucose consumption, burrowing, and nest building as early as 12–13 weeks into disease progression, two months before the onset of overt clinical signs. Hyperactivity in the open field appears at about 14 weeks, followed by deficits in several cognitive tasks, which in turn are followed by deficits in motor strength and coordination at about 18 weeks. The behavioral tasks allow us to follow the spread of the disease through the brain. Prion diseases share a fascinating property in common with AD, namely, that the pathology spreads in a predictable fashion along anatomically connected pathways from one brain region to the next. Using the morphological changes and upregulation of antigens expressed by activated microglia as an indicator of pathology, we have followed the spread of disease from a focal injection in the dorsal hippocampus through the limbic system and then to other regions of the brain, including the cortex and cerebellum (Betmouni et al., 1996).

The early behavioral deficits in burrowing and nesting, behaviors that depend on the integrity of the hippocampus, and the presence of activated microglia in the hippocampus led us to investigate whether microglia were synthesizing cytokines or inflammatory mediators that might impair synaptic signaling. We found that rather than a pro-inflammatory profile in the hippocampus, there was an anti-inflammatory profile (see Perry et al., 2002, for references). With hindsight, it is perhaps not surprising that the microglia did not have an inflammatory phenotype since the accumulation of misfolded PrP^{Sc} and the degeneration of neurons or their processes had presumably accumulated over a period of many weeks leading to the adaptation or tolerance of the microglia. Macrophage tolerance to repeated exposure of endotoxin is a well-studied phenomenon and might well be expected of microglia continuously exposed to misfolded protein fibrils or slowly degenerating neurons. We have addressed whether the exposure of other tissue macrophages to the same misfolded PrP^{Sc} protein might lead to their activation or generation of a pro-inflammatory phenotype. This is conveniently done in prion disease where misfolded PrP^{Sc} accumulates not only in the brain but also in the spleen. Spleen macrophages do not appear to be activated by the presence of the PrP^{Sc} (Cunningham et al., 2005b), in keeping with observations on other systemic amyloidoses where macrophages are very inefficient at phagocytosing amyloid.

Characterization of the cytokine milieu in the prion diseased hippocampus revealed that there were high levels of the anti-inflammatory cytokine transforming growth factor $-\beta1$(TGF-$\beta1$), prostaglandin E2, and the chemokine CCL-2/macrophage chemotactic protein-1 (Perry et al., 2002). The former two mediators are of interest since they are associated with macrophages that have phagocytosed apoptotic cells (Serhan and Savill, 2005): cells undergoing apoptosis have been described in the brain in advanced stages of murine prion disease. However, the early hippocampal pathology is associated with a loss of synapses from the stratum radiatum prior to evidence of neuronal apoptosis (Cunningham et al., 2003). The vast majority of the synapses in stratum radiatum arise from the CA3 pyramidal cells, and these cells survive throughout the course of the disease although the cell soma shrinks (Gray et al., 2009).

One function that has been ascribed to microglia is the removal of synapses from the cell surface of axotomized neurons undergoing chromatolysis, so-called "synaptic stripping" (Moran and Graeber, 2004). We investigated whether microglia were involved in the removal of the degenerating CA3 Schaffer collateral synapses from the dendrites of CA1 pyramidal neurons and whether phagocytosis of synapses may account for the anti-inflammatory phenotype. Electron microscopy revealed that there were large numbers of synapses lost from the stratum radiatum at 13 weeks into the disease, and synaptic degeneration increased as the disease progressed (Siskova et al., 2009). In contrast to the relatively linear appearance of the postsynaptic density

(PSD) adjacent to the presynaptic bouton in normal hippocampus, we observed that in diseased brains the PSDs were progressively curved around the dark degenerating synapses. Using serial sections from both conventional and dual-beam electron microscopy, we found that the PSD of the dendritic spine almost completely enwrapped the degenerating presynaptic element (Siskova et al., 2009). There was no evidence that the processes of microglia or astrocytes were directly involved in the removal of the degenerating synapses. The enwrapping, and perhaps even internalization, of presynaptic boutons has been described previously in developing neurons (Ronnevi, 1979).

If the microglia are not involved in the removal of synapses early in disease evolution, what might be the consequence of their activated but anti-inflammatory phenotype? There is much interest in the possibility that inflammation in the brain may play a role in protection or repair from chronic neurodegeneration (Rivest, 2009). We investigated the impact of neutralizing the TGF-β1 in prion diseased brain by using an adenovirus vector to deliver decorin, a scavanger of TGF-β1 (Boche et al., 2006). The virus alone had little impact on the pathology, but the delivery of decorin resulted in a dramatic increase in the extent of the microglia activation and significant cell loss of CA1 pyramidal cells. It appears that the TGF-β1 plays an important anti-inflammatory role and is protective. However, in the absence of an additional manipulation, we have little evidence that the activated microglia play any significant role in disease progression, and we suggest that rather than describing the inflammation as positive or negative it is best described as "benign."

As described above, the innate inflammatory response in the prion diseased brain is somewhat different from that described in postmortem material from patients who have died with AD. The results beg the question as to whether this mouse model of chronic neurodegeneration can really tell us anything about the pathogenesis of a human disease. Why are there no pro-inflammatory cytokines in the prion diseased brain despite the massive loss of neurons? Why does the inflammatory response appear benign? One major difference between mice with prion disease and AD patients is that unlike our mice, many people who die with AD also have significant co-morbidities such a vascular disease and diabetes, and a large proportion of patients die from systemic infectious diseases such as pneumonia.

Systemic Inflammation and Chronic Neurodegeneration

We are all aware that a systemic infection communicates with the brain: this is why we feel ill and show the spectrum of metabolic and behavioral changes referred to as sickness behavior when we get an infection. The pathways by which signals from peripheral infection or inflammation communicate with the brain have been identified and include both neural and humoral routes (Dantzer et al., 2008; Teeling and Perry, 2009). An important feature of this signaling is that there is signaling across an intact blood-brain barrier involving endothelial cells, perivascular macrophages, and microglia. The signaling to the brain from a systemic infection is part of our normal homeostasis, and there is no evidence that this leads to permanent changes in brain structure or function, except perhaps during sepsis. In contrast, there is evidence that systemic infections may have a profound effect on the diseased brain. The majority of patients with multiple sclerosis suffer from a relapsing–remitting form of the disease, at least in the initial stages, with the clinical signs waxing and waning (Compston and Coles, 2008). Approximately one-third of relapses are associated with a systemic infection, and infection-induced relapses are associated with significant and prolonged disability (Buljevac et al., 2002). In elderly individuals or patients with AD who contract a systemic infection, this may lead to delirium, which is an acute failure of cognition and attention (Fong et al., 2009). The impact of an episode of delirium is a significant risk factor for either the progression to dementia or progression of ongoing underlying dementing disease (Fong et al., 2009).

Systemic Inflammation in Neurodegeneration

We studied the impact of systemic inflammation on the innate inflammatory response in the prion diseased brain by injecting mice with lipopolysaccharide (LPS) to mimic aspects of a systemic infection. The acute effects of LPS in naive mice have been extensively studied and lead to fever, reduced activity, and loss of body weight in addition to other aspects of sickness behavior (Dantzer et al., 2008; Teeling and Perry, 2009). The mice with prion disease showed exaggerated sickness behavior, and increased levels of pro-inflammatory cytokines were present in the brain when compared to naive animals challenged with the same dose of LPS (Combrinck et al., 2002; Cunningham et al., 2005a). The differences in brain cytokine production and behavioral changes cannot be attributed to differences in systemic cytokine response (Cunningham et al., 2005b). Further analysis of the microglia phenotype by immunocytochemistry revealed that microglia in the prion diseased mice were not morphologically distinguishable between those that had a systemic LPS challenge and those that had not (Perry et al., 2007). Further staining revealed that the cytokine interleukin-1β (IL-β) could be detected in the perivascular macrophages of naive mice challenged with LPS and could not be detected in microglia of prion diseased mice: but IL-1β could be readily detected in microglia of prion diseased mice challenged with LPS. We proposed that in prion disease the microglia are "primed" by the ongoing neuropathology and morphologically activated but systemic inflammation then switches the microglia from an anti-inflammatory to a pro-inflammatory profile (Cunningham et al., 2005a; Cunningham et al., 2009; Perry et al., 2007). The switch in microglia phenotype in the prion diseased animals is also associated with an acute increase in the number of neurons undergoing apoptosis (Cunningham et al., 2005a) and acceleration in the onset of cognitive and motor deficits (Cunningham et al., 2009). The change in the innate immune response in the prion diseased brain is further highlighted by experiments in which an LPS challenge was made directly into the brain. In naive animals, LPS injection into the brain parenchyma led to little neutrophil recruitment and no detectable inducible nitric oxide synthase (iNOS) in microglia, but in animals with prion disease, there was dramatic recruitment of neutrophils to the brain parenchyma and readily detectable iNOS expression in microglia (Cunningham et al., 2005a).

The priming of microglia by ongoing neurodegeneration has profound consequences for the impact of a secondary inflammatory challenge, be it in the periphery or in the brain itself.

The impact of systemic inflammation on neurodegeneration has now been investigated in a number of different mouse models. Systemic inflammation has been shown to increase proinflammatory cytokine synthesis in a model of AD (Sly et al., 2001), accelerate motor neuron degeneration in a model of amyotrophic lateral sclerosis (Nguyen et al., 2004), exacerbate neuronal loss in a model of Parkinson's disease (Godoy et al., 2008), and switch the microglia phenotype in Wallerian degeneration (Palin et al., 2008). Microglia in aged animals also adopt an activated morphology and show an exaggerated response to systemic inflammation with an accompanying exaggeration of LPS-induced sickness behaviors (Godbout et al., 2005). The impact of systemic inflammation on the phenotype of microglia primed by ongoing pathology appears to be a generic response and is likely to be of consequence in diverse diseases of the CNS.

Systemic Infections in Alzheimer's Disease Patients

The observations described above in animal models show that interactions between systemic inflammation and the microglia might have a profound influence on the acute and chronic phases of a neurodegenerative disease. Although systemic inflammation may exacerbate the acute symptoms of a chronic neurodegenerative disease in patients, there is little information as to whether systemic inflammation or infections influence the long-term progression of disease in the absence of overt delirium. We carried out a prospective study in a relatively large cohort of AD patients to test the hypothesis that systemic inflammation associated with increased serum cytokine levels would be associated with long-term cognitive decline independent of acute delirium (Holmes et al., 2009). Three hundred patients with mild to severe AD were studied over a six-month interval. At baseline, patients were cognitively assessed and a blood sample was taken for evidence of systemic inflammation, and then at two monthly intervals, the subjects were reassessed for their cognitive status and further blood samples were taken. Carers kept a diary of systemic inflammatory events (SEIs) with an SEI defined as a short-lived transient infection or trauma not directly involving the CNS with a minimum C-reactive protein level of 1 ug/mL after the event.

At baseline, there were patients who were classified as having low levels of serum tumor necrosis factor α (TNF-α less than 2.4pg/ml) and those who had high levels (more than 2.4pg/ml). Approximately half of the subjects had an SEI over the six-month period, and these included those typical of these elderly subjects, urinary tract infections, gastrointestinal infections, and upper respiratory tract infections. Increased levels of serum TNF-α were associated with a four-fold increase in the rate of cognitive decline relative to the low serum TNF-α subjects. It is not known whether the raised TNF-α levels are associated with occult infections or other comorbidities, for example, atherosclerosis, periodontitis, diabetes, smoking, and obesity, all known to be risk factors for disease progression in AD (see Blennow et al., 2006, and Holmes et al., 2009, for references). The effect of having both raised TNF-α at baseline and an SIE over the next six months was profound with a 10-fold rate of decline in those with raised TNF-α at baseline and SIEs relative to those with low TNF-α and no SIEs over the period of study.

At the present time, this is only an association between systemic inflammation and cognitive decline, and it is thus possible that patients with impaired cognition are more susceptible to infections or trauma that lead to systemic inflammation. However, we found no evidence that the more cognitively impaired had a greater frequency of SEIs at or preceding baseline. The evidence supports the hypothesis that systemic inflammation may accelerate the rate of cognitive decline in patients with AD although further prospective or intervention studies will be required to advance this hypothesis.

Environmental Factors and Opportunities

If systemic inflammation plays a part in driving the progression of dementia, it offers a route to therapeutic intervention either by pharmaceutical intervention to treat the infection and inflammation or by manipulating other aspects of lifestyle or environment to reduce systemic inflammation. Other possible factors that may influence the development of AD include education, occupation, and diet although much needs to be done to confirm this (Blennow et al., 2006). In the laboratory it is well established that environmental enrichment can have a profound impact on the developing and diseased brain, as recently reviewed by Lamberto Maffei and colleagues (Sale et al., 2009), but how and whether similar concepts can be used to alleviate the symptoms and progression of AD in the community remain to be investigated. In a disease where the major risk factor is old age, the concept of a "cure" is not so easy to define, but the opportunities to delay disease onset and progression are waiting to be grasped.

Acknowledgments

The work carried out in the author's laboratory was funded by the Wellcome Trust and Medical Research Council (UK).

Note

This chapter is based on a lecture given at a seminar at the Scuola Normale Superiore di Pisa, September 2008, in honor of Professor Lamberto Maffei, a wonderful and generous friend of many years.

References

Akiyama H, Barger S, Barnum S, Bradt B, Bauer J, Cole GM, Cooper NR, et al. 2000. Inflammation and Alzheimer's disease. *Neurobiol Aging* 21: 383–421.

Betmouni S, Perry VH, Gordon JL. 1996. Evidence for an early inflammatory response in the central nervous system of mice with scrapie. *Neuroscience* 74: 1–5.

Blennow K, de Leon MJ, Zetterberg H. 2006. Alzheimer's disease. *Lancet* 368: 387–403.

Boche D, Cunningham C, Docagne F, Scott H, Perry VH. 2006. TGFbeta1 regulates the inflammatory response during chronic neurodegeneration. *Neurobiol Dis* 22: 638–650.

Bruce ME. 1993. Scrapie strain variation and mutation. *Br Med Bull* 49: 822–838.

Buljevac D, Flach HZ, Hop WC, Hijdra D, Laman JD, Savelkoul HF, van Der Meché FG, van Doorn PA, Hintzen RQ. 2002. Prospective study on the relationship between infections and multiple sclerosis exacerbations. *Brain* 125(Pt 5): 952–960.

Combrinck MI, Perry VH, Cunningham C. 2002. Peripheral infection evokes exaggerated sickness behaviour in pre-clinical murine prion disease. *Neuroscience* 112: 7–11.

Compston A, Coles A. 2008. Multiple sclerosis. *Lancet* 372: 1502–1517.

Cunningham C, Campion S, Lunnon K, Murray CL, Woods JF, Deacon RM, Rawlins JN, Perry VH. 2009. Systemic inflammation induces acute behavioral and cognitive changes and accelerates neurodegenerative disease. *Biol Psychiatry* 65: 304–312.

Cunningham C, Deacon R, Wells H, Boche D, Waters S, Diniz CP, Scott H, Rawlins JN, Perry VH. 2003. Synaptic changes characterize early behavioural signs in the ME7 model of murine prion disease. *Eur J Neurosci* 17: 2147–2155.

Cunningham C, Wilcockson DC, Campion S, Lunnon K, Perry VH. 2005a. Central and systemic endotoxin challenges exacerbate the local inflammatory response and increase neuronal death during chronic neurodegeneration. *J Neurosci* 25: 9275–9284.

Cunningham C, Wilcockson DC, Boche D, Perry VH. 2005b. Comparison of inflammatory and acute-phase responses in the brain and peripheral organs of the ME7 model of prion disease. *J Virol* 79: 5174–5184.

Dantzer R, O'Connor JC, Freund GG, Johnson RW, Kelley KW. 2008. From inflammation to sickness and depression: when the immune system subjugates the brain. *Nat Rev Neurosci* 9: 46–56.

Edison P, Archer HA, Gerhard A, Hinz R, Pavese N, Turkheimer FE, Hammers A, et al. 2008. Microglia, amyloid, and cognition in Alzheimer's disease: An [11C](R)PK11195-PET and [11C]PIB-PET study. *Neurobiol Dis* 32: 412–419.

Etminan M, Gill S, Samii A. 2003. Effect of non-steroidal anti-inflammatory drugs on risk of Alzheimer's disease: systematic review and meta-analysis of observational studies. *BMJ* 327: 128.

Ferri CP, Prince M, Brayne C, Brodaty H, Fratiglioni L, Ganguli M, Hall K, et al., and the Alzheimer's Disease International. 2005. Global prevalence of dementia: a Delphi consensus study. *Lancet* 366: 2112–2117.

Fong TG, Jones RN, Shi P, Marcantonio ER, Yap L, Rudolph JL, Yang FM, Kiely DK, Inouye SK. 2009. Delirium accelerates cognitive decline in Alzheimer disease. *Neurology* 72: 1570–1575.

Gasparini L, Ongini E, Wenk G. 2004. Non-steroidal anti-inflammatory drugs (NSAIDs) in Alzheimer's disease: old and new mechanisms of action. *J Neurochem* 91: 521–536.

Godbout JP, Chen J, Abraham J, Richwine AF, Berg BM, Kelley KW, Johnson RW. 2005. Exaggerated neuroinflammation and sickness behavior in aged mice following activation of the peripheral innate immune system. *FASEB J* 19: 1329–1331.

Godoy MC, Tarelli R, Ferrari CC, Sarchi MI, Pitossi FJ. 2008. Central and systemic IL-1 exacerbates neurodegeneration and motor symptoms in a model of Parkinson's disease. *Brain* 131(Pt 7): 1880–1894.

Gray BC, Siskova Z, Perry VH, O'Connor V. 2009. Selective presynaptic degeneration in the synaptopathy associated with ME7-induced hippocampal pathology. *Neurobiol Dis* 35(1): 63–74.

Guenther K, Deacon RM, Perry VH, Rawlins JN. 2001. Early behavioural changes in scrapie-affected mice and the influence of dapsone. *Eur J Neurosci* 14: 401–409.

Hardy J, Singleton A. 2009. Genomewide association studies and human disease. *N Engl J Med* 360: 1759–1768.

Holmes C, Cunningham C, Zotova E, Woolford J, Dean C, Kerr S, Culliford D, Perry VH. 2009. Systemic inflammation and disease progression in Alzheimer disease. *Neurology* 73: 768–774.

Lawson LJ, Perry VH, Gordon S. 1992. Turnover of resident microglia in the normal adult mouse brain. *Neuroscience* 48: 405–415.

McGowan E, Eriksen J, Hutton M. 2006. A decade of modeling Alzheimer's disease in transgenic mice. *Trends Genet* 22: 281–289.

Menken M, Munsat TL, Toole JF. 2000. The global burden of disease study: implications for neurology. *Arch Neurol* 57: 418–420.

Moran LB, Graeber MB. 2004. The facial nerve axotomy model. *Brain Res Brain Res Rev* 44(2–3): 154–178.

Mosser DM, Edwards JP. 2008. Exploring the full spectrum of macrophage activation. *Nat Rev Immunol* 8: 958–969.

Nguyen MD, D'Aigle T, Gowing G, Julien JP, Rivest S. 2004. Exacerbation of motor neuron disease by chronic stimulation of innate immunity in a mouse model of amyotrophic lateral sclerosis. *J Neurosci* 24: 1340–1349.

Nimmerjahn A, Kirchhoff F, Helmchen F. 2005. Resting microglial cells are highly dynamic surveillants of brain parenchyma in vivo. *Science* 308: 1314–1318.

Palin K, Cunningham C, Forse P, Perry VH, Platt N. 2008. Systemic inflammation switches the inflammatory cytokine profile in CNS Wallerian degeneration. *Neurobiol Dis* 30(1): 19–29.

Perry VH, Cunningham C, Boche D. 2002. Atypical inflammation in the central nervous system in prion disease. *Curr Opin Neurol* 15: 349–354.

Perry VH, Cunningham C, Holmes C. 2007. Systemic infections and inflammation affect chronic neurodegeneration. *Nat Rev Immunol* 7(2): 161–167.

Ransohoff RM, Perry VH. 2009. Microglial physiology: unique stimuli, specialized responses. *Annu Rev Immunol* 27: 119–145.

Rivest S. 2009. Regulation of innate immune responses in the brain. *Nat Rev Immunol* 9: 429–439.

Ronnevi LO. 1979. Spontaneous phagocytosis of C-type synaptic terminals by spinal alpha-motoneurons in newborn kittens: an electron microscopic study. *Brain Res* 162(2): 189–199.

Sale A, Bernardi N, Maffei L. 2009. Enrich the environment to empower the brain. *Trends Neurosci* 34: 233–239.

Serhan CN, Savill J. 2005. Resolution of inflammation: the beginning programs the end. *Nat Immunol* 6: 1191–1197.

Siskova Z, Page A, O'Connor V, Perry VH. 2009. Degenerating synaptic boutons in prion disease: microglia activation without synaptic stripping. *Am J Pathol* 175: 1610–1621.

Sly LM, Krzesicki RF, Brashler JR, Buhl AE, McKinley DD, Carter DB, Chin JE. 2001. Endogenous brain cytokine mRNA and inflammatory responses to lipopolysaccharide are elevated in the Tg2576 transgenic mouse model of Alzheimer's disease. *Brain Res Bull* 56: 581–588.

Stout RD, Jiang C, Matta B, Tietzel I, Watkins SK, Suttles J. 2005. Macrophages sequentially change their functional phenotype in response to changes in microenvironmental influences. *J Immunol* 175: 342–349.

Teeling JL, Perry VH. 2009. Systemic infection and inflammation in acute CNS injury and chronic neurodegeneration: underlying mechanisms. *Neuroscience* 158: 1062–1073.

Vlad SC, Miller DR, Kowall NW, Felson DT. 2008. Protective effects of NSAIDs on the development of Alzheimer disease. *Neurology* 70: 1672–1677.

26 Nerve Growth Factor and Alzheimer's Disease: New Twists to an Old Story

Antonino Cattaneo

The Debate around the Mechanisms Leading to Alzheimer's Disease

Progressive synaptic and neuronal loss in Alzheimer's disease (AD) leads to cognitive decline. No cure and no early diagnosis are presently available for AD. An early and predominant loss of basal forebrain cholinergic neurons (BFCNs) is the major functional basis for the cognitive impairment in AD, laying the grounds for the "cholinergic hypothesis" of AD (Bartus et al., 1982). At the neuropathological level, amyloid plaques and neurofibrillary tangles are the histological hallmarks, made from Aβ peptide, a cleaved product of the amyloid precursor protein (APP) and from hyperphosphorylated Tau, a microtubule binding protein, respectively.

Despite intensive research in the past two decades, no generally accepted mechanism has yet been formulated causally linking the AD triad (cholinergic deficit, amyloid Aβ, and Tau pathologies) into one unified conceptual scheme. Following the discovery that mutations in genes encoding APP and Tau cause dementing illnesses, the cholinergic hypothesis was abandoned, and the Alzheimer's field was dominated by disputes over whether Aβ or Tau abnormalities represented an upstream pivotal pathogenic cause driving the disease (the Baptist vs. Taoist confrontation).

Genetic studies of rare monogenic forms of the disease (early onset Alzheimer's disease; EOAD), which recapitulate the neuropathological and clinical profile of sporadic, late onset Alzheimer's disease (LOAD), provided the main driving force in the debate on AD mechanisms. Mutations in APP (Goate et al., 1991) and in presenilin PS-1 and PS-2 genes (Levy-Lahad et al., 1995; Rogaev et al., 1995; Sherrington et al., 1995), determining an increased Aβ processing, were found to underlie EOAD. In contrast, mutations in the gene encoding Tau, although found to cause Tau hyperphosphorylation, lead to frontotemporal dementia (FTD; Hutton et al., 1998), which is histologically distinct from AD and has no amyloid plaques. These findings reinforced the case for a serial model of causality in AD, with elevation of Aβ as the prime pathogenic driver of AD, the "amyloid hypothesis" (Hardy and Selkoe, 2002; Tanzi and Bertram, 2005; see figure 26.1a). Because EOAD and LOAD phenocopy each other clinically (except for the age of onset) and histologically, the amyloid hypothesis, although based on EOAD genetic data, was de facto extended to underlie LOAD as well. Indeed, bridging the knowledge of the molecular

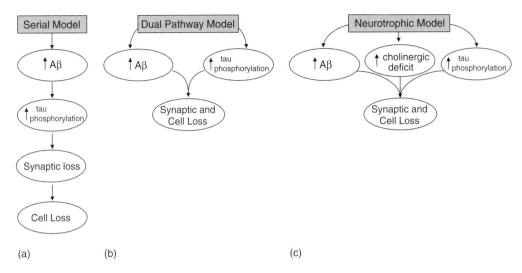

Figure 26.1
Hypothesized models linking core features of Alzheimer's disease (AD). (a) The amyloid hypothesis assumes a serial model of causality, whereby abnormal elevations of Aβ drive Tau hyperphosphorylation and other downstream manifestations of the disease. (b) Dual pathway model postulates Aβ elevation and Tau hyperphosphorylation to be linked by separate mechanisms driven by a common upstream molecular defect. (c) In this model, the common upstream driver of AD neurodegeneration is represented by alterations in neurotrophic signaling, linking the AD triad into one multiple mechanism.

mechanisms of EOAD to the etiology of sporadic LOAD is a great challenge to unraveling AD mechanisms.

The Amyloid Hypothesis Failed to Deliver Effective Therapeutic Treatments

Largely because of the strong genetic data, the amyloid hypothesis has been the driving force in guiding pharmaceutical efforts toward new treatments. Accordingly, pharmacological agents reducing brain Aβ levels should act as effective drugs for AD. However, it is noteworthy that, to date, the results of many clinical studies testing new amyloid-lowering treatments failed to deliver the expected results and have been largely disappointing. Among the different anti-Aβ-agents tested in LOAD patients, Aβ immunization is the most innovative approach (Wisniewski and Konietzko, 2008). Anti-Aβ antibodies are either elicited by active immunization or directly delivered as human recombinant antibodies (passive immunization). Despite preclinical studies in mouse models showing effective clearing of Aβ from the brain, Aβ42 immunization clinical trials (as well as those with other anti-Aβ pharmacological treatments) failed to show any clinical efficacy whatsoever. One study for all (Holmes et al., 2008), documenting the long-term effects of active Aβ42 immunization, illustrates well the case. The clinical trial was halted because of lethal meningoencephalitis in a small number of subjects, but the study followed a group of patients free of the drug's negative side effects. The immunized patients showed no significant effect of immunization on any clinical measure over a six-year period. On the other hand, immunized patients, with high titers of anti-Aβ antibodies, had a significant reduction of brain Aβ, while Tau pathology was heavily disseminated across the cortex. Thus, effectively clearing amyloid plaques from the patients' brains had no effect whatsoever on their cognitive decline. A range of possible explanations were put forward to explain these incontrovertible negative results (Holmes et al., 2008; St George-Hyslop and Morris, 2008). The amyloid hypothesis could be defended by assuming that Aβ acts as a "trigger" of downstream events, so that, once initiated, neurodegeneration might progress even if Aβ levels are reduced. One could also assume that the truly neurotoxic forms of Aβ, such as oligomers, might not have been reduced in that clinical setting. Thus, the adjourned version of the amyloid hypothesis puts the accent on "early" and on "Aβ oligomers" and considers synapses the earliest target for these "more toxic" Aβ species (Selkoe, 2002). Nevertheless, the unequivocally negative results of the clinical studies targeting Aβ call for alternative models of causality, linking Aβ and Tau pathology to an upstream common molecular or cellular driver (see figure 26.1b; Small and Duff, 2008). Therefore, there is great interest to take into consideration the "nongenetic elevators of Aβ," and in the following I will present data from our group and from the literature that led us some time ago to propose neurotrophic deficits as a common upstream mechanism linking cholinergic, Aβ, and Tau abnormalities into one comprehensive "multiple pathway" mechanism of neurodegeneration (see figure 26.1c; reviewed in Capsoni and Cattaneo, 2006; Cattaneo et al., 2008). From this framework, any therapy aimed at reestablishing a correct balance between ligands (and receptors) of the nerve growth factor (NGF) pathway appears to have a clear and strong rationale, and I will describe recent attempts from our group to proceed in this direction.

Nerve Growth Factor and Alzheimer's Disease: An Old Connection

NGF (Levi-Montalcini, 1987) has been classically connected to AD (Hefti and Weiner, 1986), on a purely correlative basis, because of the selective vulnerability of BFCNs in AD (cholinergic connection) and of the retrograde transport of NGF in these neurons (retrograde transport connection).

BFCNs provide major projections to the cerebral cortex and the hippocampus, subserving cognitive functions and memory. NGF is BFCN principal target-derived neurotrophic factor, protecting them from various insults and from their aging dependent atrophy. Accordingly, a decreased trophic support, due to a reduced amount of NGF available to BFCNs, could contribute to the cholinergic cells loss observed in AD.

NGF is produced in the cortex and hippocampus and retrogradely transported to BFCN. NGF expression is not altered in AD. Several findings collectively support the view that a diminished retrograde transport of NGF can determine a reduced neurotrophic support to BFCNs. A reduced capacity of TrkA-dependent retrograde transport of NGF may lead to the loss of

BFCNs observed in early AD (Counts et al., 2004; Mufson et al., 2000) and explains why, in AD postmortem brains, NGF and proNGF proteins are increased in the cortex and hippocampus and are diminished in basal forebrain (Fahnestock et al., 1996).

Cytoskeletal transport dysfunctions, and a reduced axonal transport of NGF, represent a common link between NGF trophic deficits, cholinergic dysfunction, and neurodegeneration (Salehi et al., 2003; Schindowski et al., 2008), so that neurons in AD cannot take full advantage of NGF, since both APP and Tau are involved in axonal transport. In partial trisomy 16 Ts65Dn mice, increased APP expression is directly linked to reduced retrograde transport of NGF in BFCN, resulting in cholinergic neuronal degeneration, which can be reversed by exogenous NGF delivery to BFCN cell bodies (Salehi et al., 2003). However, in this view, a reduced neurotrophic support would be downstream of APP (or Tau) alterations.

Nerve Growth Factor and Alzheimer's Disease: The Emerging Complexity of proNGF/NGF Equilibrium

Other mechanisms, besides neuronal transport defects, could account for a reduced neurotrophic support to BFCN in AD. The emerging complexity of the proNGF/NGF system adds another correlative element to this picture

NGF is translated as a pre-pro-protein, which is cleaved by furin in the trans-Golgi network to yield mature NGF (reviewed in Shooter, 2001). ProNGF was initially thought to be a chaperone to assists folding and secretion of mature NGF. proNGF can also be released as such and cleaved extracellularly by plasmin and matrix metalloprotease-7 (Bruno and Cuello, 2006). proNGF and NGF turned out to have distinct biological activities (Lee et al., 2001): proNGF has a higher affinity for p75^{NTR} and a lower one for TrkA compared to mature NGF and induces p75^{NTR}-dependent apoptosis. ProNGF can also induce TrkA-dependent neuronal survival, although less effectively than NGF (Fahnestock et al., 2004). We recently reported the first structural study on proNGF, showing that the propeptide domain is an intrinsically unstructured domain and providing a structural interpretation to the distinct receptor binding profile of proNGF versus NGF (Paoletti et al., 2009). The prodomain of NGF interacts with sortilin, a neuronal type-1 VPS10-domain receptor, a coreceptor with p75^{NTR} for proNGF (Nykjaer et al., 2004). Sortilin, together with the VPS10-containing protein sorLA, binds the retromer complex in neurons. Converging evidence, including genetic data, implicates the retromer sorting pathway in LOAD (reviewed in Small and Duff, 2008). The levels of proNGF and its coreceptor sortilin increase in mild cognitive impairment and early AD brains (Counts et al., 2004; Fahnestock et al., 2001), paralleling the progressive decline in TrkA receptors. A diminished conversion of proNGF to mature NGF and an increased NGF degradation in AD brains was recently reported (Bruno et al., 2009).

Thus, the biological effects of proNGF *versus* NGF influence the balance between cell death and cell survival (Nykjaer et al., 2005; Hempstead, 2006), and an imbalance in this complex ligand/receptor system has been correlatively linked to AD neurodegeneration, although no causally direct proof in vivo is available so far.

Nerve Growth Factor and Alzheimer's Disease: The First Cause–Effect Demonstration. Anti-NGF AD11 Mice as a Comprehensive Model for Sporadic Alzheimer's Disease

The multiple correlative links between NGF and AD, described above, do not, however, provide evidence for a cause–effect mechanism leading to AD neurodegeneration and do not explain what activates the aberrant processing of APP and of Tau in sporadic AD.

The first demonstration that NGF deficits could have consequences beyond a direct interference with the cholinergic system came from our studies in the anti-NGF AD11 mouse model (Capsoni et al., 2000; Ruberti et al., 2000). These mice express a recombinant, highly specific anti-NGF antibody in the adult brain and allow study of the effects of a chronic neutralization of NGF in the adult brain after normal development. Quite unexpectedly, these mice progressively develop a comprehensive AD-like neurodegeneration, more severe than the expected cholinergic deficit per se, with functional and behavioral impairments, encompassing several features of human AD. The progressive impairment of working memory, revealed by a number of behavioral tasks (Berardi et al., 2007; De Rosa et al., 2005) is accompanied by synaptic plasticity deficits in the cortex (Origlia et al., 2006) and the hippocampus (Sola et al., 2006). At the neuropathological level, besides the expected deficit in BFCNs, AD11 mice show an intracellular and extracellular accumulation of β-amyloid in the hippocampus and a progressive neuronal expression of hyperphosphorylated and truncated Tau (Capsoni et al., 2002a).

The neurodegeneration in AD11 mice is NGF dependent, since it can be fully reverted by NGF administration (Capsoni et al., 2002b; De Rosa et al., 2005), demonstrating that NGF sequestration by antibodies results in Alzheimer's neurodegeneration. Cholinergic drugs fail to substantially revert neurodegeneration in AD11 mice, confirming that the cholinergic neurotransmission deficit is not a primary event of the neurodegeneration cascade in AD11. Breeding AD11 mice under environmental enrichment (EE) conditions rescues their memory and neuropathological deficits (Berardi et al., 2007). EE is a complex stimulus, and its effectiveness in rescuing AD11 neurodegeneration confirms this neurodegeneration to be a multifactorial process.

In summary, AD11 mice display a comprehensive neurodegeneration reminiscent of LOAD. Unlike other transgenic AD models, and similarly to LOAD, in AD11 mice beta-amyloid pathology arises from endogenous APP in the absence of a mutation in APP/APP processing genes. The phenotype of AD11 mice has uncovered a new mechanism whereby neurotrophic deficits are an upstream driver, causally linked to altered APP processing and Tau pathology, in addition to determining a cholinergic deficit (Capsoni and Cattaneo, 2006; Cattaneo et al., 2008).

The Mechanism of Neurodegeneration in AD11 Mice

How can we explain this neurodegenerative process, in mechanistic terms? What have we learned from this mouse model that could be translated to mechanisms operating in human LOAD?

"Too Little NGF—Too Much ProNGF"

The NGF binding properties of anti-NGF mAb αD11, expressed in the brain of AD11 mice, provided a first clue (Paoletti et al., 2009). It turns out that the anti-NGF mAb αD11, expressed in AD11 brains, binds NGF with a three orders of magnitude higher affinity than that for proNGF ($K_D = 10^{-12}$ M and 10^{-9} M for NGF and proNGF, respectively), with binding to NGF being virtually irreversible.

The preferential binding of mAb αD11 to mature NGF, with respect to proNGF, would determine, under limiting concentrations in the mouse brain, an experimentally induced functional imbalance between NGF and proNGF by irreversibly "sequestering" mature NGF while leaving proNGF free to act in the functional "absence" of mature NGF. proNGF would activate the proneurodegeneration, proamyloidogenic pathways, interacting with sortilin and p75^{NTR} receptors. A first test of this mechanism (Capsoni and Cattaneo, 2006; Cattaneo et al., 2008) comes from studies in which AD11 mice have been crossed to p75NTR knock-out mice (p75NTR –/–). The resulting offspring (AD12 mice) shows a complete reversion of the Aβ phenotype, confirming that amyloidogenesis in the AD11 model involves proNGF/p75 signaling.

Accordingly, the main determinant of neurodegeneration in anti-NGF mice would be the selective neutralization of NGF versus proNGF by an antibody in the brain: "too little NGF-too much proNGF" (Cattaneo et al., 2008; see figure 26.2). This provides a missing link for a proNGF/NGF centered vicious cycle, integrating data on amyloid Abeta inducing dysmetabolism of proNGF (Bruno and Cuello, 2006; Bruno et al., 2009) and on proNGF increase in AD brains (Fahnestock et al., 2001).

Nerve Growth Factor Signaling and Amyloid Precursor Protein Processing: Linking NGF Deficits to the Activation of the Amyloidogenic Cascade

The AD11 model establishes direct links between alterations in NGF signaling and aberrant APP/Tau processing. Further evidence supporting this concept comes from recent studies in cultured neurons. In differentiated PC12 and hippocampal neurons, rendered NGF dependent, NGF deprivation provokes an aberrant production of Aβ and apoptotic cell death, these effects being prevented by β- and γ-secretase inhibitors and by anti-Aβ antibodies (Matrone et al., 2008a, 2008b). Intriguingly, 24 hours after NGF withdrawal, TrkA phosphorylation rebounds to levels higher than those elicited by NGF, with a downstream activation of PLC-1γ, pointing to a novel, NGF-independent mechanism linking TrkA signaling to abnormal APP processing and neuronal death (Matrone et al., 2009). Neurotrophin actions are local. In cultured neurons, NGF deprivation determines axonal degeneration by a caspase-6 local mechanism, locally activating Death Receptor 6 by an inactive surface ligand that is released in an active form after trophic factor deprivation. The DR6 ligand was identified as APP, whose shedding in a β-secretase-dependent manner is induced by NGF deprivation (Nikolaev et al., 2009).

Thus, one of the consequences of trophic factor deprivation (or other NGF signaling and processing alterations) of BFCN could be a local action on their synaptic axonal terminals,

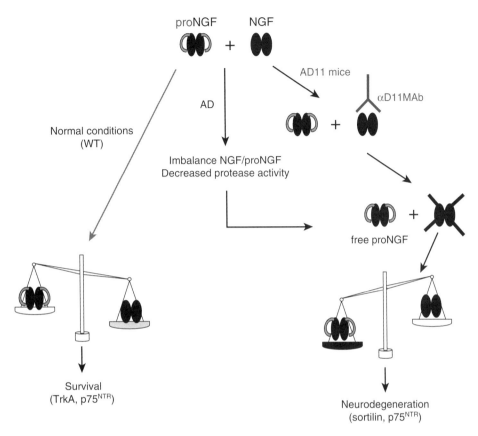

Figure 26.2
Schematic representation of the proNGF/NGF imbalance model. On the left side is the "normal" condition, when nerve growth factor (NGF) signaling is achieved mainly through the NGF/TrkA/p75NTR system. In the middle-right part of the scheme is a representation of the pathological conditions (middle, AD conditions; right, AD11 model): in both cases, an imbalance in the proNGF/NGF ratio takes place.

leading to an intra- and intercellular relay of APP-peptide-mediated local neurodegeneration that would extend the neurodegeneration to other cells/synaptic terminals.

NGF can therefore be considered as an anti-amyloidogenic factor that normally keeps the amyloidogenic pathway under control. Whenever a normal neurotrophic supply of NGF to target neurons is interrupted or altered, the amyloidogenic pathway is activated and a negative feedback, toxic loop is activated (see figure 26.3).

Synaptic Remodeling: Alterations in the Excitatory versus Inhibitory Balance
Mounting evidence suggests that AD is a synaptic failure and begins with subtle alterations of hippocampal synaptic efficacy, prior to frank neuronal degeneration (Selkoe, 2002). In AD11

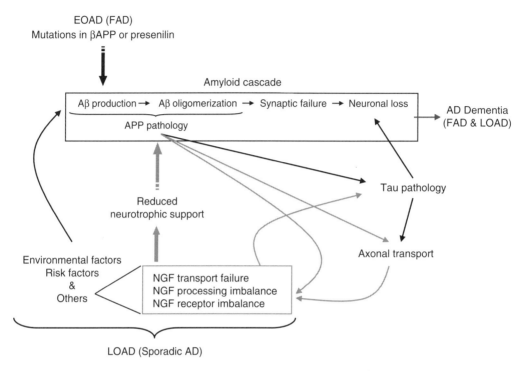

Figure 26.3
The NGF-APP and the NGF-Tau loops in sporadic late onset Alzheimer's disease (LOAD). Genetic predisposition and mutations can affect the metabolism of Aβ in early onset AD (EOAD; familial AD [FAD]), while environmental and other risk factors can lead to sporadic AD. Among the "other factors," we suggest an emerging role for (1) inflammation/immunotrophic disequilibrium (see figure 26.4) and (2) a disequilibrium in the NGF system (transport, processing, and receptor interactions), establishing a negative loop between the neurotrophic system, the amyloid cascade, and Tau pathology. APP, amyloid precursor protein.

mice, recent evidence demonstrated a major early synaptic remodeling, involving functional changes in the excitatory versus inhibitory drive in the hippocampus. GABAergic signaling shifts to an "immature" state, from hyperpolarizing to depolarizing, due to an alteration of chloride homeostasis and a downregulation of chloride transporter KCC2 expression (Lagostena et al., 2010). This major reorganization of the GABAergic circuitry within the AD11 hippocampal network may represent a homeostatic response to counterbalance neurodegeneration, or it may itself contribute to the progressive neurodegeneration. The developmental shift of GABA from depolarizing to hyerpolarizing is known to exert a critical control on the refinement of synaptic connections. The observed abnormal excitatory to inhibitory imbalance in the AD11 hippocampus shows that extensive synaptic remodeling is a major event in early neurodegeneration that could contribute to profoundly altering hippocampal circuits.

The Earliest Events in the Progression of Anti-NGF-Induced Neurodegeneration

What are the earliest events involved in the neurodegeneration mechanism, following the initial expression of anti-NGF antibodies in AD11 brains?

Global changes of gene expression were investigated, by microarray mRNA analysis, in the AD11 brain, during the earliest phases of incipient neurodegeneration (D'Onofrio et al., 2009). Postnatal days P30 to P60 are a "presymptomatic" phase of the progressive neurodegeneration. Surprisingly, wide changes in gene expression profiles occur even at P30, when no overt neuropathology is evident. The most significant differentially regulated mRNAs cluster in three gene families (D'Onofrio et al., 2009): inflammation and immune response, Wnt signaling, and synaptic neurotransmission. In the first cluster, mRNAs encoding for complement factor proteins, major histocompatibility complex, autophagic proteins, and cytokines/chemokines, show the largest differential expression. This parallels the involvement of inflammatory molecules in early stages of AD (Parachikova et al., 2007). Proteins of the innate immune system, such as complement proteins, have a "nonimmune" role in the physiological, developmentally regulated synapse elimination, a mechanism possibly reactivated in neurodegenerative diseases (Stevens et al., 2007). The early overexpression of complement cascade factors in the AD11 mouse model could contribute, very early on, to the synaptic deficits in this model, a prediction presently being tested.

The early massive modulation of Wnt pathway mRNAs is also noteworthy, in light of the independent, growing evidence showing the Wnt signaling pathway to be at the center of a dual pathway driving A-beta and Tau pathology in AD, also linked to APOE isoforms, GSK-3/Tau hyperphosphorylation, and the retromer sorting pathway (Small and Duff 2008).

This gene expression study shows that an early event in AD11 neurodegeneration is represented by a striking overall "immunotrophic," neurotrophic, and synaptic imbalance (D'Onofrio et al., 2009), broader than what would be expected on the basis of the simple, direct NGF/cholinergic connection. What does this teach us?

We believe the answer is in the specific mode of NGF neutralization, with anti-NGF antibodies in the brain. We propose that in AD11 mice the disease-causing event(s) is a direct selective neutralization of NGF versus-proNGF, combined with a response to the expression of an antibody in the brain, that might induce a neuroinflammatory and immunotrophic imbalance (see figure 26.4).

How could this mechanism relate to LOAD?

In a human AD setting, the two postulated pathological processes, NGF deficit(s) and presence of antibodies in the brain, need not be physically linked into one anti-NGF molecule, as in AD11 mice, and may or may not be causally linked. Thus, one could envisage that, in (a subset of) sporadic AD, the NGF system might be altered by one of several possible reasons (signaling alterations, processing imbalance, axonal transport defects, etc.; Capsoni and Cattaneo, 2006; Cattaneo et al., 2008; Salehi et al., 2003; Schindowski et al., 2008), while for related, or unrelated causes, systemic antibodies might diffuse into the brain, across a defective blood-brain barrier (Zlokovic, 2008), and determine neuroinflammation and immunotrophic imbalance.

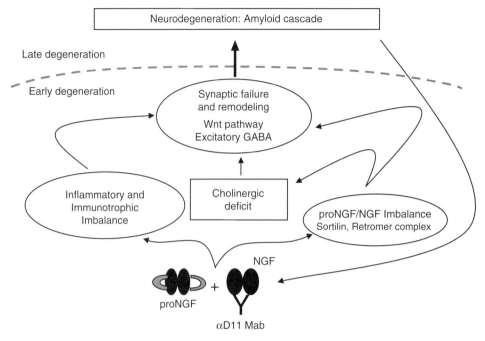

Figure 26.4
Early prodromal events in AD11 neurodegeneration: neurotrophic and immunotrophic imbalance. In the AD11 mouse brain, alongside with an "NGF-specific" stream, deriving from neutralization of NGF activity in cholinergic neurons, and a proNGF/NGF imbalance, antibodies in the brain may activate an "immune/inflammatory" stream, through activation of Fc receptors on neurons and microglia, inducing proinflammatory cytokine secretion and complement system activation, raising local neuroinflammation and contributing to the neurodegeneration process and to synaptic deficits.

Nerve Growth Factor and Alzheimer's Disease: The "New" Story

The experimental study of AD11 neurodegeneration demonstrated a novel causal link between neurotrophic signaling deficits and Alzheimer's neurodegeneration. Around these results, a new NGF hypothesis could be built, with neurotrophic deficits of various types representing an upstream driver of core AD triad pathology (see figure 26.3). Thus, AD neurodegeneration would arise from alterations of the homeostatic equilibrium of the NGF system leading, through a series of interconnected loops, to the activation of local and global neurodegeneration processes, ultimately determining the central core of AD hallmarks (see figure. 26.3). These neurotrophic deficits would be "located" upstream of the "amyloid cascade," as currently described, but would be part of a negative feedback loop that involves several feedback steps from the downstream process itself (e.g., links between APP, Tau, and axonal transport). Also, the cellular targets for NGF/proNGF actions, in this negative loop, could be more widespread than envisaged so far.

Essential elements of this mechanism, besides the "classical" NGF/TrkA/p75NTR system, are the proNGF/sortilin pathway, the retromer sorting complex, the Wnt signaling and immune and inflammatory effectors (see figure 26.4) acting on microglia and synapses, this progressively broadening the cellular basis of the pathology. Intercellular relay mechanisms for local neuro-degeneration events determine cell-to-cell, or synapse-to-synapse, spread of local neurodegen-eration and the broad cell involvement observed.

The "new" NGF hypothesis for LOAD (see figure 26.3) has significant therapeutical implica-tions. Any therapy aimed at reestablishing the correct balance between ligands (and receptors) of the NGF pathway appears to have a clear and strong rationale, as being truly able to interfere directly with a neurodegeneration mechanism involved in the disease process.

Nerve Growth Factor Based Therapies for Alzheimer's Disease: Taking Pain out of NGF

In this framework, the first therapeutic choice would be to use NGF itself as a drug. Clinical application of NGF requires solving two major problems: effective CNS delivery and limitation of adverse effects (most notably, pain). It is indeed a challenge to deliver NGF into the brain in a safe and efficient manner. First, NGF does not readily cross the blood-brain barrier. A second major issue is represented by the pronociceptive actions of NGF. Thus, NGF is a key pain mediator, controlling both the neural and the inflammatory components of pain (Pezet and McMahon, 2006).

The capacity of NGF to cause pain has been demonstrated in humans in the course of pilot clinical trials in AD patients (Eriksdotter Jonhagen et al., 1998), as well as during clinical trials undertaken to explore the potential use of NGF in peripheral polyneuropathies (Apfel, 2002). This has severely limited, in previous clinical trials, the dosage administrable to patients, jeopardizing the efficacy of the treatment (Apfel, 2002).

The clinical application of NGF in AD is therefore limited by a double constraint, of achieving a pharmacologically adequate concentration in target brain areas while preventing its adverse pain effects. For this reason, clinical trials evaluating NGF for AD have used invasive approaches, such as neurosurgery for the implant of autologous fibroblasts, engineered to secrete NGF, directly in the brain (Tuszynski et al., 2005), the direct stereotactic delivery into the brain of adeno-associated viral vectors encoding human NGF, or the chronic neurosurgical implant into the brain of biopolymer capsules filled with NGF-producing cells.

These invasive clinical approaches of NGF gene/cell therapy provide an independent valida-tion of the therapeutic potential of NGF in AD, and their outcome will provide insights into the safety, efficacy, and liabilities of NGF therapies. However, the approach is highly impractical for its extension to large numbers of AD patients. Therefore, a safe route for an effective, non-invasive delivery of NGF to the brain is required.

We have shown that the intranasal route allows a noninvasive, safe, and pharmacologically effective delivery of NGF to the brain (Capsoni et al., 2002b; De Rosa et al., 2005; Capsoni et al., 2009). NGF intranasal delivery represents an effective compromise to meet the required therapeutic window for NGF, leading to NGF buildup in target brain areas while minimizing its biodistribution to nontargeted districts where it induces pain (CSF and bloodstream).

The ideal NGF molecule for an NGF-based therapy should be traceable against endogenous NGF, to facilitate optimal dosing, and should have a reduced ability to activate nociceptive pathways while retaining identical neurotrophic activities. Thus, we designed a modified human NGF (hNGFP61S), "tagged" with a single distinctive residue, that can be easily traced against endogenous NGF and has a potency and bioactivity identical to hNGF (Covaceuszach et al., 2009). hNGFP61S constitutes a backbone whereby additional desirable functions, such as antinociceptive properties, could be further engineered into the therapeutic NGF molecule.

Is it possible to take pain out of NGF, engineering an NGF mutein having neurotrophic properties identical to hNGF but lacking its nociceptive pain-inducing activity?

Toward this aim, genetic data on a rare human syndrome, hereditary sensory and autonomic neuropathy, type V (HSAN V), were a source of inspiration. Two rare forms of human congenital insensitivity to pain are due to mutations in genes related to NGF signaling: hereditary sensory and autonomic neuropathy, type IV (HSAN IV), is due to mutations in the gene for TrkA (Indo et al., 1996, Indo, 2001), while HSAN type V is associated with a mutation (R100W) in the NGF gene (Einarsdottir et al., 2004). Both HSAN IV and V are characterized by profound loss of pain sensitivity and perception, accompanied, in HSAN IV, by severe mental retardation and learning problems (De Andrade et al., 2008). On the other hand, HSAN V patients show no mental retardation and have most neurological functions intact. The HSAN V mutation NGFR100W separates, from a clinical point of view, the neurodevelopmental effects of NGF from those involved in the activation of peripheral pain pathways, after development. This mutation could form the rational basis for the design of a "painless" NGF variant, that, while displaying a full neurotrophic activity, shows a reduced nociceptive activity. We therefore studied mechanistic aspects of the R100W mutation (Covaceuszach et al., 2010). Receptor binding measurements, with NGF recombinant proteins, demonstrated that while the affinity of NGF R100 mutants for the TrkA receptor was substantially unchanged, the binding for $p75^{NTR}$ was disrupted (1.5–2.2 nM for hNGF against 125–200 nM for hNGF R100; see figure 26.5; Capsoni et al., 2008; Covaceuszach et al., 2010). The neurotrophic potency of hNGF R100 mutants was indistinguishable from that of wild type hNGF. Interestingly, mutants hNGFR100 and hNGFP61S/R100 were equally effective as hNGF and hNGFP61S in activating, through TrkA, downstream shc and Akt pathways but failed to activate PLC-1γ. This selective TrkA signaling failure is noteworthy since the PLC-1γ pathway has been implicated in TrkA-mediated sensitization of sensory nociceptors (Chuang et al., 2001; Prescott and Julius, 2003). Thus, HSAN V-related hNGFR100 mutants have a decreased binding to the $p75^{NTR}$ receptor and an altered signaling of pronociceptive pathways (see table 26.1) Ongoing in vivo studies in pain and neurodegeneration models will confirm the therapeutic potential of these painless NGF molecules, displaying full neurotrophic activity and reduced pain-related signaling capability.

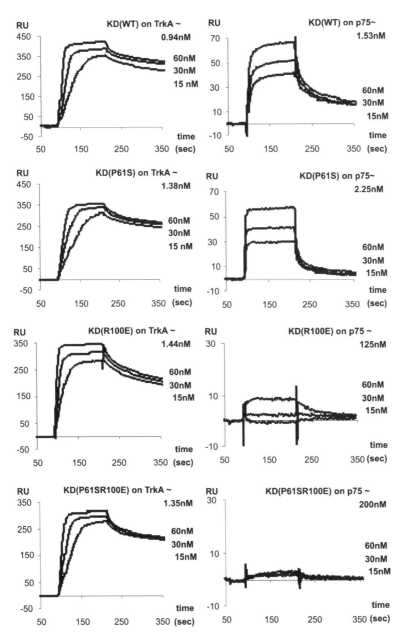

Figure 26.5
Binding affinity of painless NGF R100 mutants to TrkA and p75NTR receptors. Surface plasmon resonance receptor binding curves of hNGF, hNGFP61S, hNGFR100E, and hNGFP61S/R100E to immobilized TrKA (8400 RU) and p75NTR (4300 RU). K_D values (calculated from the full range of curves in the 15–640 nM range) are indicated (Covaceuszach et al., 2010), showing that binding to p75NTR by hNGF R100 mutants is abolished.

Table 26.1
Summary properties of hNGF R100 mutants

hNGF mutant	Binding to TrkA	Binding to P75NTR	Neurotrophic activity (cell assays)	PLC1γ activation	Nociceptive activity
hNGF	+	+	+	+	+
hNGFP61S	+	+	+	+	+
hNGFR100W	+	−	+	−	−
hNGFR100E	+	−	+	−	−
hNGFP61SR100E	+	−	+	−	n.d.

Concluding Personal Remarks

It has been for me a great and unique opportunity to be a student of Lamberto Maffei, back in 1977–1980, working on the primary visual cortex, a period of great intellectual excitement. Lamberto had created in the lab a scientific environment where discussing general topics and wild ideas was greatly encouraged, and he was always ready to listen, comment, suggest experiments, and ask questions that went to the root of the problem. My interest in neurotrophic factors dates back to those times, fostered by discussions with Lamberto, postulating a role for a hypothetical neurotrophic factor in shaping the horizontal organization of the visual cortex and the distribution of ocularity and ocular dominance columns. I like thinking that those discussions bore fruit a decade later when the fields of neurotrophins and the visual system were finally brought together. Thank you, Lamberto, for letting and helping your students' minds run free.

Acknowledgments

I am grateful to all the members of my lab at EBRI (Rome) and SNS for their enthusiasm, their hard work, and discussions.

References

Apfel SC. 2002. Nerve growth factor for the treatment of diabetic neuropathy: what went wrong, what went right, and what does the future hold? *Int Rev Neurobiol* 50: 393–413.

Bartus RT, Dean RL, 3rd, Beer B, Lippa AS. 1982. The cholinergic hypothesis of geriatric memory dysfunction. *Science* 217: 408–414.

Berardi N, Braschi C, Capsoni S, Cattaneo A, Maffei L. 2007. Environmental enrichment delays the onset of memory deficits and reduces neuropathological hallmarks in a mouse model of Alzheimer-like neurodegeneration. *J Alzheimers Dis* 11: 359–370.

Bruno MA, Cuello AC. 2006. Activity-dependent release of precursor nerve growth factor, conversion to mature nerve growth factor, and its degradation by a protease cascade. *Proc Natl Acad Sci USA* 103: 6735–6740.

Bruno MA, Leon WC, Fragoso G, Mushynski WE, Almazan G, Cuello AC. 2009. Amyloid –induced NGF dysmetabolism in Alzheimer disease. *J Neuropathol Exp Neurol* 68: 857–869.

Capsoni S, Ugolini G, Comparini A, Ruberti F, Berardi N, Cattaneo A. 2000. Alzheimer-like neurodegeneration in aged antinerve growth factor transgenic mice. *Proc Natl Acad Sci USA* 97: 6826–6831.

Capsoni S, Giannotta S, Cattaneo A. 2002a. Beta-amyloid plaques in a model for sporadic Alzheimer's disease based on transgenic anti-nerve growth factor antibodies. *Mol Cell Neurosci* 21: 15–28.

Capsoni S, Giannotta S, Cattaneo A. 2002b. Nerve growth factor and galantamine ameliorate early signs of neurodegeneration in anti-nerve growth factor mice. *Proc Natl Acad Sci USA* 99: 12432–12437.

Capsoni S, Cattaneo A. 2006. On the molecular basis linking nerve growth factor (NGF) to Alzheimer's disease. *Cell Mol Neurobiol* 26: 619–633.

Capsoni S, Covaceuszach S, Ugolini G, Spirito F, Vignone D, Stefanini B, Amato G, Cattaneo, A. 2009. Delivery of NGF to the brain: intranasal versus ocular administration in anti-NGF transgenic mice. *J Alzheimers Dis* 16: 371–388.

Capsoni S, Covaceuszach S, Marinelli S, Ugolini G, Vignone D, Spirito F, Amato G, Pavone F, Cattaneo A. Development of human nerve growth factor muteins with reduced algesic properties. *38th Annual Meeting Society for Neuroscience*, Washington DC, November 15–19, 2008. Abstract 340.4.

Cattaneo A, Capsoni S, Paoletti F. 2008. Towards noninvasive nerve growth factor therapies for Alzheimer's disease. *J Alzheimers Dis* 15: 255–283.

Chuang HH, Prescott ED, Kong H, Shields S, Jordt SE, Basbaum AI, Chao MV, Julius D. 2001. Bradykinin and nerve growth factor release the capsaicin receptor from PtdIns(4,5)P2-mediated inhibition. *Nature* 411: 957–962.

Counts SE, Nadeem M, Wuu J, Ginsberg SD, Saragovi HU, Mufson EJ. 2004. Reduction of cortical TrkA but not p75(NTR) protein in early-stage Alzheimer's disease. *Ann Neurol* 56: 520–531.

Covaceuszach S, Capsoni S, Ugolini G, Spirito F, Vignone D, Cattaneo A. 2009. Development of a non-invasive NGF-based therapy for Alzheimer's disease. *Curr Alzheimer Res* 6: 158–170.

Covaceuszach S, Capsoni S, Marinelli S, Pavone F, Ceci M, Ugolini G, Vignone D, Amato G, Paoletti F, lamba D, Cattaneo A. 2010. In vitro receptor binding properties of a "painless" NGF mutein linked to hereditary sensory autonomic neuropathy type V. *Biochem Biophys Res Commun* 391: 824–829.

De Andrade DC, Baudic S, Attal N, Rodrigues CL, Caramelli P, Lino AMM, Marchiori PE, et al. 2008. Beyond neuropathy in hereditary sensory and autonomic neuropathy type V: cognitive evaluation. *Eur J Neurol* 15: 712–719.

De Rosa R, Garcia AA, Braschi C, Capsoni S, Maffei L, Berardi N, Cattaneo A. 2005. Intranasal administration of nerve growth factor (NGF) rescues recognition memory deficits in AD11 anti-NGF transgenic mice. *Proc Natl Acad Sci USA* 102: 3811–3816.

D'Onofrio M, Arisi I, Brandi R, Di Mambro A, Felsani A, Capsoni S, Cattaneo A. 2009. Early inflammation and immune response mRNAs in the brain of AD11 anti−NGF mice. *Neurobiol Aging* Jul 13. [Epub ahead of print] PMID: 19604602.

Einarsdottir E, Carlsson A, Minde J, Toolanen G, Svensson O, Solders G, Holmgren G, Holmberg D, Holmberg M. 2004. A mutation in the nerve growth factor beta gene (NGFB) causes loss of pain perception. *Hum Mol Genet* 13: 799–805.

Eriksdotter Jonhagen M, Nordberg A, Amberla K, Backman L, Ebendal T, Meyerson B, Olson L, et al. 1998. Intracerebroventricular infusion of nerve growth factor in three patients with Alzheimer's disease. *Dement Geriatr Cogn Disord* 9: 246–257.

Fahnestock M, Scott SA, Jette N, Weingartner JA, Crutcher KA. 1996. Nerve growth factor mRNA and protein levels measured in the same tissue from normal and Alzheimer's disease parietal cortex. *Brain Res Mol Brain Res* 42: 175–178.

Fahnestock M, Michalski B, Xu B, Coughlin MD. 2001. The precursor pro-nerve growth factor is the predominant form of nerve growth factor in brain and is increased in Alzheimer's disease. *Mol Cell Neurosci* 18: 210–220.

Fahnestock M, Yu G, Coughlin MD. 2004. ProNGF: a neurotrophic or an apoptotic molecule? *Prog Brain Res* 146: 101–110.

Goate A, Chartier-Harlin MC, Mullan M, Brown J, Crawford F, Fidani L, Giuffra L, et al. 1991. Segregation of a missense mutation in the amyloid precursor protein gene with familial Alzheimer's disease. *Nature* 349: 704–706.

Hardy J, Selkoe D. 2002. The amyloid hypothesis of Alzheimer's disease: progress and problems on the road to therapeutics. *Science* 297: 353–356.

Hefti F, Weiner WJ. 1986. Nerve growth factor and Alzheimer's disease. *Ann Neurol* 20: 275–281.

Hempstead BL. 2006. Dissecting the diverse actions of pro- and mature neurotrophins. *Curr Alzheimer Res* 3: 19–24.

Holmes C, Boche D, Wilkinson D, Yadegarfar G, Hopkins V, Bayer A, Jones RW, et al. 2008. Long term effects of Abeta 42 immunization in Alzheimer's disease: follow-up of a randomized placebo-controlled phase I trial. *Lancet* 372: 216–223.

Hutton M, Lendon CL, Rizzu P, Baker M, Froelich S, Houlden H, Pickering-Brown S, et al. 1998. Association of missense and 5'-splice-site mutations in Tau with the inherited dementia FTDP-17. *Nature* 393: 702–705.

Indo Y, Tsuruta M, Hayashida Y, Karim MA, Ohta K, Kawano T, Mitsubuchi H, Tonoki H, Awaya Y, Matsuda I. 1996. Mutations in the TRKA/NGF receptor gene in patients with congenital insensitivity to pain with anhidrosis. *Nat Genet* 13: 485–488.

Indo Y. 2001. Molecular basis of congenital insensitivity to pain with anhidrosis (CIPA): mutations and polymorphisms in TRKA (NTRK1) gene encoding the receptor tyrosine kinase for nerve growth factor. *Hum Mutat* 18: 462–471.

Lagostena L, Rosato-Siri M, D'Onofrio M, Brandi R, Arisi I, Capsoni S, Franzot J, Cattaneo A, Cherubini E. 2010. In the adult hippocampus, chronic nerve growth factor deprivation shifts GABAergic signaling from the hyperpolarizing to the depolarizing direction. *J Neurosci* 30: 885–893.

Lee R, Kermani P, Teng KK, Hempstead BL. 2001. Regulation of cell survival by secreted proneurotrophins. *Science* 294: 1945–1948.

Levi-Montalcini R. 1987. The nerve growth factor 35 years later. *Science* 237: 1154–1162.

Levy-Lahad E, Wasco W, Poorkaj P, Romano DM, Oshima J, Pettingell WH, Yu CE, et al. 1995. Candidate gene for the chromosome 1 familial Alzheimer's disease locus. *Science* 269: 973–977.

Matrone C, Di Luzio A, Meli G, D'Aguanno S, Severini C, Ciotti MT, Cattaneo A, Calissano P. 2008a. Activation of the amyloidogenic route by NGF deprivation induces apoptotic death in PC12 cells. *J Alzheimers Dis* 13: 81–96.

Matrone C, Ciotti MT, Mercanti D, Marolda R, Calissano P. 2008b. NGF and BDNF signaling control amyloidogenic route and Abeta production in hippocampal neurons. *Proc Natl Acad Sci USA* 105: 13139–13144.

Matrone C, Marolda R, Ciafre S, Ciotti MT, Mercanti D, Calissano P. 2009. Tyrosine kinase nerve growth factor receptor switches from prosurvival to proapoptotic activity via Abeta-mediated phosphorylation. *Proc Natl Acad Sci USA* 106: 11358–11363.

Mufson EJ, Ma SY, Cochran EJ, Bennett DA, Beckett LA, Jaffar S, Saragovi HU, Kordower JH. 2000. Loss of nucleus basalis neurons containing trkA immunoreactivity in individuals with mild cognitive impairment and early Alzheimer's disease. *J Comp Neurol* 427: 19–30.

Nikolaev A, McLaughlin T, O'Leary DD, Tessier-Lavigne M. 2009. APP binds DR6 to trigger axon pruning and neuron death via distinct caspases. *Nature* 457: 981–989.

Nykjaer A, Lee R, Teng KK, Jansen P, Madsen P, Nielsen MS, Jacobsen C, et al. 2004. Sortilin is essential for proNGF-induced neuronal cell death. *Nature* 427: 843–848.

Nykjaer A, Willnow TE, Petersen CM. 2005. p75NTR—live or let die. *Curr Opin Neurobiol* 15: 49–57.

Origlia N, Capsoni S, Domenici L, Cattaneo A. 2006. Time window in cholinomimetic ability to rescue long-term potentiation in neurodegenerating anti-nerve growth factor mice. *J Alzheimers Dis* 9: 59–68.

Paoletti F, Covaceuszach S, Konarev PV, Gonfloni S, Malerba F, Schwarz E, Svergun DI, Cattaneo A, Lamba D. 2009. Intrinsic structural disorder of mouse proNGF. *Proteins* 75: 990–1009.

Parachikova A, Agadjanyan MG, Cribbs DH, Blurton-Jones M, Perreau V, Rogers J, Beach TG, Cotman CW. 2007. Inflammatory changes parallel the early stages of Alzheimer disease. *Neurobiol Aging* 28: 1821–1833.

Pezet S, McMahon SB. 2006. Neurotrophins: mediators and modulators of pain. *Annu Rev Neurosci* 29: 507–538.

Prescott ED, Julius DA. 2003. Modular PIP2 binding site as a determinant of capsaicin receptor sensitivity. *Science* 300: 1284–1288.

Rogaev EI, Sherrington R, Rogaeva EA, Levesque G, Ikeda M, Liang Y, Chi H, et al. 1995. Familial Alzheimer's disease in kindreds with missesnse mutations in a gene on chromosome 1 related to the Alzheimer's disease type 3 gene. *Nature* 376: 775–778.

Ruberti F, Capsoni S, Comparini A, Di Daniel E, Franzot J, Gonfloni S, Rossi G, Berardi N, Cattaneo A. 2000. Phenotypic knockout of nerve growth factor in adult transgenic mice reveals severe deficits in basal forebrain cholinergic neurons, cell death in the spleen, and skeletal muscle dystrophy. *J Neurosci* 20: 2589–2601.

Salehi A, Delcroix JD, Mobley WC. 2003. Traffic at the intersection of neurotrophic factor signaling and neurodegeneration. *Trends Neurosci* 26: 73–80.

Schindowski K, Belarbi K, Buee L. 2008. Neurotrophic factors in Alzheimer's disease: role of axonal transport. *Genes Brain Behav* 7: 43–56.

Selkoe DJ. 2002. Alzheimer's disease is a synaptic failure. *Science* 298: 789–791.

Sherrington R, Rogaev EI, Liang Y, Rogaeva EA, Levesque G, Ikeda M, Chi H, et al. 1995. Cloning of a gene bearing missense mutations in early-onset familial Alzheimer's disease. *Nature* 375: 754–760.

Shooter EM. 2001. Early days of the nerve growth factor proteins. *Annu Rev Neurosci* 24: 601–629.

Small SA, Duff K. 2008. Linking A and Tau in late-onset Alzheimer's disease: a dual pathway hypothesis. *Neuron* 60: 534–542.

Sola E, Capsoni S, Rosato-Siri M, Cattaneo A, Cherubini E. 2006. Failure of nicotine-dependent enhancement of synaptic efficacy at Schaffer-collateral CA1 synapses of AD11 anti-nerve growth factor transgenic mice. *Eur J Neurosci* 24: 1252–1264.

Stevens B, Allen NJ, Vazquez LE, Howell GR, Christopherson KS, Nouri N, Micheva KD, Mehalow AK, Huberman AD, Stafford B, et al. 2007. The classical complement cascade mediates CNS synapse elimination. *Cell* 131: 1164–1178.

St George-Hyslop PH, Morris JC. 2008. Will anti-amyloid therapies work for Alzheimer's disease? *Lancet* 372: 180–182.

Tanzi RE, Bertram L. 2005. Twenty years of the Alzheimer's disease amyloid hypothesis: a genetic perspective. *Cell* 120: 545–555.

Tuszynski MH, Thal L, Pay M, Salmon DP, U HS, Bakay R, Patel P, Blesch A, Vahlsing HL, Ho G, Tong G, Potkin SG, Fallon J, Hansen L, Mufson EJ, Kordower JH, Gall C, Conner J. 2005. A phase 1 clinical trial of nerve growth factor gene therapy for Alzheimer disease. *Nat Med* 11: 551–555.

Wisniewski T, Konietzko U. 2008. Amyloid-beta immunization for Alzheimer's disease. *Lancet Neurol* 7: 805–811.

Zlokovic BV. 2008. The blood-brain barrier in health and chronic neurodegenerative disorders. *Neuron* 57: 178–201.

27 Neurotrophins as Regulators of Visual Cortical Plasticity

Eero Castrén and José Fernando Maya Vetencourt

A major part of the understanding of how neurotrophins regulate plasticity in cortical circuits has come out from the groundbreaking studies conducted over several years by Lamberto Maffei and his coworkers.

The work of the Maffei lab, and that of other groups, has revealed the critical role of the activity-dependent synthesis and release of neurotrophic factors in the formation, maturation, and plasticity of the nervous system. These studies not only have introduced the rodent visual cortex as a model to study how experience sculpts the architecture of the nervous system but they also suggest far-reaching implications to pathological conditions where plasticity is compromised. We will here review the literature on the role of neurotrophins in the development and plasticity of the visual cortex and introduce a recent series of experiments where the visual system has been successfully used as a model of pharmacologically induced plasticity. Physiological mechanisms of developmental and pharmacologically induced plasticity are likely to resemble those that underlie the recovery of sensory functions after brain injury. Therefore, the work initiated at the Maffei lab is likely to continue to bear fruit during the years to come, including clinical applications.

Neurotrophins are a family of neurotrophic factors consisting of nerve growth factor (NGF), brain-derived neurotrophic factor (BDNF), neurotrophin-3 (NT-3), and neurotrophin-4 (NT-4). Neurotrophins support the survival and phenotypic differentiation of neurons by binding to and activating tyrosine kinase receptors of the trk family: NGF binds to trkA, BDNF and NT-4 to trkB, and NT-3 preferentially activates trkC (Huang and Reichardt, 2003). All neurotrophins are produced in a proform, which is cleaved intra- or extracellularly to produce the mature neurotrophins. While the mature, cleaved forms preferentially bind to trk receptors, the proneurotrophins bind to a common low-affinity neurotrophin receptor p75NTR, which has been reported to promote apoptosis and neurite retraction (Lu et al., 2005). Therefore, the single molecule, depending on its proteolytic processing, can activate opposite processes on neuronal properties.

In addition to supporting survival, neurotrophins are critically involved in activity-dependent neuronal plasticity (Huang and Reichardt, 2003). Neuronal activity increases the synthesis and secretion of neurotrophins, and particularly BDNF in hippocampus and cerebral cortex

(Thoenen, 1995). BDNF stimulates axon outgrowth and dendritic arborization, enhances synaptic stabilization, and is required for long-term potentiation (LTP). These findings have made BDNF and NGF popular candidate molecules for synaptic plasticity.

Neurotrophins and the Visual Cortex

Nerve Growth Factor and TrkA

Lamberto Maffei's lab was the first to investigate the role of neurotrophins in the context of plasticity in the visual cortex. Their initial attention was directed to the role of NGF, the only neurotrophin available at the time. They showed that intraventricular or intracerebral administration of NGF prevented the loss of visual acuity and contrast sensitivity caused by monocular deprivation (MD) in the rat visual cortex (Domenici et al., 1991). They also demonstrated that exogenous NGF administration prevented the ocular dominance (OD) shift of visual cortical neurons in response to MD (Maffei et al., 1992). These findings led them to propose the hypothesis that ocular dominance plasticity is based on the competition between the inputs from the two eyes for a neurotrophic factor, which is produced and released by the visual cortical neurons in an activity-dependent manner. This hypothesis is analogous to the classical model of neurotrophic factor action in the development of the peripheral nervous system (Levi-Montalcini, 1987).

Several findings from Maffei's lab and other labs have subsequently supported this very influential hypothesis: NGF is expressed in the visual cortex, and its expression is reduced by MD (Bozzi et al., 1995; Lodovichi et al., 2000). NGF administration increases neurotransmitter release within the visual cortex (Sala et al., 1998), acting predominantly on the glutamatergic and cholinergic neurotransmitter systems (Cotrufo et al., 2003). The NGF-induced regulation of OD plasticity is dependent on afferent electrical activity (Caleo et al., 1999). Inactivation of NGF by the administration of specific antibodies into the visual cortex interferes with the functional and anatomical development of the visual cortex (Berardi et al., 1994) and prolongs the critical period beyond its normal limits (Domenici et al., 1994a). Importantly, both NGF administration and the activation of trkA receptors prevent the effects of MD (Pizzorusso et al., 1999; Caleo et al., 1999), which demonstrates that NGF action in visual cortex plasticity is mediated by trkA receptors. NGF administration converts LTP to long-term depression after high-frequency stimulation in rat visual cortical slices whereas depletion of NGF by antibodies or trkA-immunoadhesin rescues LTP (Brancucci et al., 2004; Pesavento et al., 2000). These effects appear to be mediated by the cholinergic afferents (Pesavento et al., 2000).

The effectiveness of NGF to prevent the effects of MD has been consistently observed in rodents (Caleo et al., 1999), whereas the NGF action is not as clear in the cat visual system, in which case it seems to depend on the mode of neurotrophin delivery. Intraventricular NGF infusion attenuates the effects of MD in kittens, as assessed electrophysiologically and behaviorally (Carmignoto et al., 1993; Fiorentini et al., 1995). In contrast, intracortical NGF administration does not exert the same effects during the critical period (Galuske et al., 1996; Silver et al., 2001), although it appears to reactivate OD plasticity in the adult cat visual system (Galuske et al., 2000; Gu et al., 1994). These findings indicate that NFG does not act directly on visual cortical neurons but affects other systems instead. The intraventricular NGF delivery is likely to activate subcortical structures bearing NGF receptors such as afferents from the cholinergic system in the basal forebrain. The primary NGF receptor trkA is, indeed, mostly although not exclusively expressed in the cholinergic fibers; some trkA expression has been detected also in glutamatergic neurons in the visual cortex, at least during the critical period (Rossi et al., 2002; Tropea et al., 2002). Consistently, radioactive NGF infused into the visual cortex is not retrogradely transported by the thalamocortical fibers but only by the cholinergic axons (Domenici et al., 1994b). These findings show that the major site of action of NGF is on the cholinergic afferents, although some of its effects are mediated directly by the glutamatergic neurons within the visual cortex (Caleo and Maffei, 2002). The expression of trkA in the visual cortex is developmentally regulated and is increased during the critical period, whereas the p75 NTR is expressed at a constant level during cortical development (Rossi et al., 2002; Tropea et al., 2002).

Brain-Derived Neurotrophic Factor and TrkB

Since the distribution of both BDNF and its receptor trkB are widespread in brain, including the visual cortex, BDNF has become the favorite candidate as a mediator of the activity-dependent plasticity in the cortex. However, the elucidation of the role of BDNF is complicated by the fact that it has numerous different effects on the physiology of the visual cortex, including spontaneous and visually evoked neuronal activity (Lodovichi et al., 2000). Furthermore, BDNF acts on several different neuron classes in the visual cortex.

The expression of BDNF and its receptor trkB are widespread in the visual system (Castrén et al., 1992; Allendoerfer et al., 1994; Schoups et al., 1995; Bozzi et al., 1995; Tropea et al., 2001). BDNF expression in the visual cortex is activity-dependently regulated by visual stimuli through retinal activity (Castrén et al., 1992; Schoups et al., 1995; Lein et al., 2000) and increases during postnatal development after eye-opening, a phenomenon which is prevented by dark rearing (Castrén et al., 1992; Schoups et al., 1995; Capsoni et al., 1999) and MD (Bozzi et al., 1995; Rossi et al., 1999; Lein and Shatz, 2000). In adult rats, light deprivation strongly reduces the expression of BDNF mRNA and protein as well as the autophosphorylation of the trkB receptors, which are all restored back to basal levels already within an hour after light exposure (Castrén et al., 1992; Tropea et al., 2001; Capsoni et al., 1999; Viegi et al., 2002).

TrkB receptors are widely expressed in many cell types in the visual cortex, including the glutamatergic principal neurons, GABAergic interneurons, and thalamocortical axon terminals as well as in the terminals of the ascending modulatory neurotransmitter systems, such as serotonergic fibers (Tongiorgi et al., 1999; Allendoerfer et al., 1994; Cabelli et al., 1996). The expression of the full-length, tyrosine kinase containing trkB isoform is expressed in the rat visual cortex at a relatively constant level during postnatal development (Bozzi et al., 1995; Tropea and Domenici, 2001). In contrast, the expression of the truncated dominant-negative isoform of trkB increases with development in the ferret visual system, suggesting a mechanism by which the ability of BDNF to activate its receptors may be restricted with advancing maturity (Allendoerfer et al., 1994; Knüsel et al., 1994).

Infusion of BDNF into the kitten visual cortex was found to prevent the segregation of thalamocortical fibers into eye-specific columns (Cabelli et al., 1995), which suggested that competition for a limited amount of BDNF regulates the formation of OD columns. A similar effect was produced by the infusion of NT-4, which also binds to the trkB receptor, but not with NGF or NT-3 (Cabelli et al., 1995). Infusion of BDNF into the rat visual cortex blocks the physiological effects of MD (Lodovichi et al., 2000), and the same phenomenon is observed during the critical period in the kitten visual system, where even a shift in favor of the deprived eye was observed (Galuske et al., 1996; Galuske et al., 2000). Furthermore, depletion of trkB ligands by the trkB-IgG interfered with the anatomical segregation of OD columns in kittens while trkA-IgG and trkC-IgG were not effective (Cabelli et al., 1997). Interestingly, the anatomical and functional maturation of processes that underlie OD plasticity is normal in mice heterozygous for the BDNF null allele, which have about half of the normal BDNF levels in the brain (Bartoletti et al., 2002). Furthermore, recent experiments using the chemical-genetic approach to inhibit trkB function indicate that the shift of OD caused by MD during the critical period does not require trkB activity, but that the recovery of visual functions after brief MD are trkB dependent, at least in mice (Kaneko et al., 2008).

Genetic overexpression of BDNF in the visual cortex during postnatal development leads to the precocious maturation of the visual system and an accelerated time course of the critical period for OD plasticity (Huang et al., 1999). These effects were found to be mediated by a precocious maturation of cortical inhibitory circuitries, as indicated by the accelerated decline of LTP induced by stimulation of the white matter (WM-LTP), a form of synaptic plasticity that is sensitive to the maturation of inhibition in the visual system. In agreement with this notion, functional maturation of the visual system is accelerated by environmental enrichment, which promotes the maturation of inhibitory processes during development (Cancedda et al., 2004). These data indicate that the activity-dependent expression of BDNF regulates visual cortex plasticity by acting on the inhibitory interneuron system (Huang et al., 1999; Berardi et al., 2000). This is consistent with the fact that maturation of intracortical inhibitory circuitries sets the start and the end of the critical period for visual cortex plasticity (Fagiolini and Hensch, 2000; Fagiolini et al., 2004; Hensch, 2005).

In visual cortical slices, arborization of the basal dendrites is stimulated by trkB ligands BDNF and NT-4 whereas growth of the apical dendrite is stimulated by all neurotrophins (McAllister et al., 1995). BDNF acts as a local source to stimulate the dendritic growth of nearby neurons within a short distance (Horch and Katz, 2002), and the effects of BDNF on dendritic arborization depend on the neuronal activity: inhibition of the spontaneous activity abolished the effects of BDNF (McAllister et al., 1996). These data suggest that BDNF specifically acts on those dendrites and synapses that are activated by the presynaptic transmission, providing a mechanism for selectively stabilizing active synapses (McAllister et al., 1999). The enhanced dendritic sprouting induced by BDNF was accompanied by a regression of dendritic spines such that the newly formed spines exposed to BDNF were highly unstable (Horch et al., 1999). Local BDNF production may therefore promote morphological changes within dendrites and spines by enhancing the spine turnover, thereby increasing the probability that the most active spines are stabilized.

Neurotrophins also influence the afferent innervation of the thalamocortical axons from the lateral geniculate nucleus (LGN). Intraventricular or intracortical infusion of NGF icv or into the visual cortex prevents the shrinkage of LGN neurons in response to MD (Domenici et al., 1993). Among the trkB ligands, NT-4 appears to be more active on the afferent LGN neurons than BDNF (Riddle et al., 1995). NGF and NT-4 also promote the LGN axon growth and soma development during the early critical period whereas BDNF is ineffective (Wahle et al., 2003). Furthermore, cortical infusion of NT-4 promotes the growth of neurons within the superior colliculus, apparently through an anterograde transport from the visual cortex (Wahle et al., 2003).

BDNF is also expressed in the retina and anterogradely transported along retinal ganglion neurons (von Bartheld et al., 1996). Remarkably, intravitreal injection of BDNF influences not only development of the retina and the targets of retinal ganglion neurons, the LGN and the superior colliculus (Caleo et al., 2000; Lom and Cohen-Cory, 1999; Caleo et al., 2003; Menna et al., 2003), but also the OD plasticity within the visual cortex (Mandolesi et al., 2005). MD reduces BDNF levels in the deprived retina, and intravitreal injection of BDNF into the deprived eye counteracts the plastic effects of MD. This phenomenon appears to be mediated by effects on the LGN cell bodies since labeled BDNF injected into the eye is not transsynaptically transported to the visual cortex but to the LGN (Mandolesi et al., 2005). Recent experiments revealed that retinally produced transcription factor Otx-2 is anterogradely and transsynaptically transported from the retina to the visual cortex where it accumulates predominantly into the parvalbumin-containing GABAergic interneurons and thereby regulates visual cortical plasticity during the critical period (Sugiyama et al., 2008). Together, these findings suggest a new concept where anterogradely transported molecules within a sensory system influence the development and plasticity of sensory cortex.

Antidepressants, Neurotrophins, and Visual Cortical Plasticity

The data reviewed above highlight a concept that neurotrophins, and in particular BDNF, are critical regulators of neuronal plasticity in the brain. This concept suggests that if BDNF release or signaling could be regulated pharmacologically, then such pharmacological treatment could also regulate cortical plasticity. Pharmacological regulation of plasticity might be of clinical relevance in several disorders: for instance, rehabilitation after stroke might be facilitated if critical period plasticity could be transiently reactivated in adulthood by drug treatment.

Several findings suggest that antidepressant drugs increase BDNF synthesis and signaling in hippocampus and cortex (Duman et al., 1997; Duman and Monteggia, 2006; Castrén, 2004).

Infusion of BDNF into hippocampus or midbrain area or genetic overexpression of trkB receptors in neurons (Castrén, 2004) mimic the behavioral effects of antidepressants in rodents whereas inhibition of BDNF and trkB activity blocks these behavioral effects of antidepressants in mice (Saarelainen et al., 2003). Together, these data suggest the hypothesis that antidepressant drugs might increase neuronal plasticity in the cortex at least partially by activating BDNF signaling in brain (Castrén, 2005).

We have recently used rat visual cortex as a model to test the hypothesis that antidepressant drugs might activate neuronal plasticity in the brain. Using visual evoked potential (VEPs), we tested the possibility that the antidepressant drug fluoxetine might reactivate OD plasticity in adult visual cortex. Strikingly, the OD distribution in the visual cortex contralateral to the deprived eye shifted in favor of the open eye in adult MD animals chronically treated with fluoxetine but not in controls (Maya Vetencourt et al., 2008). No change of binocularity was observed with the drug treatment alone without the concomitant MD. A more detailed electrophysiological analysis revealed that fluoxetine treatment restores a degree of plasticity that is similar to that observed during the critical period, as indicated by the fact that the shift of OD was due to a reduction of the deprived eye strength following the period of MD (Maya Vetencourt et al., 2008).

We further evaluated whether the plastic outcome induced by fluoxetine could promote the recovery of visual functions in adult amblyopic animals. Remarkably, a full recovery of visual acuity and binocularity, both at electrophysiological and behavioral levels, was evident in fluoxetine-treated animals that were reverse-sutured during the last two weeks of antidepressant treatment (Maya Vetencourt et al., 2008). No rescue of visual functions was observed in reverse-sutured control animals. These data suggest that chronic antidepressant treatment allows a reorganization of neural networks miswired during development and suggest that fluoxetine might be clinically useful in the treatment of human amblyopia.

Chronic fluoxetine administration altered the inhibitory–excitatory balance in the visual system while promoting BDNF expression and WM-LTP occurrence (Maya Vetencourt et al., 2008). Interestingly, environmental enrichment, another strategy that restores plasticity in the adult, similarly decreases the excitatory–inhibitory ratio and stimulates BDNF expression as well as the occurrence of the WM-LTP (Sale et al., 2007). The relevance of the interplay between the GABAergic system and BDNF-trkB signaling in the process of plasticity reactivation is highlighted by two recent observations: (1) intracortical administration of BDNF restores OD plasticity in the rat visual system (Maya Vetencourt et al., 2008), and (2) the reinstatement of plasticity induced by both fluoxetine and environmental enrichment is prevented by cortical infusion of the benzodiazepine agonist diazepam (Maya Vetencourt et al., 2008; Sale et al., 2007). Since both of these experimental paradigms increase serotonergic transmission in the nervous system (van Praag et al., 2000), these data suggest that an enhanced 5-HT signaling set in motion an initial cascade of molecular and cellular events that trigger plasticity in the visual system (see figure 27.1). The activation of intracellular signal transduction pathways might eventually promote changes of chromatin structure (e.g., histone posttranslational modi-

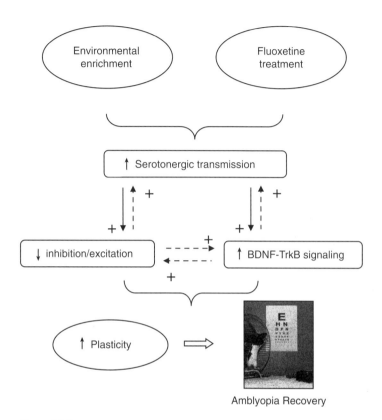

Figure 27.1

A hypothetical scheme of recovery from amblyopia in adult rats. Environmental enrichment and chronic treatment with fluoxetine increase serotonergic (5HT) transmission in the adult visual cortex, which might initiate a cascade of molecular and cellular events contributing to altering the excitation–inhibition balance and promoting brain-derived neurotrophic factor (BDNF) signaling. Together, these processes reinstate susceptibility to monocular deprivation in adulthood and promote the recovery of vision in adult amblyopic animals. In keeping with this, direct infusion of 5HT in the visual cortex restores plasticity in the adult (Maya Vetencourt, Castren, Maffei, unpublished data). Continuous arrows represent established interactions between the cellular processes indicated (boxes). Dashed lines represent interactions that remain to be ascertained.

fications) that in turn modulate gene expression patterns associated with the process of plasticity reactivation. In keeping with this, we have recently found that intracortical 5-HT infusion reactivates susceptibility to MD in adulthood and promotes the recovery of vision in adult amblyopic animals. This plastic phenomenon in the visual system was accompanied by a transitory increase of BDNF expression, which was paralleled by an increased histone acetylation status at the activity-dependently regulated BDNF promoter regions and by a decreased expression of the histone deacetylase enzyme 5 (Maya Vetencourt, Castrén, Maffei, unpublished data). These observations are also consistent with the facilitatory role of diffuse projection systems in critical period plasticity (Kasamatsu and Pettigrew, 1976; Bear and Singer, 1986; Gu and

Singer, 1995). In this context, BDNF may be a downstream target, whose expression is necessary for the occurrence of these plastic phenomena. This is supported by our recent finding that inhibition of BDNF-trkB signaling produced by intracortical infusion of trkB-IgG prevents the effects induced by fluoxetine in visual cortex plasticity (Maya Vetencourt, Castrén, Maffei, unpublished data).

Chronic antidepressant treatment enhances experience-dependent plasticity not only in rat visual cortex but also in the human visual system. Increased amplitude of neuronal firing in response to repeated presentation of visual stimuli was recently recorded in area 17 of healthy, antidepressant-treated subjects (Normann et al., 2007). These data suggest a previously unexpected degree of plasticity in the adult brain, a phenomenon that may be of clinical relevance in the treatment of pathological conditions where neuronal plasticity is compromised (Fernandez et al., 2007; Rubenstein and Merzenich, 2003).

The idea that antidepressant drugs might reactivate critical-period-like plasticity in the adult brain and allow reorganization of neuronal networks miswired by abnormal early life experiences suggests a completely new concept for the mechanism through which antidepressant drugs alleviate symptoms of depression (Castrén, 2005). It is important to note that antidepressant treatment per se does not lead to the functional recovery; environmental guidance or rehabilitation (e.g., manipulations of visual stimuli) is also required to bring about the desired effects. The role of antidepressants as enhancers of plasticity is consistent with the fact that these drugs are successfully used for the treatment of many neuropsychiatric disorders in addition to depression, including anxiety, obsessive–compulsive disorder, chronic pain, eating disorders, and many others (Wong and Licinio, 2004).

Conclusions and Implications

The groundbreaking work of Lamberto Maffei's lab has provided strong evidence that neurotrophic factors NGF and BDNF are critical regulators of OD plasticity in the visual cortex both during development and in adults. The recent data on the ability of antidepressant drugs and environmental enrichment to reactivate OD plasticity also in the adult brain suggests that the critical period is not a fixed structure that cannot be altered once terminated but a much more plastic process which can be reactivated in the adult by pharmacological treatments or environmental manipulations. Since visual cortex is commonly used as a model system to understand the development and plasticity of other cortical areas, these observations have far-reaching medical and psychological implications.

The recent series of reports from Maffei's lab that an enriched environment, and in particular somatosensory stimulation of human preterm infants, produces beneficial effects for the development of another sensory modality, the visual system (Guzzetta et al., 2009), suggests that stimulation of all the sensory modalities is beneficial and adds up to balanced development during early life and beyond (Sale et al., 2009). These findings have powerful implications for the development of psychological disturbances and their treatment and are opening up a completely novel, exciting line of research where the well-characterized visual system is used as a model to understand and assess the environmental effects in other neuronal systems.

References

Allendoerfer KL, Cabelli RJ, Escandon E, Kaplan DR, Nikolics K, Shatz CJ. 1994. Regulation of neurotrophin receptors during the maturation of the mammalian visual system. *J Neurosci* 14: 1795–1811.

Bartoletti A, Cancedda L, Reid SW, Tessarollo L, Porciatti V, Pizzorusso T, Maffei L. 2002. Heterozygous knock-out mice for brain- derived neurotrophic factor show a pathway-specific impairment of long-term potentiation but normal critical period for monocular deprivation. *J Neurosci* 22: 10072–10077.

Bear MF, Singer W. 1986. Modulation of visual cortical plasticity by acetylcholine and noradrenaline. *Nature* 320: 172–176.

Berardi N, Cellerino A, Domenici L, Fagiolini M, Pizzorusso T, Cattaneo A, Maffei L. 1994. Monoclonal antibodies to nerve growth factor affect the postnatal development of the visual system. *Proc Natl Acad Sci USA* 91: 684–688.

Berardi N, Pizzorusso T, Maffei L. 2000. Critical periods during sensory development. *Curr Opin Neurobiol* 10: 138–145.

Bozzi Y, Pizzorusso T, Cremisi F, Rossi FM, Barsacchi G, Maffei L. 1995. Monocular deprivation decreases the expression of messenger RNA for brain-derived neurotrophic factor in the rat visual cortex. *Neuroscience* 69: 1133–1144.

Brancucci A, Kuczewski N, Covaceuszach S, Cattaneo A, Domenici L. 2004. Nerve growth factor favours long-term depression over long-term potentiation in layer II-III neurones of rat visual cortex. *J Physiol* 559: 497–506.

Cabelli RJ, Hohn A, Shatz CJ. 1995. Inhibition of ocular dominance column formation by infusion of NT-4/5 or BDNF. *Science* 267: 1662–1666.

Cabelli RJ, Allendoerfer KL, Radeke MJ, Welcher AA, Feinstein SC, Shatz CJ. 1996. Changing patterns of expression and subcellular localization of TrkB in the developing visual system. *J Neurosci* 16: 7965–7980.

Cabelli RJ, Shelton DL, Segal RA, Shatz CJ. 1997. Blockade of endogenous ligands of trkB inhibits formation of ocular dominance columns. *Neuron* 19: 63–76.

Caleo M, Lodovichi C, Maffei L. 1999. Effects of nerve growth factor on visual cortical plasticity require afferent electrical activity. *Eur J Neurosci* 11: 2979–2984.

Caleo M, Medini P, von Bartheld CS, Maffei L. 2003. Provision of brain-derived neurotrophic factor via anterograde transport from the eye preserves the physiological responses of axotomized geniculate neurons. *J Neurosci* 23: 287–296.

Caleo M, Menna E, Chierzi S, Cenni MC, Maffei L. 2000. Brain-derived neurotrophic factor is an anterograde survival factor in the rat visual system. *Curr Biol* 10: 1155–1161.

Caleo M, Maffei L. 2002. Neurotrophins and plasticity in the visual cortex. *Neuroscientist* 8: 52–61.

Cancedda L, Putignano E, Sale A, Viegi A, Berardi N, Maffei L. 2004. Acceleration of visual system development by environmental enrichment. *J Neurosci* 24: 4840–4848.

Capsoni S, Tongiorgi E, Cattaneo A, Domenici L. 1999. Differential regulation of brain-derived neurotrophic factor messenger RNA cellular expression in the adult rat visual cortex. *Neuroscience* 93: 1033–1040.

Carmignoto G, Canella R, Candeo P, Comelli MC, Maffei L. 1993. Effects of nerve growth factor on neuronal plasticity of the kitten visual cortex. *J Physiol* 464: 343–360.

Castrén E. 2004. Neurotrophic effects of antidepressant drugs. *Curr Opin Pharmacol* 4: 58–64.

Castrén E. 2005. Is mood chemistry? *Nat Rev Neurosci* 6: 241–246.

Castrén E, Zafra F, Thoenen H, Lindholm D. 1992. Light regulates expression of brain-derived neurotrophic factor mRNA in rat visual cortex. *Proc Natl Acad Sci USA* 89: 9444–9448.

Cotrufo T, Viegi A, Berardi N, Bozzi Y, Mascia L, Maffei L. 2003. Effects of neurotrophins on synaptic protein expression in the visual cortex of dark-reared rats. *J Neurosci* 23: 3566–3571.

Domenici L, Berardi N, Carmignoto G, Vantini G, Maffei L. 1991. Nerve growth factor prevents the amblyopic effects of monocular deprivation. *Proc Natl Acad Sci USA* 88: 8811–8815.

Domenici L, Cellerino A, Berardi N, Cattaneo A, Maffei L. 1994. Antibodies to nerve growth factor (NGF) prolong the sensitive period for monocular deprivation in the rat. *Neuroreport* 5: 2041–2044.

Domenici L, Cellerino A, Maffei L. 1993. Monocular deprivation effects in the rat visual cortex and lateral geniculate nucleus are prevented by nerve growth factor (NGF). II. Lateral geniculate nucleus. *Proc Biol Sci* 251: 25–31.

Domenici L, Fontanesi G, Cattaneo A, Bagnoli P, Maffei L. 1994. Nerve growth factor (NGF) uptake and transport following injection in the developing rat visual cortex. *Vis Neurosci* 11: 1093–1102.

Duman RS, Heninger GR, Nestler EJ. 1997. A molecular and cellular theory of depression. *Arch Gen Psychiatry* 54: 597–606.

Duman RS, Monteggia LM. 2006. A neurotrophic model for stress-related mood disorders. *Biol Psychiatry* 59: 1116–1127.

Fagiolini M, Fritschy JM, Low K, Mohler H, Rudolph U, Hensch TK. 2004. Specific GABAA circuits for visual cortical plasticity. *Science* 303: 1681–1683.

Fagiolini M, Hensch TK. 2000. Inhibitory threshold for critical-period activation in primary visual cortex. *Nature* 404: 183–186.

Fernandez F, Morishita W, Zuniga E, Nguyen J, Blank M, Malenka RC, Garner CC. 2007. Pharmacotherapy for cognitive impairment in a mouse model of Down syndrome. *Nat Neurosci* 10: 411–413.

Fiorentini A, Berardi N, Maffei L. 1995. Nerve growth factor preserves behavioral visual acuity in monocularly deprived kittens. *Vis Neurosci* 12: 51–55.

Galuske RA, Kim DS, Castrén E, Singer W. 2000. Differential effects of neurotrophins on ocular dominance plasticity in developing and adult cat visual cortex. *Eur J Neurosci* 12: 3315–3330.

Galuske RA, Kim DS, Castrén E, Thoenen H, Singer W. 1996. Brain-derived neurotrophic factor reversed experience-dependent synaptic modifications in kitten visual cortex. *Eur J Neurosci* 8: 1554–1559.

Gu Q, Liu Y, Cynader MS. 1994. Nerve growth factor-induced ocular dominance plasticity in adult cat visual cortex. *Proc Natl Acad Sci USA* 91: 8408–8412.

Gu Q, Singer W. 1995. Involvement of serotonin in developmental plasticity of kitten visual cortex. *Eur J Neurosci* 7: 1146–1153.

Guzzetta A, Baldini S, Bancale A, Baroncelli L, Ciucci F, Ghirri P, Putignano E, et al. 2009. Massage accelerates brain development and the maturation of visual function. *J Neurosci* 29: 6042–6051.

Hensch TK. 2005. Critical period plasticity in local cortical circuits. *Nat Rev Neurosci* 6: 877–888.

Horch HW, Katz LC. 2002. BDNF release from single cells elicits local dendritic growth in nearby neurons. *Nat Neurosci* 5: 1177–1184.

Horch HW, Kruttgen A, Portbury SD, Katz LC. 1999. Destabilization of cortical dendrites and spines by BDNF. *Neuron* 23: 353–364.

Huang EJ, Reichardt LF. 2003. Trk receptors: roles in neuronal signal transduction. *Annu Rev Biochem* 72: 609–642.

Huang ZJ, Kirkwood A, Pizzorusso T, Porciatti V, Morales B, Bear MF, Maffei L, Tonegawa S. 1999. BDNF regulates the maturation of inhibition and the critical period of plasticity in mouse visual cortex. *Cell* 98: 739–755.

Kaneko M, Hanover JL, England PM, Stryker MP. 2008. TrkB kinase is required for recovery, but not loss, of cortical responses following monocular deprivation. *Nat Neurosci* 11: 497–504.

Kasamatsu T, Pettigrew JD. 1976. Depletion of brain catecholamines: failure of ocular dominance shift after monocular occlusion in kittens. *Science* 194: 206–209.

Knüsel B, Rabin SJ, Hefti F, Kaplan DR. 1994. Regulated neurotrophin receptor responsiveness during neuronal migration and early differentiation. *J Neurosci* 14: 1542–1554.

Lein ES, Hohn A, Shatz CJ. 2000. Dynamic regulation of BDNF and NT-3 expression during visual system development. *J Comp Neurol* 420: 1–18.

Lein ES, Shatz CJ. 2000. Rapid regulation of brain-derived neurotrophic factor mRNA within eye-specific circuits during ocular dominance column formation. *J Neurosci* 20: 1470–1483.

Levi-Montalcini R. 1987. The nerve growth factor: thirty-five years later. *EMBO J* 6: 1145–1154.

Lodovichi C, Berardi N, Pizzorusso T, Maffei L. 2000. Effects of neurotrophins on cortical plasticity: same or different? *J Neurosci* 20: 2155–2165.

Lom B, Cohen-Cory S. 1999. Brain-derived neurotrophic factor differentially regulates retinal ganglion cell dendritic and axonal arborization in vivo. *J Neurosci* 19: 9928–9938.

Lu B, Pang PT, Woo NH. 2005. The yin and yang of neurotrophin action. *Nat Rev Neurosci* 6: 603–614.

Maffei L, Berardi N, Domenici L, Parisi V, Pizzorusso T. 1992. Nerve growth factor (NGF) prevents the shift in ocular dominance distribution of visual cortical neurons in monocularly deprived rats. *J Neurosci* 12: 4651–4662.

Mandolesi G, Menna E, Harauzov A, von Bartheld CS, Caleo M, Maffei L. 2005. A role for retinal brain-derived neurotrophic factor in ocular dominance plasticity. *Curr Biol* 15: 2119–2124.

Maya Vetencourt JF, Sale A, Viegi A, Baroncelli L, De Pasquale R, O'Leary F, Castrén E, Maffei L. 2008. The antidepressant fluoxetine restores plasticity in the adult visual cortex. *Science* 320: 385–388.

McAllister AK, Katz LC, Lo DC. 1996. Neurotrophin regulation of cortical dendritic growth requires activity. *Neuron* 17: 1057–1064.

McAllister AK, Katz LC, Lo DC. 1999. Neurotrophins and synaptic plasticity. *Annu Rev Neurosci* 22: 295–318.

McAllister AK, Lo DC, Katz LC. 1995. Neurotrophins regulate dendritic growth in developing visual cortex. *Neuron* 15: 791–803.

Menna E, Cenni MC, Naska S, Maffei L. 2003. The anterogradely transported BDNF promotes retinal axon remodeling during eye specific segregation within the LGN. *Mol Cell Neurosci* 24: 972–983.

Normann C, Schmitz D, Furmaier A, Doing C, Bach M. 2007. Long- term plasticity of visually evoked potentials in humans is altered in major depression. *Biol Psychiatry* 62: 373–380.

Pesavento E, Margotti E, Righi M, Cattaneo A, Domenici L. 2000. Blocking the NGF-TrkA interaction rescues the developmental loss of LTP in the rat visual cortex: role of the cholinergic system. *Neuron* 25: 165–175.

Pizzorusso T, Berardi N, Rossi FM, Viegi A, Venstrom K, Reichardt LF, Maffei L. 1999. TrkA activation in the rat visual cortex by antirat trkA IgG prevents the effect of monocular deprivation. *Eur J Neurosci* 11: 204–212.

Riddle DR, Lo DC, Katz LC. 1995. NT-4-mediated rescue of lateral geniculate neurons from effects of monocular deprivation. *Nature* 378: 189–191.

Rossi FM, Bozzi Y, Pizzorusso T, Maffei L. 1999. Monocular deprivation decreases brain-derived neurotrophic factor immunoreactivity in the rat visual cortex. *Neuroscience* 90: 363–368.

Rossi FM, Sala R, Maffei L. 2002. Expression of the nerve growth factor receptors TrkA and p75NTR in the visual cortex of the rat: development and regulation by the cholinergic input. *J Neurosci* 22: 912–919.

Rubenstein JL, Merzenich MM. 2003. Model of autism: increased ratio of excitation/inhibition in key neural systems. *Genes Brain Behav* 2: 255–267.

Saarelainen T, Hendolin P, Lucas G, Koponen E, Sairanen M, MacDonald E, Agerman K, et al. 2003. Activation of the TrkB neurotrophin receptor is induced by antidepressant drugs and is required for antidepressant-induced behavioral effects. *J Neurosci* 23: 349–357.

Sala R, Viegi A, Rossi FM, Pizzorusso T, Bonanno G, Raiteri M, Maffei L. 1998. Nerve growth factor and brain-derived neurotrophic factor increase neurotransmitter release in the rat visual cortex. *Eur J Neurosci* 10: 2185–2191.

Sale A, Berardi N, Maffei L. 2009. Enrich the environment to empower the brain. *Trends Neurosci* 32: 233–239.

Sale A, Maya Vetencourt JF, Medini P, Cenni MC, Baroncelli L, De Pasquale R, Maffei L. 2007. Environmental enrichment in adulthood promotes amblyopia recovery through a reduction of intracortical inhibition. *Nat Neurosci* 10: 679–681.

Schoups AA, Elliott RC, Friedman WJ, Black IB. 1995. NGF and BDNF are differentially modulated by visual experience in the developing geniculocortical pathway. *Brain Res Dev Brain Res* 86: 326–334.

Silver MA, Fagiolini M, Gillespie DC, Howe CL, Frank MG, Issa NP, Antonini A, Stryker MP. 2001. Infusion of nerve growth factor (NGF) into kitten visual cortex increases immunoreactivity for NGF, NGF receptors, and choline acetyltransferase in basal forebrain without affecting ocular dominance plasticity or column development. *Neuroscience* 108: 569–585.

Sugiyama S, Di Nardo AA, Aizawa S, Matsuo I, Volovitch M, Prochiantz A, Hensch TK. 2008. Experience-dependent transfer of Otx2 homeoprotein into the visual cortex activates postnatal plasticity. *Cell* 134: 508–520.

Thoenen H. 1995. Neurotrophins and neuronal plasticity. *Science* 270: 593–598.

Tongiorgi E, Cattaneo A, Domenici L. 1999. Co-expression of TrkB and the N-methyl-D-aspartate receptor subunits NR1-C1, NR2A and NR2B in the rat visual cortex. *Neuroscience* 90: 1361–1369.

Tropea D, Capsoni S, Tongiorgi E, Giannotta S, Cattaneo A, Domenici L. 2001. Mismatch between BDNF mRNA and protein expression in the developing visual cortex: the role of visual experience. *Eur J Neurosci* 13: 709–721.

Tropea D, Capsoni S, Covaceuszach S, Domenici L, Cattaneo A. 2002. Rat visual cortical neurones express TrkA NGF receptor. *Neuroreport* 13: 1369–1373.

Tropea D, Domenici L. 2001. Expression of TrkB receptors in developing visual cortex is not regulated by light. *Cell Mol Neurobiol* 21: 545–552.

van Praag H, Kempermann G, Gage FH. 2000. Neural consequences of environmental enrichment. *Nat Rev Neurosci* 1: 191–198.

Viegi A, Cotrufo T, Berardi N, Mascia L, Maffei L. 2002. Effects of dark rearing on phosphorylation of neurotrophin Trk receptors. *Eur J Neurosci* 16: 1925–1930.

von Bartheld C, Byers MR, Williams R, Bothwell M. 1996. Anterograde transport of neurotrophins and axodendritic transfer in the developing visual system. *Nature* 379: 830–833.

Wahle P, Di Cristo G, Schwerdtfeger G, Engelhardt M, Berardi N, Maffei L. 2003. Differential effects of cortical neurotrophic factors on development of lateral geniculate nucleus and superior colliculus neurons: anterograde and retrograde actions. *Development* 130: 611–622.

Wong ML, Licinio J. 2004. From monoamines to genomic targets: a paradigm shift for drug discovery in depression. *Nat Rev Drug Discov* 3: 136–150.

28 Plasticity in the Developing Brain: Functional Reorganization after Early Brain Damage

Giovanni Cioni, Giulia D'Acunto, and Andrea Guzzetta

Plasticity of the Young Brain

Mechanisms of cerebral plasticity are thought to be more powerful during development. For example, children are more fast-paced than adults in learning a new language or in achieving complex skills such as playing a musical instrument. In a classic experiment on string players, the extent of the cortical representation of the left digits was found to be inversely correlated with the age at which the person had begun to play, indicating a larger amount of cerebral plasticity in subjects with earlier exposure to training (Elbert et al., 1995). Similarly, children lacking proper environmental inputs early in life are more prone to have abnormal development of the functions related to those inputs (the concept of critical periods; Lewis and Maurer, 2005). The presence of more powerful mechanisms of neuronal plasticity during early phases of development should imply that recovery from brain damage is more effective for early lesions compared to similar lesions occurring later in life. This principle was first suggested by Paul Broca in 1865 (Berker et al., 1986) and then more systematically explored by Margaret Kennard in the late 1930s (Kennard and Fulton, 1942). Since then, most of the studies carried out in different species have not denied this general principle although describing a more complex picture, which takes into consideration several other aspects beyond the timing of the insult, including the location and extent of injury (e.g., focal vs. diffuse), the clinical correlates (e.g., presence of seizures), or the genetic susceptibility of the subject (Anderson et al., 2009).

One of the most important predictors of the efficacy of functional reorganization seems to be the distribution, diffuse versus focal, of the damage (Kolb, 1995; Lidzba et al., 2009). Most strikingly, children with early unilateral left-hemisphere damage can develop normal language abilities, while lesions of similar site and extent in the adult brain would produce obvious patterns of aphasia (Bates et al., 2001). Even if an entire hemisphere is removed at an early stage of development (for instance, for the treatment of severe epilepsy), children can develop normal language and cognitive function (Liegeois et al., 2008). Also, children with unilateral ischemic stroke are able to develop normal cognitive functions and maintain them over time (Ballantyne et al., 2008). In contrast, evidence suggests that sustaining an early generalized cerebral insult (e.g., global hypoxia or traumatic brain injury) is usually associated with slower recovery and poorer outcome, compared to what is observed in adults with similar lesions (Anderson et al., 2005). The mechanism most often invoked for this higher vulnerability of early damage is that, at an early stage, cognitive development is highly dependent on the integrity of diffuse neural networks, and so the transient disruption of the developing attention, memory, and learning functions undermines the efficient acquisition of new abilities (Kolb, 1995). Conversely, at an older age, the general, already acquired cognitive abilities can be spared and the impairment is limited to functions directly related to the final area of damage.

The time boundaries of early brain damage have never been clearly defined. This is probably due not to the absence of effort but rather to the complexity of the task. Changes in cerebral plasticity, which influences the effects of brain damage, are gradual during development, and the sensitive periods are now known to be different for the various functional subsystems (Lewis and Maurer, 2005). Also, the types of brain insult are extremely variable during development and affect the nervous system in ways that are directly dependent on the level of maturation at the moment they occur. For these and other reasons, the boundaries between early and late lesions are necessarily blurry. As here we are interested in exploring how different the young brain can be in response to damage, we will focus on lesions occurring before or around birth (also called congenital lesions), which are more frequent and have been more extensively studied compared to later ones.

Specificity of Brain Injury in the Young Brain: A Few Weeks Matter

A relevant aspect of the pathophysiology of congenital brain insult is the stage of cerebral development at the moment of the insult, either prenatal or perinatal (Krageloh-Mann and Horber, 2007). Because of the complexity and speed of the maturational phenomena occurring during gestation, the response to a harmful event varies significantly according to gestational age and leads to different pictures both from the neuropathological and the clinical point of view. For the understanding of these mechanisms, an essential contribution is provided by noninvasive neuroimaging techniques, first with ultrasonography, and more recently with computed tomography and magnetic resonance imaging. These new methodologies, increasingly applied also in children, allow researchers to perform in vivo investigations of cerebral lesions, monitoring their evolution and so providing further insight on the relation between lesion and function and on the different types of reorganization.

In broad terms, types of congenital brain damage can be grouped according to timing (see figure 28.1). Lesions occurring during the first half of gestation (and in particular the first trimester) give rise to malformations of cortical development. These lesions are very complex in terms of their characterization as they can be extremely variable in size, location, and distribution, resulting in completely different clinical pictures. The underlying mechanisms of cerebral plasticity are likely to be similarly complex and variable. The second group of lesions are those occurring around the early third trimester of gestation (<25–34 weeks of gestation). The most typical of this group are periventricular leukomalacia and intraventricular hemorrhage. The first

| MALFORMATIONS OF CORTICAL DEVELOPMENT | PERIVENTRICULAR WHITE MATTER DAMAGE | CORTICO/SUBCORTICAL GREY MATTER DAMAGE |

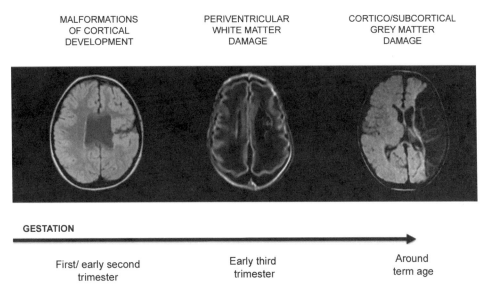

GESTATION

| First/ early second trimester | Early third trimester | Around term age |

Figure 28.1
Correlation between timing of insult and type of brain injury. Three examples are shown of typical congenital brain lesions on MRI, in which the correlation between the timing and the characteristics of the lesion are clear. In the left column, a case of schizencephalia, a malformation of cortical development secondary to an insult, occurred during the early phases of brain development. In the central column, a case of periventricular white matter damage secondary to an intraventricular hemorrhagic insult occurred at the beginning of the third trimester of gestation. In the right column, a case of ischemic infarction of the territory of the middle cerebral artery occurred around birth in a term born infant.

is an ischemic, bilateral, and diffuse lesion, while the second is a hemorrhagic lesion, usually limited inside the ventricles, but that sometimes complicates into a periventricular parenchymal infarction, usually unilateral. Finally, the third group includes lesions around term (typically lesions of the term infant at around birth). The most relevant are the hypoxic–ischemic encephalopathy and the focal cerebral stroke, of arterial origin. The first is an ischemic lesion, bilateral and diffuse, while the second is a focal lesion, similar from the neuropathological point of view to the stroke observed in adults.

As previously mentioned, the distribution of the lesion, namely, focal unilateral versus diffuse bilateral, is likely to be the single most relevant factor to influence the efficacy of plastic reorganization of brain functions. In this sense, congenital lesions provide an interesting model for studying cerebral reorganization as they naturally encompass the different combinations of distribution (focal, diffuse) and timing (early gestation, late gestation, and term) of damage.

Reorganization of Function after Early Brain Damage: The Special Case of the Motor System

The effects of a cerebral lesion are clearly connected with the site of the lesion. This implies a different involvement of the various systems in different subjects, with complex and

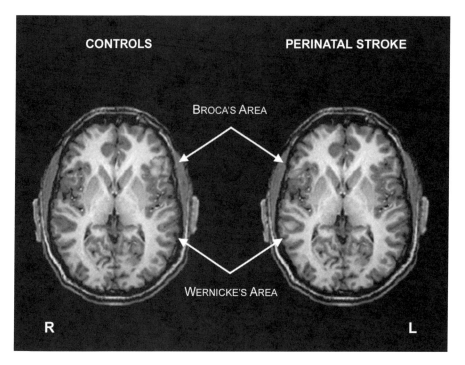

Figure 28.2 (plate 13)
Language representation in patients with left perinatal stroke and right hemispheric reorganization of language. Functional magnetic resonance imaging shows the activation of regions of the right hemisphere which are contralateral and homotopic to the regions of the language circuit activated in normal controls (group analysis performed on 8 patients and 10 normal controls). See Guzzetta et al., 2008.

heterogeneous functional correlates. Some systems are known to be extremely plastic, such as, for example, the network for language. There is now evidence not only that subjects with congenital brain damage to the dominant hemisphere are able to organize linguistic functions in the nondominant one but also that the resulting representation involves areas that are exactly homotopic to the ones active in normal controls (Staudt et al., 2002; Guzzetta et al., 2008; see figure 28.2, plate 13). Other systems, however, show a different response to lesions and are differentially affected by the timing at which damage occurs. In fact, in some cases the increased plastic potential of the brain environment at the early stages of development can induce types of reorganization that are maladaptive, in the sense that they lead to overall worse long-term outcomes. This is certainly the case with the sensorimotor system, which will be the main argument of this chapter. An increasing amount of evidence has been obtained very recently suggesting that the reorganization of the motor system is extremely dependent on the timing of an injury.

When a cerebral lesion, either cortical or subcortical, involves the motor system, neuroplastic mechanisms should be able to drive recovery of voluntary movements, restoring an adequate cortical impulse to the spinal motor neurons and interneurons. In adults, one major mechanism is available to restore a connection of the motor cortex with the spinal cord circuitry in case of a cerebral lesion. That is the reorganization of function within the ipsilesional cortex, within the primary motor cortex or in nonprimary motor areas. When damage occurs early in life, an additional mechanism becomes available. This is based on the existence, during the first weeks of life, of bilateral motor projections originating in the primary motor areas, which connect each hemisphere with both sides of the body. The ipsilateral fibers generally withdraw during development, but they can persist in case of cerebral damage, giving rise to a contralesional reorganization of motor function, exclusive of early brain damage (Eyre et al., 2007). Summarizing, after early brain damage the reorganization of motor function can follow two completely different directions. The first one consists in the reorganization within the tissue of the damaged hemisphere and is thus called ipsilesional reorganization. The second one consists in a complete shift to the unaffected hemisphere, and it is thus called contralesional reorganization. However, what are the functional correlates of these types of reorganization, and how can we influence them?

We have recently provided some evidence indicating how, in patients with early brain damage, the pattern of motor reorganization (ipsilesional vs. contralesional) is already determined during the first year of life, and possibly even within the first few months (Eyre et al., 2007). This is not a mere consequence of the size and site of the lesion but is strongly influenced by the experience following damage (action-dependent reorganization), in the sense of the complex interaction between residual motor output from the affected hemisphere and somatosensory feedback from the affected limb (hypothesis of the "amblyopia of the corticospinal system"; Eyre et al., 2007). These findings are extremely well supported by animal studies. In a series of papers, Martin and colleagues explored the development of the corticospinal system of the cat in normal conditions and following unilateral brain damage (see Martin, 2005, for a review). They found that the refinement of corticospinal terminals occurs during a protracted postnatal period and is driven by neural activity in the motor cortical areas. More active neurons are more competitive and are able to secure more synaptic space than their less active counterparts. When a unilateral cortical inactivation is produced, animals show permanent impairments in skilled distal movement during prehension, as a result of the loss of corticospinal terminal postsynaptic space. Conversely, if the inactivation is followed by bursts of transcranial magnetic stimulation of the motor cortex, spinal terminations are maintained (Salimi and Martin, 2004; see figure 28.3).

In the light of these data, the importance of an early time window (first months of life) for therapeutic intervention is greatly emphasized. This is especially true when considering that children with contralesional reorganization, that is, with the unaffected hemisphere directly controlling both hands, reach lower levels of hand motor performance, making this pattern of reorganization potentially maladaptive (Staudt et al., 2004). However, before getting to the relevance of these findings for early intervention, we have to explore the role, in this framework, of the somatosensory system.

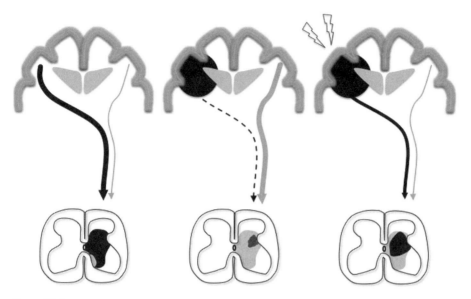

Figure 28.3
Schematic representation of the corticospinal tract in three different conditions. In case of normal development of the corticospinal tract, spinal gray matter is connected to a great extent to the contralateral motor cortex, and very little to the ipsilateral one, due to a large withdrawal of the ipsilateral corticospinal fibers (left). Following early brain damage, the lesion and the secondary reduction of brain activity can induce a withdrawal of the crossing fibers and the mainte-nance of the ipsilateral ones (center). An early intervention aimed at stimulating the activity of the affected brain (e.g., early motor training or action observation) can potentially rebalance the development of the corticospinal tract in favor of the crossing fibers (right).

The Reorganization of the Somatosensory System and Why It Does Not Always Follow the Motor System

Cerebral lesions involving the motor system often encroach upon the sensory system as well and may lead to somatosensory deficits of different severity. These functions can be studied in vivo with techniques like somatosensory evoked potentials, magnetoencephalography, and func-tional magnetic resonance imaging (fMRI) with sensorial tasks. With these means, we have recently demonstrated that, at variance with the motor system, the intrahemispheric (ipsilesional) reorganization of primary sensory function is the principal compensatory mechanism of brain damage of the sensory system, even when occurring very early during development (Guzzetta et al., 2007; see figure 28.4). The mechanisms underlying this phenomenon are not fully under-stood; however, two elements seem to be of special relevance. The first is the lack of an ana-tomical substrate for contralesional reorganization, even in the early stages of development, at variance with what happens for the motor system. The second is the possibility that thalamocorti-cal fibers, at least for some types of early lesions, are still developing when the insult occurs, thus allowing an actual bypass of the lesion and reconnection with the sensory cortex (Staudt et al., 2006).

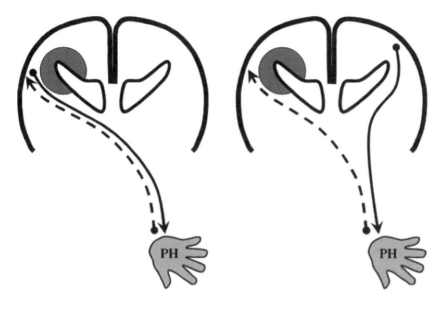

MOTOR: Ipselesional reorganization
SENSORY: Ipsilesional reorganization

(a)

MOTOR: Contralesional reorganization
SENSORY: Ipsilesional reorganization

(b)

Figure 28.4
Schematic representation of the main types of reorganization of sensorimotor function following early brain damage. (a) Ipsilesional reorganization of motor and sensory function. Both functions are reorganized in the affected hemisphere, in regions around the lesion. In this case, functional impairment is mainly related to the extent of the damage to the sensorimotor system. (b) Contralesional reorganization of motor function and ipsilesional reorganization of sensory function. Motor and sensory function of the affected limb are processed by different hemispheres. In this case, functional impairment is related not only to the extent of the damage to the sensorimotor system but also to the presence of the functional dissociation. PH, paretic hand.

It is known that during early brain development, and in particular during the early third trimester of gestation, the white matter can be particularly vulnerable to insult, exposing to injury the forming thalamocortical fibers, including the geniculostriate pathway. However, at this time of development plasticity of thalamocortical afferents is conspicuous. The afferents from the subplate zone are still migrating into the cortical plate, and there are a significant number of growth-promoting molecules and axonal guidance cues, related to a significant expression of genes coding for such molecules (Kostovic and Judas, 2006). This particular environment gives the brain additional potential strategies for plastic reorganization (see figure 28.5).

Of great interest is the fact that the different reorganizational potential of the sensory and the motor systems leads in many cases to an interhemispheric dissociation of these functions, with the first being reorganized within the affected hemisphere and the second being shifted contralaterally (see figure 28.4b). Some evidence seems to support the hypothesis that such a

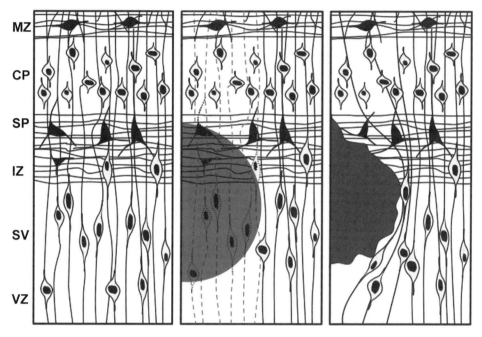

Figure 28.5
Schematic representation of the transient fetal organization of the developing cerebral wall during the eary third trimester of gestation. The thalamocortical fibers grow from the ventricular and the subventricular zones toward the subplate, where they accumulate and "wait." Synaptic contacts with subplate neurons provide interaction with endogenous cortical circuitry and regulate migration of thalamic fibers into the cortical plate (left). In case of brain injury of the periventricular white matter, growing thalamocortical fibers within the damaged tissue degenerate (center). New thalamocortical fibers can develop within the surviving tissue, establishing functional connections with the cortical target of the degenerated fibers, thus bypassing the lesion (right). MZ, marginal zone; CP, cortical plate; SP, subplate; IZ, intermediate zone; SV, subventricular zone; VZ, ventricular zone.

dissociation could determine some functional deficits in tasks requiring a strong sensorimotor integration (such as stereognosia). It is also of great interest that when motor and sensory functions are not dissociated, that is, they both share an intrahemispheric reorganization, they seem to be significantly correlated. Conversely, if interhemispheric (sensorimotor) dissociation occurs, the quality of motor function is usually more affected, irrespective of the degree of sensory impairment.

Plasticity of the Sensorimotor System and Early Intervention

In the light of these findings, the specific target of an early therapeutic intervention should be the activation of the sensorimotor cortex of the affected hemisphere, to enhance the competitive ability of a damaged corticospinal system during development and thus mitigate the consequences of the lesion on motor outcome. Ideally, such intervention should begin soon after the damage has occurred, but unfortunately stimulating a voluntary activation of the motor cortex is hard to achieve during the first weeks of life when voluntary reaching is still absent or immature. Different approaches can be imagined to overcome these limitations.

The resilience of the somatosensory system to damage, as outlined above, supports the utilization of this input as a potential window of opportunity for early intervention. We have recently demonstrated that tactile stimulation of the body is a powerful means to accelerate brain maturation in the newborn infant, with mechanisms that are not fully understood but are likely to be both local and systemic (and thus potentially transmodal; Guzzetta et al., 2009). This study was carried out with the group of Professor Lamberto Maffei exploring in parallel the effects of somatosensory stimulation in newborn rats and preterm infants. We found with some surprise that massage accelerated visual development in both humans and animals, likely through a mechanism mediated by the increase of blood levels of insulin-like growth factor-1. Also, massage seemed to affect more globally the maturation of brain development, as expressed by qualitative and quantitative measures of cortical electrical activity on the EEG. These findings further emphasize the importance of early sensory stimulation and, more generally, of environmental enrichment to allow a better start to life in newborns at risk. Still, evidence needs to be gathered before this type of intervention can be proposed as an early therapeutic program in infants with congenital brain damage.

A new, more targeted approach might be represented by the stimulation of the motor cortex through a training based on action observation (theory of the mirror neuron system). An increasing number of experiments support the existence of a mirror neuron system also in newborns (both in humans and in nonhuman primates; see Lepage and Theoret, 2007, for a review). In animal studies and human adult studies, action observation was shown to be an effective method to increase cortical excitability of the sensorimotor cortex. Based on the hypothesis that the same activation can be induced in young infants, it might be predicted that a training based on movement observation, coupled with actual hand motor activity (handling, reaching for a toy), will enhance the excitability of the sensorimotor cortex and will accelerate the maturation of the corticospinal tract and the shaping of spinal motor circuits. The activation of the motor cortex related to action observation might represent a unique opportunity for therapeutic intervention in this early period, eventually supplemented or followed by more standard rehabilitative approaches, as soon as voluntary reaching can be reliably elicited.

Conclusions

In conclusion, how can we summarize present knowledge on cerebral plasticity and reorganization following early brain damage? The concept that is clearly emerging, both from human and nonhuman studies, is that functional reorganization in children is neither better nor worse than in adults. It is simply different—and gives rise to a really different brain. Full knowledge of how different the young brain becomes (after damage), that is the specific mechanisms of cerebral plasticity in infancy, is far from being achieved. The effort is, however, highly meritorious as this knowledge will be essential to the definition and tuning of therapeutic programs based on solid neurobiological and neurophysiological principles. This approach has the potential to contribute to identifying not only the type of treatment that would be effective but also its timing, its dosage, and its means of administration. Brain mapping techniques developed over the last few years—in particular, fMRI—have provided answers to many questions that had been at the center of scientific debate for long periods. Next implementations of these techniques, as, for example, the dissemination of ultra high field MRI machines, will provide new insight into the remaining questions.

References

Anderson V, Catroppa C, Morse S, Haritou F, Rosenfeld J. 2005. Functional plasticity or vulnerability after early brain injury? *Pediatrics* 116: 1374–1382.

Anderson V, Spencer-Smith M, Leventer R, Coleman L, Anderson P, Williams J, Greenham M, Jacobs R. 2009. Childhood brain insult: can age at insult help us predict outcome? *Brain* 132(Pt 1): 45–56.

Ballantyne AO, Spilkin AM, Hesselink J, Trauner DA. 2008. Plasticity in the developing brain: intellectual, language and academic functions in children with ischaemic perinatal stroke. *Brain* 131(Pt 11): 2975–2985.

Bates E, Reilly J, Wulfeck B, Dronkers N, Opie M, Fenson J, Kriz S, et al. 2001. Differential effects of unilateral lesions on language production in children and adults. *Brain Lang* 79: 223–265.

Berker EA, Berker AH, Smith A. 1986. Translation of Broca's 1865 report: Localization of speech in the third left frontal convolution. *Arch Neurol* 43: 1065–1072.

Elbert T, Pantev C, Wienbruch C, Rockstroh B, Taub E. 1995. Increased cortical representation of the fingers of the left hand in string players. *Science* 270: 305–307.

Eyre JA, Smith M, Dabydeen L, Clowry GJ, Petacchi E, Battini R, Guzzetta A, Cioni G. 2007. Is hemiplegic cerebral palsy equivalent to amblyopia of the corticospinal system? *Ann Neurol* 62: 493–503.

Guzzetta A, Baldini S, Bancale A, Baroncelli L, Ciucci F, Ghirri P, Putignano E, et al. 2009. Massage accelerates brain development and the maturation of visual function. *J Neurosci* 29: 6042–6051.

Guzzetta A, Bonanni P, Biagi L, Tosetti M, Montanaro D, Guerrini R, Cioni G. 2007. Reorganisation of the somatosensory system after early brain damage. *Clin Neurophysiol* 118: 1110–1121.

Guzzetta A, Pecini C, Biagi L, Tosetti M, Brizzolara D, Chilosi A, Cipriani P, et al. 2008. Language organisation in left perinatal stroke. *Neuropediatrics* 39(3): 157–163.

Kennard M, Fulton JF. 1942. Age and reorganization of central nervous system. *Mt Sinai J Med* 9: 594–606.

Kolb B. 1995. *Brain Plasticity and Behavior.* Mahwah, NJ: Lawrence Erlbaum Associates.

Kostovic I, Judas M. 2006. Prolonged coexistence of transient and permanent circuitry elements in the developing cerebral cortex of fetuses and preterm infants. *Dev Med Child Neurol* 48: 388–393.

Krageloh-Mann I, Horber V. 2007. The role of magnetic resonance imaging in furthering understanding of the pathogenesis of cerebral palsy. *Dev Med Child Neurol* 49: 948.

Lepage JF, Theoret H. 2007. The mirror neuron system: grasping others' actions from birth? *Dev Sci* 10: 513–523.

Lewis TL, Maurer D. 2005. Multiple sensitive periods in human visual development: evidence from visually deprived children. *Dev Psychobiol* 46(3): 163–183.

Lidzba K, Wilke M, Staudt M, Krägeloh-Mann I. 2009. Early plasticity versus early vulnerability: the problem of heterogeneous lesion types. *Brain* 132(Pt 10): e128; author reply e129.

Liegeois F, Cross JH, Polkey C, Harkness W, Vargha-Khadem F. 2008. Language after hemispherectomy in childhood: contributions from memory and intelligence. *Neuropsychologia* 46: 3101–3107.

Martin JH. 2005. The corticospinal system: from development to motor control. *Neuroscientist* 11(2): 161–173.

Salimi I, Martin JH. 2004. Rescuing transient corticospinal terminations and promoting growth with corticospinal stimulation in kittens. *J Neurosci* 24: 4952–4961.

Staudt M, Erb M, Braun C, Gerloff C, Grodd W, Krägeloh-Mann I. 2006. Extensive peri-lesional connectivity in congenital hemiparesis. *Neurology* 66: 771.

Staudt M, Gerloff C, Grodd W, Holthausen H, Niemann G, Krägeloh-Mann I. 2004. Reorganization in congenital hemiparesis acquired at different gestational ages. *Ann Neurol* 56: 854–863.

Staudt M, Lidzba K, Grodd W, Wildgruber D, Erb M, Krägeloh-Mann I. 2002. Right-hemispheric organization of language following early left-sided brain lesions: functional MRI topography. *Neuroimage* 16: 954–967.

29 Suppression of Nogo-A to Enhance CNS Repair

Roman Willi and Martin E. Schwab

The adult mammalian central nervous system (CNS) is characterized by a substantial, yet limited capacity for axon regeneration and structural plasticity. Spontaneous plastic rearrangements of neuronal circuits and connections following CNS injuries can occur at different levels such as cortex, thalamus, and brainstem, as well as spinal cord. Functional recovery after injury to the spinal cord (SCI) or the brain is highly contingent on the extent of CNS damage. Smaller lesions can induce notable structural modifications and behavioral recovery, whereas large lesions of the CNS are usually associated with poor functional improvements. In contrast to the processes in the adult CNS, plastic rearrangements and regeneration of lesioned axons in the CNS of lower vertebrates, and in the peripheral nervous system and the developing CNS of higher vertebrates, occur much more successfully. It is therefore of fundamental biological interest and crucial therapeutic relevance to understand the molecular and cellular basis for the restriction of plasticity and regeneration of adult CNS axons. Major factors for the restricted repair in the adult CNS comprise the lack of sufficient cell-autonomous growth promoters and the presence of a multitude of environmental neurite growth inhibitors (Schwab, 2004; Yiu and He, 2006). Over the past years, several neurite growth inhibitory molecules have been identified, in particular in degenerating myelin and the astroglial scar. The current list of such myelin- and scar-associated inhibitors of axonal growth ranges from Nogo-A, myelin-associated glycoprotein (MAG), oligodendrocyte myelin glycoprotein (OMgp), and chondroitin sulfate proteoglycans (CSPGs) to specific members of the families of ephrins, semaphorins, and netrins (Schwab, 2004; Carulli et al., 2005; Liu et al., 2006; Maier and Schwab, 2006; Pasterkamp and Verhaagen, 2006; Yiu and He, 2006; Low et al., 2008). For most of these candidates, however, understanding of their in vivo function in the normal CNS and their relevance in the injured adult CNS is still lacking. To date, Nogo-A is the most potent and best-studied inhibitor contributing to axon growth failure. In this chapter, we focus on the characteristics of Nogo-A and its signaling pathway components in neurite growth inhibition and discuss mechanisms of CNS repair after Nogo-A blockade and its implications for clinical application.

The Neurite Growth Inhibitory Protein Nogo-A

More than 20 years ago, Nogo-A (initially called NI-250 or IN-1 antigen) was detected as the first inhibitor of neurite growth in the adult CNS (Caroni and Schwab, 1988a, 1988b). Full purification of Nogo-A was achieved in 1998 and yielded amino acid sequences of six peptides from this protein (Spillmann et al., 1998). The peptide sequence information subsequently led to the successful cloning of its full-length cDNA (Chen et al., 2000; GrandPre et al., 2000; Prinjha et al., 2000).

Nogo-A is one of at least three major protein products that originate from the *nogo* gene by both alternative splicing and promoter usage. All three Nogo variants share a common carboxyl terminal domain of 188 amino acids that is homologous to proteins of the small family of reticulons, a family with largely unknown functions (Oertle et al., 2003a, 2003b). Nogo-A is a protein of 1,163 amino acids (200 kDa) and is predominantly expressed by oligodendrocytes in the adult mammalian CNS (Huber et al., 2002; Wang et al., 2002). Neuronal Nogo-A expression is pronounced during development but relatively low in the adult nervous system (Huber et al., 2002; Wang et al., 2002). The isoform Nogo-B (360 amino acids, 55 kDa) is found in many tissues and cell types, whereas Nogo-C (190 amino acids, 25 kDa) is primarily expressed in muscle (Huber et al., 2002). Functions of the short isoforms Nogo-B and -C are unknown so far. At least two active regions of Nogo-A are associated with neurite outgrowth inhibition and growth cone collapse and are exposed to the extracellular space. One inhibitory site, termed Δ20, is located in the middle of the Nogo-A specific sequence, a second one (Nogo-66) in a short loop between the two hydrophobic domains of the common carboxyl terminal region (GrandPre et al., 2002; Oertle et al., 2003b).

Nogo-A Signaling Pathways in Neurite Growth Inhibition

So far, two putative receptor subunits for Nogo have been characterized: the 443-residue glycosyl-phosphatidylinositol-linked, leucine-rich repeat glycoprotein NgR (Fournier et al., 2001; Barton et al., 2003; He et al., 2003) and the paired immunoglobulin-like receptor B (PirB; mouse ortholog to human leukocyte immunoglobulin-like receptor B2, LILRB2; Atwal et al., 2008). Both receptors bind to the Nogo-66 region in the carboxyl terminal domain. Although high-affinity binding to the Nogo-A specific active region (Nogo Δ20) has been shown biochemically, a receptor for this site has not been molecularly identified so far. Interestingly, NgR and PirB also bind to the myelin-associated growth inhibitors MAG and OMgp (Liu et al., 2002; Wang et al., 2002b; Atwal et al., 2008). The mechanism by which PirB signals to inhibit axon growth in response to myelin inhibitors is not clear, however. NgR interacts with transmembrane coreceptors such as p75, TROY, and LINGO-1 in a receptor complex in order to transduce the myelin inhibitory signals (Wang et al., 2002a; Wong et al., 2002; Mi et al., 2004; Park et al., 2005; Shao et al., 2005; Yiu and He, 2006). One major intracellular signaling mechanism involves the activation of Rho-A and its effector Rho kinase (ROCK), which in turn is associated with phosphorylation and activation of the actin depolimerization factor cofilin through LIM kinase to regulate cytoskeleton stability (Niederost et al., 2002; Fournier et al., 2003; Hsieh et al., 2006; Yiu and He, 2006; Montani et al., 2009). Transactivation of two other mediators, epidermal growth factor receptor (EGFR) and protein kinase C (PKC), and intracellular calcium changes may also be involved in mediating axonal growth inhibition (Bandtlow et al., 1993; Wong et al., 2002; Sivasankaran et al., 2004; Koprivica et al., 2005; Yiu and He, 2006; see figure 29.1). As reviewed in the following paragraphs, targeting these signaling components by appropriate blockers can prevent growth cone collapse and growth inhibition induced by Nogo-A and several other inhibitors.

Nogo-A as Growth Regulator in the Intact Mammalian CNS

In the developing CNS, Nogo-A has been proposed to play a role in neuronal migration in early cortex and neuronal maturation (Mingorance-Le Meur et al., 2007; Mathis et al., 2010). In postnatal development, the Nogo-Nogo receptor system was shown to be involved in restricting experience-driven plasticity during the critical period (McGee et al., 2005). In intact adult rats, Nogo-A neutralization in vivo using monoclonal antibodies induces a transitory growth response and profuse sprouting of fibers (Zagrebelsky et al., 1998; Buffo et al., 2000; Bareyre et al., 2002). In addition, neurons from adult Nogo-A knockout mice show increased growth cone motility and neurite outgrowth, presumably by regulation of the actin cytoskeleton through modulation of the Rho-GTPase/LIM kinase/cofilin pathway (Montani et al., 2009). Collectively, Nogo-A may act as a suppressor of growth and plasticity in the intact CNS both in adulthood and during development, thus stabilizing the wiring of the highly complex fiber network and acting as a repulsive cue for cell migration and fiber growth in development. The fact that blockade or lack of Nogo-A function in the uninjured CNS leads to elevation of the neuronal growth machinery (Buffo et al., 2000; Bareyre et al., 2002; Craveiro et al., 2008; Montani et al., 2009; Willi et al., 2010) immediately brings up the question of potential effects of Nogo-A inactivation after CNS lesion.

Nogo-A Inactivation: Regeneration and Functional Recovery after CNS Injury

Neuronal circuits of the brain and spinal cord retain a limited capacity for reorganization and structural plasticity throughout life. After CNS injuries such as stroke and SCI, spontaneous compensatory adaptations in intact and damaged neuronal networks may contribute in a pivotal way to the spontaneous functional improvements observed in animals and human patients (Sanes and Donoghue, 2000; Payne and Lomber, 2001; Raineteau and Schwab, 2001; Blesch and Tuszynski, 2002; Bareyre et al., 2004; Edgerton et al., 2004). For example, recovery following small cortical lesions was shown to be associated with adjacent spared cortical areas or alternative descending pathways functionally compensating for the damaged areas both in animal models and stroke patients (Nudo, 1999; Raineteau and Schwab, 2001; Calautti and Baron,

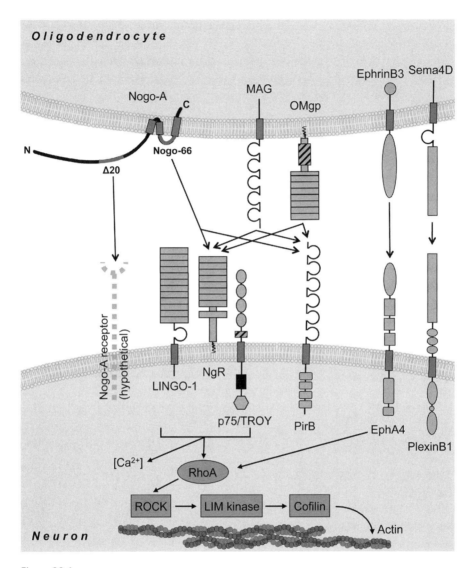

Figure 29.1
Myelin-associated inhibitors and intracellular mechanisms. The neuronal receptors for specific inhibitors and down-stream signaling pathways known to be involved in transducing these inhibitory signals are shown. Nogo-A (its Nogo-66 region), myelin-associated glycoprotein (MAG), and oligodendrocyte myelin glycoprotein (Omgp) interact with a receptor complex comprising NgR, LINGO-1, p75 (or TROY). Alternatively, these inhibitory molecules also bind to paired immunoglobulin-like receptor B (PirB). Note that the amino-terminal region of Nogo-A can also inhibit neurite outgrowth in a NgR-independent manner; the receptor for amino-Nogo is still unknown, however.

2003). Anatomical reorganization of spared descending fibers and formation of new intraspinal detour circuits after corticospinal tract (CST) lesion in rats have also been documented, and circuit formation apparently correlates with the observed improvement of hindlimb function (Bareyre et al., 2004; Courtine et al., 2008). However, such spontaneous recovery after stroke or SCI is usually partial and largely depends on the amount of spared tissue, particularly in the adult. One key reason for this restriction appears to be active inhibition of growth and plasticity by myelin (Savio and Schwab, 1990; Schwegler et al., 1995). The identification of Nogo-A as a highly potent myelin-associated inhibitor of axonal growth (Caroni and Schwab, 1988a, 1988b; Spillmann et al., 1998; Chen et al., 2000; GrandPre et al., 2000; Prinjha et al., 2000) has opened up the potential for designing and testing Nogo-targeted intervention strategies in the context of CNS injuries.

Regeneration, Sprouting, and Plasticity after Functional Blockade of Nogo-A

Neutralization of Nogo-A function is thought to trigger specific axonal repair mechanisms following injury to the CNS: regeneration of cut axons over long distances and localized plastic responses from intact fibers, as well as collateral sprouting of both damaged and spared fibers (Yiu and He, 2003; Schwab, 2004; Cafferty et al., 2008). Indeed, application of three different function-blocking monoclonal antibodies against Nogo-A has shown increased regenerative growth of injured CST axons after incomplete experimental SCI in vivo (see figure 29.2). In first experiments, lesioned CST fibers in young adult rats were reported to regenerate several millimeters beyond the site of injury when hybridoma cells producing anti-Nogo-A antibodies (IN-1) were implanted into their brain (Schnell and Schwab, 1990; Schnell et al., 1994). These promising findings were confirmed by a study using two newer highly purified monoclonal immunoglobulin G antibodies (11C7 and 7B12) delivered directly into the cerebrospinal fluid of adult rats via small intrathecal lumbar catheters (Liebscher et al., 2005). Likewise, two different Nogo-A knockout mouse lines displayed enhanced regenerative elongation after SCI (Kim et al., 2003; Simonen et al., 2003; Dimou et al., 2006), and blocking Nogo-A function through other approaches, for example, by therapies that antagonize NgR activation or by targeting downstream effectors of Nogo-NgR signaling with blocking compounds, yielded remarkably similar results with respect to CST regeneration (Dergham et al., 2002; GrandPre et al., 2002; Fournier et al., 2003).

The CST is so far the best studied spinal tract in the context of axonal regeneration after spinal cord lesion. Another descending pathway with important modulatory function for spinal cord circuits, the serotonergic raphespinal tract, also substantially responds to anti-Nogo-A antibody or NgR blocker treatment after SCI; the density of 5-HT fibers below the injury recovers, and this serotonergic re-innervation occurs in a highly lamina-specific manner (Bregman et al., 1995; GrandPre et al., 2002; Li and Strittmatter, 2003; Mullner et al., 2008). The regenerative potential after Nogo-A inactivation of other descending pathways originating from the brainstem, such as the rubrospinal, reticulospinal, and vestibulospinal tract, has not been investigated in detail yet, despite their crucial role in locomotor functions.

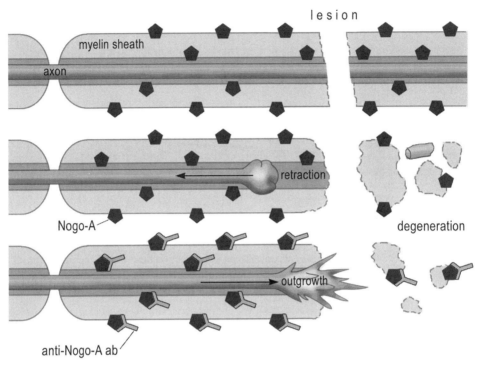

Figure 29.2
Growth-inhibitory proteins such as Nogo-A are present mainly in oligodendrocyte myelin surrounding central nervous system axons. Nogo-A signaling leads to retraction and degeneration of injured nerve fibers. Treatment with antibodies against Nogo-A after CNS injury induces growth cone formation and promotes axonal regeneration.

The observed long-distance axon growth of damaged fibers seems to correlate well with functional recovery after SCI. This relationship is, however, not exclusive, as local sprouting responses of injured and uninjured fibers are also thought to functionally compensate for the lost connections. In fact, the presence of Nogo-A blocking antibodies after unilateral transection of the CST at the level of the medulla oblongata (pyramidotomy) induces compensatory sprouting and plastic events (Thallmair et al., 1998; Z'Graggen et al., 1998). In the brainstem, sprouts of axons from the lesioned side cross the midline and innervate contralateral brainstem nuclei. The sprouting of these newly formed corticofugal fibers across the brainstem midline is topographically appropriately organized, and the newly established synaptic contacts feature characteristics of normal corticobrainstem terminals (Blochlinger et al., 2001). In the spinal cord, fibers from the intact side sprout collaterals across the spinal cord midline at various spinal levels and branch into the denervated dorsal and ventral part of the spinal cord (Thallmair et al., 1998). Interestingly, complete bilateral CST transection (by bilateral pyramidotomy) can be compensated by descending fibers from the rubrospinal system that send new collateral projections to deafferented spinal cord areas in a targeted manner in response to antibodies against

Nogo-A. These rubrospinal sprouts grow into the ventral gray matter where they build new appositions onto distal limb motoneurons which are normally not directly innervated by rubrospinal axons but receive CST input (Raineteau et al., 2001, 2002). Cortical and red nucleus microstimulations confirmed the functionality of these new connections.

Similar to conditions after SCI, blocking Nogo-A function by Nogo-A neutralization or NgR antagonism after large unilateral strokes greatly enhances collateral sprouting of corticofugal fibers from the intact to the denervated side, even when the treatment is delayed for several days. Formation of new projections originating from neurons in the contralesional intact sensorimotor cortex and targeting denervated subcortical or spinal regions results in a bilateral corticoefferent innervation pattern (Papadopoulos et al., 2002; Emerick et al., 2003; Wiessner et al., 2003; Lee et al., 2004; Seymour et al., 2005). Cortical neurons also show a higher degree of dendritic arborization and increased spine density following anti-Nogo-A antibody application (Papadopoulos et al., 2002).

Taken together, this demonstrates that lesioned and intact neurons in the injured CNS are capable of collateral sprouting, axonal regeneration, and the formation of new supraspinal and intraspinal circuits. Moreover, parallel, anatomically separate descending motor systems are able to reorganize and innervate new targets. Blocking Nogo-A signaling significantly enhances the distance of fiber growth and the often low spontaneous plastic potential.

Functional Recovery after Blockade of Nogo-A Signaling

The increased potential of fibers to grow in the injured CNS after experimental treatments decreasing Nogo-A/Nogo receptor activity is promising, but it is of utmost importance to know whether such interventions are also associated with improved recovery of sensorimotor function. Indeed, behavioral assessments were conducted in parallel with the anatomical evaluations in many of the studies done on SCI and stroke. Adult rats treated with anti-Nogo-A antibodies display enhanced functional recovery after both SCI and large strokes. For example, interruptions of the CST by large incomplete spinal cord lesions or unilateral pyramidotomy severely affect hindlimb and/or forelimb precision movements, depending on the level of the injury, and functional recovery is limited. In rats receiving Nogo-A neutralizing antibodies, however, impaired motor functions recover faster and to a much higher degree across various tests: for example, swimming, walking on a narrow beam, or crossing a horizontal ladder, but also performing precision movements such as skilled reaching and rope climbing (Bregman et al., 1995; Thallmair et al., 1998; Z'Graggen et al., 1998; Liebscher et al., 2005; see figure 29.3). Blocking Nogo-A by a soluble function-blocking NgR ectodomain, or targeting NgR or the intracellular mediators of Nogo-A signaling Rho-A and ROCK, is also effective in increasing functional recovery after SCI (Dergham et al., 2002; GrandPre et al., 2002; Li et al., 2004). Similarly, substantial functional recovery after unilateral pyramidotomy and Nogo-A or NgR knockout in mice is observed (Cafferty and Strittmatter, 2006).

An equivalent picture emerges in animal models for ischemic stroke. Middle cerebral artery occlusion or photothrombotic lesion of the sensorimotor cortex produce large unilateral strokes

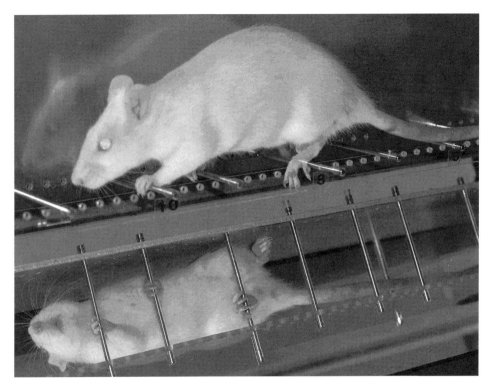

Figure 29.3
Neutralization of the myelin-associated inhibitory activity using intrathecal application of Nogo-A antibodies in vivo enhances fiber regeneration and plasticity after spinal cord injury. Animals treated with these Nogo-A function-blocking antibodies display significant functional improvement in a wide range of behavioral tests like the horizontal irregular ladder shown here.

in rodents, which are accompanied by sensorimotor deficits such as impaired skilled forelimb use (Farr and Whishaw, 2002; Gharbawie et al., 2005). As in humans, spontaneous functional recovery after large strokes is very limited. However, treatment with anti-Nogo-A antibodies or NgR receptor antagonists markedly and permanently increases the improvement of motor functions (Papadopoulos et al., 2002; Wiessner et al., 2003; Lee et al., 2004; Seymour et al., 2005).

Fibers that grow either spontaneously or through experimental manipulations in the adult CNS would have no function if they were not able to find their right targets; establishment of meaningful connections is a prerequisite for functional improvement. On the other hand, aberrant growth of primary afferent fibers and formation of random or even wrong synaptic connections could lead to pathological outcomes, such as neuropathic pain or spastic cramps (Woolf and Salter, 2000). Importantly, there is no indication of any malfunction like hypersensitivity or hyperalgesia after SCI and therapeutic treatment with reagents blocking the Nogo-A pathway

(Thallmair et al., 1998; Merkler et al., 2001; Liebscher et al., 2005). Spasticity, which develops also in rats with time after large, incomplete spinal cord lesions, was less frequent and less pronounced after anti-Nogo-A antibody treatment (Gonzenbach et al., 2010). The fact that therapeutic interventions targeting the Nogo–NgR pathway significantly enhance both regeneration and functional recovery after CNS injury is therefore intriguing, as it strongly suggests that growing fibers form new, functionally meaningful and correct connections. How these fibers find and recognize their appropriate targets and new connections are built is largely unknown as yet. Fiber tracts may initially sprout in a profuse pattern, and refinement and stabilization of the new synaptic contacts may follow in an activity-dependent manner. This would imply mechanisms of axonal guidance and target recognition as well as mechanisms of stabilization and differentiation of axonal arbors highly similar to the ones operating during development. Expression of several developmental axon guidance molecules and neurotrophic factors in the adult CNS in response to an injury can be observed, but their functional correlates in an adult tissue environment remain to be fully elucidated (Bareyre et al., 2002; Zhou et al., 2003; Zhou and Shine, 2003).

Inactivation of Nogo-A as a Clinical Avenue for Treating Spinal Cord Injury and Stroke

Traumatic spinal cord or brain injury is associated with dramatic long-term consequences, pointing to the urgency of the development of new treatment strategies. Research in rodent models has provided considerable insight into potential reparative interventions to enhance recovery after experimental SCI or stroke (Fawcett, 2002; Schwab, 2004; Silver and Miller, 2004; Thuret et al., 2006; Dobkin, 2007). Many of these studies, however, carry limitations for clinical trials, particularly with regard to ensuring the efficacy and safety of treatments for human patients. The primary reasons for that are based on differences between rodents and humans in various aspects, including anatomical, neurophysiological, and behavioral characteristics, as well as inflammatory and immune responses. The motor cortex and its descending output, the CST, for example, feature different anatomical properties and are less pronounced and important in rodents than in primates (Nudo and Frost, 2006). An increased ability to control hand musculature emerges in primates, and interruption of the CST causes more severe impairments in fine motor function of hands and feet, accordingly. The tissue reaction differs in nature and extent between these species in response to a lesion, and the time course of regenerative processes is also different (Tuszynski et al., 2002; Courtine et al., 2007). An essential step for translating entirely novel therapeutic approaches from rodents to humans therefore lies in their investigation in nonhuman primates, as this might provide a better prediction of the potential and dangers of specific therapies to mediate recovery in human patients suffering from CNS injury (Courtine et al., 2007).

A recent proof-of-concept study in adult macaque monkeys confirmed the efficacy of Nogo-A immunotherapy after SCI in primates. Unilateral cervical hemisection resulted in substantial loss of ipsilateral manual dexterity. Application of anti-Nogo-A antibodies delivered intrathecally over a period of four weeks led to increased reinnervation of the lower cervical spinal cord by regenerating CST fibers and an almost complete recovery of fine hand and finger movements of the affected hand. The improvements were stable over up to six months after the four-week antibody treatment. Importantly, there was no indication of pain or any other side effects following this therapeutic intervention (Freund et al., 2006, 2009).

Together, work on rodent models of SCI or stroke over more than a decade has critically enhanced our understanding of the detrimental mechanisms underlying these types of CNS injury. In conjunction with translational studies in nonhuman primates, this has led to the development of promising treatments that are currently under consideration for clinical trials, some of which are already ongoing. The design and organization of such clinical trials require certain prerequisites and high-level standards (Fawcett et al., 2007; Lammertse et al., 2007; Steeves et al., 2007; Tuszynski et al., 2007). As the population of injured patients is very heterogeneous with respect to lesion anatomy and, in turn, functional deficits and expected functional recovery, various factors have to be considered for inclusion and exclusion criteria, including severity, level, type, or size of the injury, as well as potentially confounding effects such as preexisting or concomitant medical conditions, other medications, and surgical interventions. In addition, outcome measures have to be analyzed on multiple levels: clinical tests, functional evaluations, and neurophysiological assessments have to be combined in order to thoroughly evaluate the effects of interventional therapies.

A currently ongoing clinical trial in acute SCI using a human anti-human Nogo-A antibody treatment (ATI 355; Novartis: NCT00406016) comprises a multinational, multicenter study design to obtain sufficient patient numbers. Networks in Europe (European Multicenter Study about Spinal Cord Injury) and North America (North American Clinical Trials Network) collecting clinical data of spinal cord injured patients serve as basis and control database for this clinical study. Highly standardized diagnosis and functional assessment protocols between different medical centers are being applied (Curt et al., 2004; Dietz and Curt, 2006). Ample initial toxicological studies related to the antibody application, particularly in nonhuman primates, have been performed and yielded no adverse effects. The ongoing Phase I of the clinical anti-Nogo-A trial coordinated by Novartis is carried out on subjects with functionally complete thoracic and cervical injuries (ASIA A; according to the American Spinal Injury Association impairment scale) primarily investigating safety, tolerance, and correct dosage of the antibody. Application for varying time periods lasting up to four weeks indicated excellent tolerance and the absence of adverse side effects so far. The near future will hopefully tell us whether therapeutic use of anti-Nogo-A antibodies in spinal cord injured patients is associated with significant regaining of sensory and motor function and may thus constitute a promising therapeutic option.

Mainly in patients with incomplete SCI, specific intense physical training during rehabilitation is crucial and may contribute to activity-dependent fine-tuning of newly formed neural circuits. Future treatment regimes for patients with SCI will thus most likely require a multidisciplinary approach, involving a combination of rehabilitative training and drugs overcoming the inhibition of growth and enhancing regeneration and plasticity. The differential mechanisms leading to recovery during training and antibody-based interventions have to be taken into account in designing these combinatorial therapies (Maier et al., 2009). The challenge for the design of optimal treatment protocols will be that potential positive interactive effects of each treatment can be fully exerted to get maximal functional recovery.

Some alternative treatment strategies targeting different molecular and cellular aspects after SCI are under development (Hawryluk et al., 2008; Rowland et al., 2008). Given that the Rho–ROCK signaling pathway is an important downstream mediator of the Nogo receptor, it represents an important point of convergence for multiple inhibitory signals. Blocking Rho by pharmacological intervention through a compound called Cethrin (Alseres Pharmaceuticals, Inc.: NCT00500812 and NCT00610337) is currently being evaluated as a potential therapeutic approach in a Phase II clinical study. Inhibitory CSPGs around the glial scar in the days following an injury prevent axons from growing through or around the spinal cord lesion site. Strategies to overcome this glial barrier focus on digestion of CSPGs with chondroitinase ABC (chABC). Other therapeutic interventions are based on application of neurotrophic factors to prevent neuronal atrophy and stimulate growth. In addition, cellular transplantation therapies are being applied to override the limited substrate for neural repair by directly replacing cells lost due to injury and by influencing the environment in order to support axonal regeneration and myelin repair and to provide neuroprotection. Such cellular approaches include transplantation of a diverse range of cell types, including glial cells and their progenitors, as well as embryonic and adult neural and bone marrow-derived stem cell populations. Future interventional strategies may involve combinatorial regimes that integrate neuroprotective, neuroregenerative, and rehabilitative approaches in the hope of optimizing the recovery of individuals with traumatic SCI.

Conclusions

Large injuries to the CNS are accompanied by profound lifelong consequences for the affected subject. Spontaneous repair mechanisms, including structural changes, rewiring processes, and circuit rearrangements, can contribute to spontaneous functional recovery—this is, however, limited, and there is a tremendous need for new medical strategies to enhance axonal regeneration and, in turn, improve the quality of the patient's life. Identification of inhibitors of regeneration and neuronal plasticity has allowed the development of specific therapeutic agents targeting these restrictors. Neutralization of the most potent of these inhibitory molecules, Nogo-A, in animal models of SCI and stroke has been shown to be effective in triggering axonal repair mechanisms and behavioral improvements. A currently ongoing clinical trial using anti-Nogo-A antibodies in paraplegic patients will tell us whether such antibody application will provide a major breakthrough with regard to treatment of humans suffering from CNS injuries.

Acknowledgments

Our work is supported by grants from the Swiss National Science Foundation, the National Center for Competence in Research "Neural Plasticity & Repair" of the Swiss National Science

Foundation, the Spinal Cord Consortium of the Christopher and Dana Reeve Foundation (Springfield, NJ), the EU–Network of Excellence NeuroNE (FP6), and the EU Collaborative Projects SPINAL CORD REPAIR (FP7) and ARISE (FP7). The authors thank Roland Schöb and Eva Hochreutener for help with the illustrations.

References

Atwal JK, Pinkston-Gosse J, Syken J, Stawicki S, Wu Y, Shatz C, Tessier-Lavigne M. 2008. PirB is a functional receptor for myelin inhibitors of axonal regeneration. *Science* 322: 967–970.

Bandtlow CE, Schmidt MF, Hassinger TD, Schwab ME, Kater SB. 1993. Role of intracellular calcium in NI-35-evoked collapse of neuronal growth cones. *Science* 259: 80–83.

Bareyre FM, Haudenschild B, Schwab ME. 2002. Long-lasting sprouting and gene expression changes induced by the monoclonal antibody IN-1 in the adult spinal cord. *J Neurosci* 22: 7097–7110.

Bareyre FM, Kerschensteiner M, Raineteau O, Mettenleiter TC, Weinmann O, Schwab ME. 2004. The injured spinal cord spontaneously forms a new intraspinal circuit in adult rats. *Nat Neurosci* 7: 269–277.

Barton WA, Liu BP, Tzvetkova D, Jeffrey PD, Fournier AE, Sah D, Cate R, Strittmatter SM, Nikolov DB. 2003. Structure and axon outgrowth inhibitor binding of the Nogo-66 receptor and related proteins. *EMBO J* 22: 3291–3302.

Blesch A, Tuszynski MH. 2002. Spontaneous and neurotrophin-induced axonal plasticity after spinal cord injury. *Prog Brain Res* 137: 415–423.

Blochlinger S, Weinmann O, Schwab ME, Thallmair M. 2001. Neuronal plasticity and formation of new synaptic contacts follow pyramidal lesions and neutralization of Nogo-A: a light and electron microscopic study in the pontine nuclei of adult rats. *J Comp Neurol* 433: 426–436.

Bregman BS, Kunkel-Bagden E, Schnell L, Dai HN, Gao D, Schwab ME. 1995. Recovery from spinal cord injury mediated by antibodies to neurite growth inhibitors. *Nature* 378: 498–501.

Buffo A, Zagrebelsky M, Huber AB, Skerra A, Schwab ME, Strata P, Rossi F. 2000. Application of neutralizing antibodies against NI-35/250 myelin-associated neurite growth inhibitory proteins to the adult rat cerebellum induces sprouting of uninjured purkinje cell axons. *J Neurosci* 20: 2275–2286.

Cafferty WB, Strittmatter SM. 2006. The Nogo–Nogo receptor pathway limits a spectrum of adult CNS axonal growth. *J Neurosci* 26: 12242–12250.

Cafferty WB, McGee AW, Strittmatter SM. 2008. Axonal growth therapeutics: regeneration or sprouting or plasticity? *Trends Neurosci* 31: 215–220.

Calautti C, Baron JC. 2003. Functional neuroimaging studies of motor recovery after stroke in adults: a review. *Stroke* 34: 1553–1566.

Caroni P, Schwab ME. 1988a. Antibody against myelin-associated inhibitor of neurite growth neutralizes nonpermissive substrate properties of CNS white matter. *Neuron* 1: 85–96.

Caroni P, Schwab ME. 1988b. Two membrane protein fractions from rat central myelin with inhibitory properties for neurite growth and fibroblast spreading. *J Cell Biol* 106: 1281–1288.

Carulli D, Laabs T, Geller HM, Fawcett JW. 2005. Chondroitin sulfate proteoglycans in neural development and regeneration. *Curr Opin Neurobiol* 15: 116–120.

Chen MS, Huber AB, van der Haar ME, Frank M, Schnell L, Spillmann AA, Christ F, Schwab ME. 2000. Nogo-A is a myelin-associated neurite outgrowth inhibitor and an antigen for monoclonal antibody IN-1. *Nature* 403: 434–439.

Courtine G, Bunge MB, Fawcett JW, Grossman RG, Kaas JH, Lemon R, Maier I, et al. 2007. Can experiments in nonhuman primates expedite the translation of treatments for spinal cord injury in humans? *Nat Med* 13: 561–566.

Courtine G, Song B, Roy RR, Zhong H, Herrmann JE, Ao Y, Qi J, Edgerton VR, Sofroniew MV. 2008. Recovery of supraspinal control of stepping via indirect propriospinal relay connections after spinal cord injury. *Nat Med* 14: 69–74.

Craveiro LM, Hakkoum D, Weinmann O, Montani L, Stoppini L, Schwab ME. 2008. Neutralization of the membrane protein Nogo-A enhances growth and reactive sprouting in established organotypic hippocampal slice cultures. *Eur J Neurosci* 28: 1808–1824.

Curt A, Schwab ME, Dietz V. 2004. Providing the clinical basis for new interventional therapies: refined diagnosis and assessment of recovery after spinal cord injury. *Spinal Cord* 42: 1–6.

Dergham P, Ellezam B, Essagian C, Avedissian H, Lubell WD, McKerracher L. 2002. Rho signaling pathway targeted to promote spinal cord repair. *J Neurosci* 22: 6570–6577.

Dietz V, Curt A. 2006. Neurological aspects of spinal-cord repair: promises and challenges. *Lancet Neurol* 5: 688–694.

Dimou L, Schnell L, Montani L, Duncan C, Simonen M, Schneider R, Liebscher T, Gullo M, Schwab ME. 2006. Nogo-A-deficient mice reveal strain-dependent differences in axonal regeneration. *J Neurosci* 26: 5591–5603.

Dobkin BH. 2007. Curiosity and cure: translational research strategies for neural repair-mediated rehabilitation. *Dev Neurobiol* 67: 1133–1147.

Edgerton VR, Tillakaratne NJ, Bigbee AJ, de Leon RD, Roy RR. 2004. Plasticity of the spinal neural circuitry after injury. *Annu Rev Neurosci* 27: 145–167.

Emerick AJ, Neafsey EJ, Schwab ME, Kartje GL. 2003. Functional reorganization of the motor cortex in adult rats after cortical lesion and treatment with monoclonal antibody IN-1. *J Neurosci* 23: 4826–4830.

Farr TD, Whishaw IQ. 2002. Quantitative and qualitative impairments in skilled reaching in the mouse (Mus musculus) after a focal motor cortex stroke. *Stroke* 33: 1869–1875.

Fawcett J. 2002. Repair of spinal cord injuries: where are we, where are we going? *Spinal Cord* 40: 615–623.

Fawcett JW, Curt A, Steeves JD, Coleman WP, Tuszynski MH, Lammertse D, Bartlett PF, et al. 2007. Guidelines for the conduct of clinical trials for spinal cord injury as developed by the ICCP panel: spontaneous recovery after spinal cord injury and statistical power needed for therapeutic clinical trials. *Spinal Cord* 45: 190–205.

Fournier AE, GrandPre T, Strittmatter SM. 2001. Identification of a receptor mediating Nogo-66 inhibition of axonal regeneration. *Nature* 409: 341–346.

Fournier AE, Takizawa BT, Strittmatter SM. 2003. Rho kinase inhibition enhances axonal regeneration in the injured CNS. *J Neurosci* 23: 1416–1423.

Freund P, Schmidlin E, Wannier T, Bloch J, Mir A, Schwab ME, Rouiller EM. 2006. Nogo-A-specific antibody treatment enhances sprouting and functional recovery after cervical lesion in adult primates. *Nat Med* 12: 790–792.

Freund P, Schmidlin E, Wannier T, Bloch J, Mir A, Schwab ME, Rouiller EM. 2009. Anti-Nogo-A antibody treatment promotes recovery of manual dexterity after unilateral cervical lesion in adult primates—re-examination and extension of behavioral data. *Eur J Neurosci* 29: 983–996.

Gharbawie OA, Gonzalez CL, Whishaw IQ. 2005. Skilled reaching impairments from the lateral frontal cortex component of middle cerebral artery stroke: a qualitative and quantitative comparison to focal motor cortex lesions in rats. *Behav Brain Res* 156: 125–137.

Gonzenbach RR, Gasser P, Zorner B, Hochreutener E, Schwab ME. 2010. Muscle spasms in spinal cord injured rats are reduced by training or neurite growth enhancing treatment. *Ann Neurol.* 68: 48–57.

GrandPre T, Nakamura F, Vartanian T, Strittmatter SM. 2000. Identification of the Nogo inhibitor of axon regeneration as a Reticulon protein. *Nature* 403: 439–444.

GrandPre T, Li S, Strittmatter SM. 2002. Nogo-66 receptor antagonist peptide promotes axonal regeneration. *Nature* 417: 547–551.

Hawryluk GW, Rowland J, Kwon BK, Fehlings MG. 2008. Protection and repair of the injured spinal cord: a review of completed, ongoing, and planned clinical trials for acute spinal cord injury. *Neurosurg Focus* 25: E14.

He XL, Bazan JF, McDermott G, Park JB, Wang K, Tessier-Lavigne M, He Z, Garcia KC. 2003. Structure of the Nogo receptor ectodomain: a recognition module implicated in myelin inhibition. *Neuron* 38: 177–185.

Hsieh SH, Ferraro GB, Fournier AE. 2006. Myelin-associated inhibitors regulate cofilin phosphorylation and neuronal inhibition through LIM kinase and Slingshot phosphatase. *J Neurosci* 26: 1006–1015.

Huber AB, Weinmann O, Brosamle C, Oertle T, Schwab ME. 2002. Patterns of Nogo mRNA and protein expression in the developing and adult rat and after CNS lesions. *J Neurosci* 22: 3553–3567.

Kim JE, Li S, GrandPre T, Qiu D, Strittmatter SM. 2003. Axon regeneration in young adult mice lacking Nogo-A/B. *Neuron* 38: 187–199.

Koprivica V, Cho KS, Park JB, Yiu G, Atwal J, Gore B, Kim JA, Lin E, Tessier-Lavigne M, Chen DF, He Z. 2005. EGFR activation mediates inhibition of axon regeneration by myelin and chondroitin sulfate proteoglycans. *Science* 310: 106–110.

Lammertse D, Tuszynski MH, Steeves JD, Curt A, Fawcett JW, Rask C, Ditunno JF, et al. 2007. Guidelines for the conduct of clinical trials for spinal cord injury as developed by the ICCP panel: clinical trial design. *Spinal Cord* 45: 232–242.

Lee JK, Kim JE, Sivula M, Strittmatter SM. 2004. Nogo receptor antagonism promotes stroke recovery by enhancing axonal plasticity. *J Neurosci* 24: 6209–6217.

Li S, Strittmatter SM. 2003. Delayed systemic Nogo-66 receptor antagonist promotes recovery from spinal cord injury. *J Neurosci* 23: 4219–4227.

Li S, Liu BP, Budel S, Li M, Ji B, Walus L, Li W, et al. 2004. Blockade of Nogo-66, myelin-associated glycoprotein, and oligodendrocyte myelin glycoprotein by soluble Nogo-66 receptor promotes axonal sprouting and recovery after spinal injury. *J Neurosci* 24: 10511–10520.

Liebscher T, Schnell L, Schnell D, Scholl J, Schneider R, Gullo M, Fouad K, et al. 2005. Nogo-A antibody improves regeneration and locomotion of spinal cord-injured rats. *Ann Neurol* 58: 706–719.

Liu BP, Fournier A, GrandPre T, Strittmatter SM. 2002. Myelin-associated glycoprotein as a functional ligand for the Nogo-66 receptor. *Science* 297: 1190–1193.

Liu BP, Cafferty WB, Budel SO, Strittmatter SM. 2006. Extracellular regulators of axonal growth in the adult central nervous system. *Philos Trans R Soc Lond B Biol Sci* 361: 1593–1610.

Low K, Culbertson M, Bradke F, Tessier-Lavigne M, Tuszynski MH. 2008. Netrin-1 is a novel myelin-associated inhibitor to axon growth. *J Neurosci* 28: 1099–1108.

Maier IC, Schwab ME. 2006. Sprouting, regeneration and circuit formation in the injured spinal cord: factors and activity. *Philos Trans R Soc Lond B Biol Sci* 361: 1611–1634.

Maier IC, Ichiyama RM, Courtine G, Schnell L, Lavrov I, Edgerton VR, Schwab ME. 2009. Differential effects of anti-Nogo-A antibody treatment and treadmill training in rats with incomplete spinal cord injury. *Brain* 132: 1426–1440.

Mathis C, Schroter A, Thallmair M, Schwab ME. 2010. Nogo-A regulates neural precursor migration in the embryonic mouse cortex. *Cereb Cortex* 20: 2380–2390.

McGee AW, Yang Y, Fischer QS, Daw NW, Strittmatter SM. 2005. Experience-driven plasticity of visual cortex limited by myelin and Nogo receptor. *Science* 309: 2222–2226.

Merkler D, Metz GA, Raineteau O, Dietz V, Schwab ME, Fouad K. 2001. Locomotor recovery in spinal cord-injured rats treated with an antibody neutralizing the myelin-associated neurite growth inhibitor Nogo-A. *J Neurosci* 21: 3665–3673.

Mi S, Lee X, Shao Z, Thill G, Ji B, Relton J, Levesque M, et al. 2004. LINGO-1 is a component of the Nogo-66 receptor/p75 signaling complex. *Nat Neurosci* 7: 221–228.

Mingorance-Le Meur A, Zheng B, Soriano E, del Rio JA. 2007. Involvement of the myelin-associated inhibitor Nogo-A in early cortical development and neuronal maturation. *Cereb Cortex* 17: 2375–2386.

Montani L, Gerrits B, Gehrig P, Kempf A, Dimou L, Wollscheid B, Schwab ME. 2009. Neuronal Nogo-A modulates growth cone motility via Rho-GTP/LIMK1/cofilin in the unlesioned adult nervous system. *J Biol Chem* 284: 10793–10807.

Mullner A, Gonzenbach RR, Weinmann O, Schnell L, Liebscher T, Schwab ME. 2008. Lamina-specific restoration of serotonergic projections after Nogo-A antibody treatment of spinal cord injury in rats. *Eur J Neurosci* 27: 326–333.

Niederost B, Oertle T, Fritsche J, McKinney RA, Bandtlow CE. 2002. Nogo-A and myelin-associated glycoprotein mediate neurite growth inhibition by antagonistic regulation of RhoA and Rac1. *J Neurosci* 22: 10368–10376.

Nudo RJ. 1999. Recovery after damage to motor cortical areas. *Curr Opin Neurobiol* 9: 740–747.

Nudo RJ, Frost SB. 2006. The evolution of motor cortex and motor systems. In: *Evolution of Nervous Systems in Mammals* (Krubitzer LA, Kaas JH, eds), pp 373–395. Oxford: Academic Press.

Oertle T, Klinger M, Stuermer CA, Schwab ME. 2003a. A reticular rhapsody: phylogenic evolution and nomenclature of the RTN/Nogo gene family. *FASEB J* 17: 1238–1247.

Oertle T, van der Haar ME, Bandtlow CE, Robeva A, Burfeind P, Buss A, Huber AB, et al. 2003b. Nogo-A inhibits neurite outgrowth and cell spreading with three discrete regions. *J Neurosci* 23: 5393–5406.

Papadopoulos CM, Tsai SY, Alsbiei T, O'Brien TE, Schwab ME, Kartje GL. 2002. Functional recovery and neuroanatomical plasticity following middle cerebral artery occlusion and IN-1 antibody treatment in the adult rat. *Ann Neurol* 51: 433–441.

Park JB, Yiu G, Kaneko S, Wang J, Chang J, He XL, Garcia KC, He Z. 2005. A TNF receptor family member, TROY, is a coreceptor with Nogo receptor in mediating the inhibitory activity of myelin inhibitors. *Neuron* 45: 345–351.

Pasterkamp RJ, Verhaagen J. 2006. Semaphorins in axon regeneration: developmental guidance molecules gone wrong? *Philos Trans R Soc Lond B Biol Sci* 361: 1499–1511.

Payne BR, Lomber SG. 2001. Reconstructing functional systems after lesions of cerebral cortex. *Nat Rev Neurosci* 2: 911–919.

Prinjha R, Moore SE, Vinson M, Blake S, Morrow R, Christie G, Michalovich D, Simmons DL, Walsh FS. 2000. Inhibitor of neurite outgrowth in humans. *Nature* 403: 383–384.

Raineteau O, Schwab ME. 2001. Plasticity of motor systems after incomplete spinal cord injury. *Nat Rev Neurosci* 2: 263–273.

Raineteau O, Fouad K, Noth P, Thallmair M, Schwab ME. 2001. Functional switch between motor tracts in the presence of the mAb IN-1 in the adult rat. *Proc Natl Acad Sci USA* 98: 6929–6934.

Raineteau O, Fouad K, Bareyre FM, Schwab ME. 2002. Reorganization of descending motor tracts in the rat spinal cord. *Eur J Neurosci* 16: 1761–1771.

Rowland JW, Hawryluk GW, Kwon B, Fehlings MG. 2008. Current status of acute spinal cord injury pathophysiology and emerging therapies: promise on the horizon. *Neurosurg Focus* 25: E2.

Sanes JN, Donoghue JP. 2000. Plasticity and primary motor cortex. *Annu Rev Neurosci* 23: 393–415.

Savio T, Schwab ME. 1990. Lesioned corticospinal tract axons regenerate in myelin-free rat spinal cord. *Proc Natl Acad Sci USA* 87: 4130–4133.

Schnell L, Schwab ME. 1990. Axonal regeneration in the rat spinal cord produced by an antibody against myelin-associated neurite growth inhibitors. *Nature* 343: 269–272.

Schnell L, Schneider R, Kolbeck R, Barde YA, Schwab ME. 1994. Neurotrophin-3 enhances sprouting of corticospinal tract during development and after adult spinal cord lesion. *Nature* 367: 170–173.

Schwab ME. 2004. Nogo and axon regeneration. *Curr Opin Neurobiol* 14: 118–124.

Schwegler G, Schwab ME, Kapfhammer JP. 1995. Increased collateral sprouting of primary afferents in the myelin-free spinal cord. *J Neurosci* 15: 2756–2767.

Seymour AB, Andrews EM, Tsai SY, Markus TM, Bollnow MR, Brenneman MM, O'Brien TE, Castro AJ, Schwab ME, Kartje GL. 2005. Delayed treatment with monoclonal antibody IN-1 1 week after stroke results in recovery of function and corticorubral plasticity in adult rats. *J Cereb Blood Flow Metab* 25: 1366–1375.

Shao Z, Browning JL, Lee X, Scott ML, Shulga-Morskaya S, Allaire N, Thill G, et al. 2005. TAJ/TROY, an orphan TNF receptor family member, binds Nogo-66 receptor 1 and regulates axonal regeneration. *Neuron* 45: 353–359.

Silver J, Miller JH. 2004. Regeneration beyond the glial scar. *Nat Rev Neurosci* 5: 146–156.

Simonen M, Pedersen V, Weinmann O, Schnell L, Buss A, Ledermann B, Christ F, Sansig G, van der Putten H, Schwab ME. 2003. Systemic deletion of the myelin-associated outgrowth inhibitor Nogo-A improves regenerative and plastic responses after spinal cord injury. *Neuron* 38: 201–211.

Sivasankaran R, Pei J, Wang KC, Zhang YP, Shields CB, Xu XM, He Z. 2004. PKC mediates inhibitory effects of myelin and chondroitin sulfate proteoglycans on axonal regeneration. *Nat Neurosci* 7: 261–268.

Spillmann AA, Bandtlow CE, Lottspeich F, Keller F, Schwab ME. 1998. Identification and characterization of a bovine neurite growth inhibitor (bNI-220). *J Biol Chem* 273: 19283–19293.

Steeves JD, Lammertse D, Curt A, Fawcett JW, Tuszynski MH, Ditunno JF, Ellaway PH, et al. 2007. Guidelines for the conduct of clinical trials for spinal cord injury (SCI) as developed by the ICCP panel: clinical trial outcome measures. *Spinal Cord* 45: 206–221.

Thallmair M, Metz GA, Z'Graggen WJ, Raineteau O, Kartje GL, Schwab ME. 1998. Neurite growth inhibitors restrict plasticity and functional recovery following corticospinal tract lesions. *Nat Neurosci* 1: 124–131.

Thuret S, Moon LD, Gage FH. 2006. Therapeutic interventions after spinal cord injury. *Nat Rev Neurosci* 7: 628–643.

Tuszynski MH, Grill R, Jones LL, McKay HM, Blesch A. 2002. Spontaneous and augmented growth of axons in the primate spinal cord: effects of local injury and nerve growth factor-secreting cell grafts. *J Comp Neurol* 449: 88–101.

Tuszynski MH, Steeves JD, Fawcett JW, Lammertse D, Kalichman M, Rask C, Curt A, et al. 2007. Guidelines for the conduct of clinical trials for spinal cord injury as developed by the ICCP Panel: clinical trial inclusion/exclusion criteria and ethics. *Spinal Cord* 45: 222–231.

Wang KC, Kim JA, Sivasankaran R, Segal R, He Z. 2002a. P75 interacts with the Nogo receptor as a co-receptor for Nogo, MAG and OMgp. *Nature* 420: 74–78.

Wang KC, Koprivica V, Kim JA, Sivasankaran R, Guo Y, Neve RL, He Z. 2002b. Oligodendrocyte-myelin glycoprotein is a Nogo receptor ligand that inhibits neurite outgrowth. *Nature* 417: 941–944.

Wang X, Chun SJ, Treloar H, Vartanian T, Greer CA, Strittmatter SM. 2002. Localization of Nogo-A and Nogo-66 receptor proteins at sites of axon–myelin and synaptic contact. *J Neurosci* 22: 5505–5515.

Wiessner C, Bareyre FM, Allegrini PR, Mir AK, Frentzel S, Zurini M, Schnell L, Oertle T, Schwab ME. 2003. Anti-Nogo-A antibody infusion 24 hours after experimental stroke improved behavioral outcome and corticospinal plasticity in normotensive and spontaneously hypertensive rats. *J Cereb Blood Flow Metab* 23: 154–165.

Willi R, Weinmann O, Winter C, Klein J, Sohr R, Schnell L, Yee BK, Feldon J, Schwab ME. 2010. Constitutive genetic deletion of the growth regulator Nogo-A induces schizophrenia-related endophenotypes. *J Neurosci* 30: 556–567.

Wong ST, Henley JR, Kanning KC, Huang KH, Bothwell M, Poo MM. 2002. A p75(NTR) and Nogo receptor complex mediates repulsive signaling by myelin-associated glycoprotein. *Nat Neurosci* 5: 1302–1308.

Woolf CJ, Salter MW. 2000. Neuronal plasticity: increasing the gain in pain. *Science* 288: 1765–1769.

Yiu G, He Z. 2003. Signaling mechanisms of the myelin inhibitors of axon regeneration. *Curr Opin Neurobiol* 13: 545–551.

Yiu G, He Z. 2006. Glial inhibition of CNS axon regeneration. *Nat Rev Neurosci* 7: 617–627.

Zagrebelsky M, Buffo A, Skerra A, Schwab ME, Strata P, Rossi F. 1998. Retrograde regulation of growth-associated gene expression in adult rat Purkinje cells by myelin-associated neurite growth inhibitory proteins. *J Neurosci* 18: 7912–7929.

Z'Graggen WJ, Metz GA, Kartje GL, Thallmair M, Schwab ME. 1998. Functional recovery and enhanced corticofugal plasticity after unilateral pyramidal tract lesion and blockade of myelin-associated neurite growth inhibitors in adult rats. *J Neurosci* 18: 4744–4757.

Zhou L, Shine HD. 2003. Neurotrophic factors expressed in both cortex and spinal cord induce axonal plasticity after spinal cord injury. *J Neurosci Res* 74: 221–226.

Zhou L, Baumgartner BJ, Hill-Felberg SJ, McGowen LR, Shine HD. 2003. Neurotrophin-3 expressed in situ induces axonal plasticity in the adult injured spinal cord. *J Neurosci* 23: 1424–1431.

30 New Perspectives in the Treatment of Amblyopia

Dennis M. Levi

Amblyopia (from the Greek, *amblyos*—blunt; *opia*—vision) is a developmental abnormality that results from physiological alterations in the visual cortex and impairs form vision (Ciuffreda, Levi, and Selenow, 1991). Amblyopia is clinically important because, aside from refractive error, it is the most frequent cause of vision loss in infants and young children, occurring naturally in about 2% to 4% of the population (see Ciuffreda, Levi, and Selenow, 1991), and it is of basic interest because it reflects the neural impairment which can occur when normal visual development is disrupted. The damage produced by amblyopia is generally expressed in the clinical setting as a loss of visual acuity in an apparently healthy eye, despite appropriate optical correction; however, there is a great deal of evidence showing that amblyopia results in a broad range of neural, perceptual, and clinical abnormalities (for reviews, see Kiorpes, 2006; Levi, 2006).

Amblyopia can easily be reversed or eliminated when diagnosed and treated early in life. Thus, there is a premium on early detection of amblyopia and its risk factors. It has been estimated that perhaps as many as three quarters of a million preschoolers are at risk for amblyopia in the United States, and roughly half of those may not be detected before school age. Moreover, detection is likely to be more delayed in low socioeconomic areas. Improved vision screening and access to treatment could, in principle, eliminate amblyopia as a public health issue (Wu and Hunter, 2006).

There has been a sea change in our thinking about amblyopia in the last decade based on a new understanding of the underlying pathophysiology (based in part on new brain-imaging methods such as functional magnetic resonance imaging) and a massive shift in our thinking about adult plasticity and the treatment of amblyopia fueled by a number of important clinical trials and by pioneering work by Lamberto Maffei and his colleagues in a rodent model of amblyopia.

Critical Periods in Perceptual Development

Critical periods for experience-dependent plasticity are ubiquitous. They occur in virtually every species from *Drosophila* to human (Berardi et al., 2000) and for a wide range of sensory functions. Hubel and Wiesel's Nobel Prize-winning work showing the importance of sensory experience in shaping neural connections during a critical period early in life was inspired, in large measure, by the 18th-century notion that early visual deprivation (e.g., blindness at birth) resulted in brain changes that led, in turn, to defective visual perception (Wiesel, 1982). Based in good measure on the work of Hubel and Wiesel and subsequent anatomical and physiological studies, it is now clear that while the visual cortex is by no means a tabula rasa, there is a good deal of specification at birth. However, it is also clear that there is an important role for maturation and experience.

It is now clear that that there are different critical periods for different functions, even within the same sensory system (e.g., Harwerth et al., 1987, 1990), different critical periods for different parts of the brain, even within different layers of the primary visual cortex (LeVay et al., 1980), and different critical periods for recovery than for induction of sensory deprivation (Berardi et al., 2000).

It has long been held that there is a close correspondence between sensory development and the critical period (e.g., Teller and Movshon, 1986), and the idea that experience-dependent plasticity is closely linked with the development of sensory function is still widely held (Berardi et al., 2000). However, as we shall discuss later, there is also growing evidence for plasticity in the adult nervous system.

Critical Periods and Neural Plasticity in Human Vision

Much of the evidence for critical periods stems from work on the effects of altered sensory input in the cat and the monkey, in particular, monocular visual deprivation, strabismus, or unequal refractive error (Wiesel, 1982; for a recent review, see Mitchell, 2004). If the sensory deprivation occurs early, the animal is left with a permanent visual impairment—with amblyopia and with permanent alterations in primary visual cortex.

In humans, the presence of amblyopia is almost always associated with an early history of abnormal visual experience: binocular misregistration (strabismus) or image degradation (high refractive error, anisometropia, cataract, or form deprivation). The severity of the amblyopia appears to be associated with the degree of imbalance between the two eyes (e.g., dense unilateral cataract results in severe loss) and with the age at which the amblyogenic factor occurred. Precisely how these factors interact is as yet unknown, but it is now clear that different early visual experiences result in different functional losses in amblyopia (McKee, Levi, and Movshon, 2003), and a clear and significant factor that distinguishes performance among amblyopes is the presence or absence of binocular function.

Critical Periods for the Development of Amblyopia

Clinicians are well aware that amblyopia does not develop after 6 to 8 years of age (Worth, 1903; von Noorden, 1981), suggesting that there is a "sensitive period" for the development of amblyopia; however, in humans with naturally occurring amblyopia, the age of onset of the amblyogenic condition(s) is difficult to ascertain, and the effects of intervention combine to make it difficult to obtain a clear picture of the "natural history" of amblyopia development. Thus, much of our current understanding of the development of amblyopia accrues from animal studies (see Boothe et al., 1985, for a review) and from retrospective studies of clinical records (e.g., von Noorden, 1981). Technological improvements in infant testing have also provided more direct data on the development of naturally occurring amblyopia in humans (Mohindra et al., 1979; Maurer et al., 1983; Jacobson et al., 1981; Birch, 1983; Maurer et al., 1999) and monkeys (Kiorpes and Boothe, 1981; Kiorpes et al., 1984, 1989). All of these studies provide strong evidence for amblyopia induced by early deprivation.

An attractive hypothesis is that structures and functions which develop earliest are most robust to the effects of abnormal visual input while those that develop more slowly seem most suscep-tible. Levi and Carkeet (1993) called this the "Detroit model"—a biological analog of the "last hired, first fired" philosophy. This hypothesis suggests that different structures and/or functions may be susceptible to the effects of visual deprivation at different times during development. As noted above, there is clear evidence from anatomical and physiological studies that the sensi-tive period in layer IVc (the input layer) of the cortex of monkeys is considerably shorter than that of other layers (LeVay et al., 1980). Behavioral studies of lid-sutured monkeys (Harwerth et al., 1987, 1990) provide strong evidence that different psychophysical functions are affected by lid suture at different times. For example, they found that early lid suture (age 3–6 months) had a marked influence upon scotopic and photopic spectral sensitivity and essentially abolished pattern and binocular vision. A later onset of deprivation (up to about 25 months) had no influ-ence upon spectral sensitivity, but it resulted in reduced contrast sensitivity at high spatial fre-quencies, and reduced binocular summation. Lid suture beyond 25 months had no effect on contrast sensitivity but still disrupted binocular functioning. There are several points worth noting. First, to extrapolate these results to monocular pattern deprivation in humans, the 1:4 rule should be applied (i.e., 1 monkey year is equivalent to about 4 human years; Boothe, Dobson, and Teller, 1985). Second, the effects of deprivation seem to be the "mirror image" of the developmental sequence. Thus, as noted above, different visual functions (and presumably their underlying anatomical and physiological structures) develop at different rates. Those which develop earliest seem most robust to the influences of pattern deprivation while those that develop last are most at risk and remain susceptible for the longest time.

While the upper limit for susceptibility of excitatory binocular interactions is not yet certain, it appears to be later than that for acuity or contrast sensitivity in monkeys and may extend to at least 7 or 8 years (and possibly more) in humans. Psychophysical studies of interocu-lar transfer in humans with a history of strabismus (Banks et al., 1975; Hohmann and Creutzfeldt, 1975) provide an indirect estimate of the period of susceptibility of binocular connections. The results of both studies suggest that binocular connections are highly vulnerable during the first 18 months of life and remain susceptible to the effects of strabismus until at least age 7 years.

Is There a Critical Period for Treatment of Amblyopia?

The notion that there is a critical period(s) for the development of amblyopia has often been taken to indicate that there is also a critical period for the treatment of amblyopia. This concept grew out of the work of Claude Worth (1903). Worth suggested that the presence of a "sensory obstacle" (e.g., unilateral strabismus) arrested the development of visual acuity ("amblyopia of arrest"), so that the patient's acuity remained at the level achieved at the time of onset of strabismus. In this view, the depth of amblyopia is a direct function of the age of onset of the "sensory obstacle." Worth further suggested that if amblyopia of arrest were allowed to persist, that "amblyopia of extinction" could occur as a result of binocular inhibition. In Worth's view, only this "extra" loss of sensory function (i.e., the amblyopia of extinction) could be recovered by treatment. Although this latter notion is open to question in the light of present knowledge, the ideas of Worth (1903) have had a powerful influence upon both clinicians and basic scientists. Thus, many of our currently held concepts of amblyopia, such as plasticity, sensitive periods, and abnormal binocular interaction, were already described more than a century ago and gained currency with the work of Hubel and Wiesel (1970) and the many anatomical and physiological studies that followed. Thus, while amblyopia can often be reversed when treated early, treatment is generally not undertaken in older children and adults. Below, we consider both experimental and clinical evidence for plasticity in the adult visual system that calls into question the notion of a sensitive period for treatment.

For centuries, the primary treatment for amblyopia has consisted of patching or penalizing the fellow preferred eye, thus "forcing" the brain to use the weaker amblyopic eye. It is often stated that humans with amblyopia cannot be treated beyond a certain age; however a review of the literature suggests otherwise. Recent clinical trials suggest that treatment may be just as effective in older (13 to 17 years) patients who have not been previously treated as in younger (7 to 12 years) children (Pediatric Eye Disease Investigator Group, 2005).

Plasticity in adults with amblyopia is also dramatically evident in the report of amblyopic patients whose visual acuity spontaneously improved in the wake of visual loss due to macular degeneration in the fellow eye (El Mallah, Chakravarthy, and Hart, 2000; Rahi et al., 2002). There are also reports suggesting that some adult amblyopes recover vision in their amblyopic eye following loss of vision in their fellow (nonamblyopic) eye (Vereecken and Brabant, 1984). These studies are consistent with the notion that the connections from the amblyopic eye may be suppressed rather than destroyed. Loss of the fellow eye would allow these existing connections to be unmasked, as occurs in adult cats with retinal lesions.

Learning and Plasticity in the "Mature" Visual System

Recent work suggests that there is a good deal more plasticity in the adult sensory nervous system than previously suspected. Sensory cortex is topographically organized: in visual cortex, the world is mapped retinotopically, in auditory cortex tonotopically, and in somatosensory cortex, the skin surface is mapped somatotopically. What we have learned over the past 20 years or so is that in the adult these sensory maps are plastic—reorganizing within limits in response to injury and experience. While we still do not fully understand the mechanisms, it is clear that there is plasticity at the synaptic and cellular level and at the level of cortical representation. When the somatsosensory, auditory, or visual cortex is deprived of its normal sensory input, the area reorganizes (see Buonomano and Merzenich, 1998, for a review). In the visual system, for example, Chino and his colleagues made a small lesion in the retina of an adult cat, depriving the primary visual cortex of activating input. After enucleating the nonlesioned eye, they found substantial and rapid reorganization of receptive fields around the cortical area corresponding to the lesion (Chino et al., 1992). Similar reorganization occurs in primate cortex following bilateral lesions (Heinen and Skavenski, 1991). This reorganization is interesting because the new receptive fields support visual function and, therefore, act to "fill in" the blind spots in the perceptual world. They also provide some important clues about the mechanisms of adult neural plasticity that have important implications for understanding amblyopia. Chino et al. (1992) actually measured function immediately before as well as after enucleating the fellow eye and found that the reorganization occurred only after enucleation, and then occurred within hours. This suggests that the reorganization may have involved adaptive alterations in the effectiveness of existing connections that were suppressed by the fellow eye. In this scenario, removing the intact fellow eye may have "unmasked" these existing (but perhaps weak) connections. Later we'll discuss the implications of this for understanding plasticity in amblyopia.

Human adults are capable of improving performance on sensory tasks though repeated practice or perceptual learning (PL—yes, you can teach old dogs new tricks!—for a recent review, see Fine and Jacobs, 2002), and this learning also has consequences in the cortex (Buonomano and Merzenich, 1998). Eleanor Gibson (1963) defined perceptual learning as "Any relatively permanent and consistent change in the perception of a stimulus array following practice or experience with this array." Over the last half-century or so, perceptual learning has been studied intensively. It has formed the basis of thousands of articles, chapters, and books (a Google search results in close to a million hits) and for two recent Special Issues of *Vision Research*. Indeed, advertising for the book *Perceptual Learning* (Fahle and Poggio, 2002) states: "A familiar example is the treatment for a 'lazy' or crossed eye. Covering the good eye causes gradual improvement in the weaker eye's cortical representations. If the good eye is patched too long, however, it learns to see less acutely."

The focus here is on a rather narrower definition of perceptual learning—specifically, the notion that practicing visual tasks can lead to dramatic and long-lasting improvements in performing them, that is, practice makes perfect! In adults with normal vision, practice can improve performance on a variety of visual tasks, and this learning can be quite specific (to the trained task, orientation, eye, etc.—see Fahle, 2005).

The strong interest in visual learning stems from the possibility that the learning takes place in early stages of visual processing. Indeed the finding that learning with simple patterns shows nontransfer to different locations, different orientations, or the untrained eye has been taken as evidence that the learning might take place in early stages of processing. However, as noted by Mollon and Danilova (1996), nontransfer of learning, often thought to be early, can sometimes be explained by central mechanisms, and the massive interconnectedness of cortex makes it difficult to separate early and late stages of processing. Moreover, recent work (Xiao et al., 2008) shows complete transfer of learning from one location to another if the second location has been sensitized with an irrelevant stimulus and task. The complete transfer of perceptual learning to new retinal locations revealed by Xiao et al. calls into question both location specificity as a key property of visual perceptual learning and the well-received belief by many researchers that the retinotopic early visual cortex is the neuronal basis of perceptual learning. Rather, it points to a crucial role for nonretinotopic higher brain areas that engage attention and decision making for perceptual learning, and this may have important implications for perceptual learning in individuals with amblyopia.

Experimental Treatment of Amblyopia beyond the Sensitive Period

While amblyopia can often be reversed when treated early, conventional treatment (patching) is generally not undertaken in older children and adults. Moreover, patching itself may lead to a reduction in binocular vision and stereopsis and to psychosocial problems such as a loss of self-esteem (Webber, Wood, Gole, and Brown, 2008). Thus, it is desirable to minimize the duration and extent of patching. A number of studies in our lab and others over the last fifteen years or so suggest that perceptual learning (PL) may provide an important new method for treating amblyopia (see Levi and Li, 2009, for a review). Indeed, one strong appeal of the PL approach for treating amblyopia is the widely held notion that PL can lead to permanent changes in both performance and in neural processing at an early stage of visual coding, perhaps as early as V1. The extant evidence suggests that the primary neural damage in the amblyopic visual system takes place in the visual cortex (Kiorpes, 2006; Levi, 2006).

Our own recent work, and that of others, suggests that substantial neural plasticity exists in the visual system of adults and older children with naturally occurring amblyopia due to high levels of astigmatism, anisometropia, strabismus, and/or form-deprivation, suggesting that PL may be a very useful approach for amblyopia treatment (see Levi and Li, 2009, for an extensive review and meta-analysis). As of this writing, there have been 14 studies of PL in amblyopia published to date. These studies cover a range of tasks including Vernier acuity, contrast detection, letter identification (both first- and second-order) and position discrimination. Most of the almost 200 amblyopic observers showed improvement in the trained task, and some showed a degree of transfer to visual acuity, although the amount of improvement varied substantially both between tasks and between individuals.

PL generally results in a fairly rapid improvement that occurs over a time scale of a few thousand trials in normal foveal vision. Figure 30.1 shows data from SC, an adult (30 years of age) anisometropic amblyope who practiced a position discrimination task (Li et al., 2008) with his amblyopic eye over a course of 50 sessions (i.e., 50,000 trials). The observer's task was to

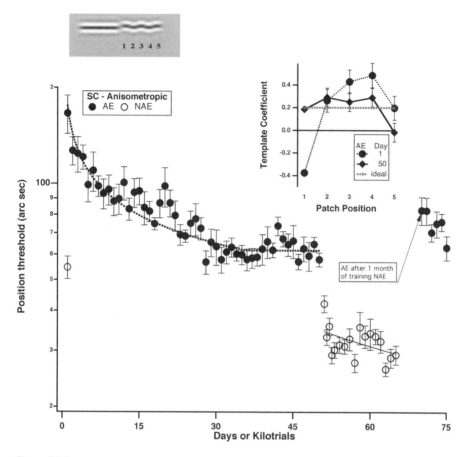

Figure 30.1
Slow learning in an adult amblyope. The inset shows his template on day 1 and day 50. AE, amblyopic eye; NAE, nonamblyopic eye. Replotted from Li et al., 2008.

judge the position of the left (reference) segment relative to the right segment. Positional noise was produced by shifting the position of each Gabor patch in the vertical direction around the intended mean line position of the test (right) segment according to a discrete binary probability function. We designed this stimulus to ask how positional information is integrated along the length of the stimulus in normal fovea, but it is especially appropriate for studying amblyopic vision where position integration along the length of the stimulus is abnormal (Levi and Klein, 1986). SC's initial threshold was 166 arc sec., but improved, over the course of ≈ 35 sessions (35 kilotrials) to 58 arc sec.—an improvement of 65%. This improvement is accompanied by a substantial change in his classification images (inset). The classification image shows how each of the five segments (numbered 1 to 5 in figure 30.1, corresponding to the numbers along the abscissa) are weighed by the visual system. An ideal observer would weigh each of the five segments equally (gray circles and line at 0.2 on the ordinate). SC's classification image (circles) is markedly inefficient on day 1. Indeed, patch 1 is weighted in the wrong direction, and most of the weighting is on patch 4. In contrast, by day 50 (diamonds) he is using the first four patches efficiently, and his template efficiency improved from ≈30% to 73%! This improvement in efficiency was accompanied by an almost 60% reduction in internal noise. These results are all the more remarkable because SC was a regular (5 days/week) observer in the lab for three years and had participated in dozens of experiments, clocking in hundreds of thousands of trials on a variety of different tasks prior to this experiment.

Over the course of these experiments, his visual acuity improved from 20/63 when he first came to the lab to 20/40. Note that his performance on the position task following practice approached (but did not quite reach) the level of his dominant eye on day 1 (open circle). There are several other striking features in figure 30.1. After 50,000 trials with the amblyopic eye, we retested SC's dominant eye and found a small but significant (≈23%) transfer of improvement.

One month of practice with his dominant yielded a further improvement, along with a deterioration of the amblyopic eye, which quickly returned to its day 50 level after a few sessions of training. The deterioration in the amblyopic eye points to a genuine neural plasticity. This slow learning is unprecedented in normal vision; however, we believe that understanding the time course, limits, and mechanisms involved is essential to understanding the neural changes that occur both in PL and in the course of treatment of amblyopia

The specificity of PL noted above poses some interesting difficulties. If the improvement following practice was solely limited to the trained stimulus, condition, and task, then the type of plasticity documented here would have very limited (if any) therapeutic value for amblyopia since amblyopia is defined primarily on the basis of reduced Snellen acuity. Importantly, PL of many tasks (Vernier acuity, position discrimination, contrast sensitivity) appears to transfer, at least in part, to improvements in Snellen acuity, as does practicing contrast detection. In addition to visual acuity improvement, other degraded visual functions such as stereoacuity and visual counting may improve as well.

Beyond Perceptual Learning—Resetting the Excitatory–Inhibitory Balance

Although much of the original work on critical periods was done in cats and monkeys, recent work in rodents, where genetic manipulations are possible and the life span is brief, have provided a number of new insights into the mechanisms of plasticity and the potential for recovery in adults (for a recent review, see Morishita and Hensch, 2008). Lamberto Maffei has been one of the pioneers in this endeavor. Specifically, through chronic administration of the antidepressant fluoxetine (Prozac), Maffei and colleagues (Maya Vetencourt et al., 2008) were able to reduce intracortical inhibition and increase expression of brain-derived neurotrophic factor in adult rats that had been monocularly deprived during the critical period. Most importantly, fluoxetine also restored visual acuity in these "amblyopic" adult rats. Other rodent studies suggest that reverse suture coupled with environmental enrichment (Sale et al., 2008) or 10 days of dark exposure (He et al., 2007) all result in substantial recovery of visual acuity (Morishita and Hensch, 2008) in adult rodents.

Over the centuries, there have been numerous attempts to increase the effectiveness of treatment. These attempts have a long and checkered history, ranging from the sublime to the ridiculous, and include subcutaneous injection of strychnine, electrical stimulation of the retina and optic nerve, flashing lights, red filters and rotating gratings (Revell, 1971), administration of Levodopa/Carbidopa (Leguire et al., 1993, and see Levi, 1994) and shocks to the brain via transcranial magnetic stimulation (Thompson et al., 2008). Few were subjected to rigorous scrutiny, and those that were often failed to stand up to it. Thus, any "promising" new method should be examined critically, and there is a clear need for careful, controlled studies.

Conclusions

Amblyopia is, aside from refractive error, the most common cause of visual loss in children. Thus, amblyopia is a serious public health issue. When diagnosed and treated early, the visual losses may be easily reversed. With early detection and treatment, amblyopia could conceivably be eliminated. Treatment for amblyopia is generally undertaken only in children; however, as discussed above, there is now considerable evidence that treatment of amblyopia may also be effective in adults. These findings, along with the results of new clinical trials, suggest that it might be time to reconsider our notions about neural plasticity in amblyopia.

References

Banks MS, Aslin RN, Letson RD. 1975. Sensitive period for the development of human binocular vision. *Science* 190: 675–677.

Berardi N, Pizzorusso T, Maffei L. 2000. Critical periods during sensory development. *Curr Opin Neurobiol* 10: 138–145.

Birch EE. 1983. Assessment of binocular function during infancy. *Ophthalmic Paediatr Genet* 2: 43–50.

Boothe RG, Dobson V, Teller DY. 1985. Postnatal development of vision in human and non-human primates. *Annu Rev Neurosci* 8: 495–545.

Buonomano DV, Merzenich MM. 1998. Cortical plasticity: from synapses to maps. *Annu Rev Neurosci* 21: 149–186.

Chino YM, Kaas JH, Smith EL, Langston AL, Cheng H. 1992. Rapid reorganization of cortical maps in adult cats following restricted deafferation in retina. *Vision Res* 32: 789–796.

Ciuffreda KJ, Levi DM, Selenow A. 1991. *Amblyopia: Basic and Clinical Aspects.* Stoneham, MA: Butterworth-Heinemann,

El Mallah MK, Chakravarthy U, Hart PM. 2000. Amblyopia: is visual loss permanent? *Br J Ophthalmol* 84: 952–956.

Fahle M, Poggio T. 2002. *Perceptual Learning.* Cambridge, MA: MIT Press.

Fahle M. 2005. Learning to tell apples from oranges. *Trends Cogn Sci* 9: 455–457.

Fine I, Jacobs RA. 2002. Comparing perceptual learning tasks: a review. *J Vis* 2: 190–203.

Gibson E. 1963. Perceptual learning. *Annu Rev Psychol* 14: 29–56.

Harwerth RS, Smith EL, III, Duncan GC, Crawford MLJ, von Noorden GK. 1987. Multiple sensitive periods in the development of the primate visual system. *Science* 232: 235–238.

Harwerth RS, Smith EL, III, Duncan GC, Crawford MLJ, von Noorden GK. 1990. Behavioral studies of the sensitive periods of development of visual functions in monkeys. *Behav Brain Res* 41: 179–198.

He HY, Ray B, Dennis K, Quinlan EM. 2007. Experience-dependent recovery of vision following chronic deprivation amblyopia. *Nat Neurosci* 10: 1134–1136.

Heinen SJ, Skavenski AA. 1991. Recovery of visual responses in foveal V1 neurons following bilateral foveal lesions in adult monkey. *Exp Brain Res* 83: 670–674.

Hohmann A, Creutzfeldt OD. 1975. Squint and the development of binocularity in humans. *Nature* 254: 613–614.

Hubel DH, Wiesel TN. 1970. The period of susceptibility to the physiological effects of unilateral eye closure in kittens. *J Physiol* 206: 419–436.

Jacobson SG, Mohindra I, Held R. 1981. Age of onset of amblyopia in infants with esotropia. In *Pathophysiology of the Visual System* (Maffei L, ed). Documenta Ophthalmologica Proceedings Series 30: 210–216.

Kiorpes L. 2006. Visual processing in amblyopia: animal studies. *Strabismus* 14: 3–10.

Kiorpes L, Boothe RG. 1981. Naturally occurring strabismus in monkeys (Macaca nemestrina). *Invest Ophthalmol Vis Sci* 20: 257–263.

Kiorpes L, Boothe RG, Carlson MR. 1984. Acuity development in surgically strabismic monkeys. *Invest Ophthalmol Vis Sci (Suppl.)* 25: 216.

Kiorpes L, Carlson MR, Alfi D, Boothe RG. 1989. Development of visual acuity in experimentally strabismic monkeys. *Clin Vis Sci* 4: 95–106.

Leguire LE, Rogers GL, Bremer DL, Walson PD, McGregor ML. 1993. Levodopa/carbidopa for childhood amblyopia. *Invest Ophthalmol Vis Sci* 34: 3090–3095.

LeVay S, Wiesel TN, Hubel DH. 1980. The development of ocular dominance columns in normal and visually deprived monkeys. *J Comp Neurol* 191: 1–5.

Levi DM. 1994. Pathophysiology of binocular vision and amblyopia. *Curr Opin Ophthalmol* 5: 3–10.

Levi DM. 2006. Visual processing in amblyopia: human studies. *Strabismus* 14: 11–19.

Levi DM, Carkeet A. 1993. Amblyopia: A consequence of abnormal visual development. In: *Early Visual Development, Normal and Abnormal* (Simons K, ed), pp 391–408. Oxford, UK: Oxford University Press.

Levi DM, Klein SA. 1986. Sampling in spatial vision. *Nature* 320: 360–362.

Levi DM, Li RW. 2009. Perceptual learning as a potential treatment for amblyopia: a mini-review. *Vision Res* 49: 2535–2549.

Li RW, Klein SA, Levi DM. 2008. Prolonged perceptual learning of positional acuity in adult amblyopia: perceptual template retuning dynamics. *J Neurosci* 28: 14223–14229.

Maurer D, Lewis TL, Tytla ME. 1983. Contrast sensitivity in cases of unilateral congenital cataract. *Invest Ophthalmol Vis Sci* 24(Suppl.): 21.

Maurer D, Lewis TL, Brent HP, Levin AV. 1999. Rapid improvement in the acuity of infants after visual input. *Science* 286: 108–110.

Maya Vetencourt JF, Sale A, Viegi A, Baroncelli L, De Pasquale R, O'Leary OF, Castrén E, Maffei L. 2008. The antidepressant fluoxetine restores plasticity in the adult visual cortex. *Science* 320: 385–388.

McKee SP, Levi DM, Movshon JA. 2003. The pattern of visual deficits in amblyopia. *J Vis* 3: 380–405.

Mitchell DE. 2004. The effects of early forms of visual deprivation on perception. In: *The Visual Neurosciences.* Vol. 1 (Chalupa LM, Werner JS, eds), pp 189–204. Cambridge MA: MIT Press.

Mohindra I, Jacobson SG, Thomas J, Held R. 1979. Development of amblyopia in infants. *Trans Ophthalmol Soc U K* 99: 344–346.

Mollon JD, Danilova MV. 1996. Three remarks on perceptual learning. *Spat Vis* 10: 51–58.

Morishita H, Hensch TK. 2008. Critical period revisited: impact on vision. *Curr Opin Neurobiol* 18: 101–107.

Pediatric Eye Disease Investigator Group. 2005. Randomized trial of treatment of amblyopia in children aged 7 to 17 years. *Am J Ophthalmol* 143: 1634–1642.

Rahi JS, Logan S, Borja MC, Timms C, Russell-Eggitt I, Taylor D. 2002. Prediction of improved vision in the amblyopic eye after visual loss in the non-amblyopic eye. *Lancet* 360: 621–622.

Revell MJ. 1971. *Strabismus: A History of Orthoptic Techniques*. London: Barrie and Jenkins.

Sale A, Maya-Vetencourt JF, Medini P, Cenni MC, Baroncelli L, De Pasquale R, Maffei L. 2008. Environmental enrichment in adulthood promotes amblyopia recovery through a reduction of intracortical inhibition. *Nat Neurosci* 10: 679–681.

Teller DY, Movshon JA. 1986. Visual development. *Vision Res* 26: 1483–1506.

Thompson B, Mansouri B, Koski L, Hess RF. 2008. Brain plasticity in the adult: modulation of function in amblyopia with rTMS. *Curr Biol* 18: 1067–1071.

Vereecken EP, Brabant P. 1984. Prognosis for vision in amblyopia after the loss of the good eye. *Arch Ophthalmol* 102: 220–224.

von Noorden GK. 1981. New clinical aspects of stimulus deprivation amblyopia. *Am J Ophthalmol* 92: 416–421.

Webber AL, Wood JM, Gole GA, Brown B. 2008. Effect of amblyopia on self-esteem in children. *Optom Vis Sci* 85: 1074–1081.

Wiesel TN. 1982. Postnatal development of the visual cortex and the influence of environment. *Nature* 299: 583–591.

Worth CA. 1903. *Squint: Its Causes, Pathology and Treatment*. Philadelphia: The Blakiston Co.

Wu C, Hunter DG. 2006. Amblyopia: diagnostic and therapeutic options. *Am J Ophthalmol* 141: 175–184.

Xiao LQ, Zhang JY, Wang R, Klein SA, Levi DM, Yu C. 2008. Complete transfer of perceptual learning across retinal locations enabled by double training. *Curr Biol* 18: 1922–1926.

Contributors

Laura Baroncelli   Laboratory of Neurobiology, Scuola Normale Superiore, Pisa, Italy

Nicoletta Berardi   Department of Psychology, Florence University, and CNR Institute of Neuroscience, Pisa, Italy

Giovanni Berlucchi   National Institute of Neuroscience–Italy, and Department of Neurological Sciences, Section of Physiology and Psychology, University of Verona, Italy

David C. Burr   CNR Institute of Neuroscience, Pisa, Italy, Scientific Institute Stella Maris, Pisa, Italy, and Department of Psychology, Università Degli Studi di Firenze, Firenze, Italy

Matteo Caleo   CNR Institute of Neuroscience, Pisa, Italy

Giorgio Carmignoto   CNR Institute of Neuroscience, Padova, Italy, and Department of Experimental Biomedical Sciences, University of Padova, Padova, Italy

Eero Castrén   Neuroscience Center, University of Helsinki, Helsinki, Finland

Antonino Cattaneo   Scuola Normale Superiore, Pisa, Italy, and European Brain Research Institute (EBRI)–Rita Levi Montalcini Foundation, Rome, Italy,

Leo M. Chalupa   Department of Neurobiology, Physiology, and Behavior, University of California, Davis, Davis, CA, and Department of Pharmacology and Physiology, School of Medicine and Office of Vice President of Research, The George Washington University, Washington, DC

Barbara Chapman   Center for Neuroscience, University of California, Davis, Davis, CA

Bidisha Chattopadhyaya   CHU Ste. Justine/Université de Montréal, Montréal, Canada

Chinfei Chen   Children's Hospital, Boston, and Division of Neuroscience and F.M. Kirby Neurobiology Center, Harvard Medical School, Boston, Massachusetts

Giovanni Cioni   Division of Child Neurology and Psychiatry, University of Pisa, Pisa, Italy, and Department of Developmental Neuroscience, IRCCS Stella Maris

Julie L. Coombs   Department of Neurobiology, Physiology, and Behavior, University of California, Davis, Davis, California

Giulia D'Acunto   Division of Child Neurology and Psychiatry, University of Pisa, Pisa, Italy

Colette Dehay   Stem Cell and Brain Research Institute, INSERM U846, Bron, France, and Université Lyon I, Lyon, France

Graziella Di Cristo   CHU Ste. Justine/Université de Montréal, Montréal, Canada

Maria-Magdolina Ercsey-Ravasz   Interdisciplinary Center for Network Science and Applications, Department of Physics, University of Notre Dame, South Bend, Indiana

David Fitzpatrick   Department of Neurobiology, Duke University School of Medicine, Duke University, and Duke Institute for Brain Sciences, Duke University, Durham, North Carolina

Leonardo Fogassi   Dipartimento di Neuroscienze, Università di Parma, and Istituto Italiano di Tecnologia (IIT), Unità di Parma, Italy

Lucia Galli-Resta   CNR Institute of Neuroscience, Pisa, Italy

Marie-Alice Gariel   Stem Cell and Brain Research Institute, INSERM U846, Bron, France, and Université Lyon I, Lyon, France

Marta Gómez-Gonzalo   CNR Institute of Neuroscience and Department of Experimental Biomedical Sciences, University of Padova, Padova, Italy

Alessandro Graziano   Center for Neuroscience, University of California, Davis, Davis, California; present address: Department of Pharmacology and Physiology, Drexel University College of Medicine, Philadelphia, Pennsylvania

Andrea Guzzetta   Department of Developmental Neuroscience, IRCCS Stella Maris, and Queensland Cerebral Palsy and Rehabilitation Research Centre, Royal Children's Hospital, University of Queensland, Brisbane, Australia

Andrew Hamilton   Center for Neuroscience, University of California, Davis, Davis, California

Z. Josh Huang   Cold Spring Harbor Laboratory, Cold Spring Harbor, New York

Edward G. Jones   Center for Neuroscience, University of California, Davis, Davis, California

Henry Kennedy   Stem Cell and Brain Research Institute, INSERM U846, Bron, France, and Université Lyon I, Lyon, France

In-Jung Kim   Department of Molecular and Cellular Biology and Center for Brain Science, Harvard University, Cambridge, Massachusetts; currently, Department of Ophthalmology, Yale University School of Medicine, New Haven, Connecticut

Kenneth Knoblauch   Stem Cell and Brain Research Institute, INSERM U846, Bron, France, and Université Lyon I, Lyon, France

Dennis M. Levi   School of Optometry and Helen Wills Neuroscience Institute, University of California, Berkeley, Berkeley, California

Ye Li   Department of Neurobiology, Duke University School of Medicine, Duke University, Durham, North Carolina

Giuseppe Luppino Dipartimento di Neuroscienze, Università di Parma, and Istituto Italiano di Tecnologia (IIT), Unità di Parma, Italy

Lamberto Maffei CNR Institute of Neuroscience, and Laboratory of Neurobiology, Scuola Normale Superiore, Pisa, Italy

Georgia Mandolesi Santa Lucia Foundation (IRCCS), Rome, Italy

Nikola T. Markov Stem Cell and Brain Research Institute, INSERM U846, Bron, France, and Université Lyon I, Lyon, France

Jean-Marc Melgari Clinical Neurology, Campus Bio-Medico University, Rome, Italy

M. Concetta Morrone CNR Institute of Neuroscience, Scientific Institute Stella Maris, and Department of Physiological Sciences, Università di Pisa, Pisa, Italy

John G. Partridge Department of Physiology and Biophysics, Georgetown University School of Medicine, Washington, DC

Thomas Perrault, Jr. Department of Neurobiology and Anatomy, Wake Forest University School of Medicine, Winston-Salem, North Carolina

V. Hugh Perry CNS Inflammation Group, School of Biological Sciences, University of Southampton, Southampton, England

Tommaso Pizzorusso Department of Psychology, Florence University, and CNR Institute of Neuroscience, Pisa, Italy

Josef P. Rauschecker Laboratory of Integrative Neuroscience and Cognition, Departments of Physiology and Biophysics, Neurology and Psychology, Georgetown University, Washington, DC

Gregg H. Recanzone Center for Neuroscience and Department of Neurobiology, Physiology and Behavior, University of California, Davis, Davis, California

Giacomo Rizzolatti Dipartimento di Neuroscienze, Università di Parma, and Istituto Italiano di Tecnologia (IIT), Unità di Parma, Italy

Paolo Maria Rossini Clinical Neurology, Campus Bio-Medico University, Rome, Italy, and Casa di Cura San Raffaele, Cassino, Italy

Benjamin A. Rowland Department of Neurobiology and Anatomy, Wake Forest University School of Medicine, Winston-Salem, North Carolina

Alessandro Sale CNR Institute of Neuroscience, Pisa, Italy

Joshua R. Sanes Department of Molecular and Cellular Biology and Center for Brain Science, Harvard University, Cambridge Massachusetts

Martin E. Schwab Brain Research Institute, University of Zurich, and Department of Biology, ETH Zurich, Zurich, Switzerland

Wolf Singer Max Planck Institute for Brain Research, Frankfurt am Main, Germany

Maria Spolidoro   Laboratory of Neurobiology, Scuola Normale Superiore, Pisa, Italy

Terrence R. Stanford   Department of Neurobiology and Anatomy, Wake Forest University School of Medicine, Winston-Salem, North Carolina

Barry E. Stein   Department of Neurobiology and Anatomy, Wake Forest University School of Medicine, Winston-Salem, North Carolina

Piergiorgio Strata   Department of Neuroscience and National Institute of Neuroscience—Italy, University of Turin, Turin, Italy

Mriganka Sur   Department of Brain and Cognitive Sciences and Picower Institute for Learning and Memory, Massachusetts Institute of Technology, Cambridge, Massachusetts

Zoltán Toroczkai   Interdisciplinary Center for Network Science and Applications, Department of Physics, University of Notre Dame, South Bend, Indiana

Stephen D. Van Hooser   Department of Neurobiology, Duke University School of Medicine, Duke University, Durham, North Carolina

José Fernando Maya Vetencourt   Scuola Normale Superiore, Pisa, Italy

Stefano Vicini   Department of Physiology and Biophysics, Georgetown University School of Medicine, Washington, DC

Leonard E. White   Department of Community and Family Medicine, Department of Neurobiology, Duke University School of Medicine, and Duke Institute for Brain Sciences, Duke University, Durham, North Carolina

Roman Willi   Brain Research Institute, University of Zurich, and Department of Biology, ETH Zurich, Zurich, Switzerland

Nathan R. Wilson   Department of Brain and Cognitive Sciences and Picower Institute for Learning and Memory, Massachusetts Institute of Technology, Cambridge, Massachusetts

Karen Zito   Center for Neuroscience, University of California, Davis, Davis, California

Index